17 Update in Intensive Care and Emergency Medicine

Edited by J.-L. Vincent

D. W. Wilmore Y. A. Carpentier (Eds.)

Metabolic Support of the Critically Ill Patient

With 89 Figures and 68 Tables

Springer-Verlag
Berlin Heidelberg New York
London Paris Tokyo
Hong Kong Barcelona
Budapest

Series Editor

Prof. Dr. Jean-Louis Vincent
Clinical Director, Department of Intensive Care, Erasme Hospital
Free University of Brussels, Route de Lennik 808
1070 Brussels, Belgium

Volume Editors

Prof. Dr. Douglas W. Wilmore
Laboratory for Surgical Metabolism,
Brigham and Women's Hospital
75 Francis Street, Boston Massachussetts 02115, USA

Prof. Dr. Yvon A. Carpentier
L. Deloyers Laboratory for Experimental Surgery,
Free University of Brussels, Avenue J. Wybran 40,
1070 Brussels, Belgium

ISBN-13:978-3-642-85013-4 e-ISBN-13:978-3-642-85011-0
DOI: 10.1007/978-3-642-85011-0

Softcover reprint of the hardcover 1st edition 1993

19/3130-5 4 3 2 1 0 – Printed on acid-free paper

Contents

Monitoring Compositional Changes and Biochemical Functions

What Type of Metabolic Support?

Organ Specific Nutrients and Associated Therapy

Preventing Complications

Disease/Nutrients Interactions

List of Contributors

Bihari D.
Department of Intensive Care,
Guy's Hospital, St Thomas Street,
London SE1 9RT, United Kingdom

Boermeester M.A.
Department of Surgery, Free
University Hospital, De Boelelaan
1117, 1081 HV Amsterdam,
The Netherlands

Boeynaems J.M.
Institute of Interdisciplinary
Research, School of Medicine, Free
University of Brussels, 808 Route
de Lennik, 1070 Brussels, Belgium

Bracco D.
Institute of Physiology, University
of Lausanne, Lausanne, Switzerland

Byrne T.A.
Laboratories of Nutrition and
Metabolism, Brigham and Women's
Hospital, 75 Francis Street, Boston
MA 02115, USA

Carpentier Y.A.
L. Deloyers Laboratory for
Experimental Surgery and Clinical
Nutrition Unit, Free University of
Brussels, 40 Avenue J. Wybran,
1070 Brussels, Belgium

Cerra F.B.
Department of Critical Care and
Clinical Nutrition, University of
Minnesota, Minneapolis MN 55455,
USA

Chang R.
Department of Intensive Care,
Guy's Hospital, St. Thomas Street,
London SE1 9RT, United Kingdom

Chioléro R.
Intensive Care Unit, CHU Vaudois,
1011 Lausanne, Switzerland

Dulloo A.G.
Institute of Physiology, University
Hospital, Geneva, Switzerland

Esterbauer H.
Institute of Biochemistry,
University of Graz, Schubertstrasse 1,
8010 Graz, Austria

Fink M.P.
Division of Trauma and Surgical
Critical Care, Beth Israel Hospital,
330 Brookline Avenue, Boston
MA 02215, USA

Fürst P.
Institute for Biological Chemistry
and Nutrition, University of
Hohenheim, Garbenstrasse 30,
70599 Stuttgart, Germany

Garlick P.
Rowett Research Institute,
Aberdeen, Scotland,
United Kingdom

Gilpin D.A.
Shriners Burns Institute, 815
Market Street, Galveston
TX 77550-2725, USA

Grimble R.F.
Department of Human Nutrition,
University of Southampton,
Biomedical Sciences Building,
Bassett Crescent East,
Southampton SO9 3TU,
United Kingdom

Herndon D.N.
Shriners Burns Institute,
815 Market Street, Galveston
TX 77550-2725, USA

Hill G.L.
Department of Surgery, Auckland
Hospital, Auckland 3, New Zealand

Houdijk A.P.J.
Department of Surgery, Free
University Hospital, De Boelelaan
1117, 1081 HV Amsterdam,
The Netherlands

Iapichino G.
Intensive Care Unit, Ospedale
Maggiore, Via F. Sforza 33,
20122 Milano, Italy

Jacobs D.O.
Division of General and
Gastrointestinal Surgery, Brigham
and Women's Hospital, 75 Francis
Street, Boston MA 02115, USA

Jeejeebhoy K.N.
Department of Medicine, St
Michaels Hospital, 30 Bond Street,
Toronto Ontario, Canada

Lerebours E.
Service des Maladies de l'Appareil
Digestif et de la Nutrition, Hôpital
Charles Nicolle, 1 rue de Germont,
76031 Rouen, France

Lew J.I.
Department of Surgery, University
Hospital, 4 Silverstein Pavilion,
Philadelphia PA 19104, USA

Lowry, S.F.
Department of Surgery, New York
Hospital-Cornell Medical Center,
525 E. 68th Street, New York
NY 10021, USA

Mitchell I.
Department of Intensive Care,
Guy's Hospital, St Thomas Street,
London SE1 9RT, United Kingdom

Monk D.
Department of Surgery, Auckland
Hospital, Auckland 3, New Zealand

Muller M.J.
Shriners Burns Institute,
815 Market Street, Galveston
TX 77550-2725, USA

Newsholme E.A.
Department of Biochemistry,
University of Oxford, South Park
Road, Oxford OX1 3QU,
United Kingdom

Pichard C.
Clinical Nutrition Dietetics,
Division of Gastroenterology,
University Hospital, Geneva,
Switzerland

Plank L.D.
Department of Surgery, Auckland
Hospital, Auckland 3, New Zealand

Radrizzani D.
Intensive Care Unit, Ospedale
Maggiore, Via F. Sforza 33,
20122 Milano, Italy

Revelly J.P.
Intensive Care Unit, Department
of Anesthesiology, University
Hospital, Lausanne, Switzerland

Robinson M.K.
Division of General and
Gastrointestinal Surgery, Brigham
and Women's Hospital, 75 Francis
Street, Boston MA 02115, USA

Rombeau J.L.
Department of Surgery, University
Hospital, 4 Silverstein Pavilion,
Philadelphia PA 19104, USA

Slosman D.
Department of Nuclear Medicine,
University Hospital, Geneva,
Switzerland

Stehle P.
Institute for Biological Chemistry
and Nutrition, University of
Hohenheim, Garbenstrasse 30,
70599 Stuttgart, Germany

Takala J.
Department of Intensive Care,
Kuopio University Hospital,
70210 Kuopio, Finland

Van Leeuwen P. A. M.
Department of Surgery, Free University Hospital, De Boelelaan 1117, 1081 HV Amsterdam, The Netherlands

Vinnars E.
Kabi Pharmacia Infusion, 112 87 Stockholm, Sweden

Wernerman J.
Department of Anesthesiology, Metabolic Research Laboratory, Karolinska Institute, St Göran's Hospital, 112 81 Stockholm, Sweden

Wilmore D. W.
Laboratories of Nutrition and Metabolism, Brigham and Women's Hospital, 75 Francis Street, Boston MA 02115, USA

Young L. S.
Laboratories of Nutrition and Metabolism, Brigham and Women's Hospital, 75 Francis Street, Boston MA 02115, USA

Zaloga G. P.
Section of Critical Care, Department of Anesthesiology, Bowman Gray School of Medicine, Medical Center Boulevard, Winston Salem NC 27157-1009, USA

Ziegler T. R.
Department of Medicine, Brigham and Women's Hospital, Joslin Diabetes Center, 1 Joslin Place, Boston MA 02215, USA

Abbreviations

AIDS	Acquired immuno-deficiency syndrome
ARDS	Adult respiratory distress syndrome
ATP	Adenosine triphosphate
BCCA	Branched-chain amino acids
BCM	Body cell mass
BPI	Bactericidal/permeability increasing protein
BW	Body weight
CNS	Central nervous system
COPD	Chronic obstructive pulmonary disease
DNA	Deoxyribonucleic acid
ECW	Extracellular water
EE	Energy expenditure
EN	Enteral nutrition
FA	Fatty acids
GALT	Gut associated lymphoid tissue
GH	Growth hormone
GI	Gastro-intestinal
GSH	Gluthatione
HDL	High density lipoprotein
HPLC	Human plasma lipid chromatography
ICU	Intensive care unit
ICW	Intracellular water
IFN-	Interferon-
IGF	Insulin-like growth factor
IL	Interleukin
IV	Intravenous
LBP	Lipopolysaccharide binding protein
LDH	Lactate dehydrogenase
LDL	Low density lipoproteins
LPS	Lipopolysaccharide

MLN	Mesenteric lymph nodes
MOF	Multiple organ failure
MRS	Magnetic resonance spectroscopy
MV	Mechanical ventilation
N	Nitrogen
NMR	Nuclear magnetic resonance
NO	Nitric oxide
PAF	Platelet activating factor
PCM	Protein-calorie malnutrition
PCr	Phosphocreatine
PDE	Phosphodiesterase
pHi	Intramucosal pH
PME	Phosphomonoester
REE	Resting energy expenditure
RES	Reticulo-endothelial system
rhGS	Recombinant human growth hormone
RNA	Ribonucleic acid
SMF	Skeletal muscle function
SOD	Superoxide dismutase
TBARS	Thiobarbituric acid reactive substances
TBSA	Total body surface area
TBW	Total body water
TNF	Tumor necrosis factor
TPN	Total parenteral nutrition
VLDL	Very low density lipoproteins
VO_2	Oxygen consumption/uptake

Monitoring Compositional Changes and Biochemical Functions

Measuring Body Composition in Intensive Care Patients

G. L. Hill, D. Monk, and L. D. Plank

Introduction

Body composition research has led to a better understanding of the molecular structure of the body which has enhanced clinical care in many areas including critical care medicine. For many years, body composition measuring technology has not been adequate to enable its practical use in intensive care environments. However, new advances have opened the possibility for body composition measurements to be obtained not only for the evaluation of therapies used in intensive care patients, but also for the daily care of critically ill patients.

Body composition is a growing and expanding science, the definiton of which has been helped by the presentation recently of a "Model" by Wang and his colleagues from the obesity research centre at Columbia University in New York [1]. They have proposed a model comprising levels of body composition of increasing complexity (Fig. 1). The *atomic model* describes the body in terms of approximately 50 elements of which 9 (O, C, H, N, Ca, P, K, Na, Cl) account for greater than 98% of body weight. Although these

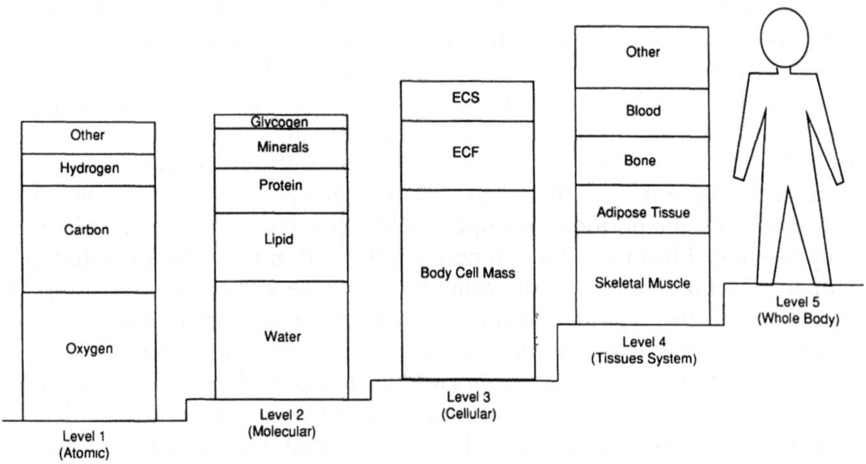

Fig. 1. Five levels of human body composition: ECS and ECF, extracellular solids and fluid, respectively. (From [1] with permission)

elements can be measured in the critically ill: O, C, Na, Ca and P by delayed gamma neutron activation analysis; H, Cl and N by prompt gamma neutron activation analysis; and K by whole body counting; the clinical or scientific usefulness of such measurements has not yet been demonstrated in the critical care setting although there are some theoretical bases for them becoming so in the future. For instance, changes in total body carbon may be a useful way of assessing changes in body energy stores in critically ill patients [2], and measurements of total body chlorine may prove to be valuable for estimating changes in extracellular water [3].

The Molecular Model of Body Composition

Wang et al.'s second level of body composition has been called the *molecular model* of body composition. Although, as these authors point out, it is not helpful to consider the body in terms of its thousands of chemical compounds, it has proved to be of considerable clinical value to break down the body into terms of closely related molecular species. We [4] and others [1] have described a 5 compartment model comprising water, protein, glycogen, mineral, and fat (lipid). These compartments can be measured in ICU patients in the following ways.

Water

Measurements in human subjects of total body water (TBW) by tritium dilution have been available for nearly 60 years [5]. Body water measurements in ICU patients, however, are much more difficult to obtain than in normal subjects or even the vast majority of sick patients because of several factors. First, such patients often have greatly expanded TBW at the end of the phase of fluid sequestration with accumulations of more than 10 L being not uncommon. Furthermore, such water expansion often includes collections of free fluid within body cavities (ascites, pleural effusions, intraluminal gut fluid, etc) where mixing of isotope via the circulation is slow. Under these circumstances, the period of isotope equilibration can be expected to be variably prolonged from the 2 to 3 h period sufficient in normally hydrated individuals. During this period of equilibration, there will be loss of isotope in urine, nasogastric aspirates, and from fluid via surgical drains and by evaporation. The patients are all receiving IV fluids at moderate infusion rates as well. These fluids cannot be withheld over the period of isotope equilibration, and by virtue of their non-instantaneous mixing with body water lead to a dilution effect in plasma water. Finally, the total body water itself may be changing during the period of isotope equilibration due to imbalance between gains and losses.

In order to study the effects of the above mentioned factors, we measured total body water in 11 ICU patients [6]. All had major emergency surgery or severe blunt trauma and were receiving inotropic drug infusions during the measurement of TBW. Sixteen studies were performed in 11 patients. Each was given 3.7 MBq of tritiated water in 10 mL of sterile water intravenously from a syringe which was weighed before and after injection. Samples of blood were taken from indwelling arterial lines every hour for 6h. Urine and other drain volumes were recorded and sampled for isotope each hour. The volume of fluids given IV each hour was also recorded.

At each hour (t) after injection, the volume of distribution of the isotope (TBW_t) was determined as:

$$TBW_t = \frac{\text{Isotope dose injected} - \text{Losses } (t=0 \text{ to } t=t)}{\text{Specific activity in serum water at time t}}$$

In order to take some account of the changes in TBW over the 6 h period, the TBW at the time of isotope injection (TBW_0) was derived from each of the 6 hourly results, thus:

$$TBW_0 = TBW_1 - (\text{Fluid input minus output from } t=0 \text{ to } t=t)$$

For each study, there were thus a series of estimates of TBW_0 and the final value of TBW_0 chosen for the patient was usually the mean of the 4, 5 and 6 h estimates.

Table 1 shows the values of TBW_0 obtained at 1–6 h after injection of tritium in 16 studies in the 11 critically ill patients. It can be seen that, in general, values of TBW_0 thus obtained rise by about 6% over the first 3 h after isotope injection and are fairly stable from the fourth hour. Repeated measures analysis of variance with analysis of the differences between adjacent water measurements indicates that there are significant increases in the volume of dilution of the isotope over the first 3 h but not thereafter in this group of patients. The extent of measured isotope losses (as urine, nasogastric fluid and surgical drain loss) at 4 h after injection varied from 0.53 to 3.29% of the administered dose with a mean value of 1.24%.

An estimate of the precision (SD) of the measurement of TBW_0 in the group of patients was obtained by analysis of the 4, 5 and 6 h results from the table and was found to vary from 0.4 to 3.0% with a mean value of 1.2%. The experimental precision on a single estimate on the basis of counting statistics alone is approximately 0.8%. Clearly, a better estimate of the TBW at the time of isotope injection is obtained by making repeated measurements during the period 4–6 h after injection. Because of the persistent uncertainty surrounding the size of the nonaqueous exchangeable hydrogen in humans during the 4–6 h equilibration period, the systematic error that results is likely to be approximately 3% or better [7].

Table 1. Values of total body water in litres obtained 1–6 h after isotope injection together with the weight (kg) of each patient at the time of study

Patient	Weight	Time after injection (hours)					
		1	2	3	4	5	6
RO1	89.3	48.05	50.98	50.83	51.76	51.51	51.33
WH1	70.4	44.06	47.04	48.59	50.66	49.19	49.54
FL1	81.5	48.50	50.22	51.07	49.82	50.45	51.24
FL2	79.4	48.65	49.15	49.73	49.80	48.85	49.34
PE1	89.9	51.18	51.62	52.92	52.60	54.91	52.92
PE2	93.4	50.05	53.29	54.84	53.67	54.17	53.47
PE3	96.9	53.37	54.42	55.89	56.39	56.62	57.68
MC2	71.6	39.09	41.83	42.27	43.45	42.40	42.54
NI2	89.9	48.06	49.19	49.89	49.73	48.97	49.93
MO1	83.5	46.16	50.84	50.92	51.42	50.14	52.41
MO2	88.2	56.63	58.39	55.95	57.45	57.73	57.97
HI1	72.9	39.10	42.62	42.38	43.67	43.32	43.02
BL1	68.6	40.25	42.93	44.03	44.51	44.56	43.84
TU1	93.7	55.05	60.84	59.47	63.77	63.81	64.20
RS1	117.0	70.69	74.16	75.52	76.34	75.79	76.75
2RS2	122.1	71.95	75.50	78.73	78.51	77.78	82.22
Mean TBW_0		50.68	53.31	53.94	54.59	54.38	54.90

Significance of differences between 1-hour values of TBW_0

Comparison	1 v 2	2 v 3	3 v 4	4 v 5	5 v 6
P value	0.00003	0.07	0.07	0.38	0.17

Protein

To date, there are very few facilities in the world which are equipped to measure total body nitrogen (protein) in critically ill patients, and in which changes in total body protein can be measured even in the presence of multiple organ failure (MOF) and while the patient is receiving intensive care.

Our own, unique facility comprises a prompt gamma *in vivo* neutron activation scanner (Fig. 2) situated alongside a dual-energy X-ray absorptiometer both of which have been specially adapted for use in studies of critically ill patients. The facility is situated in the hospital, alongside the surgical wards and near the department of Critical Care Medicine. Even with this specially constructed prompt gamma scanner, measurements of total body protein in critically ill patients with fluid overload is fraught with complex methodological difficulties and requires special calibration of the equipment to avoid the confounding effects of excessive hydrogen background (from the fluid expansion) and varying ratios of total body hydrogen to total body nitrogen which may occur with massive overhydration.

Table 2 shows the results of our recent studies of the accuracy and precision of the measurement of total body protein in such situations. We obtained measurements of total body protein from our prompt gamma neutron

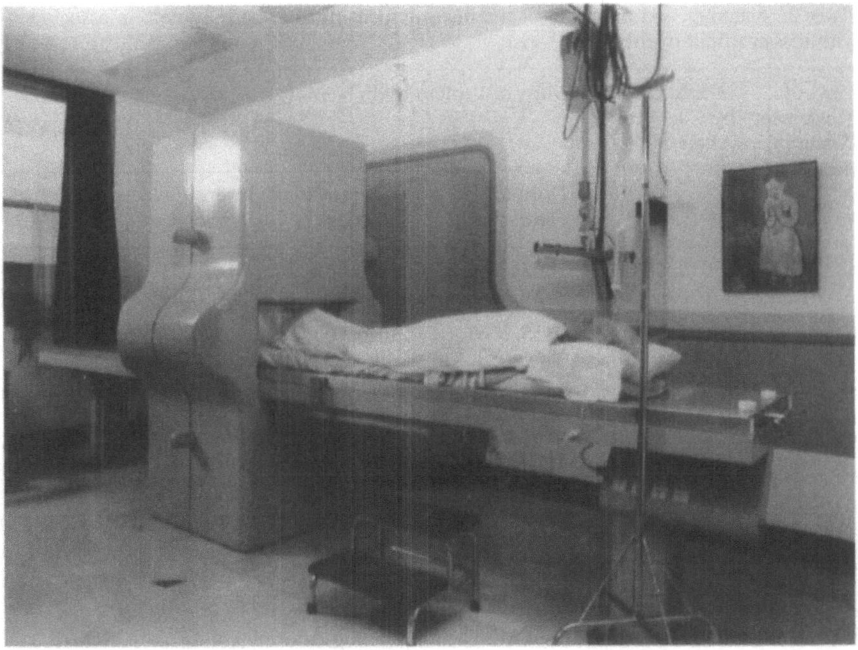

Fig. 2. The prompt gamma in vivo neutron activation analysis scanner in the University Department of Surgery at Auckland Hospital

activation analysis facility in phantoms constructed of mince meat which underwent increasing degrees of fluid overload. The protein and fat content of each phantom was adjusted to correspond approximately to the average values we have observed in 733 patients studied (that is, 12% protein, 25% fat) and contained a skeleton made from calcium phosphate (approximately 6% by weight). Each phantom was scanned in its entirety over approximately 2000 sec to give total counts of nitrogen. After substraction of the background contribution to the signal, the total body protein (total body nitrogen × 6.25) was calculated from an experimentally derived relationship between observed count rate per gram of nitrogen and subject dimensions. Each phantom was scanned 15 times, repositioning being carried out before each scan. 15 scans were performed again when the phantoms were moderately overhydrated (administration of 3–6 L of physiological saline depending on phantom size) and 15 more times after fluid overload (6–12 L of physiological saline). It can be seen from Table 2 that the total body protein measured by prompt gamma IVNAA is within 4% of the value measured directly by chemical analysis and the precision of the estimates of total body protein was between 2.7 and 4.5% depending on phantom size (95% confidence limits 1.6%–6.1%.

Table 2. Accuracy and precision of the measurement of total body protein in association with massive fluid overload

Mass of Mincemeat Phantom (kg)	Mass of Protein by Chemical Analysis (g)	Mass of Protein by IVNAA (g)			
		Normal Hydration	Moderate Fluid Overload	Severe Fluid Overload	ANOVA[a]
43[b]	5918±126[c]	6036±54 3.4% (2.1–4.8)[d]	6017±65 4.2% (2.5–5.8)	6163±51 3.4% (2.1–4.8)	ns
62[e]	8624±177	8552±65 3.4% (2.3–4.6)	8640±66 3.4% (2.3–4.5)	8597±87 4.5% (3.0–6.1)	ns
75	10348±211	9977±80 3.1% (1.9–4.4)	10176±87 3.3% (2.0–4.6)	10217±73 2.7% (1.6–3.8)	ns
87	11744±253	11530±106 3.6% (2.1–5.0)	11382±79 2.7% (1.6–3.8)	11521±116 3.9% (2.3–5.5)	ns

[a] F test for IVNAA protein measurements
[b] This phantom received 3200 s scans
[c] Mean ± S.E.M.
[d] CV with 95% confidence interval
[e] This phantom received 20 IVNAA scans at each degree of hydration

Fat (Lipid)

Lipid by Difference: Fat or triglyceride forms approximately 90% of the total lipid content of the body. The other 10% comprises "essential lipids" such as sphingomyelin and phospholipids which form cell membranes. It is total body lipid that is measured by the combined neutron activation/tritiated water approach – i.e., the so called difference technique [4]. With this technique total body water measurements are combined with measurements of total body protein, minerals and glycogen, and the total body lipid is obtained by difference:

$$\text{Total body lipid} = BW - (TBP + TBW + TBM + TBG)$$

where BW = body weight, TBP = total body protein, TBW = total body water, TBM = total body mineral, TBG = total body glycogen, respectively.

The problem with estimates of total body lipid by the difference technique is that there is currently no way of directly measuring TBG which is estimated from skeletal size [4].

Fat by Dual-Energy X-ray Absorptiometry (DXA): Total body fat can be measured by DXA although it is not clear how much essential lipid is measured as well with this technique. In Table 3, the results of our recent study

Table 3. Accuracy and precision of the measurement of total body fat in association with massive fluid overload

Mass of Mincemeat Phantom (kg)	Mass of Fat by Chemical Analysis (g)	Mass of Fat by DXA[a] (g)			
		Normal Hydration	Moderate Fluid Overload	Severe FLuid Overload	ANOVA[a]
43	11262±97[c]	9805±32 1.3% (0.8–1.8)[d]	10184±49 1.9% (1.2–2.6)	10125±34 1.3% (0.8–1.8)	$p<0.0001$
62[e]	16411±140	14641±36 1.1% (0.7–1.5)	14798±37 1.1% (0.7–1.5)	15005±36 1.1% (0.7–1.5)	$p<0.0001$
75	19691±168	19518±67 1.3% (0.8–1.8)	19777±75 1.2% (0.6–1.8)	19926±84 1.6% (1.0–2.2)	$p<0.002$

[a] Fat result dependent on composition of material used as bone equivalent so comparison with chemical analysis in this study does not reflect the *in vivo* situation
[b] F test for DXA fat measurements
[c] Mean±S.E.M.
[d] CV with 95% confidence interval
[e] This phantom received 20 DXA scans at each degree of hydration

of the accuracy and precision of the measurement of total body fat in three phantoms with increasing degrees of fluid overload can be seen. We obtained measurements of total body fat from our DXA facility (15 replicate scans) in phantoms constructed of mincement and lard which underwent moderate fluid overload (3–6 L of isotonic saline) and massive fluid overload (6–12 L of isotonic saline). Total body fat was also measured chemically in multiple samples from the phantoms by ether extraction to remove fat but not essential lipid. From these data, it can be seen that the precision (short-term) of the estimates of total body fat was between 1.1% and 1.9% (95% confidence limits 0.6%–2.6%).

Mineral

Osseous mineral, the larger component of which is calcium hydroxyapatite, comprises by weight most of the mineral in the body. It can be measured with high accuracy and precision by DXA [8–11]. There is also non-bone mineral amounting to about 600 g in Reference Man [12] and which we calculate in critically ill patients by its relationship with total body protein using the equation

$$\mathrm{NBM} = 0.06\ \mathrm{TBP}.$$

Glycogen

The principal distribution of glycogen is in skeletal muscle and liver which together contain about 500 g in Reference Man [12]. However, there may be considerably more glycogen accumulation in intensive care patients receiving high carbohydrate infusions [13]. While indirect methods have allowed estimates of body glycogen to be made [14], the recent ability to measure total body fat by DXA enables estimates of body glycogen to be made by difference according to the following equation:

$$TBG = BW - (TBF + TBW + TBP + TBM)$$

Although we have made estimates of total body glycogen in septic ward patients [15], there are few data available which give estimates of glycogen in critically ill patients [16]. With present techniques, errors are of such magnitude that only group data are meaningful [17, 18].

State of the Art Body Composition Measurements in Intensive Care Patients

An integrated system for measuring the major molecular compartments of the body in intensive care patients has been developed but its use at present is confined to research applications. The system as used in the University Department of Surgery at Auckland Hospital is as follows.

The patient is taken from the ICU to the scanning room which is equipped as an intensive care environment. He is injected with tritiated water to measure TBW and then is weighed on a hoist weighing system consisting of an electrically operated block and tackle attached to a load cell and to a frame that supports a canvas sheet on which the patient lies; the system transfers the patient from the bed to the scanning couch and the body weight is measured during the transfer. The patient enters the scanners 'feet first' with all lines (catheter drains, EKG leads, etc.) following, the monitors placed at the head of the couch and with the respiratory trolley following alongside. The patient is first scanned in the prompt gamma facility (30 min) and then is

Table 4. Precision and accuracy of body composition assessment

Component	Method	Precision (95% confidence limits) (%)	Accuracy (%)	Reference
Protein	IVNAA	3.5 (1.6–6.1)	4	–
Fat	DXA	1.3 (0.6–2.6)	5	[10]
Water	Tritium dilution	1.2 (0.0–2.8)	<5	[7]

moved to the DXA scanner which is in the same room. From tritium dilution, the TBW is estimated, from the prompt gamma *in vivo* neutron activation scan values for total body protein and non-osseous mineral are obtained, and DXA gives values for total osseous mineral and total body lipid or fat. These measurements, together with measurements of body weight (via the hoist), give values for total body glycogen by difference. Thus, the clinically relevant molecular components of the body in terms of protein, lipid, water, mineral and glycogen are obtained from a procedure which takes about 60 min, involving 0.50 mSv of radiation (about 25% of the radiation from natural sources per year). The accuracy and precision of the major components is shown in Table 4.

Use of the Molecular Model of Body Composition in Sudies of Intensive Care Patients

These methods requiring very expensive equipment and a very specialized staff are obviously not for everyday patient care. Their use is however particularly valuable in assessing the effects of new therapies which are currently being proposed for enhancing recovery in intensive care patients. At the University of Auckland, using this methodology, we are currently conducting clinical trials of nutrients as pharmacological agents in patients after major trauma, perioperative treatment with growth factors in patients undergoing rectal excision, and immunotherapeutic agents in patients with serious sepsis.

The Cellular Model of Body Composition

The body has been described by Wang et al [1] as being composed of 4 main compartments at the cellular level, that is, the body cell mass, extracellular fluid, extracellular solids, and fat.

The Body Cell Mass (BCM)

Moore's concept that the body contains a central active core that determines its work capacity, nutritional requirements, protein synthetic capability, oxygen consumption and carbon dioxide output has been immensely valuable and not the least in studies of patients in the ICU [19]. He described this "core" as the body cell mass and its measurement was based on the measurement of total body potassium. By assuming an average ratio for the intracellular K to intracellular N of 3 mmol K/g N and that one quarter of wet cell weight is protein, he pointed out that the body cell mass could be derived from total exchangeable potassium as follows:

$$BCM = 6.25 \times 4 \times (K_e\text{-}ECK)/3$$

$$BCM = K_e \times 8.33$$

where K_2 = total exchangeable potassium, ECK = extracellular potassium (about 2% of body potassium and neglected in the final expression).

Thus, the quantification of the body cell mass is dependent on the assumptions that it has an average K/N ratio of 3 in all states of sickness and health, and that protein comprises 25% of cell mass even in intensive care patients. Although Moore's description and extensive use of the "body cell mass" has proven fundamental to our understanding of the body composition changes in intensive care patients and has aided our understanding of critical illness, the assumptions which allow total body potassium to be used to quantify body cell mass in this way cannot always be made in such patients without resort to complicated tables or nomograms [20].

Extracellular Solids

Almost half of the body protein is an extrusion from cells and spends its life outside cells as structural protein or as soluble protein or as enzymes. These proteins, which are synthesized within cells and live their lives outside cells, form most of what is called extracellular solids; they include the fibrous supporting structures of the body, including collagen, elastin, the dermis, hair, teeth, cartilage and joint capsules. These substances probably do not contribute in any way to the active metabolic processes of the body and are usually assumed to be stable in critically ill patients. This may not be correct, however, and because of this, attempts have been made to divide total body protein into that which is contained within cells and that which is present outside cells. The most widely used model was developed by Burkinshaw et al. [21] who presented data in sick patients in which total body protein was divided into that which was contained in skeletal muscle and that which was contained in the rest of the body. Cohn et al. [22] extending this concept further separated body protein into that contained within viscera and that which was extracellular.

Such models are in an early stage of refinement and cannot at present cope with the changes accompanying critical illness, particularly fluctuations in cellular volumes in tissues as cell contents are consumed by the catabolic process or expanded by excess intracellular water.

Extracellular Fluid

Dilution Methods: Although extracellular water forms a fairly constant proportion of TBW in healthy adults, in sickness extracellular water invariably expands particularly so after resuscitation where it may increase by 50% or more [23, 24]. Traditionally, extracellular water has been measured by radio-sulphate or bromide dilution [25–28] but there are enormous difficulties in interpreting isotope dilution studies in critically ill patients [29]. In normal subjects, an allowance of 10% for bromide penetration of cells and 3% for sulphate is adequate to compensate for losses from the circulation. However, little is known of the kinetics of these substances in intensive care patients and recent work suggests that penetration of these substances into cells is quite different in the critically ill [30].

Neutron Activation: It is possible to measure total body chlorine by neutron activation analysis with reasonable precision (about 5%) [3, 31] and the results of such measurements in sickness (but not critical illness) compared with measurements of extracellular water derived from bromide dilution are shown in Table 5. Clearly the application of measurements of total body chlorine to intensive care patients awaits future work.

In summary, it must be said that the cellular model of body composition poses major practical difficulties for intensive care patients. Not only are difficulties presented by overhydration but alterations in osmolality and alterations in intracellular concentration of K and N make the practical application of this model using present technology extraordinarily difficult.

Other Methods

Whole Body Methods

There are also other ways described by Wang et al. [1] for conceptualizing body composition in terms of the whole body.

Computed Tomographic (CT) body scanning has been used to measure volumes of subcutaneous and adipose tissue [32]. **Magnetic Resonance Imaging** (MRI) has similarly been presented as a tool for measuring the composition of the whole body [33, 34]. There are no data describing use of either CT or MRI for measurements of body composition in intensive care patients.

Table 5. Comparison of extracellular water derived from TBCl with ECW measured by bromide in 10 elective surgical patients

	Extracellular Water (L)	
	TBCl	Bromide
Mean ± SD	16.53 ± 4.08	19.01 ± 2.51
Range	12.12–25.44	16.01–25.08

Dual-energy X-ray Absorptiometry

Dual-energy X-ray absorptiometry (DXA) is being developed to measure not only fat and minerals but also the total lean tissues of the body. With this technology, the tissue content of different regions of the body can also be measured [35], and quite recently, the appendicular muscle mass has been estimated by this technique [36]. The accuracy and precision of such measurements in intensive care patients are being researched at the moment. This technology, which is increasingly available in many hospitals, may open a new era in the measurement of body composition in intensive care patients.

Multifrequency Bioelectrical Impedance Analysis

Multiple frequency bioelectrical impedance analysis (BIA) is an experimental technology. Single frequency (50 kHz) impedance devices have been utilized to estimate both fat-free mass, TBW and its compartments for many years in healthy populations [37–40]. Recent reports indicate that the clinical usefulness of single frequency measurements on individuals who are experiencing fluid status changes is controversial [41–45]. Multifrequency impedance measurements which allow differential current flow through the intra- and extracellular spaces to be assessed may improve the accuracy with which hydration status and fluid distribution may be determined [46, 47]. Carefully controlled clinical trials comparing multifrequency BIA with other methods of measurement of fluid spaces in clinical populations are being conducted.

Combined DXA/BIA

We feel that the combination of DXA and multifrequency BIA may prove ultimately to be the most practical and least expensive method to measure body composition in intensive care patients. For instance, over a period of less than 30 min and with minimal radiation exposure, the combined measurement could break down the body into terms of fat and bone mineral, and subdivide the lean tissues of the body into terms of extracellular and intracellular fluid and quantify the remaining tissues (by difference from body mass) composed of protein, glycogen and non-bone mineral.

Anthropometric Indices

On the whole body level, anthropometric indices such as body weight, body volume, stature, trunk and limb circumferences, and skinfold thicknesses can be estimated directly. We have investigated the value of measuring 2 anthropometric indices in intensive care patients and have as a result come to the following conclusions:

Weight change in intensive care patients is nearly all water change: In intensive care patients, weight changes cannot be used to estimate tissue changes. Changes in body mass are predominantly due to large changes in TBW greatly in excess of protein and fat, and often in the opposite direction. In order to study the relationship between weight change and water change, we studied the changes in body composition over a 10 day period in 10 trauma and 8 septic patients in our ICU (Table 6) [48]. Thus, for both groups of patients, the observed weight changes were predominantly due to changes in body water.

Skinfold anthropometry cannot accurately measure fat in intensive care patients: We have shown that skinfold anthropometry is an inaccurate method of assessing total body fat in patients presenting for nutritional support in the surgical ward [49]. We found that skinfold anthropometry underestimated body fat by about 3 kg in such patients. Because of large changes in weight, use of skinfold anthropometry is even more inappropriate in the patient in intensive care. We measured total body fat by the neutron activation/tritiated water dilution method and also derived total body fat from skinfold anthropometry in 8 ICU patients (Table 7). The highly significant mean difference between total body fat measured by the neutron activation technique and that derived from skinfold anthropometry can be seen.

Conclusion

Simple assessment of body composition such as body weight and anthropometric measurements are not applicable to intensive care patients. A molecular model of the body can be constructed in such patients by using State-of-the-Art technology such as *in vivo* neutron activation analysis combined with dual-energy X-ray absorptiometry and tritium dilution. In this way, the total body contents of fat, protein, glycogen, minerals and water can be mea-

Table 6. Body composition changes over 10 days in patients after severe blunt trauma and serious sepsis

	Trauma	Sepsis
Weight (kg)	-4.2 ± 1.2^{2}	-6.2 ± 2.9
Water (kg)	-3.3 ± 1.4^{1}	-6.8 ± 2.6^{1}
Protein (kg)	-1.1 ± 0.2^{4}	-1.5 ± 0.3^{3}
Fat (kg)	$+0.2 \pm 0.6$	$+2.2 \pm 0.8^{1}$

All values as mean ± SEM
Paired *t*-test: $^{1}p<0.05$, $^{2}p<0.01$, $^{3}p<0.002$, $^{4}p<0.001$, all other changes not significant.

Table 7. Total body fat measured by IVNAA and by skinfold anthropometry

Patient	Weight	TBF (IVNAA) (kg)	TBF (Anthropometry) (kg)
1	79.4	24.0	21.7
2	81.5	14.0	23.4
3	79.4	13.5	26.3
4	83.5	15.6	26.7
5	68.6	9.8	19.3
6	65.0	12.3	16.4
7	72.9	17.4	30.8
8	59.7	20.7	22.5
9	89.9	22.0	29.6
Mean ± SE		16.6 ± 1.6	24.1 ± 1.6
Differences Mean ± SE 7.5 ± 1.8 (p = 0.003)			

sured with sufficient accuracy and precision to allow clinical trials of therapeutic agents which may enhance recovery in critically ill patients.

Using measurements of total body potassium, total body fat (DXA), and extracellular water (bromide or sulphate dilution), a cellular model of the body can also be applied to ICU patients but the interpretative difficulties appear to be insurmountable. Other whole body techniques such as CT scanning and MRI are extremely expensive and as yet untried, and their future is uncertain. On the other hand, the use of multifrequency bioelectrical impedance analysis to measure body fluid compartments and DXA to measure tissue composition may eventually prove to be the most practical and least expensive method for the measurement of body composition in intensive care patients.

References

1. Wang ZM, Pierson RN Jr, Heymsfield SB (1992) The five-level model: A new approach to organizing body-composition research. Am J Clin Nutr 56:19–28
2. Kinney JM, Moore FD (1956) Carbon balance. A clinical approach to energy exchange. Surgery 40:16–26
3. Yasumura S, Cohn SH, Ellis KJ (1983) Measurement of extracellular space by total body neutron activation. Am J Physiol 244:R360–R404
4. Beddoe AH, Streat SJ, Hill GL (1984) Evaluation of an in vivo prompt gamma neutron activation facility for body composition studies in critically ill intensive care patients: Results on 41 normals. Metabolism 33:270–280
5. von Hevesy G, Hofer E (1934) Elimination of water from the human body. Nature 134:879

6. Streat SJ, Beddoe AH, Hill GL (1985) Measurement of total body water in intensive care patients with fluid overload. Metabolism 34:688–694
7. Culebras JM, Moore FD (1977) Total body water and the exchangeable hydrogen. Theoretical calculations of nonaqueous exchangeable hydrogen in man. Am J Physiol 232:R54–R59
8. Mazess RB, Barden HS, Bisek, JP, Hanson J (1990) Dual energy X-ray absorptiometry for total body and regional bone mineral and soft tissue composition. Am J Clin Nutr 51:1106–1121
9. Mazess RB, Collick B, Trempe J, Barden H, Hanson J (1989) Performance evaluation of a dual-energy X-ray bone densitometer. Calcif Tissue Int 44:228–232
10. Haarbo J, Gotfredsen A, Hassager C, Christiansen C (1991) Validation of body composition by dual energy X-ray absorptiometry. Clin Physiol 11:331–341
11. Gotfredsen A, Borg J, Christiansen C, Mazess RB (1984) Total body bone mineral in vivo by dual photon absorptiometry. II. Accuracy. Clin Physiol 4:357–362
12. ICRP (1975) Report of the task group on reference man. ICRP Report 23. Pergamon, Oxford
13. Askanazi J, Carpentier YA, Elwyn DH, et al (1980) Influence of total parenteral nutrition on fuel utilisation in injury and sepsis. Ann Surg 191:40–46
14. Parry BR (1987) The energy needs of surgical patients. Thesis. University of Otago, New Zealand
15. Hill GL, Stokes MA, Burkinshaw L (1990) Total body glycogen – A proposed technique for measurement in severely ill patients. Aust NZ J Surg 60:715
16. Streat SJ, Beddoe AH, Hill GL (1987) Aggressive nutritional support does not prevent protein loss despite fat gain in septic intensive care patients. J Trauma 27:262–266
17. Stokes MA, Hill GL (1990) A new method for the measurement of total energy expenditure in severely ill patients. Aust NZ J Surg 60:715
18. Hill GL, Knight GS, Stokes MA, Plank LD (1992) Body composition in patient care. In: Kral JG, van Itallie TB (eds) Recent developments in body composition analysis: Methods and applications, Smith-Gordon, London, pp 129–135
19. Moore FD, Olesen KH, McMurray JD, Parker HD, Ball MR, Boyden CM (1963) The body cell mass and its supporting environment: Body composition in health and disease. WB Saunders, Philadelphia
20. Moore FD (1980) Energy and maintenance of the body cell mass. JPEN 4:228–260
21. Burkinshaw L, Hill GL, Morgan DB (1978) Assessment of the distribution of protein in the human body by in vivo neutron activation analysis. In: Nuclear activation techniques in the life sciences, International Atomic Energy Agency, Vienna pp 787–798
22. Cohn SH, Vartsky D, Yasumura S, Vaswani AN, Ellis KJ (1983) Indexes of body cell mass: Nitrogen versus potassium. Am J Physiol 244:E305–E310
23. Hill GL (1992) Disorders of nutrition and metabolism in clinical surgery – Understanding and management. Churchill Livingstone, Edinburgh
24. Moore FD (1959) Metabolic care of the surgical patient. WB Saunders, Philadelphia
25. Shires GT, Williams J, Brown F (1960) Simultaneous measurement of plasma volume, extracellular fluid volume, and red blood cell mass in man utilizing I^{131}, $S^{35}O_4$, and Cr^{51}. J Lab Clin Med 55:776–783
26. Walser M, Seldin DW, Grollman A (1953) An evaluation of radiosulfate for the determination of extracellular fluid in man and dogs. J Clin Invest 32:299–311
27. Barratt TM, Walser M (1969) Extracellular fluid in individual tissues and in whole animals: The distribution of radiosulfate and radiobromide. J Clin Invest 48:56–66
28. Brodie BB, Brand E, Leshin S (1939) The use of bromide as a measure of extracellular fluid. J Biol Chem 130:555–563
29. Moore FD, Shires GT (1967) Moderation. Ann Surg 166:300–301
30. Hannon RJ, Boston VE (1990) Fluid and ion redistribution in skeletal muscle in an animal sepsis model. J Paediat Surg 25:599–603
31. Mitra S, Plank LD, Knight GS, Hill GL (1993) In vivo measurement of total body chlorine using the 8.57 MeV prompt de-excitation following thermal neutron capture. Phys Med Biol 38:161–172

32. Tokunaga K, Matsuzawa Y, Ishikawa K, Tarui S (1988) A novel technique for the determination of body fat by computed tomography. Int J Obesity 7:437–445
33. Fuller MF, Foster MA, Hutchison JMS (1985) Estimation of body fat by nuclear magnetic resonance imaging. Proc Nutr Soc 44:108A
34. Fowler PA, Fuller MF, Glasbey CA, Cameron GG, Foster MA (1992) Validation of the in vivo measurement of adipose tissue by magnetic resonance imaging of lean and obese pigs. Am J Clin Nutr 56:7–13
35. Schlemmer A, Hassager C, Haarbo J, Christiansen C (1990) Direct measurement of abdominal fat by dual photon absorptiometry. Int J Obesity 14:603–611
36. Heymsfield SB, Smith R, Aulet M, et al (1990) Appendicular skeletal muscle mass: Measurement by dual-photon absorptiometry. Am J Clin Nutr 52:214–218
37. Lukaski HC, Johnson PE, Bolonchuk WW, Lykken GI (1985) Assessment of fat-free mass using bioelectrical impedance measurements of the human body. Am J Clin Nutr 41:810–817
38. Khaled MA, McCutcheon MJ, Reddy S, Pearman PL, Hunter GR, Weinsier RL (1988) Electrical impedance in assessing human body composition: The BIA method. Am J Clin Nutr 47:789–792
39. Segal KR, van Loan M, Fitzgerald PI, Hodgdon JA, van Itallie TB (1988) Lean body mass estimation by bioelectrical impendance analysis: A four-site cross-validation study. Am J Clin Nutr 47:7–14
40. Kushner RF, Schoeller DA (1986) Estimation of total body water by bioelectrical impedance analysis. Am J Clin Nutr 44:417—424
41. Meguid MM, Lukaski HC, Tripp MD, Rosenburg JM, Parker FB (1992) Rapid bedside method to assess changes in postoperative fluid status with bioelectrical impedance analysis. Surgery 112:502–508
42. Kurtin PS, Shapiro AC, Tomita H, et al (1990) Volume status and body composition of chronic dialysis patients: Utility of bioelectric impedance plethysmography. Am J Nephrol 10:363–367
43. Zillikens MC, van den Berg JWO, Wilson JHP, Swart GR (1992) Whole-body and segmental bioelectrical-impedance analysis in patients with cirrhosis of the liver: Changes after treatment of ascites. Am J Clin Nutr 55:621–625
44. Schroeder D, Christie PM, Hill GL (1990) Bioelectric impedance analysis for body composition: Clinical evaluation in general surgical patients. JPEN 14:129–133
45. Dal Cin S, Braga M, Molinari M, Cristallo M, Di Carlo V (1991) Reliability of bioelectrical impedance analysis in dehydrated subjects. Clin Nutr 10(Suppl):9
46. Duerenberg P, Schouten FJM (1992) Loss of total body water and extracellular water assessed by multifrequency impedance. Eur J Clin Nutr 46:247–255
47. Segal KR, Burastero S, Chun A, Coronel P, Pierson RN Jr, Wang J (1991) Estimation of extracellular and total body water by multiple-frequency bioelectrical-impedance measurement. Am J Clin Nutr 54:26–29
48. Streat SJ, Hill GL (1987) Nutritional support in the management of critically ill patients in surgical intensive care. World J Surg 11:194–201
49. Streat SJ, Beddoe AH, Hill GL (1985) Measurement of body fat and hydration of the fat-free body in health and disease. Metabolism 34:509–518

Applications of Magnetic Resonance Spectroscopy to Nutrition and Metabolism

D. O. Jacobs and M. K. Robinson

"Disease can impose an extreme short term disturbance,
which leads to a regulatory catastrophe, or instability of metabolic control,
in individual cells, whole organs, or the total organism.
All these processes and phenomena have their molecular basis in the underlying
biochemical events that are functionally expressed only in the living cells
or organisms."[1, 2]

Introduction

The development of magnetic resonance spectroscopy (MRS) has made it possible to examine cellular and organellar function non-invasively and to improve our understanding of the pathophysiological and clinical changes observed in many disease states. Various MRS techniques allow investigators to study intracellular abnormalities, their biochemical bases, and the mechanisms by which they occur. These responses are important to understand since they often antedate the development of more overt manifestations of disease and end-state organ failure. Organ systems that have been studied include muscle, heart, brain, and liver.

Background and Introduction to Magnetic Resonance Spectroscopy

Nuclear magnetic resonance (NMR) techniques are based on the response of certain nuclear species with an odd number of protons or neutrons to static magnetic fields and other energy applied in the radiofrequency range. Some diagnostically relevant nuclei are ^{1}H, ^{2}H, ^{13}C, ^{19}F, ^{23}Na, ^{31}P and ^{39}K. These nuclei behave like bar magnets and will align their poles with the direction of an externally applied static magnetic field. When energy is applied to one of these molecules as a radiofrequency pulse, its alignment with the external magnetic field is perturbed. Once the radiofrequency pulse is discontinued, the nucleus returns to its equilibrium state by dissipating the absorbed energy through interactions with the surrounding environment and with other molecules [3]. The computer-assisted capture and analysis of the dissipated energy forms the basis for nuclear MRS and imaging. Detection is largely dependent on the strength of the NMR signal which in turn is determined by 4 factors: concentration within the region of interest, natural isotopic abundance, relative sensitivity, and mobility. For example, MRS techniques are only 1/15th as sensitive to ^{31}P as they are to ^{1}H because protons are far more abundant in body tissues.

Concentration and mobility are most relevant for the clinical investigator. The higher the concentration of the element imaged, the stronger the signal. Unfortunately, the particular isotope possessing spin may not be the isotope in greatest natural abundance in the body. For example, the predominant isotope of carbon, ^{12}C, is present in reasonable concentrations in the body. However, ^{12}C has an even number of proteins and neutrons, and thus cannot be detected in NMR experiments. ^{13}C, which is NMR-visible, accounts for only 1% of the total carbon in the body. This fact has led to the use of ^{13}C enriched tracers for most carbon NMR studies. In contrast, ^{31}P is both the naturally occurring isotope and the isotope observable by NMR.

Mobility is also an important determinant of the ability of a given nucleus to generate an effective signal. Mobility is greater if the nucleus is part of a relatively small molecule in the cytoplasm rather than if it is associated with large macromolecules bound to membranes. These factors are particularly important in ^{31}P spectroscopy. *In vivo* ^{31}P magnetic resonance spectroscopy performed using static magnetic fields of the strengths currently available can detect phosphorus metabolites such as inorganic phosphate and ATP that are present in concentrations greater than 0.5 mM. Significant binding to mitochondria and other effects that reduce mobility may decrease the number of ^{31}P nuclei that can be detected to approximately 20% of the total present.

Despite these potential difficulties, a large body of information on metabolic changes in various organs and tissues has been obtained using phosphorus MRS and spectroscopy of other nuclei. In the following discussions, 31-phosphorus will be used to illustrate the utility of the MRS techniques. However, one should keep in mind that 31-phosphorus is just one of many MRS visible nuclei that may ultimately be proven to be relevant to the study of metabolism and physiology *in vivo*.

Phosphorus is a major component of the body that is present at a level which comprises approximately 1% of the lean weight of the human adult. It plays a crucial role in many metabolic processes, e.g., it is present in the sugar phosphate backbone of nucleic acids and it forms a part of the polar group of the phospholipids of various cell membranes. In general, however, the phosphorus of DNA and of most phospholipids is not observable by ^{31}P MRS of living tissue partly because of its relatively low concentration but also because of signal broadening and loss of resolution secondary to the immobility of phosphorus in these compounds.

Many of the investigations that are relevant to metabolic assessment have been performed on skeletal muscle. ATP is broken down through the activity of various ATPases (including the Na^+-K^+ ATPase) to provide energy for cellular work (Fig. 1). This ATP is provided by glycolysis, glycogenolysis, and oxidative phosphorylation but can also be provided via the breakdown of the high energy phosphate storage compound phosphocreatine (PCr). In

$$ATP \xrightarrow{ATPases} ADP + Pi^* + Energy$$

$$PCr^* + ADP \xrightarrow{Creatine\ Kinase} ATP^* + Creatine$$

* represents compounds that are MRS Visible

Fig. 1. Two metabolic pathways in skeletal muscle to assess cellular energetics using phosphorus MRS

this reaction catalyzed by creatine kinase, ADP is rephosphorylated to regenerate ATP. Thus, when phosporous (^{31}P) compounds are measured in skeletal muscle, the processes associated with the production and utilization of ATP are followed. Although absolute quantification is possible, changes in the ratios of the phosphate compounds are used to estimate changes in energy availability (ATP/Pi), the relationship between high energy phosphate stores and ATP (PCr/ATP), and thermodynamic capacity (PCr/Pi) (which represents the sum of forward flow through the two pathways). The β-ATP peak is used to represent changes in ATP since its peak, unlike those of α and γ-ATP, is not contaminated by other adenine nucleotides or ^{31}P MRS visible compounds.

Figure 2 shows a representative spectrum obtained from rat skeletal muscle at rest using a high strength magnetic field (8.45 Tesla). In skeletal muscle, 5 major peaks are readily detected representing the 3 phosphate atoms of ATP, PCr, and inorganic phosphate. Occasionally, a smaller, broader peak upfield (+ ppm) from the inorganic phosphate peak may be seen which corresponds to phosphomonoesters (PME). Muscle PME is believed to be largely comprised of gylcolytic intermediates such as glucose-6-phosphate. The distance between the PCr and the P_i peaks in skeletal muscle (chemical shift) in ppm can be used to determine intracellular pH since this

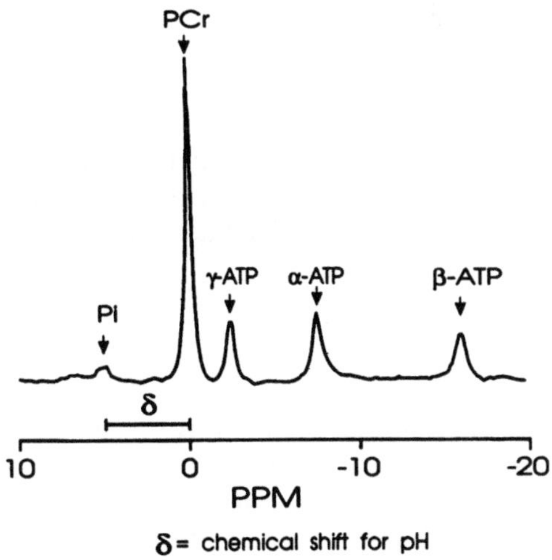

Fig. 2. A typical in vivo high resolution ^{31}P spectrum of the rat gastrocnemius muscle at rest. Five major peaks represents γ, α and β phosphates of ATP, phosphocreatine (PCr), and inorganic phosphate (Pi). The distance between PCr and Pi peaks (σ) can be used to measure intracellular pH

distance varies linearly with H^+ concentration over a wide physiological range. The intracellular pH value is obtained by comparison with a graph of chemical shifts in ppm versus pH for titrated organic phopshate solutions.

There are two primary aspects which are important in interpreting magnetic resonance spectra correctly. These are the assignment of the peaks, i.e. qualitative analysis, and the measurement of relative or absolute amounts of the various compounds, i.e. quantitative analysis. In general, the amount of tissue from which the signals are obtained varies according to the technique that is used to obtain the signals. Furthermore, determination of the concentration of the MRS visible metabolities requires the use of an internal or external standards although there are methods that do not require the use of these standards. Many investigators use ATP concentrations, measured *in vitro*, as an internal standard based either on the assumption that the concentration of this metabolite does not vary significantly under the experimental conditions and/or the demonstration that this is true using *in vitro* assays. One potential weakness of this method, especially when it is used to analyze skeletal muscle, is that it assumes that the tissue scanned is relatively homogeneous in the sense of having predominantly one fiber type. Whereas this is most likely the case for the superficial region of the gastrocnemius, it may not be true in other muscle tissues or organ beds.

In addition to the measurement of absolute or relative quantities of phosphorus containing compounds, e.g. ATP, PCr, and inorganic phosphate, and pH, MRS can also be used to measure chemical reaction rates *in vivo* and *in vitro*. Forsen and Hoffmann first described the use of NMR magnetization transfer to measure chemical fluxes in 1964 [4]. In a magnetization transfer experiment, a magnetic label is applied to one or more resonances. The transfer of the magnetic label between chemical sites is a reflection of both the chemical reaction rate and the intrinsic NMR relaxation time. Theoretically, given a reaction of the general form:

$$AX + B \underset{K_2}{\overset{K_1}{\rightleftharpoons}} BX + A$$

where A and B transfer a moiety X which contains a magnetic nucleus, between them, then k_1 and k_2 can be measured separately using magnetization transfer techniques. For example, in skeletal muscle creatine kinase catalyzes the exchange of phosphate between two distinct, MRS-visible sites, PCr and the γ-phosphate of ATP according to:

$$PCr \underset{k_{rev}}{\overset{k_{for}}{\rightleftharpoons}} [\gamma\text{-P}]ATP$$

Thus, whereas, traditional ^{31}P MRS spectroscopy can be used to obtain the concentrations of PCr and ATP, magnetization transfer experiments provide direct estimates of rate constants. In skeletal muscle, selective irradiation and saturation of PCr or [γ-P]-ATP with a long radiofrequency pulse of low power of varying durations and measurement of transfer of magnetic label (e.g.

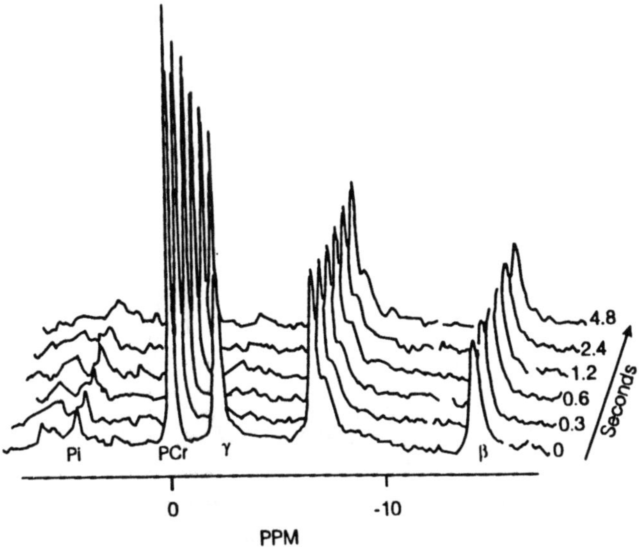

Fig. 3. Spectra from saturation transfer experiments. A surface coil was positioned over the gastrocnemius muscle of a rat and ^{31}P MRS spectra were obtained after 0 to 4.8 sec of selective saturation at the γ-ATP peak. Changes in the area under the PCr peak are used to calculate PCr breakdown rates

an exponential decrease in the area under the PCr peak when the pulse is applied at γ-P[ATP]) is used to calculate k_{for} and k_{rev} for the creatine kinase reaction, respectively(Fig. 3). Fluxes through the foward and reverse creatine kinase reaction can be calculated as k_{for}*[PCr] and k_{rev}*[ATP], respectively. Furthermore, when the inorganic phosphate signal is well discriminated, saturation at γ-P[ATP] may also be used to measure ATP synthesis from inorganic phosphate *in vivo* since its signal will also decrease exponentially with saturation time.

The measurement of chemical fluxes or the rate constants for the creatine kinase pathway may provide useful information about the metabolic status and the physiological demands being placed on a particular organ. Such measurements provide more dynamic information than the simpler measurements of high energy phosphate ratios. For example, steady state concentrations of PCr and ATP are relatively poor indicators of brain function [5]. PCr and ATP levels in a rat anesthetized with barbiturate that has low EEG activity are indistinguishable from those of controls [6]. Seizures induced by the administration of bicuculine do not reduce cerebral ATP levels despite a marked increase in EEG activity [7]. However, the forward rate constant (as a marker of ATP turnover) is a much more sensitive indicator of brain function than the measurement of steady state PCr and ATP concentration [8].

In spectra of the liver, the three phosphate atoms of ATP and inorganic phosphate are also readily visualized (Fig. 4). The PME peak is more prom-

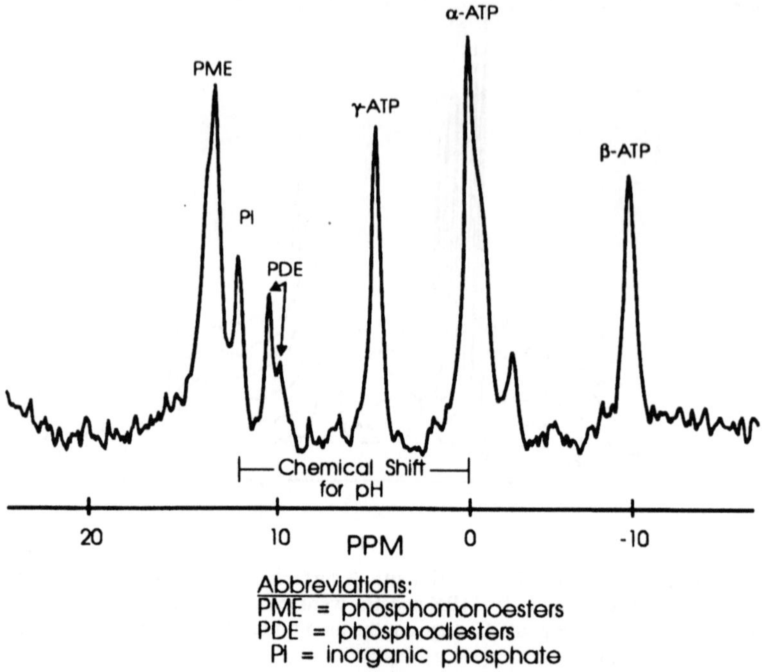

Fig. 4. The 3 phosphate atoms of ATP and inorganic phosphates are also readily identified in *in vivo* spectra of the liver. Peaks corresponding to PME and PDE can also be identified

inent and represents sugar phosphates, membrane phospholipd precursors such as phosphoethanolamine and phosphocholine, but also may include a small contribution from adenosine monophosphate as well. A peak corresponding to the phosphodiesters (PDE), i.e. phospholipid catabolites such as glycerophosphocholine and glycerophosphoethanolamine, is seen between the peaks identifying inorganic phosphate and γ-ATP. Thus, PME and phosphodiester (PDE) peaks are largely made up by membrane phospholipid precursors and breakdown products. For this reason, changes in the PME/ATP and PDE/ATP ratios correlate with changes in hepatocellular membrane synthesis or degradation if intracellular ATP concentrations do not change significantly.

A PCr peak is seen in hepatic spectra since the liver has no PCr. One can derive the ATP to Pi ratio from MRS analysis of the liver by dividing the area under the β-ATP peak by the area under the Pi peak just as is done for skeletal muscle. By convention, the ratio for liver MRS studies is usually reported as Pi/ATP (rather than ATP/Pi) and is therefore inversely related to cell energy status. Accordingly, as the Pi to ATP ratio increases, cell energy status worsens. The ATP to Pi ratio is an excellent qualitative estimate of the cell's phosphorylation potential because the concentration of ADP is much smaller (less than 5%) than the concentration of either ATP or Pi, and therefore changes in phosphorylation potential largely depend on changes in ATP and Pi. In MRS scans of the liver, the chemical shift or distance between the Pi and α-ATP peaks is linearly related to intracellular pH. An increase in the distance between these peaks indicates that the hepatocytes are becoming more alkalotic while a decrease in this distance indicates relative acidosis. Thus the information from the typical liver MRS scan can be used to assess hepatocellular energy status, hepatocyte intracellular pH, and hepatocyte membrane integrity, all of which provide basic information about liver function (Table 1).

Importance of the Phosphorylation Potential

All intracellular processes, either directly or indirectly, depend on the ability of the cell to maintain adequate production of ATP. ATP provides the energy necessary for vital cellular functions. Furthermore, many metabolic reactions are controlled changes in the cell's "energy status". There are two com-

Table 1. Explanation of commonly used liver phosphorus MRS indices

MRS parameter	Interpretation	Explanation
Pi/ATP	Inversely related to intracellular energy status	The Pi to ATP ratio is closely related to the phosphorylation potential which is a commonly used index of cell energy status.
Chemical shift between Pi and α-ATP peaks	Directly related to intracellular pH	Hydration of inorganic phosphate molecule varies according to intracellular hydrogen ion concentration. The α-phosphorus of ATP is not affected by cell hydrogen ion concentration. Thus, on MRS scans, the Pi peak shifts relative to the α-ATP peak (i.e. the distance between these peaks) changes as intracellular hydrogen ion concentration changes.
PME/ATP	Direct association with phospholipid membrane damage if no change in intracellular ATP concentration	PME region contains the peaks of phosphocholine, phosphoethanolamine, and α-glycerophosphate which are intermediary metabolites of membrane phospholipid turnover. Increase in this region is associated with membrane damage.
PDE/ATP	Direct association with phospholipid membrane damage if no change in intracellular ATP concentration	PDE region contains the peaks of glycerophosphocholine and glycerophosphoethanolamine which are intermediary metabolites of phospholipid catabolism. Increase in this region is associated with membrane damage.

monly used indices of cell energy status: Atkinson's energy charge and the phosphorylation potential.

The energy charge is defined as:

$$\frac{[ATP]+1/2[ADP]}{[ATP]+[ADP]+[AMP]}.$$

Daniel Atkinson, after whom the energy charge is named, demonstrated that a high energy charge inhibits ATP-generating pathways and stimulates ATP-utilizing pathways [9] (Malcolm's 13). Thus, under normal circumstances there is an internal mechanism which regulates energy charge within a narrow range.

Another important index of energy state which can be measured *in vivo* is the phosphorylation potential. The phosphorylation ratio of a cell is defined as [10]:

$$PR=\frac{[ATP]}{[ADP][Pi]}.$$

The phosphorylation potential is directly related to the free energy available from ATP and, in contrast to Atkinson's energy charge, varies with the concentration of inorganic phosphate. This ratio modulates a variety of metabolic processes including, for example:

1. the efficiency of cardiac work per mole of coronary O_2 delivered;
2. the oxidation-reduction state of cellular co-factors;
3. whether dietary or tissue amino acids will be synthesized into tissue protein or broken down into glucose;
4. the extent of the plasma membrane gradients of the essential electrolytes;
5. the intracellular pH; and
6. the distribution of water between the various cellular compartments.

Since the phosphorylation potential is critically related to a number of essential properties of living cells and is a critical index of cellular function, it may be monitored and perhaps manipulated by specific therapeutic metabolic interventions.

Normally, the concentration of ADP free in the cytosol (20 to 50 mmol) is below the sensitivity of typical MRS equipment. However, the phosphorylation potential in heart, brain, and muscle can be determined indirectly using the PCr present in these tissues and the creatine kinase equilibrium. Since the reactants of the creatine kinase reaction are in near equilibrium in these tissues, the free ADP concentration can be determined from the intracellular pH, PCr, ATP, and creatine concentrations and the equilibrium constant for the creatine kinase reaction according to:

$$[ADP]=\frac{[ATP][Cr]}{[PCr][H^+][K_{CK}]},$$

where $[H^+]$ is derived from the pH measurement, and K_{CK} is the equilibrium constant. The creatine concentration may be determined *in vitro* or can be estimated by assuming that any change in this substrate is equimolar to the change in phosphate. The substrate ratios and the intracellular pH are determined directly from the spectra. The phosphorylation potential or ratio, can then be derived using the calculated free ADP concentration and the ratio of ATP to inorganic phosphate (Pi) is taken directly from the phosphorus MRS spectra.

The discussion so far has emphasized the use of ^{31}P MRS as a two-dimensional (2-D) tool. However, it is important to note that localization techniques are being refined to the point where "metabolite maps" similar to traditional CT-like transverse, coronal or other anatomical images can also be constructed. It is also important to remember that 2-D and 3-D MRS are highly specialized fields which require specialized hardware and software. At this time, few centers are capable of performing these studies. However, machines capable of magnetic resonance imaging are present in most major hospital centers.

Phosphorus MRS has been used to study tissue energetics of exercising muscle. During anaerobic (ischemic) contraction, only glycogenolysis and PCr breakdown can *regenerate* ATP, though the predominant fuel for skeletal muscle in the well-fed state is free fatty acids [11]. Under aerobic conditions, especially during the early stages of dynamic exercise, both oxidative and anaerobic reactions contribute to ATP formation. The resynthesis of PCr and the return of the muscle energy state to the equilibrium conditions are thought to be dependent on oxidative processes alone. Futhermore, the maximal mitochondrial metabolic rate can be determined from the time constant of the slope of the recovery curves. Thus, the restoration of resting PCr concentrations, and the clearance of inorganic phosphate and H+ after exercise, as measured from the intracellular pH recovery, have characteristic time courses in healthy muscle.

Argov and Chance [12] has reviewed the use of phosphorus MRS during muscular exercise as a tool for nutritional and metabolic assessment, and reported how the efficiency of the coupling between ATP usage and work can be used to analyze muscle function and metabolic state. For example, Chance and associates [13] recorded wrist flexor and gastrocnemius work output while ^{31}P NMR spectra were obtained. This study and others have shown that oxidative phosphorylation can be modeled as a metabolic process which follows Michaelis-Menton kinetics for single enzyme systems. The typical phosphorus MRS experiment during exercise involves graded levels of work and the measurement of high energy phosphate ratios such as PCr/Pi under steady state or near steady state conditions. Typically, work rate per unit volume of muscle and PCr/Pi are linearly related [14]. Chance's work suggests that the slope and the extent of the linearity of the relationship between work output and NMR ratios such as PCr/Pi are indices that can be used to identify normal and abnormal muscle function and to compare changes in oxidative metabolism. Thus, theoretically, a metabolic deficiency such as fasting, might lead to a greater decrease in PCr/Pi in response to a specific work load and would decrease the slope of the line describing changes in PCr/Pi as a function of the amount of work performed.

The application of ^{31}P magnetic resonance techniques specifically to the metabolic assessment and critical care is still in its infancy. Nevertheless, there are animal studies and an increasingly large number of studies in humans which illustrate the utility of MRS methods to understand how skeletal muscle and other organs respond to nutritional deprivation and other metabolic challenges.

Animal Studies

Effects of Starvation and Refeeding

^{31}P NMR spectroscopy has great potential as a research instrument with which to investigate the effects of malnutrition on skeletal muscle. The technique is particularly attractive since one can simultaneously and in an integrated manner study functional and metabolic perturbations induced by nutrient deprivation. Data from animal studies suggest that these techniques may be valuable. For example, serial ^{31}P MRS spectra have been obtained from the hind limb of rats during 8 days of starvation and 4 days of refeeding [15]. ATP/Pi, PCr/Pi, and pH were unchanged over the study period. PCr/ATP ratios were significant lower by the 4 day of complete starvation but returned to normal by the 4th day of refeeding. This early study demonstrated that ^{31}P nuclear MRS could be used to detect changes in muscle energy metabolism associated with starvation and refeeding, and suggested that intracellular ATP concentrations were maintained at the expense of PCr during periods of starvation. Furthermore, it was hypothesized that resting PCr/ATP ratios might correlate with nutritional depletion and repletion.

Pichard and colleagues [16] examined the effect of various dietary manipulations on rat muscle energetics in a more extensive study using phosphorus NMS and *in vitro* biochemical analyses. In this study, changes in various high-energy phosphate ratios were determined in resting controls, 2-day fasted and hypocalorically fed rats, and in animals refed after hypocaloric feeding. ATP, inorganic phosphate, and intracellular magnesium levels were comparable in the 4 groups of animals. However, the ratios of PCr/Pi and ATP/Pi, the calculated PCr concentration, and the free-energy change of ATP hydrolysis were decreased, but the calculated free ADP concentration was increased in fasted and underfed animals as compared to controls. The authors concluded that their data were also consistent with the hypothesis that ATP levels are maintained at the expense of PCr during undernutrition. This occurs at a time when ATP production is altered by changes in aerobic and anaerobic metabolism. What was not clear was whether the decrease in PCr was secondary to a decreased synthesis of this compound as a result of starvation while forward flux through the creatine kinase pathway was unchanged, or whether levels decreased in association with an increased forward flux.

MRS saturation transfer studies were performed in rats during fasting and refeeding 1) to measure the forward rate constant for the creatine kinase reaction in resting gastrocnemius muscle to determine if there were physiological adjustments in the breakdown rate of PCr; i.e. flux in the direction of ATP synthesis, to maintain skeletal muscle ATP levels; and 2) to understand how skeletal muscle adapts to decreased levels of PCr [17]. A simple linear regression analysis showed that the rate constant for the forward creatine kinase reaction, k_{for}, increased linearly with fasting of up to 96 h in duration and returned to normal within 3 days of *ad libitum* refeeding. A significant increase in k_{for} was detected by 24 h of starvation. PCr/ATP but not ATP levels determined *in vitro*, also decreased with fasting. Even though PCr levels decreased in these rats, forward flux through the creatine kinase pathway (and hence ATP production via this route) was not significantly different from that measured in the normally nourished controls. In contrast, septic rats have a 20% decrease in PCr/ATP within 24 h of cecal ligation and puncture while ATP concentrations *in vitro* were unchanged [18]. The drecrease in PCr levels was associated with a greater increase in k_{for} than that seen in starvation. Furthermore, a 20% increase in the PCr breakdown rate was detected in the septic animals. These studies illustrate how the relatively simple measurement of k_{for} and PCr breakdown rates *in vivo* can provide useful information about metabolic stress within a tissue bed or organ.

Some studies performed in animals would also suggest that there are changes in skeletal muscle function that can be examined using NMR techniques. In one study, adult rats were fasted for 6 days [19]. On days 0, 3, and 6 of starvation, the animals underwent ^{31}P NMR spectroscopy during isometric exercise of the right lower limb. The limb was exercised by percutaneous supramaximal stimulation of the sciatic nerve for 10 min periods at 0.25, 0.5, 1.0, and 2.0 Hz. Increasing exercise decreased PCr/Pi in an monoexponential fashion. By day 6, PCr/Pi at each stimulation rate was significantly less than at day 0. In addition, the slope of the mean PCr/Pi-stimulation rate function at day 6 was significantly less than at day 0 (0.77 versus 0.35, $p<0.03$). The decrease in PCr/Pi was thought to be secondary to the depletion of intracellular PCr since it is hydrolyzed to resynthesize ATP consumed by muscle contraction. These data imply that skeletal muscle would become less efficient with ongoing starvation and would require a greater PCr (energy) consumption for a given stimulation rate (work load) as compared to normal controls.

This hypothesis was tested in animal experiments that modeled steady-state changes in PCr/Pi within the gastrocnemius muscle as a function of the frequency of supramaximal stimulation of the sciatic nerve. In these studies of rats fasted for 4 days, the decrease in PCr/Pi during nerve stimulation was well fitted by a single exponential equation. The mean stimulation frequency required to cause a 50% decrease in PCr/Pi was 0.41 Hz compared to 1.03 Hz for well fed controls. Thus, work was being performed at the same rate in both groups but in fasted rats, the metabolic expense was greater, and their function less efficient. In these same fasted animals, the recovery rate of PCr/Pi, i.e. return to baseline values, was approximately 6 times slower than that of controls. The latter strongly suggests that oxidative capacity was reduced.

Effects of Growth Hormone Administration on Skeletal Muscle During Fasting and Refeeding

Administering growth hormone (GH) to humans who are receiving adequate amounts of protein but insufficient calories increases their nitrogen accretion or retention by increasing protein synthesis out of proportion to protein catabolism, and by enhancing the mobilization of peripheral energy stores such as body fat. Together, these effects of GH administration minimize the body's drive to breakdown muscle protein to provide carbon skeletons for gluconeogenesis.

In order to analyze the effects of GH administration on skeletal muscle energetics and muscular function during hypocaloric refeeding after fasting, one must first understand the effect of hypocaloric nutritional repletion after a short term fast. This issue was the subject of a recent investigation. In this experiment, male Wistar rats were fasted for 4 days and then were randomized to one of two groups. Animals in the first group were refed a nutritionally complete liquid diet *ad libitum* whereas rats in the second group were refed hypocalorically. The hypocaloric diet provided only 25% of the daily caloric requirement. Both diets supplied adequate amounts of protein (3 mg of nitrogen per gram body weight per day). All of the animals were allowed water *ad libitum*. ^{31}P magnetic resonance spectra of the gastrocnemius were obtained using a surface coil in a magnet operating at a very high magnetic field strength. Scans were performed while the rats were in a well fed condition, after 4 days of fasting, and 4 days after they had resumed a normal or hypocaloric diet. These spectra were used to determine phosphate ratios, including PCr/ATP, intracellular pH, and the forward rate constant (k_f) and forward flux (which is the breakdown rate of PCr) through the creatine kinase pathway. ATP, protein content, and creatine kinase activity were determined spectrophotometrically.

The ATP levels, protein content, creatine kinase activity, and intracellular pH of skeletal muscle did not change significantly with fasting or refeeding of the control or hypocaloric diet. Rats that were fasted experienced a 30% decrease in body weight. Hypocalorically refed rats did not gain weight while the animals that were allowed to refeed *ad libitum* essentially regained the weight that was lost during the fasting period. The PCr/ATP ratio (and, therefore, PCr stores since ATP levels did not change significantly) decreased with fasting but eventually returned to normal levels in both groups of refed rats (Fig. 5).

Rats that were refed hypocalorically had a significantly larger forward rate constant than rats in the control group which were allowed to refeed *ad libi-*

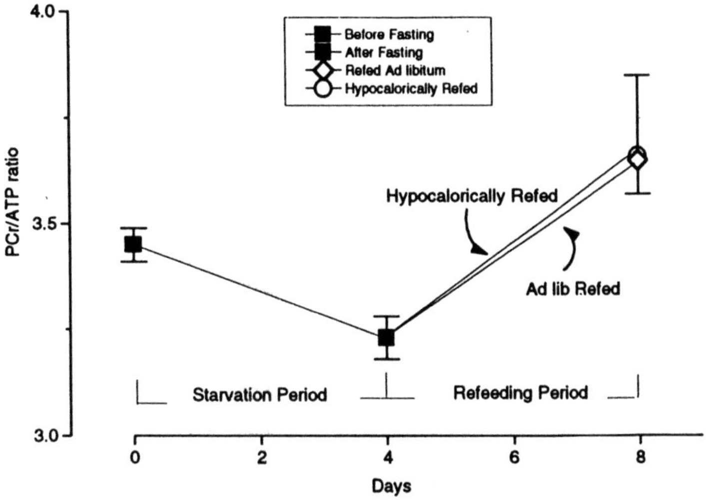

Fig. 5. PCr/ATP ratios decreased significantly with starvation and returned to normal levels in hypcalorically and ad libitum refed rats

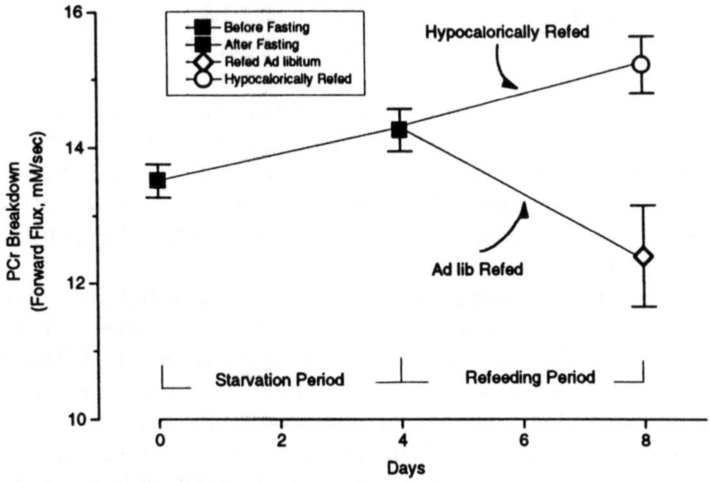

Fig. 6. PCr breakdown rates increased with fasting. In addition, after 4 days of refeeding, the breakdown of PCr was much higher in hypocalorically refed rats

tum (0.41 ± 0.02 vs 0.36 ± 0.02, $p < 0.05$). In addition, after 4 days of refeeding, the breakdown rate of PCr was much higher in hypocalorically refed rats (Fig. 6). This suggests that ATP turnover rates were much higher in these undernourished animals.

This study shows that the restoration of normal PCr/ATP ratios and therfore high energy phosphate stores in skeletal muscle does not require anabolic weight gain. A likely explanation for these findings is that the restoration or recovery of normal levels of PCr occurs as an adaptive process where a new equilibrium state of the creatine kinase pathway is achieved. In this instance, both forward and reverse flux through the creatine kinase pathway, and therefore PCr turnover, must be increased. Thus, although the hypocalorically fed rat is able to restore normal steady state levels of ATP and PCr, the turnover of high-energy phosphates is increased. This experiment shows (not surprisingly!) that hypocaloric refeeding is clearly superior to starvation in terms of maintaining normal intramuscular levels of high energy phosphates, but it further suggests that nutritional or metabolic support techniques which decrease PCr turnover may be advantageous.

The next step was to study the effects of GH administration on energetics in skeletal muscle during a short term fast. As was alluded to previously, exogenous GH administration has been shown to improve nitrogen retention in a variety of catabolic patients but its effects on energetics in skeletal muscle are unknown. In the experiment that will be described, rats were randomized to be fed a nutritionally complete diet (control) or to be fasted for 4 days with (+GH) or without growth hormone (−GH) administration. Rats in the +GH group received 5 micrograms of GH per gram body weight subcutaneously twice daily during the study period, whereas animals in the control and −GH groups received placebo injections; all were allowed to drink water *ad libitum*. Urine was collected daily so that nitrogen, phosphorus, potassium, sodium, and water balances could be calculated. *In vivo* ^{31}P MRS of the right gastrocnemius muscle was performed at baseline, and 2 and 4 days after fasting. High energy phosphate ratios, intracellular pH, and PCr breakdown rate were determined, however, the PCr breakdown rate was only measured at baseline and after 4 days of starvation. Tissue ATP levels, total creatine kinase (CK) activities, and other substrates were measured spectrophotometrically.

As expected, both groups of rats that were fasted lost weight as compared to the well fed controls that gained weight. However, GH treated rats lost 15% less weight that the rats which did not receive GH. The 15% less severe weight loss was associated with a 13% greater nitrogen retention. In addition, as has been observed in other studies, the administration of growth hormone was associated with increased phosphorus, potassium, sodium, and water balances. These findings are consistent with a less pronounced decrease in lean body mass in the GH treated rats.

ATP levels and creatine kinase activities were the same in all groups of animals. PCr/ATP levels, and therefore high energy phosphate stores, were slightly but significantly lower in the rats that were fasted for 2 days and given GH secondary to an increased consumption of PCr. However, after 4 days of fasting, PCr/ATP levels were similarly depressed in both groups of fasted animals (Fig. 7).

After 4 days of fasting, PCr breakdown rates were significantly higher in the fasted animals that did not receive GH as compared to the other two groups. PCr breakdown rates were similar in control rats and animals that

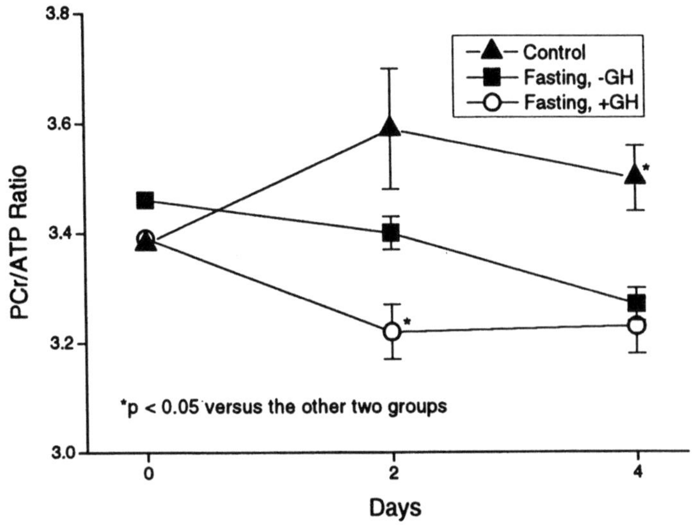

Fig. 7. PCr/ATP ratios indicative of changes in high energy stores were slightly lower in GH-treated rats which were fasted for 2 days. After 4 days of fasting, PCr/ATP levels were similarly depressed in both groups of fasted animals

were fasted and given GH (Fig. 8). These data strongly suggest that rats that are fasted and treated with GH have a decreased need for production of ATP via the breakdown of PCr. During short term fasting in the rat, GH administration improves nitrogen balance and allowed more efficient use of peripheral energy stores. Teleologically speaking, this may confer a significant advantage to the host, since the organism would have a greater ability to increase ATP synthesis from PCr breakdown when energy demands increase, such as might occur during muscular contraction. This finding may help explain why patients who are administered GH and who have undergone major surgical operations are better able to maintain grip strength as compared to patients who do not receive this anabolic agent [20].

Liver Injury and Hepatic Failure

The unexplained sequential failure of multiple organ systems in critically ill patients was first described by Tilney and associates 20 years ago [21]. As advances have been made in lifesupport systems and intensive care medicine, it has become increasingly well recognized that acutely ill patients often survive on a short term basis only to succumb later to this syndrome of progressive organ failure. Multiple organ failure syndrome (MOF) is now responsible for 50 to 80% of all deaths in critically ill surgical patients and is the leading cause of morbidity and mortality in the surgical intensive care unit.

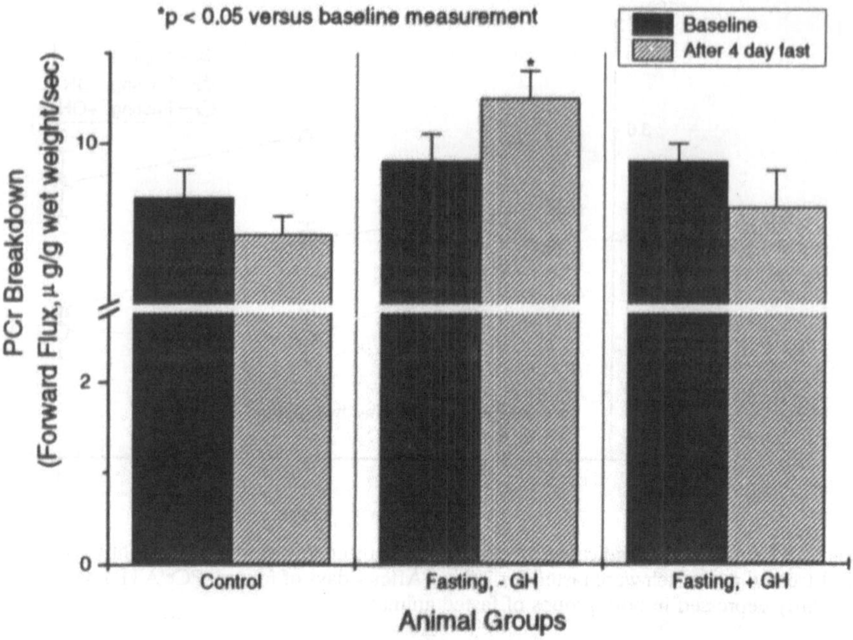

Fig. 8. PCr breakdown rates were significantly higher in fasted animals which were not treated with GH. Breakdown rates were similar in controls and GH-treated rats

In recent years, there has been intense research into the etiology of MOF. It is thought that the syndrome results from shock, infection and/or sterile inflammatory reactions which initiate a cascade of events that ultimately cause sequential failure of the host's major organs [22]. Characteristically, the liver is one of the first organs that becomes dysfunctional in those who eventually develop the complete syndrome. Because the liver plays a critical role in many vital functions of the body, failure of this organ not only hampers general reparative processes but also predisposes the host to dysfunction of other organs. Assessment of liver function is one of the first steps in identifying ways to prevent or attenuate liver failure during critical illness. Traditionally, liver function has been monitored by measuring plasma alanine and aspartate transaminases, alkaline phosphatase, and bilirubin. The liver failure found in MOF (and not related to primary liver disease such as biliary obstruction or viral hepatitis) is associated with minimally elevated hepatic transaminases and alkaline phosphatase and a progessively worsening conjugated hyperbilirubinemia. The severity of hyperbilirubinemia can be used as a predictor of survival in MOF patients [23]. While abnormalities in these parameters are relatively specific for liver dysfunction, they indicate both reversible and irreversible pathological processes and give little insight into the underlying cellular mechanisms responsible for the pathology.

Other indices used to assess liver function include measurement of hepatically synthesized serum protein levels such as transferrin and albumin. Depletion of these proteins is characteristically a late occurrence in patients with MOF and can signify liver dysfunction [23]. However, the specificity of this finding is low relative to other tests since malnourishment without liver dysfunction can also give rise to these findings [24]. It has been demonstrated that as hepatic function deteriorates, clearance of plasma aromatic amino acids such as phenylalanine is reduced. Consequently, measurement of the clearance of aromatic amino acids is one way to assess the severity of liver dysfunction. The ratio of acetoacetate to β-hydroxybutyrate which is thought to reflect hepatic mitochondrial redox potential has also been used to assess liver function. Reduction of this ratio can reflect impairment of hepatocellular energy status. In addition, Ozawa and colleagues [25] found that a decrease in this ratio below 0.4 heralds the onset of MOF and below 0.25 is associated with increased mortality.

Although there are multiple methods for the assessment of liver function, these traditional methods are suboptimal for several reasons. First, they tend to measure late manifestations of hepatocellular injury which may represent irreversible hepatocyte pathology. The ability to measure early changes in hepatic function may aid in refinement of therapeutic maneuvers that prevent progression of hepatocyte injury to cell death. Second, traditional liver function tests often lack specificity and sensitivity. Increased bilirubin in the surgical or trauma patient, for example, can represent true liver dysfunction or resorption of a large hematoma while serum hepatic transaminase level may be completely normal in the critically ill patient with clinically obvious liver failure. Third, present strategies for assessing liver function inadequately define pathological events at the cellular level and therefore limit the development of specific therapy that prevents or limits hepatic dysfunction.

As was described previously, ^{31}P MRS is a technique which allows the accurate, sensitive and non-invasive evaluation of liver function at the hepatocellular level *in vivo*. In addition, MRS can detect early, reversible changes in hepatocyte function as well as late, irreversible changes under a variety of conditions [26–28]. Several of the mediators of organ damage in MOF are thought to exact early, subtle changes in cellular metabolism which are potentially reversible. Unchecked, these changes can progress to irreversible hepatocellular damage and cell death [22]. Consequently, MRS may offer a powerful tool with which to monitor the progression of hepatic dysfunction and to determine its pathogenesis thereby directing development of therapeutic interventions. Specifically, ^{31}P MRS allows the *in vivo* determination of the concentration of hepatocyte phosphate compounds vital for normal hepatocellular function and integrity.

Several investigators have used MRS to define alterations in hepatocyte phosphate metabolism in animal models of injury. Kobayashi and colleagues [29], for example, studied animals that were subjected to cecal ligation and puncture and compared them to those that underwent a sham operation (Table 2). Twenty-four hours after operation, there was an 80% increase in the

Table 2. Liver MRS indices and substrate concentrations in rats following cecal ligation and puncture (CLP) and sham operation (sham-op, mean ± SEM)

Group	MRS Indices			β-OH-Acyl CoA (mM/g wet wt/min)	ATP (μmol/g wet wt)
	Pi/ATP	PME/ATP	pH		
CLP	0.90 ± 0.11 [a]	0.89 ± 0.15	7.36 ± 0.02	2.09 ± 1.12 [a]	3.52 ± 0.25
Sham-op	0.50 ± 0.06	0.82 ± 0.09	7.44 ± 0.04	0.42 ± 0.05	3.21 ± 0.31

[a] $p<0.05$ vs sham-op by Mann-Whitney test. (From [14] with permission)

liver Pi/ATP ratio in the cecal ligation and puncture group compared to sham operated animals. No differences in hepatocellular pH and the hepatic PME/ATP ratio were noted between groups. The authors used *in vitro* assays of liver homogenates to determine that β-hydroxyacyl Co-A dehydrogenase activity, the rate-limiting enzyme for intramitochondrial β-oxidation of fatty acids, was increased five-fold in the septic animals.Phosphofructokinase, the key enzyme in control of glycolysis, as well as citrate synthase and succinate dehydrogenase, important enzymes which catalyze reactions in the Kreb's cycle, were similar in the septic and non-septic animals. Liver ATP concentrations as determined by *in vitro* assay were similar in the two groups of animals. The authors interpreted these results to mean that hepatocyte energy status is markedly depressed during early systemic infection, and that consequently the liver may have a limited ability to fuel metabolic activities crucial for cell vitality and host defense during sepsis. Because the hepatic Pi/ATP ratio increased while ATP concentration remained unchanged, it is likely that there is accelerated Pi production, and thus ATP turnover during systemic infection. This increase in hepatic ATP consumption may be partially supported by enhanced oxidation of fatty acids as indicated by a rise in β-hydroxyacyl Co-A dehydrogenase activity. The fact that intracellular pH of the hepatocytes was similar in the two groups suggests that these observations were not secondary to a significant perfusion abnormality of the liver. The cecal ligation and puncture model used by these investigators resulted in no animal deaths within the 24 h time frame of the study, indicating that it is a relatively early sepsis model. Also of note, the derangements in liver energetics observed preceded alteration of the PME/ATP ratio, an established indicator of significant liver damage [27, 28]. Thus, it was concluded that treatment strategies that support hepatic energy needs may help prevent subsequent development of overt hepatic failure.

Hachisuka and associates [30] have recently defined changes in phosphate metabolism in ischemic liver. They clamped the porta hepatitis in mice for 15 and 30 min and used MRS analysis to monitor hepatic changes. As ischemic time increased, there was a pronounced decrease in the β-ATP peak and a significant rise in the Pi peak. Consequently, there was a marked increase in the Pi/ATP ratio. All these findings indicate a severe change in overall energy status of the hepatocytes. This is consistent with the fact that hepatocytes can only meet energy requirements under anaerobic conditions for a limited time period and demonstrates the ability of MRS to monitor and quantitate the severity of the energetic changes (Fig. 9). Hachisuka also used MRS in this study of liver ischemia to precisely characterize and quantitate changes in PME and PDE which are intermediary metabolites of membrane phospholipid turnover (Table 3) [30]. This was accomplished using a liver perchloric acid extraction technique. Perchloric acid extracts of liver homogenates have reduced contamination with alkaline earth and transitional metal cations. When these specimens undergo MRS analysis *in vitro*, there is better line resolution and an improved signal-to-noise ratio in the MRS scan. The spectra obtained in this fashion have easily discernible peaks within the PME and PDE regions. These peaks are ordinarily not identifiable with *in vivo* MRS scans. In addition, the improved resolution results in peaks that correspond to single compounds that do not overlap with the peaks of other compounds making it possible to precisely identify each chemical species. The authors found that phosphocholine and phosphoethanolamine (whose peaks occur within the PME region and are the precursors of phospholipid anabolism) did not change during ischemia. However, the PDE which are intermediary metabolites of phospholipid catabolism were markedly decreased. These metabolites are converted to α-glycerophosphate by PDE phosphodiesterase [31]. In addition, α-glycerophosphate, whose peak also occurs within the PME region and acts as both a precursor of phospholipid synthesis and an intermediary of phospholipid degradation, was found to be markedly elevated. The authors concluded that elevation of α-glycerophosphate in ischemic liver could be attributed to active phospholipid degradation of cellular membranes, since a large amount of phospholipid synthesis would not be expected given the finding of negligible increase in phosphocholine and phosphoethanolamine. No histologic evidence of liver change was noted after 30 min of liver ischemia. Thus, they were able to demonstrate degradation of membrane phospholipid before cellular morphologic changes occurred. This implies that subcellular morphologic alterations can be detected using MRS analysis.

Table 3. Phosphorus compounds in control and ischemic mouse liver (μmol/g wet wt)

Compound	Control	15-min ischemia	30-min ischemia
PME Region			
α-glycerophosphate	1.14±0.51	2.26±0.18[a]	3.04±0.60[a]
phosphocholine	1.47±0.40	1.62±0.21	1.73±0.24
phosphoethanolamine	0.73±0.08	0.88±0.21	0.87±0.22
PDE-Region			
glycerophosphocholine	0.42±0.10	Not Detected	Not Detected
glycerophosphoethanolamine	0.12±0.06	Not Detected	Not Detected

[a] $p<0.05$ vs control. (From [16] with permission)

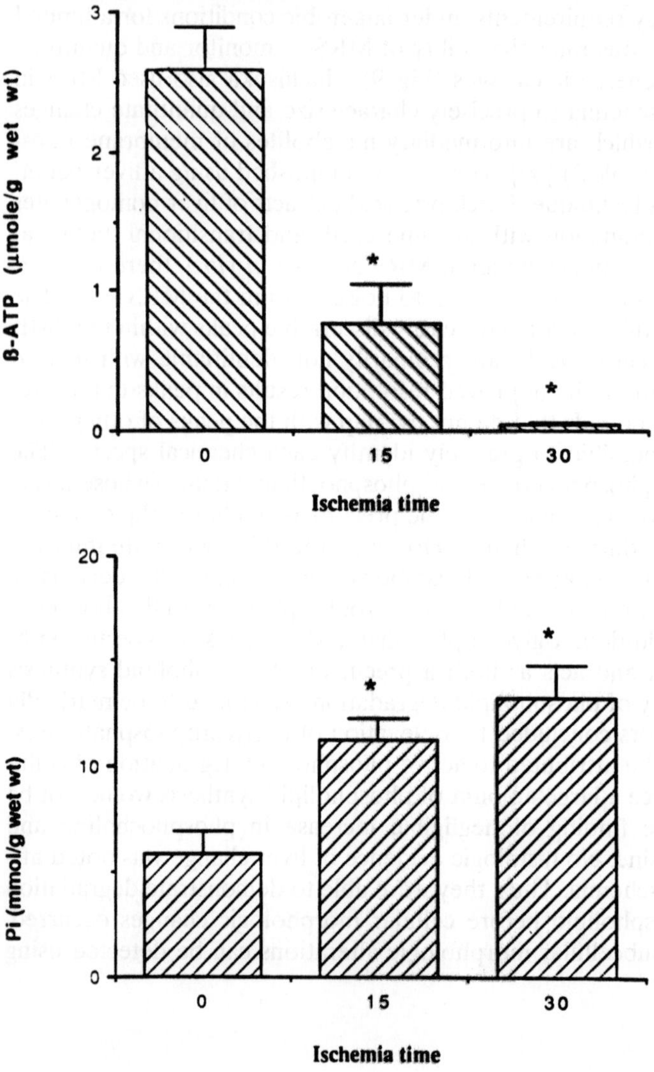

Fig. 9. Changes in Pi and β-ATP in ischemic rat liver as detected by phosphorus MRS

^{31}P MRS may also be potentially useful for examination of possible etiologies of liver dysfunction during critical illness. For example, mechanisms which protect organs from free radical mediated damage are particularly important during critical illness because production of oxygen free radicals is often accelerated under these conditions [32]. Glutathione (GSH) is crucial for the body's defense against reactive oxygen metabolites [33]. However, several experimental and clinical studies indicate that this tripeptide is depleted during serious illness [34–37]. Thus, deficiency of GSH stores may predispose the host to ongoing tissue damage from oxygen free radicals which could progress to failure of organs such as the liver [38]. Kobayashi and associates [39] examined the relationship between depletion of hepatic GSH stores, hepatocellular injury, and energetics using ^{31}P MRS. Rats were given an otherwise non-toxic dose of the drug diethylmaleate which depletes tissue GSH stores and were compared to rats with normal glutathione levels. The authors found that the GSH-deficient rats had a significant increase in the Pi/ATP ratio indicating marked impairment of hepatocyte energy status. There was also an increase in the PME/ATP ratio which is consistent with an increase in hepatocellular injury as discussed previously. Both the Pi/ATP and PME/ATP ratios were significantly correlated with the severity of GSH depletion. Thus GSH depletion alone and without an overlying stress such as sepsis or shock is associated with changes in energetics and hepatocellular membrane integrity. Even under normal conditions there is production of oxygen free radicals. Presumably, the GSH deficiency in this model was sufficient to allow oxidant induced tissue damage as evidenced by an increase in the PME/ATP ratio and impairment of hepatocyte energy status. Of note, these changes were observed in the absence of a demonstrable differences in traditional liver function tests such as alanine amino transferase, alkaline phosphatase, and bilirubin. The change in energy status could be secondary to impaired energy production (free radicals are known to inhibit glycolytic enzymes [40]) and/or secondary to an increased energy demand for reparative processes. Thus, GSH deficiency in critically ill patients may independently contribute to impaired hepatocyte energy status and altered hepatocellular integrity. This could consequently predispose individuals to the development of hepatic dysfunction and overt liver failure. Although this theory has yet to be proven beyond all doubt, this MRS study does suggest a direction for future therapeutic interventions aimed at attenuating liver dysfunction during serious illness.

Finally, ^{31}P MRS may prove to be very useful in identifying specific treatments for preventing or limiting liver dysfunction. A recent study used ^{31}P MRS to examine the effects of glutamine administration on liver energetics during sepsis [41]. Rats received glutamine-enriched or glutamine-free total parenteral nutrition (TPN) for 6 days prior to undergoing cecal ligation and puncture. The animals were continued for an additional 20h on their TPN regimens following cecal ligation and puncture and then underwent liver MRS analysis. There was a 50% reduction in the Pi/ATP in the septic rats receiving glutamine-enriched TPN compared to those receiving glutamine-free TPN. In addition, there was a 33% decrease in the PME/ATP ratio in the glutamine animals. These findings suggest that glutamine-enriched TPN enhances cellular energetics in septic rats and therefore may improve the liver's ability to meet the metabolic demands of systemic infection. In addition, glutamine-enriched TPN attenuated the hepatocellular injury associated with sepsis as assessed by the PME/ATP ratio (Fig. 10). It was concluded in this study that glutamine may be a critical fuel that is also important for prevention of hepatocellular injury during microbial invasion of the

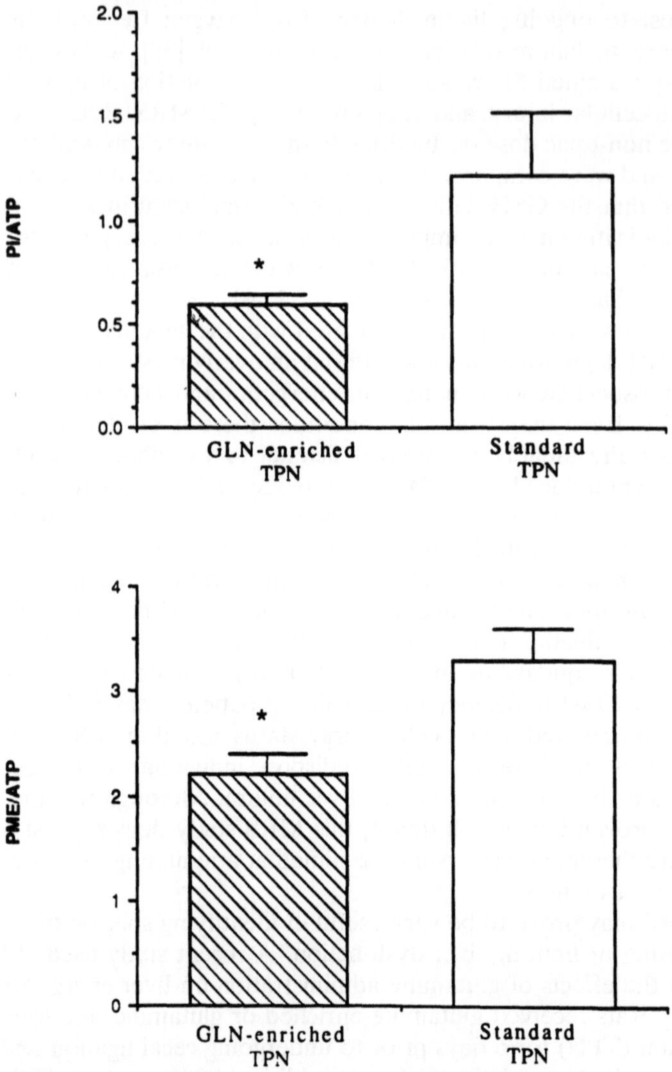

Fig. 10. Septic rats which received glutamine-supplemented parenteral nutrition had a 50% reduction in Pi/ATP and a 33% decrease in PME/ATP

host. There are several mechanisms through which glutamine could possibly exert this beneficial effect. For example, it has been shown that glutamine is an important fuel source in oxidant-injured cells [42] and it is well known that there is increased free-radical mediated liver injury in sepsis [31]. Glutmaine may supplement tissue glutathione stores in sepsis and therefore may aid in defense against oxidant injury [43]. Glutamine is an important fuel for immune cells [44] and attenuates translocation of bacteria from the intestinal tract in models of critical injury [45]. Hence, this amino acid may decrease severity of sepsis and stress on the liver. Regardless of the exact mechanism, this study suggests that provision of glutamine may be an important adjunct to the treatment of patients who are at high risk of developing liver dysfunction.

Human Studies

Reports of metabolic changes induced by diseases relevant to the practice of nutritional support are few. However, many investigations suggest that MRS studies may be an important tool for metabolic assessment in the future and will certainly improve our understanding of the metabolic response to malnutrition, stress, infection, and refeeding. For example, a fast of 72 h duration in a patient with carnitine palmitoyl transferase deficiency, who therefore could not use long chain fatty acids as an energy source, was recently reported [46]. This patient had decreased muscular efficiency after a 65 h fast as compared to his baseline. In addition, a failure to generate normal force during prolonged exercise was noted. Similarly, patients with genetic deficiencies of phosphofructokinase who have normal resting phosphorus MRS scans of skeletal muscle have a greater increase in Pi/PCr for given workload as compared to normal controls [47].

Other studies have investigated the effects of nutritional supplementation in patients with specific metabolic deficiencies. Patients with myophosphorylase deficiency, a condition known as McArdle's disease, cannot metabolize intramuscular glycogen, but the administration of glucose intravenously increases their exercise capacity. In MRS scans, this effect is readily demonstrated as a lower Pi/PCr ratio at the end of exercise as compared to the values before treatment. Changes in metabolism can also be detected using ^{31}P MRS. ^{31}P MRS studies of patients with Duchenne's muscular dystrophy demonstrate higher inorganic phosphate levels, intracellular pH, and PDE but lower PCr and PCr/Pi ratio [48]. In patients with mitochondrial complex III deficiency which induces severe exercise intolerance and muscular weakness, the oral administration of electron scavengers vitamin K_3 and C improved energy metabolism and exercise tolerance. The same is true of other mitochondrial myopathies where various vitamins and co-factors have been shown to improve clinical status and augment the energy state as determined by ^{31}P MRS.

^{13}C NMR may have wide application to the study of organ and tissue metabolism. However, ^{13}C MRS studies are restricted to the investigations of compounds present in high concentrations such as glycogen, fats, and triglycerides, or one must use ^{13}C enriched substrates. Labelling techniques similar to ^{14}C tracer methods can be used to determine the fluxes through many metabolic pathways. In many cases, the ^{13}C labelling studies are superior since the position of the label within metabolites can be easily determined. For example, normally most of the glucose taken up by muscle is metabolized non-oxidatively and is stored as glycogen. Direct measurements of glycogen synthesis in muscle are difficult, since the changes in glycogen concentration are so small that they cannot be accurately detected using muscle biopsy techniques. ^{13}C NMR allows accurate quantitation of the glycogen content of muscle (and other tissues) non-invasively [49] by measuring the signal which arises from the 1.1% of carbon nuclei which naturally occur at this isotope. The accuracy of NMR measurements of glycogen concentrations can be increased by infusing ^{13}C-enriched glucose. Using these techniques, Shulman et al. [50] showed that muscle glycogen synthesis is the principal pathway of glucose disposal in normal subjects.

Currently, ^{1}H MRS may be used to follow changes in the C-3 lactate resonance under a variety of metabolic conditions. However, fairly detailed information about other metabolites can also be obtained using these spectra. For example, in the rat brain ^{1}H MRS is able to demonstrate resonances of aspartate, glutamine, glutamate, as well as lactate [50]. The ability to monitor changes in intracellular glutamine concentrations in concert with changes in cellular energetics may prove to be especially informative in future studies of the effects of nutrient deprivation and nutritional and metabolic intervention.

Conclusion

In vivo ^{31}P MRS can be used to characterize alterations in liver phosphate metabolism in models of critical illness, to examine possible etiologies of this dysfunction, and to explore potentially useful treatments that prevent or limit organ dysfunction and ameliorate catabolic responses. Although the usefulness of MRS has been demonstrated in animal models, it has yet to be widely used as an investigative tool in humans.

In the case of hepatic injury, this is in part related to difficulties in the past with obtaining high quality MRS data from the livers of human subjects. However, new magnetic spectrometers and scanning techniques will allow determination of liver phosphate signals through overlying skin, subcutaneous tissue and skeletal muscle. Consequently, use of this technology is more feasible in human volunteers and patients. Liver failure during critical illness is thought to be secondary to a host of mediators such as oxygen free radicals and possibly a perfusion or microperfusion abnormality. Future directions in critical care research will include examining ways to block these mediators, improve perfusion of the liver and enhance the host's own defense mechanisms against hepatocyte injury. Since alteration of high-energy phosphate metabolism contributes to cellular and organ dysfunction during many serious illnesses, *in vivo* ^{31}P MRS technology is a potentially powerful tool that may be useful in the refinement of therapeutic interventions for critically ill patients with metabolic dysfunction.

References

1. Chance B, Clark BJ, Nioka S, et al (1985) Phosphorus nuclear magnetic resonance spectroscopy in vivo. Circulation 72 (Supp IV):103–110
2. Radda GK (1992) Control, bioenergetics, and adaptation in health and disease: Noninvasive biochemistry from nuclear magnetic resonance. FASEB J 6:3032–3038
3. Bore PJ (1985) Principles and applications of phosphorus magnetic resonance spectroscopy. In: Kressel HY (ed) Magnetic Resonance Annual. New York, Raven Press, pp 45–69
4. Forsen S, Hoffman RA (1963) Study of moderately rapid chemical exchange reactions by means of nuclear magnetic double resonance. J Chem Phys 39:2892–2901
5. Holtzman D, Offutt M, Tsuji M, et al (1993) Creatine kinase reaction rate in the cyanide poisoned mouse brain. J Cerebral Blood Flow and Metabolism 13:153–161
6. Carlsson C (1975) Metabolic changes in the cerebral cortex of the rat induced by intravenous pentphalsodium. Acta Anaesth Scand 57:1–17
7. Petroff OAC, Prichard JW, Behar KL, et al (1984) In vivo phosphorus nuclear magnetic resonance spectroscopy in status epilepticus. Ann Neurol 16:169–177
8. Rudin M, Sauter A (1989) The rate constants of the creatine kinase reaction in rat brain: A probe for brain function? Society for Magnetic Resonance in Medicine, Eighth Annual Scientific Meeting, vol 1:489
9. Atkinson DE (1977) Cellular energy metabolism and its regulation. Academic Press, Orlando, FL
10. Chance B, Veech RL (1988) Phosphorus magnetic resonance spectroscopy as a probe of nutritional state. In: Kinney JM, Jeejeebhoy KN, Hill GH, Owen OE (eds) Nutrition and metabolism in patient care. Philadelphia, WB Saunders Co. pp 119–128
11. Fehlig P, Warren J (1975) Fuel homeostasis in exercise. N Engl J Med 293:1078–1081
12. Argov Z, Chance B (1991) Phosphorus magnetic resonance spectroscopy in nutritional research. In: Olson RE, Bier DM, McCormick DB (eds). Annual Review of Nutrition. Annual Reviews Inc Palo Alto, California, vol 11, pp 449–464
13. Chance B, Eleff S, Leigh JS, et al (1981) Mitochondrial regulation of phosphocreatine/inorganic phosphate ratios in exercising human muscle: A gated ^{31}P NMR study. Proc Natl Acad Sci USA 68:6714–6718
14. Chance B, Leigh JS Jr, Clark B, et al (1985) Control of oxidative metabolism and oxygen delivery in human skeletal muscle: A steady state analysis of the work/energy cost transfer function. Proc Natl Acad Sci USA. 82:8384–8388
15. Jacobs DO, Whitman G, Maris J, et al (1985) ^{31}P Nuclear magnetic resonance spectroscopy of rat skeletal muscle during starvation. JPEN 9:107a (Abs)
16. Pichard C, Vaughan C, Struk R, Armstrong RL, Jeejeebhoy KN (1988) Effect of dietary manipulation (fasting, hypocaloric feeding, and subsequent refeeding) on rat muscle energetics as assessed by nuclear magnetic resonance spectroscopy. J Clin Invest 82:895–901
17. Jacobs DO, Kobayashi T, Wilmore DW (1990) Starvation alters forward flux through the creatine kinase pathway. Association for Academic Surgery (Abs)
18. Jacobs DO, Kobayashi T, Imagire J, et al (1991) Sepsis alters skeletal muscle energetics and membrane function. Surgery 110:318–326
19. Koruda MJ, Argov Z, Maris J, et al (1985) 31-Phosphorus nuclear magnetic resonance spectroscopy of stimulated muscle during starvation. Surg Forum 26:260–261
20. Jiang ZM, He GZ, Zhang SY, Wang XR, et al (1989) Low dose growth hormone and hypocaloric nutrition attenuate the protein-catabolic response after major operation. Ann Surg 210:513–524
21. Tilney NL, Bailey GL, Morgan AP (1973) Sequential system failure after rupture of abdominal aortic aneurysms: An unsolved problem in postoperative care. Ann Surg 178:117–122
22. Deitch EA (1992) Multiple organ failure. Ann Surg 216:117–134

23. Cerra FB, Walvatne C (1990) Hepatic dysfunction in multiple organ failure. in: Deitch EA (ed) Multiple organ failure: Pathophysiology and basic concepts of therapy. Thieme Medical Publishers, Inc New York, pp 241–260
24. Munro HN, Crim MC (1988) The proteins and amino acids. In: Shils ME, Young VR (eds) Modern Nutrition in Health and Disease. Lea and Febiger, Philadelphia, pp 137–150
25. Ozawa K, Aoyama H, Yasuda K, et al (1983) Metabolic abnormalities associated with postoperative organ failure. Arch Surg 118:1245–1251
26. Pelias ME, Townsend MC (1992) In vivo ^{31}P NMR assessment of early hepatocellular dysfunction during endotoxemia. J Surg Res 52:505–509
27. Angus PW, Dixon RM, Rajagopala B, et al (1990) A study of patients with alcoholic liver disease by ^{31}P nuclear magnetic resonance spectroscopy. Clin Sci 78:33–38
28. Bates TE, Williams SR, Proctor E, Gadian DG (1988) Investigation of drug induced acute liver failure by ^{31}P NMR and conventional biochemical methods: The importance of absolute concentrations. NMR in Biomed 1:67–71
29. Kobayashi T, Robinson MK, Rounds JD, et al (1992) Depression of hepatocyte energy status during systemic infection: An in vivo ^{31}P magnetic resonance spectroscopy study. Surg Forum 53:11–13
30. Hachisuka, T, Nakayama S, Tomita T, Takagi H (1992) ^{31}P Nuclear magnetic resonance study of phospholipid metabolites in ischemic liver. J Surg Res 53:251–256
31. Dawson RMC (1987) Liver glycerophosphorylcholine phosphodiesterase. Biochem J 62:689–695
32. Reilly PM, Schiller HJ, Bulkley GB (1991) Reactive oxygen metabolites in shock. In: Wilmore DW, Brenan ME, Harken AH, Holcroft JW, Meakins JL (eds) Care of the Surgical Patient. New York, Scientific American, Inc, pp 130–132
33. Meister A, Anderson ME (1983) Glutathione. Ann Rev Biochem 52:711–760
34. Martensson J (1986) The effect of fasting in leukocyte and plasma glutathione and sulfur amino acid concentration. Metabolism 35:118–121
35. Shi ECP, Fisher R, McEvoy M, Vantol R, Rose M, Ham JM (1982) Factors influencing hepatic glutathione concentrations: A study in surgical patients. Clin Sci 62:279–283
36. Corbucci GG, Gasparetto A, Candiani A, et al (1985) Shock induced damage to mitochondrial function and some cellular antioxidant mechanisms in humans. Circ Shock 15:15–26
37. Keller GA, Barke R, Harty JT, Humphrey E, Simmons RL (1985) Decreased hepatic glutathione levels in septic shock. Arch Surg 120:941–945
38. Robinson MK, Rounds JD, Jacobs DO, Wilmore DM (1992) Glutathione deficiency increases organ dysfunction after hemorrhagic shock. Surgery 112:140–149
39. Kobayashi T, Robinson MK, Robinson V, De Rosa E, Wilmore DW, Jacobs DO (1993) Hepatic glutamine depletion induces hepatocellular injury and alters high energy phosphate metabolism. J Surg Res 54:189–195
40. Hyslop PA, Hinshaw DB, Halsey WA, et al (1988) Mechanisms of oxidant-mediated cell injury. J Biol Chem 263:1665–1675
41. Robinson MK, Kobayashi T, Rounds JD, et al (1992) Glutamine enhances hepatocellular energetics during sepsis. Surg Forum 43:171–174
42. Hinshaw DB, Burger JM, Delius RE, Hyslop PA (1990) Mechanism of protection of oxidan injured endothelial cells by glutamine. Surgery 108:298–305
43. Hong RW, Robinson MK, Rounds JD, Wilmore DW (1991) Glutamine protects the liver following Corynebacterium parvum/endotoxin-induced hepatic necrosis. Surg Forum 42:1–3
44. Ardawi MS (1988) Glutamine and glucose metabolism in human peripheral lymphocytes. Metabolism 37:99–103
45. Souba WW, Klimberg S, Plumley DA, et al (1990) The role of glutamine in maintaining a healthy gut and supporting the metabolic response to injury and infection. J Surg Res 48:383–391

46. Argov Z (1989) Phosphorus magnetic resonance spectroscopy (^{31}P NMR) as a tool for in vivo monitoring of mitochondrial muscle disorders. In: Azzi A, Drahota Z, Papa S (eds) Molecular Basis of Membrane-Associated Disease. Springer-Verlag, Berlin, pp 183–199
47. Chance B, Eleff S, Bank W, et al (1982) ^{31}P NMR studies of control of mitochondrial function in phosphofructokinase-deficient human skeletal muscle. Proc Natl Acad Sci USA 79:7714–7718
48. Younkin DP, Berman P, Sladky J, et al (1987) ^{31}P NMR studies in Duchenne muscular dystrophy: Age-related metabolic changes. Neurology 37:165–169
49. Shulman GI, Rothman DL, Jue T, et al (1990) Quantitation of muscle glycogen synthesis in normal subjects and subjects with non-insulin-dependent diabetes by ^{13}C nuclear magnetic resonance spectroscopy. N Engl J Med 322:223–228
50. Behar KL, den Hollander JA, Petroff OAC, et al (1985) Effect of hypoglycemic encephalopathy upon amino acids, high-energy phosphates, and pH, in the rat brain in vivo: Detection by sequential ^{1}H and ^{31}P NMR spectroscopy. J Neurochem 44:1045–1055

Muscle Function and Energetics

K. N. Jeejeebhoy

Introduction

Lack of nutrient intake results in a loss of body fat and lean tissue [1] and hitherto the effects of nutritional depletion and repletion with refeeding have been judged by changes in body composition, especially of lean tissue. Lean tissue is composed of water, minerals, nitrogen and glycogen [2, 3], and feeding wasted individuals results in a gain of the multiple elements in lean tissue [4] as well as body fat. One of the elements responding to nutrient intake is body potassium, which has been used as an index of body cell mass [5], the metabolically active component of the lean tissue. We [6, 7] and others [8–10] have shown that in contrast to body nitrogen, body potassium responds rapidly to feeding by both oral [7] and intravenous routes [6, 8–10]. These changes have been interpreted as being due to changes in lean mass. However, the early restitution of body potassium without a rise in body nitrogen indicates that cell ion uptake occurs earlier than protein synthesis with nutritional support [9]. In support of this conclusion it has been shown, using ion selective electrodes, that hypocaloric feeding results in a fall in muscle membrane potential and in the concentration of intracellular ionic K^+ [11, 12]. The changes were specifically related to nutrient deprivation as they could not be reversed by potassium supplementation *per se* [12]. Since 5 molecules of ATP are required for the incorporation of one molecule of amino acid into protein, and 77% of the free-energy change of ATP hydrolysis is used to maintain the Na-K gradient across the cell membrane [13, 14], and energy intake limits nitrogen retention [15], these findings suggest that nutritional support initially alters cell energetics rather than mass. We have observed Z band degeneration and calcium accumulation with hypocaloric feeding in humans [16] and have suggested that it is related to changes in cell energetics. Cell energetics is also important for muscle activity and we showed [7, 17–22] that skeletal muscle function (SMF) including that of the diaphragm [20] can be altered by nutrient deprivation and restored by refeeding, observations confirmed by others [23–25]. Christie and Hill [24] also showed that nutritional support improves muscle, including diaphragmatic function before any increase in body protein or body mass. Finally, Windsor and Hill [25] demonstrated that the functional effects of nutrition are more important than subnormal body protein as an index of surgical risk. In order to understand how malnutrition influences muscle function, it is necessary to examine the effects of nutrient deprivation on individual parameters of muscle function.

Alteration of SMF by Nutrient Deprivation and Refeeding

There is a change in the force-frequency curve, slower relaxation and greater low frequency fatigue (i.e. a muscular, not neuromuscular effect) in malnourished patients, hypocaloric dieters and anorexics – all restored by refeeding [7, 17, 18]. These date were uninfluenced by non-nutritional factors such as uremia, COPD, sepsis, trauma, steroid administration and surgery [19–21]. The same effects were also seen in the diaphragm, a vital muscle, by ourselves and others [20, 23]. These changes are unrelated to physical activity since moderate exercise alter neither the tetanic force [26], nor the contractile properties of muscle [27]. Disuse atrophy results in faster relaxation [28], which is exactly opposite to that seen with hypocaloric feeding.

Changes in Muscle Biopsies in the Human and the Rat [16, 22]

In both human and rat muscle biopsie, there was a reduction in the rate-limiting enzyme of the glycolytic pathway, phosphofructokinase (PFK); and in a Krebs cycle enzyme, succinate dehydrogenase (SDH), a finding which has been confirmed [29].

Changes in Muscle Calcium

In both a human and animal studies [16, 22], we noticed that the malnourished muscle has a significantly higher intracellular calcium, and lower K^+ [11, 12] by comparison with controls.

Changes in Muscle Cell Energetics as determined by ^{31}P-NMR Spectroscopy (^{31}P-NMRS)

Our studies of muscle using ^{31}P-NMRS in the resting state [30], showed that phosphocreatine (PCr) falls, free-energy change for ATP hydrolysis (ΔG_{ATP}) and free ADP (FADP) rise in hypocalorically fed rats. The change in the ΔG_{ATP} while small, was of a magnitude which has been shown in the heart to be associated with marked changes in systolic pressure [14]. Furthermore, it was shown that exposing skinned muscle fibers [31] to a lower ΔG_{ATP}, comparable to that seen in fatigued muscle (in this paper [31] ΔG_{ATP} is referred to as affinity, with which it is synonymous [32]) resulted in a reduction of maximum force compared to fibers exposed to a higher ΔG_{ATP}. When muscle is stimulated, the Pi rises and PCr falls due to ATP hydrolysis resulting in a raised Pi/PCr ratio. Mitochondrial rephosphorylation restores the PCr levels during post-exercise rest, and correspondingly the Pi levels fall. In stimulated muscle, we have recently observed that the raised Pi/PCr ratio which occurs following muscle contraction falls much more slowly in muscles from hypocalorically fed rats as compared with controls. These findings suggest impaired mitochondrial rephosphorylation.

Analysis of Factors affecting Muscle Performance and Energetics in Hypocaloric State

Muscle Function

Fatigue: When muscle is stimulated repeatedly then the force generated with each succeeding contraction is lower than the previous one. The fall in force in this situation is called fatigue. The loss of force could be due to lack of nerve transmission but it has been shown that fatigue in the hypocaloric state at 30 Hz stimulation (human) and 100 Hz (animals) occurs because of muscular rather than neuromuscular factors [33, 34]. Since the energy cost of an isometric force increases linearly with the force-time integral [35, 36], the lower total maximal force with fatigue may indicate limited energy utilization.

Force frequency curve. *(Ratio of low frequency force to high frequency force).* As muscle is stimulated with increasing rate of stimuli ranging from 10 to 100 Hz, the force of contraction in the human adductor pollicis muscle rises. However, in muscle from malnourished humans, the force at 10 Hz (F_{10}) remains normal but the increase of force with increasing frequency of stimuli to 100 Hz (F_{100}) does not occur. Thus the F_{10}/F_{100} ratio rises in malnutrition. It has been shown that the increased F_{10}/F_{100} ratio is associated with reduced heat production in the human adductor pollicis and reduced ATP turnover in mouse soleus [37, 38], suggesting reduced energy production.

Slow relaxation rate: Muscle relaxation is an intrinsic property of muscle which is very constant. To understand the significance of slow relaxation, it is necessary to understand that during muscle relaxation, stimulation results in calcium efflux from the endoplasmic reticulum into the cytosol. The rise in cytosolic calcium causes muscle to contract. Muscle relaxation occurs because calcium is pumped against a concentration gradient back into the endoplasmic reticulum. This is an energy demanding process. In malnourished, muscle relaxation is markedly slow. This finding suggests reduced rate of calcium pumping. Slow relaxation in hypocaloric muscle is independent of fiber type [39]. Slow relaxation rate is known to be associated with fatigue [40–44]. Since relaxation depends on detachment of myosin cross-bridges following binding with ATP [45], its rate is likely to be altered by factors governing ATP hydrolysis, or actin-myosin interactions [36]. Possible mechanisms include: a) reduced energy release during ATP hydrolysis related to a fall in ΔG_{ATP} [46]; b) raised ADP levels inhibiting the Ca^{++} ATPase activity and calcium uptake into the sarcoplasmic reticulum [47]; and c) reduced rate of ATP production [48]. Thus all the physiological findings, particularly the slow relaxation which is independent of muscle stretch [49], suggest abnormal energetics. Why does this happen in the nutritionally deprived patient or animal? In order to answer this question, it is necessary to look at 1) the pH and availability of substrate; 2) cell energetics; and 3) cell calcium kinetics.

pH and Substrate Availability

As discussed in our paper [22], glycogen deficiency is not a cause of altered SMF. Fatty acids are abundant in the starved state and is unlikely to be limiting. In our model hypocaloric feeding changed in muscle pH minimally [30].

Cell Energetics

ATP production is under feedback control from ATP consumption. The ADP is a regulator of both glycolysis and mitochondrial oxygen consumption. Mitochondrial oxygen consumption increases with a rise in ADP levels thus increasing the rate of ATP production from ADP. Chance et al. [50] have shown that with increasing work load the Pi/PCr ratio rises. The relationship of work rate to the Pi/PCr ratio is a rectangular hyperbola [50]. The Pi/PCr ratio is related to the FADP levels [51–53]. Initially the relationship of Pi/PCr to work is linear until the Pi/PCr approximates 1.0. Then the relationship between Pi/PCr and muscle work alters so that a marked change in the ratio is associated with a small increase in work [52, 53]. Experimentally, the flattening of the curve of the relation between work and Pi/PCr ratio is associated with fatigue. At this point, a further rise in ADP levels will not stimulate mitochondrial oxygen consumption [52]. In order to assess the effects of malnutrition on cell energetics, we performed two different studies. First, we studied the changes in cell energetics in the rat in the resting state. Second, we studied the effect of nutrition on cell energetics as a muscle contracted and relaxed.

Muscle energetics in the resting state [30]: Control rats (CONT) were fed chow *ad libitum.* The CONT was compared to another group subjected to an acute 2 day fast (2DF) and another subjected to chronic undernutrition by a week of hypocaloric feeding (HYPO). These HYPO rats were fed 25% of CONT calories until they lost 20% of their initial weight. A group of HYPO rats were refed *ad libitum* for a week and restudied. In all groups, we measured levels of ATP, PCr, Pi and pH, using a combination of NMR and biochemical analysis. In addition, free Mg^{2+}, free ADP, and free energy change of ATP hydrolysis were calculated.

Control and refed animals: The levels of ATP, PCr, Pi and pH of control animals are similar to those published for a comparable fast twitch muscle, cat biceps [54]. In addition, in control animals, the mean ratio of PCr/total phosphorus (ATP+PCr+Pi) was 0.758, Pi/total phosphorus was 0.039, and ATP/total phosphorus was 0.202, which are almost identical to those published by Meyer et al. [54]. The calculated free ADP levels are within the range calculated by Veech et al. [54] if the assumed free Mg^{2+} of 1 mM. Our G_{ATP} for muscle of −68 kJ/m is similar to that reported for cat biceps of −72 kJ/m [54]. Animals refed after hypocaloric feeding were not different from controls.

Effect of a 2-day fast and hypocaloric feeding: The striking effect was a significant fall in PCr, which was associated with a loss of muscle creatine. Thus the reserves of energy phosphorus decreased, while the calculated G_{ATP} fell significantly. It is of interest that Dawson et al. [46] found that in fatigued muscle, a fall in G_{ATP} was related to the slow relaxation rate, such that small changes in G_{ATP} were associated with significant changes in relaxation rates. This effect of the change in the G_{ATP} on relaxation rate was hypothesized to be due to slower pumping of calcium [46], a concept supported by Kodoma [56]. We [18] and others [57] have also observed that fasted and hypocalorically-fed rats, and malnourished humans have a slower relaxation rate, perhaps due to a fall in ΔG_{ATP}.

Effect of pH and free Mg^{2+} levels on free ADP and ΔG_{ATP}: It is recognized that the above factors will alter the K_{ck} and the G_{ATP}. However, the differences in pH are small and the actual values influence the calculation to a minor extent. The free Mg^{2+} levels obtained by us from the NMR data are consistent with the recent observations of Maughan [58] and Gupta et al. [59]. Despite the uncertainty of the precise free Mg^{2+} level, it is clear that the differences between the groups remain statistically significant.

Significance of the observed changes: The changes are not due to acidosis or anoxia of the muscle because the blood pH, pCO_2 and HCO_3^- were normal and not different between the groups. Furthermore, muscle pH was not different in the 2DF, which showed a marked fall in PCr and ΔG_{ATP} and rise in free ADP. Even in hypocaloric animals, the muscle pH only fell by 0.04. Muscle biopsy data in critically ill septic subjects showed lower phosphagens [60]. These findings are similar to those related to hypocalorically fed rats in the present study. The fall in PCr and rise in free ADP have been noted in fatigue [46]. However, there are major differences. In fatigue, there is a significant fall in pH (to below 7.0), a rise in Pi, and total creatine remains constant except in severe exercise [61]. In malnutrition, the Pi was not significantly different from controls, therefore changes in Pi concentration could not be the cause of the change in the force frequency curve and relaxation rate seen in malnourished rat gastrocnemius [22]. The fall in PCr and rise in free ADP could be due to a change in fiber type [16]. NMR studies in cat muscle have shown that fast twitch fibers have a higher ATP, lower free ADP, PCr and markedly lower Pi levels compared with slow twitch fibers [54]. Since malnutrition was not associated with a rise in Pi, nor in a significant fall in ATP, an alteration in fiber type cannot entirely explain the observed findings. The changes are more likely to be due to a loss of muscle PCr relative to total creatine, resulting in a relative loss of energy reserve. Since ADP is rapidly translocated into the mitochondria and phosphorylated to ATP, a rise in the ADP could result from deficient oxidative phosphorylation. The findings are consistent with the hypothesis that the reduced phosphofructokinase (PFK) and succinic dehydrogenase (SDH) levels observed in malnutrition [16, 62] may limit the flux of glycolytic and oxidative pathways. A recent study of the effect of 5 day fasting on the ^{31}P NMR of human forearm has shown reduced lactate production, and changes in the Pi/PCr ratio consistent with a limitation of anaerobic glycolysis [63].

Effect of nutrition on muscle energetics in contracting-relaxing muscle: In this study, we had the same three different models of nutrition. However we had two different controls to correspond to the duration of the 2DF and HYPO rats (CONT) and to the longer duration of the REF rats called CREF. In addition, the study was designed to examine the question of the effect of the added energy expenditure of muscle contraction on the energetics in relation to the nutritional status. In this study, we observed two different stimulated states. First, the effect of chronic stimulation with only a 1-min recovery observed over the entire study period, and second, the acute recovery after a stimulus during the period of a minute.

Control (CONT) and Control for refed animals (CREF): Previously, we had studied muscle energetics in the unstimulated muscle in an identical model of nutritional manipulation [30]. The only difference is the inclusion of another control group (CREF) for the refed animals. The biochemical techniques used in this study are identical to those used previously [30], and the NMR techniques substantially the same but modified for the fact that these muscles required stimulation. In our previous study, we showed that in control animals, the ATP, PCr, Pi, pH, ratios of ATP, PCr and Pi/total phosphorus (ATP + PCr + Pi) were comparable to those published earlier [54] for the cat biceps, a comparable fast twitch muscle. In addition, the calculated FADP and ΔG_{ATP} were also comparable to those published by others [54, 55] if the free Mg^{2+} is assumed to be be the same as in those studies, namely 1 mM. In this study, the CONT ATP, PCr and Pi levels 42 sec after the stimulus (Figs. 1–3), the time of maximal rest prior to the next stimulus, were similar to those published earlier for unstimulated muscles [30]. Correspondingly, the mean PCr/total phosphorus of 0.768, Pi/total phosphorus 0.053, and ATP/total phosphorus were similar to those published by us earlier for unstimulated muscle in controls [30] and by Meyer et al. [54]. At time 0, just after the muscle was stimulated, while the mean ATP/total phosphorus ratio

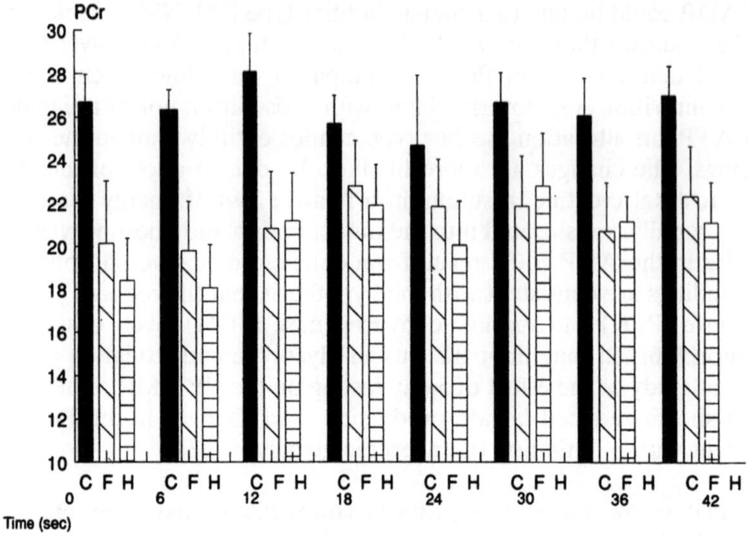

Fig. 1. ATP levels (mmol/g wet weight) of unstimulated and stimulated muscle. The unstimulated muscle was freeze-clamped from the unstimulated leg at the end of the study. The stimulated muscle was freeze-clamped during the muscle contraction at the end of the study. C = CONT, F = 2DF, H = HYPO.

(mean 0.162) was not significantly different from that at 42 sec after the stimulus, ratios of the Pi/total phosphorus (mean 0.164) and PCr/total phosphorus (mean 0.672) were significantly different. These findings show that the CONT muscles returned to the unstimulated state before the next stimulus. The results were similar in the CREF muscles. The FADP and the ΔG_{ATP} levels in controls at 42 sec after stimulation were comparable to those published by Veech et al. [55] and Meyer et al. [54]. These findings suggest that in our model, we were able to reproduce the metabolite concentrations in controls at 42 sec after stimuli comparable to those observed in unstimulated muscle.

Effect of stimulation on rats on a 2-day fast and on those receiving hypocaloric feeding: ATP, PCr and Pi levels. The PCr levels were significantly lower in the 2DF and HYPO rats (Fig. 2a). Since the total creatine (TCr) levels were not different between the groups, therefore the lower PCr is clearly due to a change in cell energetics. The regression showed that during the stimulation-recovery period the PCr levels rose in CONT, 2DF and HYPO groups at a comparable rate. Hence, the creatine kinase reaction appears to be unaltered by the nutritional manipulations. As expected, just after the stimulation (time 0), the Pi levels were comparably elevated in CONT, 2DF and HYPO groups, and subsequently fell exponentially during the stimulation recovery period (Fig. 3a). However, the rate of fall of Pi in the HYPO group was significantly slower than in CONT or 2DF showing that oxidative phosphorylation was significantly affected by hypocaloric feeding but not by an

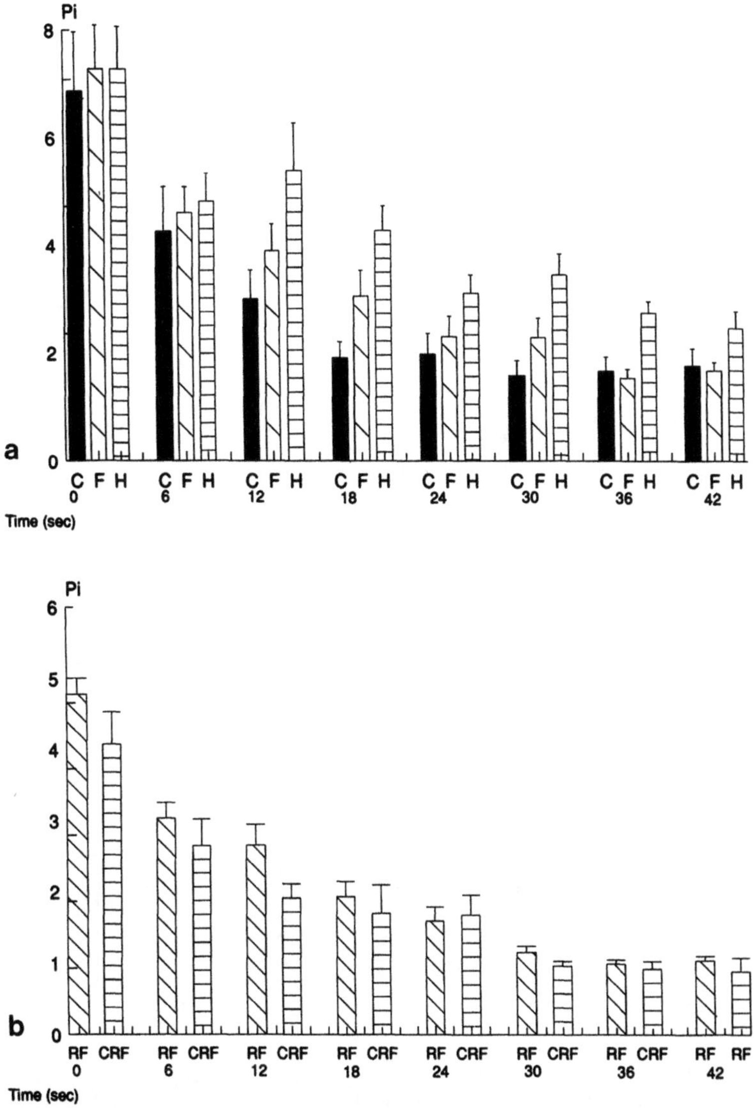

Fig. 2. a PCr levels (mmol/g wet weight) of muscle of CONT (C), 2DF (F), and HYPO (H) rats measured 200 us after the end of stimulation (time 0) and at 6 second intervals to 42 sec. **b** PCr levels (mmol/g wet weight) of muscle of CREF (CRF) and REF (RF) rats measured 200 us after the end of stimulation (time 0) and at 6 second intervals to 42 sec.

acute fast. The defect in rephosphorylation was supported by the higher FADP levels seen in 2DF and HYPO animals as compared to CONT (Fig. 4a). In addition, the FADP levels progressively rose from CONT to HYPO rats with the 2DF animals having intermediate levels (Fig. 4a). Hence, there is an abnormality of rephosphorylating ADP with 2-day fasting, and this ab-

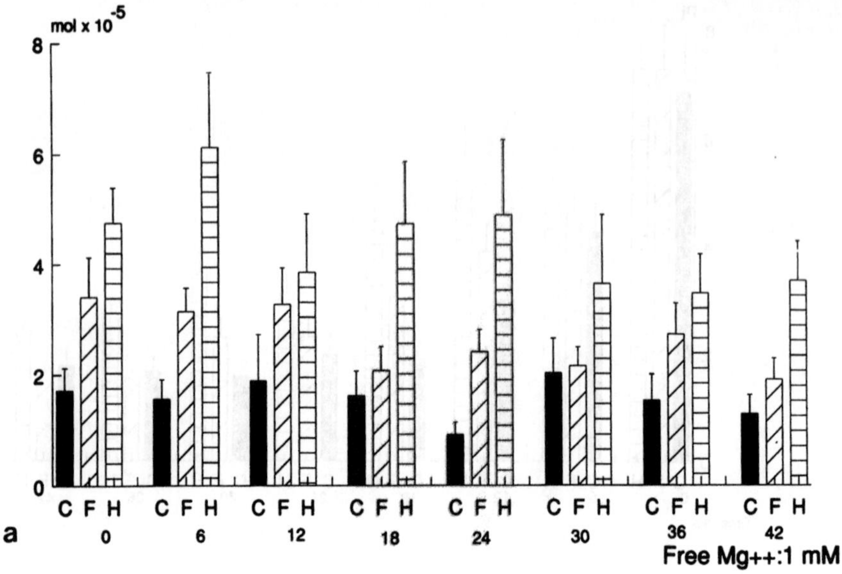

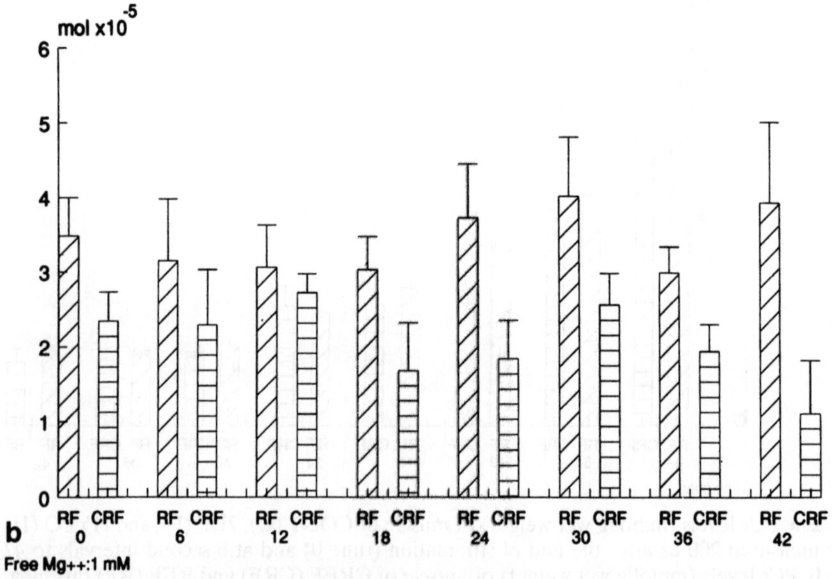

Fig. 3. a Pi levels (mmol/g wet weight) of muscle of CONT (C), 2DF (F), and HYPO (H) rats measured 200 us after the end of stimulation (time 0) and at 6 second intervals to 42 sec. **b** Pi levels (mmol/g wet weight) of muscle of CREF (CRF) and REF (RF) rats measured 200 us after the end of stimulation (time 0) and at 6 second intervals to 42 sec.

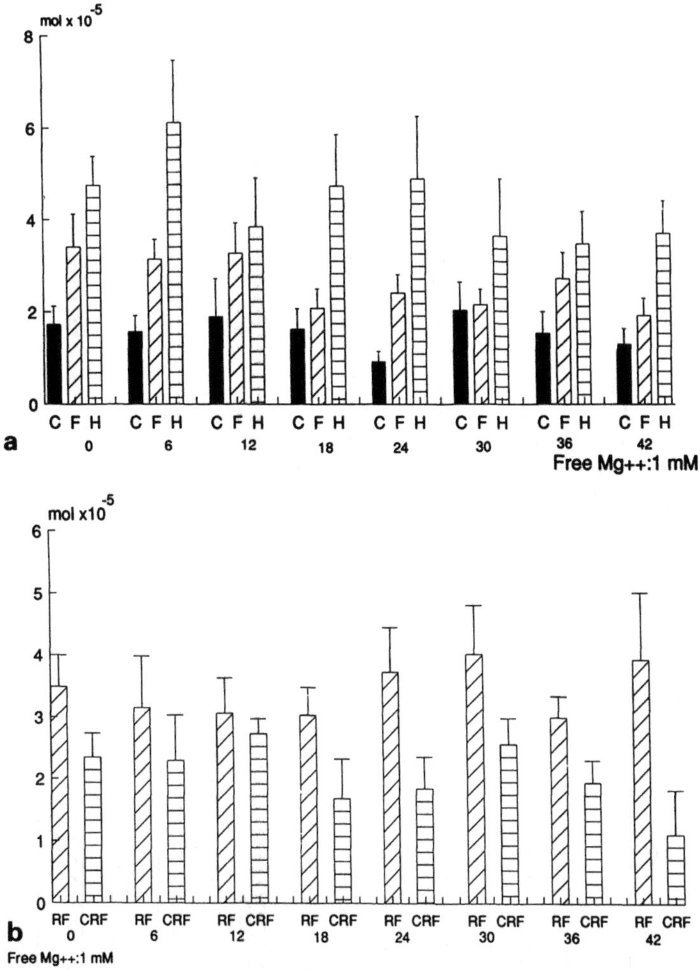

Fig. 4. a FDAP levels (mol × 10^{-5}) of muscle of CONT (C), 2DF (F), and HYPO (H) rats measured 200 us after the end of stimulation (time 0) and at 6 second intervals to 42 sec. **b** FADP levels (mol × 10^{-5}) of muscle of CREF (CRF) and REF (RF) rats measured 200 us after the end of stimulation (time 0) and at 6 second intervals to 42 sec.

normality is intensified by hypocaloric feeding over a longer term with weight loss. The data based on calculated FADP is supported by similar changes in the absolute PCr/Pi ratio and its restitution during the stimulation-recovery period. This ratio is the lowest in the HYPO muscle, and in addition, the slope of the recovery of this ratio is the slowest in the HYPO muscle. This ratio has been shown to be a function that relates work to the concentration of control chemicals, the so called transfer function [52]. Since the ATP levels were comparable to those seen in controls and there were no significant differences in ATP levels as a result of stimulation, the creatine

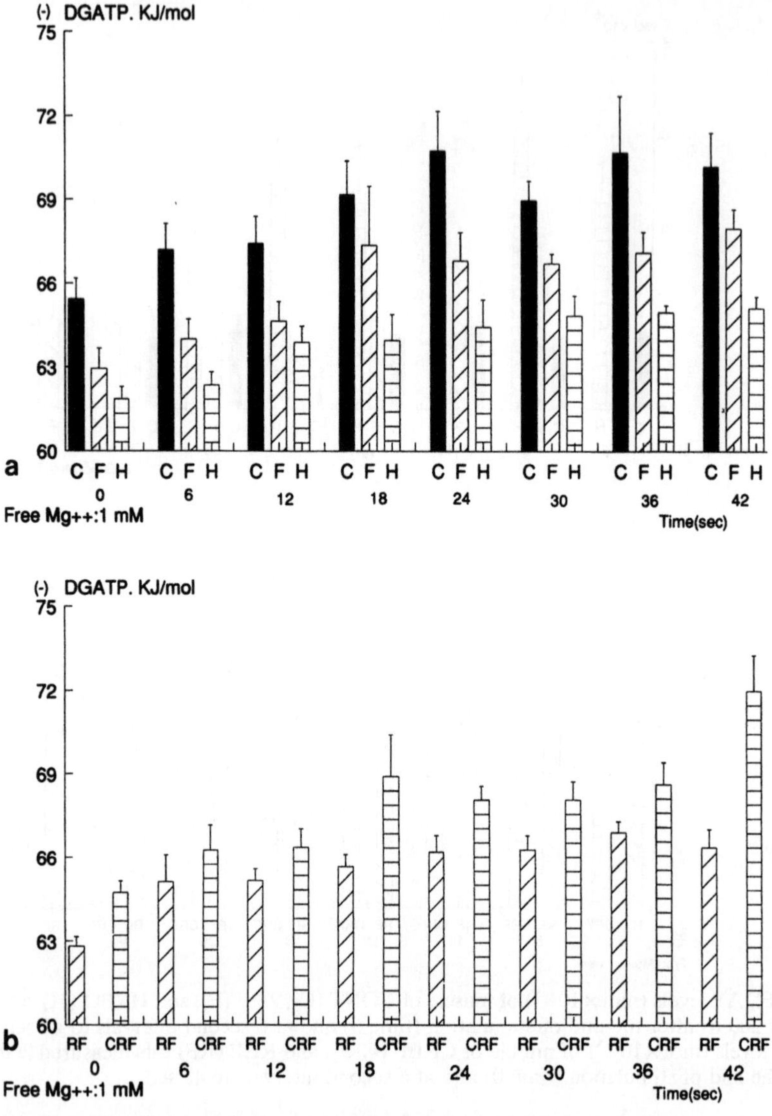

Fig. 5. a ΔGATP levels (kJ/mol of ATP) of muscle of CONT (C), 2DF (F), and HYPO (H) rats measured 200 us after the end of stimulation (time 0) and at 6 second intervals to 42 sec. **b** ΔGATP levels (kJ/mol of ATP) of muscle of CREF (CRF) and REF (RF) rats measured 200 us after the end of stimulation (time 0) and at 6 second intervals to 42 sec.

kinase reaction maintained normal ATP levels despite an abnormality of rephosphorylation of ADP. Finally, there was also a fall in the ΔG_{ATP} which was significantly higher in CONT as compared to 2DF, and lowest in the HYPO rats (Fig. 5a).

Effect of refeeding, hypocalorically fed rats: ATP, PCr and Pi levels. Refeeding did not completely restore the PCr levels but did restore the rate of fall of Pi during the stimulation-recovery period (Fig. 3b). Hence rephosphorylation of ADP appeared to have partly recovered. The higher FADP and lower ΔG_{ATP} in REF as compared with CREF suggest that rephosphorylation of ADP had not completely recovered with refeeding (Fig. 4b and 5b). Furthermore, the free energy change of ATP hydrolysis fell at the end of stimulation (ΔG_{ATP} levels increased or less negative) in both REF and CREF rats. However during the stimulation-recovery period, the REF rats did not restore the ΔG_{ATP} levels at the same rate as the CREF animals, indicating a residual abnormality (Fig. 5b).

TCr, pH and intracellular Mg^{2+}: The TCr content of muscle in relation to wet weight were not different in the groups. This finding suggests that the muscle composition in relation to the contractile elements were comparable in all groups. The pH likewise was not different in the groups, nor was the relative Mg^{2+} content. Since the K_{ck} and G° are altered by the pH and the Mg^{2+} of muscle, therefore the kinetics of the creatine kinase reaction, the calculated G° are comparable between the groups, making the relative comparison of FADP and ΔG_{ATP} between the groups possible as we had also shown previously [30].

Significance of the observed findings: The findings confirm our previous observation in unstimulated muscle that hypocaloric feeding reduces PCr levels, increases FADP levels, and reduces ΔG_{ATP} levels. In addition, by observing the effect of stimulation, it was noted that hypocaloric feeding reduces the rate of rephosphorylation during recovery. Also unlike the unstimulated muscle refeeding did not restore the lower PCr, higher FADP and lower ΔG_{ATP} levels to normal. Furthermore, the recovery of ΔG_{ATP} after stimulation was slower. The data are consistent with a reduction of oxidative phosphorylation due to mitochondrial dysfunction for the following reasons: similar changes have been observed in mitochondrial myopathies [64]. Although the reduced PCr could be due to a rise in the proportion of oxidative type I fibers noted to occur in malnutrition, the slow recovery of the PCr/Pi ratio noted herein is not consistent with this possibility. Type I fibers with a high oxidative activity show a very rapid postexercise recovery of the PCr/Pi ratio [65]. It is not due to anoxia as the muscle pH did not fall. While muscle lactate measured at the end of the experiment was significantly higher in HYPO muscles, the difference could not be due to anoxia as it was similarly raised in the unstimulated limb and was not increased by stimulation. It may be speculated that a mildly raised lactate level unchanged by stimulation (with resultant increase in oxygen consumption) may be due to a change in muscle NAD/NADH ratio. The cause of the mitochondrial abnormality remains speculative. However, in previous human studies, we showed that hypocaloric feeding with 400 kcal/d for 2 weeks resulted in vacuolation of mitochondria observed by electron microscopy in muscle biopsies [16]. Another possible cause for the observed changes may be the altered thyroid function seen in malnutrition. Malnutrition results in a decrease in T_3 and an increase in the less active reverse T_3 [66], and it has been shown that the PCr/Pi ratio is lower and is restored more slowly postexercise in hypothyroid patients [67].

Cell Calcium Kinetics

Dawson et al. [46] found a linear correlation between the relaxation rate and the ΔG_{ATP}. They postulated that the slow relaxation rate was due to a rise in ΔG_{ATP}. Since muscle relaxation is caused by uptake of calcium into the lateral cisternae of the sarcoplasmic reticulum, the total force available to drive Ca^{2+} into the sarcoplasmic reticulum during relaxation is [46]:

$$-(dG/dE)_{total} = -(dG/dE)_{ATP} - n\,(dG/dE)_{Ca} \tag{1}$$

Also the work required to pump a mole of calcium into the sarcoplasmic reticulum is:

$$(dg/dE)_{Ca} = 2.58 \ln [\text{free } Ca^{2+}] \text{ in}/[\text{free } Ca^{2+}]\text{out Kj mol}^{-1} \tag{2}$$

Since the hydrolysis of 1 mol of ATP results in the uptake of 2 mol of Ca^{2+}, therefore n=2.
Substituting (2) in (1).
When $-(dG/dE)_{total} = 0$ and calcium distribution is in equilibrium then:

$$(dG/d)_{ATP} = 5.98 \ln [\text{free } Ca^{2+}] \text{ in}/[\text{free } Ca^{2+}] \text{ out}$$

Rearranging the equation.

$$[\text{Free } Ca^{2+}]_{in}/[\text{Free } Ca^{2+}] \text{ out} = e^{(dG/dE)ATP/5.9} \tag{3}$$

Hence small changes in dG/dE of ATP (change in the free-energy change of ATP hydrolysis) may have profound effects on the regulation of free cytosolic calcium [46]. We had found a rise in calcium in hypocaloric muscle [16, 22] and have postulated that the abnormal energetics of hypocaloric muscle may increase cytosolic calcium because the steep electrochemical gradient for calcium across the sarcolemma makes the entry of calcium into the cell a passive process [68] and calcium efflux has to occur to maintain homeostasis by mechanisms which require ATP hydrolysis such as the CaMgATPase system [69] and by Na exchange [70] (the exchanged Na has to be pumped out of the cell by Na-K ATPase). Jones et al. [71] noted that muscle fatigue was followed by release of lactate dehydrogenase (LDH) and Z band degeneration preventable, by excluding calcium from the medium [72], and fatigued muscle had twice as much intracellular calcium as controls when the medium contained calcium [73]. Finally inhibiting energy metabolism by cyanide, or iodoacetate also acts synergistically with fatigue to enhance LDH release. Thus, there is evidence that fatigue associated with a reduction in available energy may induce calcium accumulation in the muscle. Z band degeneration and mitochondrial vacuolation are also observed in malnourished muscle with an increase in intracellular calcium [16]. Since increase in cytosolic calcium increases mitochondrial calcium uptake [74], our findings suggest that calcium accumulation may injure hypocaloric muscle and reduce mitochondrial function.

Conclusions

The above data show that malnutrition has profound effects at the membrane level changing the energetics of the sodium pump as well as changes in calcium kinetics affecting muscle function. The central problem appears to be limitation of aerobic and anaerobic energy production. The energetic changes are then responsible for altered function and changes in cell composition. For example the estimation of lean body mass by total body potassium probably reflects alteration in the sodium-potassium pump energetics rather than an actual change in lean tissue *per se*. Therefore the demonstration of the effects and treatment of malnutrition should be based on functional considerations.

References

1. Keys A, Brozek J, Henschel A, Mickelsen O, Taylor HL (1950) The Biology of Human Starvation. Vol I and II. Minneapolis, University of Minnesota Press
2. Heymsfeld SB, Lichtman S, Baumgartner RN, et al (1990) Body composition of humans: Comparison of two improved four-compartment models that differ in expense, technical complexity and radiation exposure. Am J Clin Nutr 52:52–58
3. Roubenoff R, Kehayias JJ (1991) The meaning and measurement of lean body mass. Nut Rev 49:165–175
4. Hill GL, King RFGJ, Smith RC (1979) Multi-element analysis of the living body by neutron activation analysis-application to critically ill patients receiving intravenous nutrition. Br J Surg 66:868–872
5. Moore FD, Olesen KH, McMurrey JD, Parker HV, Ball MR, Boyden CM (1963) The body cell mass and its supporting environment. WB Saunders, Philadelphia
6. Jeejeebhoy KN, Baker JP, Wolman SL, et al (1982) Critical evaluation of the role of clinical assessment and body composition studies in patients with malnutrition and after total parenteral nutrition. Am J Clin Nutr 35 (Suppl.):1117–1127
7. Russell DMcR, Prendergast PJ, Darby PL, Garfinkel PE, Whitwell J, Jeejeebhoy KN (1983) A comparison between muscle function and body composition in anorexia nervosa: The effect of refeeding. Am J Clin Nutr 38:229–237
8. Collins JP, Oxby CB, Hill GL (1978) Intravenous amino acids and intravenous hyperalimentation as protein-sparing therapy after major surgery: A controlled trial. Lancet 1:788–791
9. Almond DJ, King RFGJ, Burkinshaw L (1987) Potasium depletion in surgical patients: Intracellular cation deficiency is independent of loss of body protein. Clin Nutr 6:45–50

10. Almond DJ, King RFGJ, Burkinshaw L, Laughland A, McMahon MJ (1989) Influence of energy source upon body composition in patients receiving intravenous nutrition. JPEN 13:471–477
11. Fong CN, Atwood HL, Jeejeebhoy KN, Charlton MP (1987) Nutrition and muscle potassium: Differential effect in rat slow and fast muscles. Can J Physiol Pharmacol 65:2188–2190
12. Pichard C, Hoshino E, Allard JP, Charlton MP, Atwood HL, Jeejeebhoy KN (1991) Intracellular potassium and membrane potential in rat muscles during malnutrition and subsequent refeeding. Am J Clin Nutr 54:489–498
13. Newsholme E, Leech AR (1983) Biosynthesis of nucleic acids and proteins, Chap 18. In: Newsholme E, Leech AR (eds) Biochemistry for the medical sciences, 1st edn, J Wiley & Sons, Chichester, pp 651–680
14. Kammermeier H (1987) High energy phosphate of the myocardium: Concentration versus free energy. In: Jacob R, Just H, Holubarsch C (eds) Cardiac energetics. Basic research in cardiology. Springer-Verlag, New York, Vol 82 (suppl 2) pp 31–36
15. Munro HN (1964) Historical Introduction. In: Munro HN, Allison JB (eds) Mammalian protein metabolism. Academic Press, New York, Vol 1, pp 16–18
16. Russell DMcR, Walker PM, Leiter LA, et al (1984) Metabolic and structural changes in skeletal muscle during hypocaloric dieting. Am J Clin Nutr 39:503–513
17. Lopes J, Russell DMcR, Whitwell J, Jeejeebhoy KN (1982) Skeletal muscle function in malnutrition. Am J Clin Nutr 36:602–610
18. Russell DMcR, Leiter LA, Whitwell J, Marliss EB, Jeejeebhoy KN (1983) Skeletal muscle function during hypocaloric diets and fasting: A comparison with standard nutritional assessment parameters. Am J Clin Nutr 37:133–138
19. Berkelhammer CH, Leiter LA, Jeejeebhoy KN, et al (1985) Skeletal muscle function in chronic renal failure: An index of nutritional status. Am J Clin Nutr 42:845–854
20. Fraser IM, Russell DMcR, Whittaker S, et al (1984) Skeletal and diaphragmatic muscle function in malnourished chronic obstructive lung disease. Am Rev Respir Dis 129:A269
21. Brough W, Horne G, Blount A, Irving MH, Jeejeebhoy KN (1986) Effects of nutrient intake, surgery, sepsis, and long term administration of steroids on muscle function. Br Med J 293:983–988
22. Russell DMcR, Atwood HL, Whittaker JS, et al (1984) The effect of fasting and hypocaloric diets on the functional and metabolic characteristics of rat gastrocnemius muscle. Clin Sci 67:185–194
23. Dureuil B, Viires N, Veber B, Pavlovic D, et al (1989) Acute diaphragmatic changes induced by starvation in rats. Am J Clin Nutr 49:738–744
24. Christie PM, Hill GL (1990) Effect of intravenous nutrition on nutrition and function in acute attacks of inflammatory bowel disease. Gastroenterology 99:730–736
25. Windsor JA, Hill GL (1988) Weight loss with physiologic impairment: A basic indicator of surgical risk. Ann Surg 207:290–296
26. Sale DG, Martin JE, Moroz DE (1992) Hypertrophy without increased isometric strength after weight training. Eur J Appl Physiol 64:51–55
27. Barnard RJ, Edgerton VR, Peter JB (1970) Effect of exercise on skeletal muscle. II. Contractile properties. J Appl Physiol 28:767–770
28. Simard CP, Spector SA, Edgerton VR (1982) Contractile properties of rat hind limb muscles immobilized at different lengths. Exp Neurology 77:467–482
29. Sieck GC, Lewis MI, Blanco CE (1989) Effects of undernutrition on diaphragm fiber size, SDH activity, and fatigue resistance. J Appl Physiol 66:2196–2205
30. Pichard C, Vaughan C, Struk R, Armstrong RL, Jeejeebhoy KN (1988) The effect of dietary manipulations (fasting, hypocaloric feeding and subsequent refeeding) on rat muscle energetics as assessed by nuclear magnetic resonance spectroscopy. J Clin Invest 82:895–901
31. Godt R, Nosek TM (1989) Changes of intracellular milieu with fatigue or hypoxia depress contraction of skinned rabbit skeletal and cardiac muscle. J Physiol 412:155–180

32. Wilkie DR (1981) Shortage of chemical fuel as a cause of fatigue: Studies by nuclear magnetic resonance, bicycle ergometry. In: Porter R, Whelan J (eds) Human muscle fatigue: Physiological mechanisms. Pitman Medical, London pp 102–119
33. Bigland-Ritchie B (1981) EMG and fatigue of human voluntary and stimulated contractions. In: Porter R, Whelan J (eds) Human muscle fatigue: Physiological mechanisms. Pitman Medical, London, pp 130–156
34. Jones DA (1981) Muscle fatigue due to changes beyond the neuromuscular junction. In: Porter R, Whelan J (eds) Human muscle fatigue: Physiological mechanisms. Pitman Medical, London, pp 178–196
35. Rome LC, Kushmerick MJ (1983) Energetics of isometric contractions as a function of muscle temperature. Am J Physiol 244 (Cell Physiol 13): C100–C109
36. Homsher E, Kean CJ (1978) Skeletal muscle energetics and metabolism. Ann Rev Physiol 40:93–131
37. Edwards RHT, Hill DK, Jones DA (1975) Metabolic changes associated with the slowing of relaxation in fatigued mouse muscle. J Physiol (London) 251:287–301
38. Wiles CM, Edwards RHT (1982) Metabolic heat production in isometric ischaemic contractions of human adductor pollicis. Clin Physiol 2:499–512
39. Nishio ML, Jeejeebhoy KN (1991) The effect of acute fasting versus hypocaloric feeding on skeletal muscle relaxation rate. J Appl Physiol 71:204–209
40. Edwards RHT, Hill DK, Jones DA (1972) Effect of fatigue on the time course of relaxation from isometric contractions of skeletal muscle in man. J Physiol (London) 227:26P–27P
41. Wiles CM, Young A, Jones DA, Edwards RHT (1979) Relaxation rate of constituent muscle fibre types in human quadriceps. Clin Sci 56:47–52
42. Viitasalo JT, Komi PV (1981) Effects of fatigue on isometric force and relaxation time characteristics in human muscle. Acta Physiol Scand 111:87–95
43. Esau SA, Bellamare F, Grassino A (1983) Changes in relaxation rate with diaphragmatic fatigue in humans. J Appl Physiol (Respirat Environ Exercise Physiol) 54:1353–1360
44. Esau SA, Bye PTP, Pardy RL (1983) Changes in rate of relaxation of sniffs with diaphragmatic fatigue. J Appl Physiol (Respirat Environ Exercise Physiol) 55:731–735
45. Lymn RW, Taylor EW (1971) Mechanism of adenosine triphosphate hydrolysis by actomyosin. Biochemistry 10:4617–4624
46. Dawson MJ, Gadian DG, Wilkie DR (1980) Mechanical relaxation rate and metabolism studied in fatiguing muscle by phosphorus nuclear magnetic resonance. J Physiol (London) 299:465–484
47. Blinks JR, Rudel R, Taylor SR (1978) Calcium transients in isolated amphibian skeletal muscle fibres: Detection by aequorin. J Physiol (London) 277:291–323
48. Hultman E, Sjoholm H, Sahlin K, Edstrom L (1981) Energy metabolism in intact muscle. In: Porter R, Whelan J (eds) Human muscle fatigue: Physiological mechanisms. Pitman Medical, London, pp 19–40
49. Jewell BR, Wilkie DR (1960) Mechanical properties of relaxing muscle. J Physiol (London) 152:30–47
50. Chance B, Eleff S, Leigh JS (1981) Mitochondrial regulation of phosphocreatine, phosphate ratios in exercised human muscle: A gated ^{31}P NMR study. Proc Natl Acad Sci USA 78:6714–6718
51. Gyulai L, Roth Z, Leigh JS, Chance B (1985) Bioenergetic studies of mitochondrial oxidative phosphorylation using ^{31}Phosphorus NMR. J Biol Chem 260:3947–3954
52. Chance B, Leigh JS, Clark BJ (1985) Control of oxidative metabolism and oxygen delivery in human skeletal muscle: A steady-state analysis of the work/energy cost transfer function. Proc Natl Acad Sci USA 82:8384–8388
53. Chance B, Leigh JS, Kent J (1986) Multiple controls of oxidative metabolism in living tissues as studied by phosphorus magnetic resonance. Proc Natl Acad Sci USA 83:9458–9462
54. Meyer RA, Brown TR, Kushmerick MJ (1985) Phosphorus nuclear magnetic resonance of fast- and slow-twitch muscle. Am J Physiol 248 (Cell Physiol 17): C279–C287

55. Veech RL, Lawson JWR, Cornell NW, et al (1979) Cytosolic phosphorylation potential. J Biol Chem 254:6538–6547
56. Kodama T (1985) Thermodynamic analysis of muscle ATPase mechanisms. Physiol Rev 65:468–551
57. Chan STF, McLaughlin SJ, Ponting GA, et al (1986) Muscle power after glucose-potassium loading in undernourished patients. Br Med J 293:1055–1056
58. Maughan D (1983) Diffusable magnesium in frog skeletal muscle cells. Biophys J 43:75–80
59. Gupta RK, Gupta P, Yoshok WD, et al (1983) Measurement of the dissociation constant of MgATP at physiological nucleotide levels by a combination of ^{31}P NMR and optical absorbance spectroscopy. Biochem Biophys Res Commun 117:210–216
60. Liaw KY, Askanazi J, Michelson CB, et al (1980) Effect of injury and sepsis on high-energy phosphate in muscle and red cells. J Trauma 20:755–759
61. Sahlin K, Palmskog G, Hultman E (1978) Adenine nucleotide and IMP contents of the quadriceps muscle in man after exercise. Pflugers Arch 374:193–198
62. Church JM, Choong BY, Hill GL (1986) Abnormal muscle fructose bisphosphatase activity in malnourished cancer patients. Cancer 58:2448–2452
63. Lunt JA, Brauer M, Swinamer D, et al (1986) An evaluation of fasting on exercise-induced changes in pH, Pi/PCr from skeletal muscle. Mag Res Med 3:946–952
64. Argov Z, Maris J, Damico L, et al (1987) Bioenergetic heterogeneity of human mitochondrial myopathies as demonstrated by in vivo phosphorus magnetic resonance spectroscopy. Neurology 37:257–262
65. Giger U, Argov Z, Schnall M, et al (1986) Myopathy in phosphofructokinase deficient dogs studied by in vivo 31-P NMR. Muscle & Nerve 19 (Suppl 5s):187
66. Vagenakis AG (1977) Thyroid hormone in prolonged experimental starvation in man. In: Vigersky R (ed) Anorexia nervosa. Alan R Liss, New York, pp 243–252
67. Argov Z, Renshaw PF, Boden B, et al (1988) Effects of thyroid hormones on skeletal muscle bioenergetics: In vivo phosphorus-31 magnetic resonance spectroscopy study of humans and rats. J Clin Invest 81:1695–1701
68. Li CL, Shy GM, Wells J (1957) Some properties of mammalian skeletal muscle fibres with particular reference to fibrillation potentials. J Physiol 135:522–535
69. Sulakhe PV, Drummond GI, Ng DC (1973) Calcium binding by skeletal muscle sarcolemma. J Biol Chem 248:4150–4157
70. Caputo C, Balanos P (1978) Effect of external sodium and calcium on calcium efflux in frog striated muscle. J Membr Biol 41:1–14
71. Jones DA, Jackson MJ, Edwards RHT (1983) Release of intracellular enzymes from an isolated mammalian skeletal muscle preparation. Clin Sci 65:193–201
72. Jones DA, Jackson MJ, McPhail G, Edwards RHT (1984) Experimental mouse muscle damage: Importance of external calcium. Clin Sci 66:317–322
73. Jackson MJ, Jones DA, Edwards RHT (1984) Experimental skeletal muscle damage: Nature of calcium-activated degenerative process. Eur J Clin Invest 14:369–374
74. Nicholls D, Ackerman K (1982) Mitochondrial calcium transport. Biochem Biophys Acta 683:57–88

Muscle Intracellular Ions during Malnutrition and Refeeding

C. Pichard, D. Slosman, and A. G. Dulloo

Introduction

Consequences of protein-calorie malnutrition (PCM) have mostly been approached in terms of changes in body cell mass, or in body compartments as lean and fat masses. Such an approach exaggerates the relationship between tissue composition and tissue function. In addition, evidence of body compartment alterations does not provide any information about the pathophysiological consequences of such changes. For instance, does a reduction in muscle mass reduce the muscle performance in terms of power and endurance? In contrast, a function-oriented approach gives an overall appreciation of the integrity of a given mechanism which might be altered by malnutrition. Functions might be studied at different levels: a whole organism (i.e. heat production), an organ (i.e. muscle power), or an individual cell (i.e. membrane potential). At the cellular level, the relationship between ions content and membrane properties reflects that between PCM and cellular function.

This chapter will discuss the current knowledge on muscle cell physiology in relation to manipulations of nutritional intake and metabolic stress, and there will be an attempt to relate fundamental results to functional issues.

Reasons to focus on Skeletal Muscle Tissue

Skeletal muscle in normal adult is the body's major metabolically-active tissue since it represents about 40% of total body mass and consumes about 40% of total oxygen needs in resting conditions. It is not surprising therefore that significant energy balance alterations, as seen during PCM or refeeding, deeply affects mass and content of muscle [1, 2]. In addition, underfeeding and/or refeeding are related to early muscle dysfunction [2] (also see chapter by K. N. Jeejeebhoy), defined as altered contractility characteristics, at a time when body composition still remains unchanged. This suggests that significant electrophysiological cellular modifications are occurring and are related to changes in intra- and extracellular space characteristics, such as ions concentrations and membrane function. In addition, both the level of protein and calorie intake [2] and the level of stress [3, 4] interact to alter muscle cell morphology, content and function.

These observations have led to research focused on the relationship between cell electrolytes content and membrane status.

Water and Muscle Tissue

Changes in fuels and proteins during PCM alter water content of muscle tissue. Indeed clinicians accustomed to malnourished patients or subjects on prolonged stress [5–8] are familiar with an expanded total body water (TBW) and sodium content, as reflected by edema predominantly observed in lungs and limbs. Although, at the muscle tissue level, this water expansion is not so clearly apparent.

In *animal* studies of prolonged undernutrition, conflicting reports have shown either no change or an increase in total muscle water content. In case of 2 to 5 days fasting in rats, intracellular water (ICW) content remained unchanged [9]; whereas underfeeding for 21 days (25% of control food intake) resulted in an increased ICW. In contrast, Adibi et al. [10] found no change of ICW after 8 days fasting in rats, while others have found a decrease of ICW after 3 days of fasting prolonged by 3 weeks of undernutrition [11], or in case of 7 days of underfeeding in the rat [12]. Finally, Platt et al. [13] demonstrated an increase of total water content in underfed pigs.

It should be recalled that the determination of extra-(ECW) and intracellular water is based on the chloride method [14]. Briefly, chloride is freely diffusible across the skeletal muscle fiber membrane at rest and is distributed

Table 1. Total water, extracellular and intracellular water content (L/kg dry weight) in soleus and extensor digitorum longus (EDL) muscles during underfeeding and subsequent refeeding

	No of rats	Total water	Extracellular water	Intracellular water
SOLEUS				
Control 7 days	7	3.494 ± 0.036	721 ± 30	2.773 ± 0.046
Underfed	7	3.226 ± 0.041[b]	572 ± 36[a]	2.654 ± 0.042
Control 14 days	8	3.385 ± 0.040	646 ± 19	2.739 ± 0.044
Refed	7	3.418 ± 0.038	558 ± 61	2.860 ± 0.037[a]
EDL				
Control 7 days	8	3.320 ± 0.023	498 ± 30	2.822 ± 0.035
Underfed	8	3.001 ± 0.026[b]	428 ± 42	2.573 ± 0.041[b]
Control 14 days	7	3.350 ± 0.034	431 ± 15	2.919 ± 0.035
Refed	7	3.428 ± 0.058	397 ± 47	3.030 ± 0.034[a]

Mean ± SE. Control rats fed ad libitum for 7 days compared with underfed rats receiving 25% of the controls' food intake for 7 days, and control rats fed ad libitum for 14 days compared with refed rats for 7 days after being underfed.
[a] $p < 0.05$
[b] $p < 0.005$, *t*-test. (From [19] with permission.)

according to the Nernst equation [15–17]. Assuming a constant cell membrane potential of −85 mV, the extracellular chloride to intracellular chloride ratio calculated from the Nernst equation is 24/1. Such a calculation based on a *constant* membrane potential might partially be responsible for the somewhat conflicting data reported. In a further paragraph, the bias specific to the calculation methods of cellular ions will be discussed. Recent data are presented below in an animal model of malnutrition and refeeding in which actual membrane potential has been used to calculate ECW and ICW (Table 1).

In *human* studies, kwashiorkor has been associated to an increased total muscle water content resulting from an increase in both ECW and ICW [18]. Moreover, in malnourished patients, as well as in anorexic female patients [19] and in obese women on 400-kcal/day carbohydrate diet for 2 weeks [9], an increased TBW and ICW has been described [7, 20]. However, children with PCM have more unpredictable change in ICW which may increase, decrease, or remain unchanged [18]. In well-nourished acutely ill patients, who died within 3 days after admission and after having exclusively been on IV 5% dextrose, no significant change in muscle water has been observed [21]. In contrast, in chronically ill malnourished patients, who died within 2 weeks after hospital admission and lost an average of 2 additional kilograms of body weight, biceps and psoas muscles had significant expanded water content at autopsy [21]. In malnourished cancer patients, ECW is significantly larger than in controls, but this may be partially corrected by refeeding for 4 days [22]. In patients with Crohn's disease, total parenteral nutrition (TPN) for 3 weeks resulted in an increase of TBW [23]. Bergström et al. [22] have found an ECW expansion related to stress secondary to colectomy or hip replacement. During surgical stress (colectomy or hip replacement), muscle water content, both intracellular and extracellular, from biopsy samples was significantly increased ($p<0.001$) when compared to preoperative values despite of adequate enteral nutritional support. This observation highlights the role of stress on muscle water retention, and suggests that stress and PCM have synergistic effect on the water retention of muscle tissue [22]. Finally, refeeding subsequent to prolonged malnutrition has been associated with an important tissue water expansion [8, 24].

To summarize, whole body water content is expanded by PCM and normalized by refeeding. During measurements of ions, at the tissue level as well as at the intracellular level, the determination of water volume is critical because ions concentration are usually expressed per volume of water. At the extra- and intracellular level, conflicting results have been reported and are probably related to the calculation method. It seems quiet clear that proper methodology of water distribution across cell membrane should include membrane potential (E_m) determination because E_m varies with nutritional intake which in turn affects the final calculation.

Body Cell Mass and Body Electrolyte Content

Nutritional studies are regularly focused on the relationship between body cell mass and total amount of various ions, in particular potassium [7, 25, 26]. Indeed total body potassium is mostly (99%) contained in muscle tissue and is believed to reflect lean body mass which is of cardinal importance in terms of nutritional adequacy. Early work in patients on parenteral nutrition from MacNeil et al., Moore et al. and others has shown a constant relationship between total body potassium and total body nitrogen (3.0 mMoles K^+ to 1 g nitrogen) [25–28]. Subsequently, this ratio has been found to vary during malnutrition and refeeding. Total body potassium varies more rapidly than total body nitrogen, which suggests that changes in potassium concentration in tissues might occur independently of changes in nitrogen (Table 2) [29]. In addition, Almond et al. [30] have shown that in patients on refeeding, intracellular potassium repletion occurs before changes in nitrogen. Adipose or lean tissue have different electrolyte contents and are known to vary independently according to the type of energy supply and the hormonal environment [7, 21]. Thus, acute PCM tends to deplete more selectively lean tissue mass while chronic restriction decreases both lean and fat tissue masses because of the involvement of protein-sparing mechanisms. On the other hand, stress potentiates the catabolic effect of underfeeding, increasing further lean tissue catabolism [31, 32]. It is therefore logical to observe a discrepancy between total body cell mass and total body electrolyte content [7]. On this basis, a reliable approach of specific tissue composition necessitates direct measurements of the electrolytes content of muscle tissue.

Table 2. Changes in body composition during refeeding of anorexic patients

	Total body nitrogen (TBN)[a]	Total body potassium (TBK)[b]	K/N ratio
Base-line	1.21 ± 0.11	1590 ± 179	1.30 ± 0.07
2 week refeeding	1.26 ± 0.14[c]	1821 ± 205	1.42 ± 0.04
4 week refeeding	1.33 ± 0.10	1897 ± 205	1.40 ± 0.06
6 week refeeding	1.37 ± 0.09	2000 ± 205	1.45 ± 0.09
8 week refeeding	1.37 ± 0.10	2103 ± 179	1.53 ± 0.05

[a] predicted normal value (1.70 ± 0.08 kg)
[b] normal value (2462 ± 359 mmol)
[c] all increases in body composition (TBN, TBK, K/N ratio) during refeeding were significant compared with baseline ($p < 0.05$) except TBN at 2 week. (From [29] with permission.)

Muscle Tissue and Electrolyte Content

Animal Studies

In vitro muscle ions analysis have shown that nutritional imbalances lead to significant modifications of total (extra- plus intracellular), extra- and intracellular electrolyte content. There is some conflicting data on potassium alterations. Russel et al. [9] found no changes, when Pichard et al. [12] have claimed that intracellular potassium concentrations in both extensorum digitorum longus and soleus muscles are decreased after hypocaloric feeding for 7 days. In addition, Russel et al. [33] have shown increased extracellular sodium and chloride, but decreased intracellular calcium. Contrariwise acute starvation produced a rise in intracellular magnesium and a fall in phosphate [9]. Characteristic alterations related to prolonged underfeeding in rats are summarized on Tables 3, 4, and 5. These results have to be interpreted cautiously keeping in mind the following principles. To calculate ions distribution between intra- and extracellular space, the Nernst's equation [16] is applied:

$$E_s = (RT/z_sF)\ln([S]_o\text{-}[S]_i)$$

where E_s is the equilibrium potential as a function of the concentration ratio of extracellular $[S]_o$ to intracellular $[S]_i$ ion and the ionic valence, R is the gas constant, T is absolute temperature on the Kelvin scale, z_s the electrical charge of the ion S, and ln the natural logarithm, respectively.

Table 3. Total ions content (mmol/kg dry weight) in soleus and extensor digitorum longus (EDL) muscles measured by atomic or flame absorption spectrophotometry during underfeeding and subsequent refeeding

	No of rats	Potassium	Magnesium	Phosphorus
SOLEUS				
Control 7 days	7	385.1±8.0	34.7±1.4	173.9±2.9
Underfed	7	284.9±11.4[a]	29.4±1.0[a]	168.3±3.6
Control 14 days	8	385.5±8.6	35.0±1.2	177.8±4.5
Refed	7	359.8±7.4	29.8±0.6[a]	136.0±4.2[a]
EDL				
Control 7 days	8	446.7±10.0	40.4±1.5	211.9±3.0
Underfed	8	357.7±14.0[a]	39.6±1.2	208.4±3.1
Control 14 days	7	441.1±12.0	43.9±1.0	232.1±6.3
Refed	7	403.7±6.4[a]	36.6±1.1[a]	171.4±7.4[a]

Mean±SE. Control rats fed ad libitum for 7 days compared with underfed rats receiving 25% of the controls' food intake for 7 days, and control rats fed ad libitum for 14 days compared with refed rats for 7 days after being underfed.

[a] $p<0.05$, *t*-test. (From [19] with permission.)

For example, in this equation, knowing the total amount of potassium, chloride and water of a particular muscle, as well as the extracellular concentration of chloride (estimated by correcting the plasma chloride value) [3]), it is possible to calculate intracellular and extracellular K^+ by assuming a *constant* resting membrane potential, E_s [34]. This equation has been established in healthy normal cells, but a significant diminution of membrane potential has been shown in cells of malnourished [12, 33, 35] or/and stressed [3] organisms. This is the first cause of erroneous results.

In addition, tissue ions content is generally expressed per unit of ECW and ICW. As water calculation is based on the chloride method [14] which assumes a constant membrane potential of −85 mV, a second cause of error is therefore possible. For instance, underfeeding is associated with decreased membrane potential which is corrected by refeeding [12, 35]. This observation is true only in slow twitch rat fibers but not in fast-twitch fibers in which the membrane potential remains unchanged in response to underfeeding. Thus, conflicting reports mentioned above might have resulted from this erroneous assumption of a constant membrane potential. Some authors have also measured the membrane potential directly using microelectrodes in rat following diet manipulations [12, 35, 36]. This has allowed them to properly calculate the ions extra- and intracellular concentrations and to confirm a decrease in intracellular K^+ concentrations (Tables 4 & 5).

Table 4. Muscle extracellular potassium $[K^+]_e$, magnesium $[Mg^{++}]_e$ and phosphorus $[P]_e$ (mmol/kg dry weight) in soleus and extensor digitorum longus (EDL) muscles measured by atomic or flame absorption spectrophotometry during underfeeding and subsequent refeeding

	No of rats	$[K^+]_e$	$[Mg^{++}]_e$	$[P]_e$
SOLEUS				
Control 7 days	7	3.0±0.2	0.69±0.05	2.4±0.1
Underfed	7	1.8±0.1[b]	0.39±0.02[b]	1.1±0.1[b]
Control 14 days	8	2.8±0.2	0.54±0.03	1.5±0.1
Refed	7	2.8±0.4	0.37±0.06[a]	1.3±0.2
EDL				
Control 7 days	8	2.1±0.2	0.50±0.05	1.7±0.2
Underfed	8	1.4±0.2[b]	0.35±0.04[b]	1.0±0.1[b]
Control 14 days	7	2.0±0.2	0.34±0.02	0.9±0.1
Refed	7	2.0±0.3	0.28±0.04	1.0±0.2

Mean±SE. Control rats fed ad libitum for 7 days compared with underfed rats receiving 25% of the controls' food intake for 7 days, and control rats fed ad libitum for 14 days compared with refed rats for 7 days after being underfed.

[a] $p<0.002$

[b] $p<0.001$, *t*-test. (From [19] with permission.)

Table 5. Intracellular total intracellular potassium $[K^+]i$, magnesium $[Mg^{++}]i$ and phosphorus [P]i (mmol/L of intracellular water) in soleus and extensor digitorum longus (EDL) muscles measured by atomic or flame absorption spectrophotometry during underfeeding and subsequent refeeding

	No of rats	$[K^+]i$	$[Mg^{++}]i$	[P]i
SOLEUS				
Control 7 days	7	139.3±4.1	12.9±0.7	63.7±1.8
Underfed	7	106.7±4.0[a]	10.6±0.3[a]	64.7±2.0
Control 14 days	8	141.1±5.0	12.8±0.8	59.9±2.4
Refed	7	124.9±3.5[a]	10.2±0.3[b]	44.3±1.3[a]
EDL				
Control 7 days	8	158.2±4.2	14.8±0.7	77.7±1.8
Underfed	8	138.3±4.6[a]	15.2±0.5	80.2±1.9
Control 14 days	7	151.1±4.9	14.7±0.4	78.1±2.7
Refed	7	133.2±2.9[a]	12.0±0.6[a]	56.3±3.0[a]

Mean±SE. Control rats fed ad libitum for 7 days compared with underfed rats receiving 25% of the controls' food intake for 7 days, and control rats fed ad libitum for 14 days compared with refed rats for 7 days after being underfed.
[a] $p<0.005$, *t*-test. (From [19] with permission.)

Human Studies

For a long time, little was known about the human muscle electrolyte content because of the rather difficult access of muscle tissue in living individuals. It was only after the development of fine needle muscle biopsy technique that significant progress was made in the knowledge of ions content in various pathologies, including PCM and subsequent refeeding [34, 37, 38].

In anorexia nervosa and chronic PCM, the decreases in intracellular and extracellular potassium are associated with magnesium deficiency and with increases in sodium [39] and sometimes in phosphate [18]. In the case of short term underfeeding (2 weeks at 400 kcal/day), obese patients had altered intra- and extracellular ions concentrations (sodium, potassium, chloride, calcium, phosphate, magnesium) but only differences in calcium concentrations reached a statistical level of significance [9]. This increase in intracellular calcium concentration is associated with an increase in calcium urinary excretion which suggests bone calcium mobilization [32] and an increase in cellular calcium uptake [40]. This increase means that there is a net positive balance of calcium across the sarcolemma. It is likely that this effect is due largely to an increase in the mitochondrial calcium for reasons that have been reviewed elsewhere in details [41], mainly because of a reduction in the free-energy change of ATP hydrolysis and change in electrochemical gradient for calcium across the sarcolemma. In human muscle tissue, therefore, it seems that malnutrition, even in the short term, is associated with alterations of ions content. Evidence of *intracellular* potassium depletion found in animal models is not consistently found in human muscle (whereas increase in calcium has been found to be significant in both).

Bergström et al. [21] have shown that refeeding for 4 days after surgical stress was related to significant increase in muscle Na and Cl content, whereas K and Mg were decreased as expressed by weight of fat free muscle tissue. When these data were expressed as mmol per liter of intracellular water, Na was not significantly altered, K and Mg were increased ($p < 0.01$) when compared to preoperative values despite of adequate enteral nutritional support [22]. This observation highlights the importance of referring to water content rather than to muscle mass because of changes of ICW and ECW related to stress and/or PCM. This is crucial, because as changes in cellular electrolytes concentrations are occurring, alterations in cellular functioning, such as membrane polarization and excitability, can be observed by *in vivo* measurements and correlated to basic cellular electrophysiological explanations [15–17].

Muscle Cells and in vivo Ions Determination

In vitro muscle analysis have shown that any nutritional imbalances lead to significant modifications of extra- and intracellular electrolytes and water content. In some of these works, ions contents were expressed as fat-free and glycogen-free dry weight. This is important because intracellular ions concentrations are also dependent of intracellular components such as amino acids and glycogen. It has been claimed that intracellular components may also bind ions, for instance amino acids and potassium [42, 43]. In addition, potassium, as well as other intracellular ions, may be distributed between the cytosol and in intracellular microstructures such as mitochondria, a phenomenon named the ionic intracellular compartmentalization [44]. This is a critical issue, because *only* free diffusible potassium is electrophysiologically active (Fig. 1) and correlated to the cellular membrane function. Therefore, we feel that there was a case to try to measure free diffusible ion in an *in vivo* model of nutritional manipulations. As potassium is the more abundant intracellular ion, as well as the most important in term of membrane potential, free intracellular potassium activity has been measured *in vivo* using a rat model.

Animal Studies

The membrane potential (E_m) and the intracellular potassium activity (aK^+_i) of the fibers in three different rat muscles were measured by means of double-barrelled K^+-selective microelectrodes as described by Charlton et al. [45]. The advantage of a double-barrelled K^+-selective microelectrode over chemical analysis is to be able to determine *in vivo*, simultaneously with the membrane potential, the free and physiologically relevant intracellular

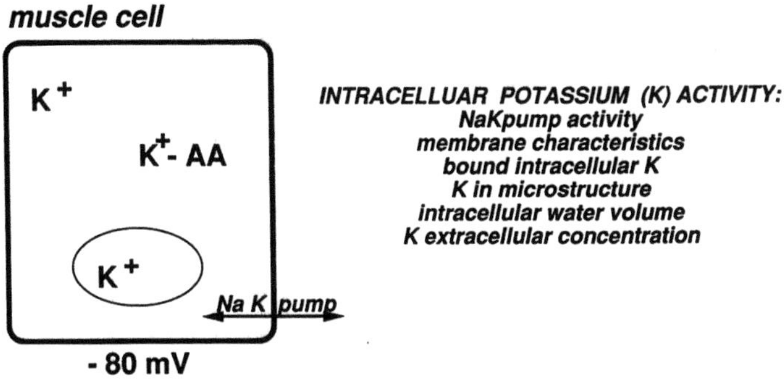

Fig. 1. Intracellular potassium concentration and activity is dependent of various factors inside and outside the cell. K^+-AA = bound potassium.

K^+ activity without contamination from the bound intracellular K^+ and the extracellular K^+ (Fig. 2).

We designed a rat study based on this technology in order to analyze the effects of short term starvation (48 h) as well as that of 1 week underfeeding corresponding to 25% of the nutritional intake of control animals. Then underfed animals were refed *ad libitum* for a full week and compared to control animals fed *ad libitum* for 2 weeks. For intracellular puncture, rats were maintained in a heated chamber (32°C) and the muscle bathed with a physiological solution. The muscle fibers were then exposed. Specific skeletal muscles consist of different percentages of slow-twitch and fast-twitch fibers [2]. The soleus muscle is representative for slow-twitch fibers (>73–75%) and extensor digitorum longus muscle for fast-twitch fibers (>93–98%) for the rats defined above. Slow-twitch fibers are responsible for posture maintenance and locomotion, while fast-twitch fibers are recruited only during vigorous activity. The slow-twitch fibers are more vulnerable to the energy deprivation of malnutrition and more responsive to refeeding. The fast-twitch fibers are more responsive to exercise. Thus the investigations of these different fiber types should provide complementary information for whole

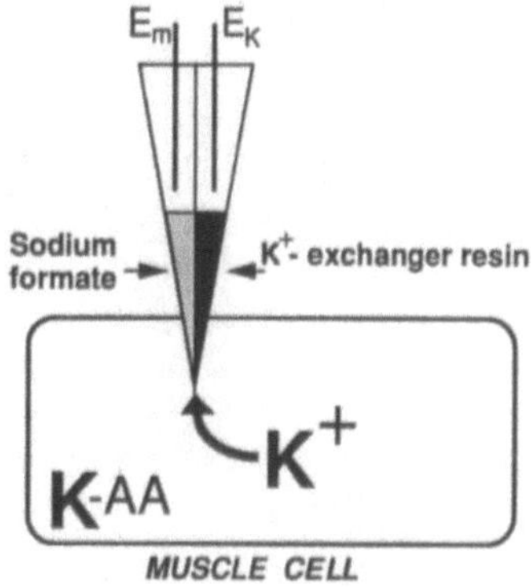

Fig. 2. The membrane potential (E_m) and the intracellular potassium potential (E_K) is measured by the mean of double-barrelled K^+-selective microelectrode. The advantage of such a microelectrode over traditional chemical analysis is to be able to determine *in vivo*, simultaneously with the membrane potential, the free and physiogically relevant intracellular K^+ activity without contamination from the bound intracellular K^+ (K-AA) and the extracellular K^+.

body skeletal muscles. Those from slow-twitch muscle fibers, as in the soleus muscle, namely those from fast-twitch muscle fibers, as in the extensorum digitorum longus muscle and finally, those in a muscle combining both slow-

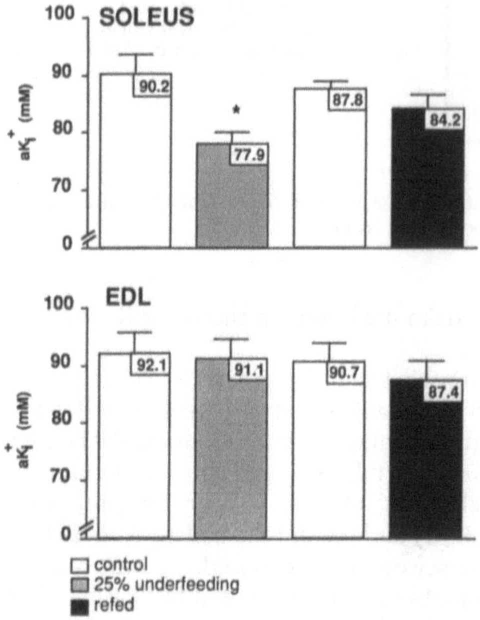

Fig. 3. The intracellular K^+ activity (aK_i^+) is shown in the soleus muscle, representative for slow-twitch fibers, and the extensor digitorum longus muscle (EDL), representative for fast-twitch fibers, in rats following 1 week of underfeeding corresponding to 25% of the nutritional intake of control animal, and in underfed animals refed *ad libitum* for a full week and compared to control animals fed *ad libitum* for 2 weeks. Mean ± SD. * $p<0.05$. (From [12] with permission.)

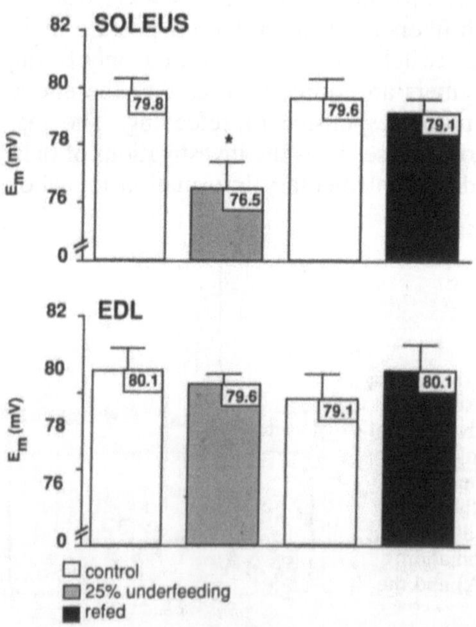

Fig. 4. Membrane potential is shown in the soleus and the extensor digitorum longus muscles (EDL) in rats following 1 week of underfeeding corresponding to 25% of the nutritional intake of control animal, and in underfed animals refed *ad libitum* for a full week and compared to control animals fed *ad libitum* for 2 weeks. Mean ± SD. * $p<0.05$. (From [12] with permission.)

and fast-twitch muscle fiber types as in the gastrocnemius muscle [35]. The K^+-selective barrel had a typical response and all microelectrodes were calibrated at the beginning and during intracellular measurements [12]. The mathematical model to calculate the values of aK^+_i has been reported elsewhere in details [45]. The changes in intracellular K^+ and membrane potential are summarized in Figures 3, 4 & 5.

Underfeeding alters the intracellular K^+ activity in all fiber types but in larger proportions in slow-twitch muscle fibers, as shown in the soleus muscle. By comparison, the gastrocnemius and extensorum digitorum longus muscles (predominantly fast-twitch fibers) are more resistant to underfeeding. This selective effect of malnutrition is not specific to intracellular K^+ since it has also been described for glucose uptake [46]. Reduced Na^+K^+ pump activity is thought to be responsible for the loss of intracellular K^+ in slow-twitch muscle fibers, an effect which Clausen et al. [15] have attributed to hypothalamic modulation of the sympathetic nervous system (SNS) and other endocrine organs. Indeed, the hypothalamus regulates both the insulin and catecholamine release, which in turn are able to influence the Na^+K^+ pump activity [15]. A role for SNS in the modulation of the Na^+K^+ pump is also suggested by Yoshimatsu et al. [47] on the basis of findings that the Na^+K^+ pump in the soleus can be modulated by peripheral sympathetic nerve activity via alpha-adreno receptors. However, direct assessment of SNS activity using labelled norepinephrine-turnover techniques in specific tissues and organs, indicates that unlike in heart, liver and adipose tissues, caloric deprivation does not influence central sympathetic outflow to various

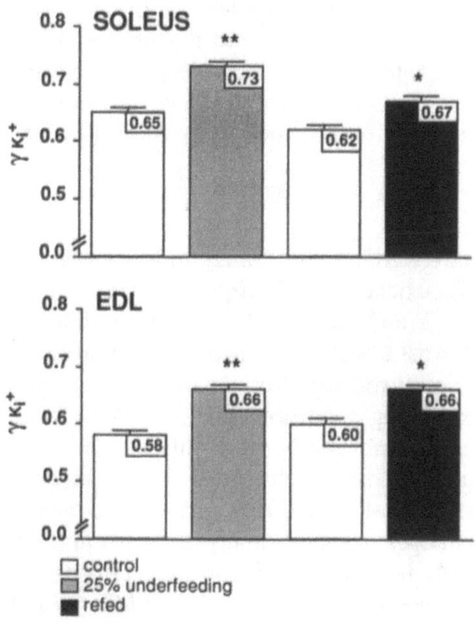

Fig. 5. Ratio of free to total intracellular K^+ (γK_i^+) is shown in the soleus and the extensor digitorum longus (EDL) muscles in rats following 1 week of underfeeding corresponding to 25% of the nutritional intake of control animal, and in underfed animals refed *ad libitum* for a full week and compared to control animals fed *ad libitum* for 2 weeks. Mean ± SD. * $p < 0.05$. (From [12] with permission.)

skeletal muscle types [48]. There is clearly a need to reassess neuro-endocrine mechanisms underlying the selective effect of undernutrition on intracellular K^+ loss in the slow-twitch muscle. To this end, further studies would need to delineate the effect of undernutrition in altering thyroid hormones and insulin levels from alterations in reduced muscle receptor sensitivity to these hormones as well as to catecholamines.

In 1986, the normalization of the muscle relaxation-contraction charactristics has been shown in malnourished patients receiving intravenously a 2 days load of potassium-glucose [49]. This observation correlates with the muscle fiber ionic content to the muscle function and highlights the crucial role of K^+ for muscle electrophysiology. It also suggests that in case of malnutrition, the refeeding process associated with protein synthesis has to be preceded by an intracellular K^+ repletion. In underfed rats, the intracellular K^+ fiber concentration obtained using chemical *in vitro* analysis is smaller than the intracellular K^+ concentration measured by the K^+-selective microelectrode. This results from the specific reading of the K^+-selective microelectrode, which measures only the free K^+, and therefore confirms that part of the intracellular K^+ is bound [15].

In addition to the reduction in intracellular K^+ concentration, a significant depolarization has been observed during underfeeding in the soleus muscle, but similar effects were not observed in the gastrocnemius nor in the extensorum digitorum longus muscle. Following the 2-day fast, the membrane potential remained stable in either muscle, and hence contrasts with the decrease K^+ mentioned above in the soleus. Refeeding for 7 days partially normalized both intracellular K^+ and membrane polarization.

It should be recalled that the resting membrane potential and excitability are ultimately dependent on the Na^+K^+ pump activity which relies on magnesium availability and is stimulated by Na^+ and K^+. The energy cost for ions pumping requires energy in quantities which are directly proportional to the electrochemical gradient between the extra- and intracellular concentration and is represented by the following equation:

$$\Delta G_i = zF(E_m\text{-}E_i)$$

where ΔG_i is the change in free-energy in joules/mole of the ion i against its electrochemical driving force (E_m-E_i). Both the resting membrane potential (E_m) and the equilibrium potential (E_i) are calculated according to the Nernst equation. Based on calculation detailed elsewhere [2, 41], both free-energy and free Mg^{++} are not limiting factors for the N^+K^+ pump activity in resting conditions [41, 50]. Therefore, this strongly suggests alterations of cell membrane permeability which explain the dissociation between K^+ loss and the lack of change in depolarization observed in the soleus muscle fiber of rats after a 2-day fast. These mechanisms may possibly be related to changes in membrane properties and constituents. In a study of hypocalorically fed animals (Fig. 6), the phosphoenergetic of rat leg muscle have been studies *in vivo* using a ^{31}P NMR [51]. The spectra generated displayed an

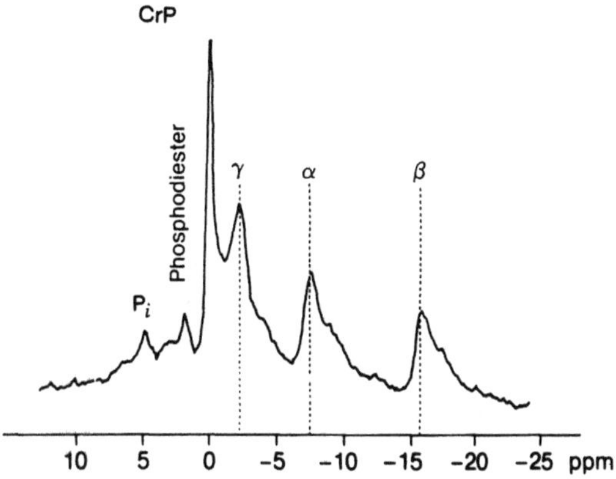

Fig. 6. Spectra obtained from ^{31}P nuclear magnetic resonance of the gastrocnemius muscle of rats following 1 week of underfeeding corresponding to 25% of the nutritional intake of control animal. The peaks shown correspond to phosphoenergy compounds, respectively inorganic phosphate, creatine phosphate, and adenosine triphosphate. Note a phosphodiester peak appears in underfed animals which suggests an alteration of membrane constituents. (From [51] with permission.)

usual peak corresponding to phosphodiester compounds, generally recognized as cell membrane constituents. Thus, malnutrition may be associated with significant changes of cell membrane constituents which are likely to alter the transmembrane ionic exchanges. The latter might be involved in the pathophysiological dissociation between membrane potential and intracellular K^+ concentration presented before (Fig. 3).

The possibility arises therefore that changes in cell membrane characteristics (due to imbalance of the intracellular ion content) could in general provide a mechanistic explanation of the perturbated muscle performance observed during malnutrition and subsequent refeeding.

Human Studies

Knowledge about the human muscle electrolyte content has been obtained on samples measured *in vitro* and hence subjected to the same criticisms formulated for animal muscle tissue.

Very few *in vivo* human studies have been reported. In a very elegant study, Legaspi et al. [36] have analyzed the effect of *unstressed* starvation for 10 days on patients muscle tissue. The resting membrane potential of muscle cell of the anterior tibial muscle was determined using a genuine technique of transdermal puncture with a microelectrode. Then a sample of the same muscle was obtained, using usual biopsy technique, for measurements of sodium, potassium and chloride. Starvation produces a decrease in membrane potential (-82 ± 1 to -76 ± 3 mVolt). When total, extra- and intracellular potassium was calculated using the Nernst equation and the actual membrane potential, no significant difference was found (87 ± 7 to 107 ± 14; 4.4 ± 0.3 to 3.9 ± 0.4; 149 ± 11 to 173 ± 29 mmol/L ICW, respectively). Nevertheless, during the same time, nitrogen balance became significantly negative and intracellular amino acids as glutamine decrease from 29.98±2.49 to 14.70±2.89 mmol/L ICW ($p<0.05$).

Cunningham et al. [3] have formulated the hypothesis that stress might significantly potentiate the effect of underfeeding. In a remarkable clinical study, they have measured the membrane potential of deltoid muscle cell in 26 normal humans, 7 ambulatory patients with minor medical problems and 21 in-hospital patients with severe illness and malnutrition. They found no difference between the two first categories (−88±3.8 to −89±2.1 mVolt), but a significantly reduced signal in severy ill patients (66.3±9.0 mVolt). This finding highlights the role of stress on cell function during malnutrition. In addition, analysis of muscle samples indicated that potassium was unchanged while sodium was increased in different muscle types.

Thus, the results found in rat models of underfeeding were not confirmed in human. There are many possible explanations for these discrepancies. First the assessment of membrane potential in human muscle is certainly much more difficult technically than in rat and is reflected by the large standard error of the mean – such problems may have contributed to obscure statistically significant differences. For instance, the depth of muscle cell punctured has a major effect on the membrane potential recorded and is much more difficult to control in a human experimental setting [3]. Second, the type of muscle under investigation might have been similar to the extensorum digitorum longus muscle in which no difference was found in the animal model. Finally, a few days starvation of a 70 kilogram man is probably quiet different from that seen in a 200 gram rat ...

Importance of Muscle Tissue Ions Content Determination during Malnutrition and Refeeding in Human

Specific muscle dysfunctions have been demonstrated in various clinical situations [2, 41, 52–57]. In addition, analysis of muscle function may be used as an indicator of nutritional status during both malnutrition progression or refeeding process [2, 41, 58–60]. As muscle function is intrinsically related to cellular function, namely polarization dependent upon ionic exchange and content, additional data are needed to understand the pathophysiological processes involved. Stress being a strong potentiator of the deleterious effects of underfeeding, animal models should be developed for further studies. Globally, it seems reasonable to encourage further research on cell membrane characteristics and energetics.

Conclusion

The pathophysiological consequences of malnutrition and refeeding, with or without stress, found in animal models have only been partially reproduced in man. The exploration of muscle function, in terms of ion concentrations at the cellular level, has provided new information regarding the relationship between malnutrition, various diseases and muscle behavior in the adult human. This functional approach provides more information about the physiologically active lean body mass than does traditional and indirect assessment. Further investigations should focus on the adverse effects of malnutrition on the permeability of the cellular membrane and special attention should be given to the respective role of ions and energetic compounds in modulating the relationship between nutrients and muscle function.

References

1. Heymsfield SB, McManus CB, Seitz SB, Nixon DW, Smith Andrew J (1984) Nutritional assessment of adult protein-energy malnutrition. In: Wright RA, Heymsfield SB, McManus CB (eds) Nutritional assessment, Blackwell Scientific Publications, Inc; Boston pp 27–83
2. Pichard C, Jeejeebhoy KN (1988) Muscle dysfunction in malnourished patients. Quarter J Int Med 260:1021–1045
3. Cunningham JN, Carter NW, Rector FC, Seldin DW (1971) Resting transmembrane potential difference of skeletal muscle in normal subjects and severely ill patients. J Clin Invest 50:49–59
4. Cuthbertson DP (1979) The metabolic response to injury and its nutritional implications: Retrospect and prospect. JPEN 3:108–129
5. Chiolero R, Gay LJ, Cotting J, Gurtner C, Schuitz Y (1992) Assessment of changes in body water by biompedance in acutely ill surgical patients. Intensive Care Med 18:322–326
6. Heymsfield SB, Head CA, McManus CB, et al (1984) Respiratory cardiovascular and metabolic effects of enteral hyperalimentation: Influence of formula dose and composition. Am J Clin Nutr 40:116–130
7. Shizgal HM, Vasilevsky CA, Gardiner PF, et al (1986) Nutritional assessment and skeletal function. Am J Clin Nutr 44:761–777
8. Solomon SM, Kirby DF (1990) The refeeding syndrome: A review. JPEN 14:90–97
9. Metcoff J, Frank S, Yoshida T, et al (1975) Protein calorie malnutrition. In. Olsen RE (ed) Protein calorie malnutrition, Academic Press, New York:pp 65–85
10. Eales L (1961) Abnormalities of fluid and electrolyte metabolism in malnutrition in adult. In: Brock JF (ed) Recent advances in human nutrition, Churchil, J. A. Ltd; London pp 198–217
11. Russell DM, Walker PM, Leiter LA, et al (1984) Metabolic and structural changes in skeletal muscle during hypocaloric dieting. Am J Clin Nutr 39:503–513
12. Lennmarken C, Sandstedt S, Croner S, Symreng T, Larsson J (1984) Muscle metabolic changes in severe malnutrition – Effect of parenteral nutrition. Clin Nutr 3:41–45
13. Heymsfield SB (1982) Biochemical composition of muscle in normal and semistarved human subjects: Relevance of anthropometric measurements. Am J Clin Nutr 36:131–142
14. Bergström J, Fürst P, Holmström B (1981) Influence of injury and nutrition on muscle water and electrolytes. Ann Surg 193:810–816
15. Jacobson S, Carlmark B (1990) Total body potassium, fat and water during total parenteral nutrition in Crohn's disease. Clin Nutr 9:272–280
16. Sitges-Serra A, Arcas G, Guirao X, Garcia-Dominho M, Gil MJ (1992) Extracellular fluid expansion during parenteral refeeding. Clin Nutr 11:63–68
17. Adibi SA (1971) Interrelationships between level of amino acids in plasma and tissue during starvation. Am J Physiol 221:829–838
18. Spence CA, Hansen-Smith FM (1978) Comparison of the chemical and biochemical composition of thirteen muscles of the rat after dietary protein restriction. Brit J Nutr 39:647–658

19. Pichard C, Hoshino E, Allard J, et al (1991) Intracellular potassium activity and membrane potential in rat muscle during malnutrition and refeeding studied in vivo by potassium-sensitive microelectrode (KISE) and atomic absorption. Am J Clin Nutr 54:489–498
20. Platt BS, Heard CRC, Stewart RJC (1964) Experimental protein-calorie deficiency. In: Munro HN, Allison JB (eds). Mammalian protein metabolsim, Academic Press; New York, pp 445–521
21. Bergstrom J, Hultman E (1974) Water, electrolyte and glycogen content of muscle tissue in patients undergoing regular dialysis therapy. Clin Nephrol 2:24–34
22. Clausen T, Kjeldsen K (1987) Effects of potassium deficiency on N,K homeostasis and Na^+,K^+-ATPase in muscle. Curr Topics Membr Transport 28:403–419
23. Hille B (1984) Potassium channels and chloride channels. In: Sunderland (ed) Ionic channels of excitable membrane. Sinauer Associates Incorporation, pp 99–114
24. Wills NK, Clausen C, Clauss WC (1987) Electrophysiology of active potassium transport across the mammalian colon. Curr Topics Membr Transport 28:441–456
25. McNeill KG, Mernagh JR, Jeejeebhoy KN, Wolman SL, Harrison JE (1979) In vivo measurements of body protein based on the determination of nitrogen by prompt gamma analysis. Am J Clin Nutr 32:1955–1961
26. McNeill KG, Harrison JE, Mernagh JR, Stewart S, Jeejeebhoy KN (1982) Changes in body protein, body potassium, and lean body mass during total parenteral nutrition. JPEN 6:106–112
27. Lukaski HC, Mendez J, Buskirk ER, Cohn SH (1981) A comparison of methods of assessment of body composition including neutron activation analysis of total body nitrogen. Metabolism 30:777–782
28. Moore FD, Oelsen KH, McMurray JD, et al (1978) The body cell mass and its supporting environment. In: N.R.C.C.o.A. Nutrition, Body Composition in Health and Disease, WB Saunders Co, Washington D.C. pp 56–116
29. Russell DM, Prendergast PJ, Darby PL, et al (1983) A comparison between muscle function and body composition in anorexia nervosa: The effect of refeeding. Am J Clin Nutr 38:229–237
30. Almond DF, King RFGJ, Burkinshaw L, Laughland A, McMahon MF (1987) Potassium depletion in surgical patients: Intracellular cation deficiency is independent of loss of body protein. Clin Nutr 6:45–50
31. Nordenström J, Carpentier YA, Askanazi J, et al (1983) Free fatty acid mobilization and oxidation during parenteral nutrition in trauma and infection. Ann Surg 198:725–735
32. Slosman DO, Casez JP, Pichard C, et al (1992) Assessment of whole-body composition using dual X-ray absorptiometry. Radiology 185:593–598
33. Russell DM, Atwood HL, Whittaker JS, et al (1984) The effect of fasting and hypocaloric diets on the functional and metabolic characteristics of rat gastrocnemius muscle. Clin Sciences 67:185–194
34. Bergström J (1962) Muscle electrolytes in man. Scand J Clin Lab Invest (Suppl) 68:14
35. Fong CN, Jeejeebhoy KN, Atwood HL, Charlton MP (1987) Nutrition and muscle potassium: Differential effect in rat slow and fast muscles. Can J Pharmacol Physiol 65:2188–2190
36. Legaspi A, Roberts JP, Albert JD, Tracey KJ, Shires GT (1988) The effects of starvation and total parenteral nutrition on skeletal muscle amino acid content and membrane potential difference in normal man. Surg Gynecol Obst 166:233–240
37. Viteri F, Behar M, Arroyave G, Scrimshaw NS (1964) Clinical aspects of protein malnutrition. In: Munro HN, Allison JB (eds) Mammalian protein metabolism. Academic Press, New York pp 381–481
38. Fisler JS, Drenick EJ (1987) Starvation and semi-starvation diets in the management of obesity. Ann Rev Nutr 7:465–484
39. Jeejeebhoy KN (1988) Bulk or bounce – The object of nutritional support. JPEN 12:539–549

40. Hummel Z (1980) Bound potassium in muscle II. Acta Biochimica Biophysica Acad Scien Hungarica 15:89–94
41. Reikeras O, Nordstrand K (1989) Effects of glucose-insulin-potassium infusion on glycogen levels in cardiac and skeletal muscles in rats. Clin Nutr 8:213–215
42. Adam WR, Korettsky AP, Weiner MV (1988) Potassium adaptation: ^{39}K-NMR evidence for intracellular compartmentalization of K^+. Am J Physiol 254:F401–F406
43. Charlton MP, Silverman H, Atwood HL (1981) Intracellular potassium activities in muscles of normal and dystrophic mice: An in vivo electrometric study. Exper Neurol 71:203–219
44. Shoji S (1986) Effects of stretch and starvation on glucose uptake of rat soleus and extensor digitorum longus muscles. Muscle Nerve 9:144–147
45. Yoshimatsu H, Oomura Y, Katafuchi T, Akaike N (1986) Hypoythalamic regulation of sodium-potassium pump activity in skeletal muscle. Brain Research 384:17–22
46. Dulloo AG, Young JB, Landsberg L (1988) Sympathetic nervous system responses to cold exposure and diet in rat skeletal muscle. Am J Physiol 255:E180–E188
47. Chan STF, McLaughlin SJ, Ponting GA, Biglin J, Dudley HAF (1986) Muscle power after glucose-potassium loading in undernourished patients. Brit Med J 293:1055–1056
48. Pichard C, Vaughan C, Struck RS, Armstrong RL, Jeejeebhoy KN (1988) The effects of fasting hypocaloric feeding and refeeding on muscle energetics studied by 31 phosphorus nuclear magnetic resonance. Am J Clin Nutr 47:773
49. Edwards R, Young A, Wiles M (1980) Needle biopsy of skeletal muscle in the diagnosis of myopathy and the clinical study of muscle function and repair. N Engl J Med 302:261–271
50. Magnusson K, Wahren J, Ekman L (1990) Protein synthesis in skeletal muscle during starvation and refeeding: Comparison of data from intact muscle and muscle biopsy material. Metabolism 39:1113–1117
51. Amundsen LR, Graves JM (1991) Testing knee extensor muscles of survivors of poliomyelitis. J Hum Muscle Performance 1:25–34
52. Berkelhammer CH, Leiter LA, Jeejeebhoy KN (1985) Skeletal muscle function in chronic renal failure: An index of nutritional status. Am J Clin Nutr 42:845–854
53. Bruce SA, Newton D, Woledge RC (1989) Effect of subnutrition on normalized muscle force and relaxation rate in human subjects using voluntary contractions. Clin Sciences 76:637–641
54. Lennmarken C, Sandstedt S, Schenck HV, Larsson J (1986) The effect of starvation on skeletal muscle function in man. Clin Nutr 5:99–103
55. Lennmarken C, Rutberg H, Jorfeldt L, Larsson J (1990) Effect of starvation on work capacity and voluntary skeletal muscle function in man. Clin Nutr 9:231–233
56. Tani H, Itoh H, Nagasaki H (1992) Dynamic properties of the knee extensor muscles in young and elderly subjects. J Hum Muscle Performance 1:41–50
57. Kalfarentzos F, Spiliotis J, Velimezis G, Dougenis D, Androulakis J (1989) Comparison of forearm muscle dynamometry with nutritional prognostic index, as a preoperative indicator in cancer patients. JPEN 13:34–36
58. Fong Y, Hesse DG, Tracey KJ, et al (1988) Submaximal exercise during intravenous hyperalimentation of depleted subjects. Ann Surg 207:297–304
59. Zeiderman MR, McMahon MJ (1989) The role of objective measurement of skeletal muscle function in the pre-operative patient. Clin Nutr 8:161–166
60. Pichard C, Vaughan C, Struck RS, Armstrong RL, Jeejeebhoy KN (1988) The effect of dietary manipulations (fasting, hypocaloric feeding and subsequent refeeding) on rat muscle energetics as assessed by nuclear magnetic resonance spectroscopy. J Clin Invest 82:895–901

Estimation of Peroxidative Damage*

H. Esterbauer

Introduction

The last decade saw an ever growing interest in deleterious effects of increased lipid peroxidation promoted by oxygen radicals. Most membrane systems in mammalian cells are rich in polyunsaturated fatty acids (PUFA) highly susceptible to oxidative stress. Oxidative stress was defined as a disturbance in the prooxidant-antioxidant balance in favor of the former [1]. Oxidative stress is not a rare event, but indeed part of our daily life. The adult human with an energy requirement of 10000 kJ per day consumes about 660 g of oxygen each day. It is estimated that approximately 90 to 95% of that oxygen is converted by mitochondrial respiration to harmless water ($O_2 + 4$ electrons $+ 4H^+ \rightarrow 2H_2O$), whereas the remaining 5 to 10% of oxygen undergo univalent and divalent reduction, yielding reactive oxygen species, such as superoxide radicals ($O_2 + 1$ electron $\rightarrow O_2^-$), hydrogen peroxide ($O_2 + 2$ electrons $+ 2H^+ \rightarrow H_2O_2$), and hydroxyl radicals ($H_2O_2 + 1$ electron $\rightarrow OH^{\cdot} + OH^-$). Extrapolated to the entire life span of about 70 years, the human body consumes the huge amount of about 17 tons of oxygen and this results in the concomitant production of 0.8 to 1.7 tons of oxygen radicals [2]. As all other aerobic organisms, human beings have numerous detoxifying mechanisms to protect cells from toxic effects of oxygen radicals and lipid peroxidation. These include an array of protective enzymes (e.g. superoxide dismutase, catalase, glutathione peroxidase, glutathione reductase, glutathione transferase) as well as low molecular weight water and lipid soluble antioxidants such as ascorbate, glutathione, α-tocopherol and carotenoids. There is increasing, though by far not conclusive evidence [3–5] that in certain pathological conditions the protective systems may be overwhelmed, and that cell damage by oxygen radicals and lipid peroxidation plays a crucial and perhaps causative role in the pathogenesis of a number of chronic and acute diseases, such as cancer, inflammation, shock, liver injury, rheumatoid arthritis, aging and atherosclerosis. TF Slater [4], one of the most prominent pioneers in this field once wrote "It is one thing to be able to detect the presence of free radical intermediates and to demonstrate free radical disturbances in a wide range of tissue injury, but it is quite another thing to be able to show that these free radical disturbances have some primary importance".

* Dedicated to Prof. Dr. Erwin Schauenstein on the occasion of his 75th birthday.

The same is fully true for lipid peroxidation. It must frankly be admitted that hitherto the evidences in support of a pathogenic role of lipid peroxidation in human diseases are not at all hard facts, but rather indirect conclusions based mainly on biochemical and experimental animal studies. Perhaps the best developed hypothesis is, that the atherogenic potential of low density lipoproteins strongly increases, if it becomes modified by lipid peroxidation [6, 7]. It was convincingly shown that oxidized LDL is present in lesions, and that prevention of oxidation by oral supplementation with antioxidants can reduce formation of lesions in animals [8]. In this context, it seems worth to note that the major contributions to the LDL oxidation hypothesis came not from scientists working on free radicals and lipid peroxidation, but rather from groups specialized on atherosclerosis research. It is probably this type of interdisciplinary endeavor, with major focus on the disease itself, which could unravel the truth of the repeatedly postulated association between free radicals/lipid peroxidation and pathogenesis of diseases. Similarly, the development of good methods for measurement of peroxidative damage *ex vivo* or *in vivo* in humans requires close collaboration of analytical chemists, pathobiochemists, and clinicians.

Problems in Assessing Lipid Peroxidation Damage in vivo

One major handicap for pathobiochemists and clinicians is that most of the methods developed for measurement of lipid peroxidation damage *in vitro* are not applicable for the *ex vivo* or *in vivo* situation. With isolated tissues (e.g. hepatocytes, macrophages, endothelial cells) or cell fragments (e.g. microsomes), it is rather easy to show whether an exposure to an oxidative stress leads to lipid peroxidation or not. In such cases, lipid peroxidation can be measured by numerous analytical chemical methods (Table 1) including loss of polyunsaturated fatty acids, loss of antioxidants, oxygen consumption, increase of lipid hydroperoxides and conjugated dienes, increase of malonaldehyde and other aldehydes, increase of lipid hydroperoxides degradation products, formation of fluorescent lipids and proteins, evolution of hydrocarbon gases, measurement of low level chemiluminescence and detection of lipid radicals. *In vivo,* increased lipid peroxidation will always be restricted to a small percentage of the tissue and consequently changes of concentration of lipid peroxidation markers in the blood, if they occur at all, will be low. Moreover, many of the lipid peroxidation products are rapidly detoxified and/or metabolized, and therefore increased plasma levels exist often only for a short time period following an oxidative burst. The fact that tissue and body fluids from healthy subjects always contain a low basal level of lipid peroxides and other lipid oxidation products also causes severe limitations in the assessment of the diagnostic value of lipid peroxidation markers. Finally, a principal problem in determining lipid peroxidation products in biological samples is the possibility of peroxides being formed during sample work up by autoxidation of PUFA. Keeping all

Table 1. Methods for measurement of lipid peroxidation damage

Assay	Comments
1. TBARS	The test material (e.g. plasma) is reacted with TBA, free MDA and MDA-precursors form a chromogen which can be measured by the absorbance at 532 nm or fluorescence at 553 nm. The specificity is significantly increased if the TBA reaction mixture is separated by HPLC [11]. The latter method gives for normal plasma values of about 0.5–1.0 μM TBARS; a rapid, sensitive and reproducible assay; assay should be the first choice.
2. Pentane, ethane	Pentane and ethane formed by metal ion catalyzed oxidative degradation of omega-6 and omega-3 PUFA respectively are in part exhaled and can be analyzed by GC [13]. Severe disturbance can come from air pollutants and gut bacteria. Rigorous control are essential.
3. 4-Hydroxynonenal (HNE)	HNE is formed during oxidative degradation of omega-6 PUFA [12, 20]. HNE in plasma or other test material can be determined after appropriate derivation by HPLC, GC/MS or GC. Normal plasma levels are in the range of 0.3–0.8 μM. Analyses tedious.
4. Antibody techniques	Some lipid peroxidation products covalently bind to proteins, monoclonal and polyclonal antibodies specific for MDA and HNE epitopes allow detection of such modified proteins in plasma (ELISA) or cells (immunostaining) [14–18]. Will become a promising technique. Antibodies commercially not yet available.
5. Fatty acids	Loss of fatty acids by lipid peroxidation can be measured by GC, *in vivo* overall loss minimal.
6. Oxygen consumption	Lipid peroxidation consumes oxygen. Rate and extent of oxygen consumption can be measured by an oxygen electrode.
7. Lipid peroxides	The overall concentration of lipid peroxides can be measured by iodometric assays [21, 22] and by enzymatic assays with glutathione peroxidase. HPLC with post-column chemiluminescence detection allows determination peroxides in the different lipid classes [23, 24]. The level of phosphatidylcholine hydroperoxides in normal plasma is 0.01–0.5 μM. Sophisticated instrumentation necessary for HPLC, but very promising method.
8. Diene conjugation	Peroxidation of PUFA results in formation of lipid hydroperoxides with conjugated double bonds with absorbance at 234 nm. The increase of 234 nm absorbance is proportional to peroxides. Assay not sensitive enough for plasma, very frequently used now to monitor susceptibility of LDL to oxidation *in vitro* [7].

Assay	Comments
9. Fluorescence	MDA and other aldehydes (e.g. HNE) formed during lipid peroxidation react with amino groups to fluorescent products (fluorescence at 430–470 nm) [25]. These products are rather long lived and accumulate *in vivo* as lipofuscin. Low levels of such fluorescent products in plasma are difficult to measure because of interference with many other fluorescent compounds. One possibility is three dimensional fluorescence spectroscopy [26].
10. HETES and HODE	Hydroperoxy fatty acids present in oxidized material can be reduced to hydroxy fatty acids, i.e. hydroxyeicosatetraenoic acid and hydroxyoctadecadienoic acid [27]. Positional isomers of HETES and HODE can be measured by GC/MS. Often difficult to distinguish between lipoxygenase pathway and lipid peroxidation pathway.
11. Antioxidants	Lipid peroxidation is usually accompanied by a loss of lipid (vitamin E) and water soluble (ascorbate) antioxidants [7]. Sensitive and specific HPLC methods for measurement of plasma levels of vitamin E and ascorbic acids are available. Plasma antioxidant levels depend on diet, a decrease must not necessarily reflect oxidative stress or lipid peroxidation.
12. ESR	Electron spin resonance techniques can detect lipid peroxyl and lipid alkoxyl radicals [3]. Method not sensitive enough for *ex vivo* investigations. Spin traps increase sensitivity. Spin traps can, however, not be used in humans.
13. Chemiluminescence	Lipid peroxidation is frequently accompanied by light emission (low level chemiluminescence), light can be measured by luminometer or a conventional liquid scintillation counters. Method can be used for monitoring lipid peroxidation in whole organs [28].

The author considers method 1 to 4 as most promising for assessment of in vivo peroxidative damage. For additional information and references see review by Gutteridge and Halliwell [5].

this in mind, only a few methods remain useful in studies in human patients (Table 1).

The favorite assay is the measurement of malonaldehyde by the classical thiobarbituric acid (TBA) test [9, 10]. The specificity of the test can be significantly improved if combined with HPLC [11]. A number of methods are now available for measuring 4-hydroxynonenal and other aldehydic lipid peroxidation products, because these assays are more specific than the TBA test, they gain increasing importance [12]. Measurement of pentane and ethane in the exhaled air by gas-chromatography is the only available noninvasive method [13]. Some authors report that this technique works well, while other criticize it as unspecific and irreproducible. Several laboratories presently develop imunological assays (ELISAs, RIA) for determining proteins modified by lipid peroxidation products [14–18] or autoantibodies against oxidatively modified proteins [19]. It can be expected that such assays will soon gain diagnostic importance.

TBARS as an Index of Lipid Peroxidation

Peroxidation of PUFA with more than two methylene interrupted double bonds (e.g. arachidonic acid, docosahexaenoic acid) results in formation of free malonaldehyde and several other products (e.g. hydroperoxy epidioxides), which can break down under thermal and acid catalyzed conditions to free malonaldehyde. Numerous assays were developed to quantify free malonaldehyde and malonaldehyde precursors as marker for lipid peroxidation [9, 12]. Among all, the most common method is the TBA test, first introduced by food chemists to measure rancidity of fats. In this assay, the test material is heated under acidic conditions with TBA [9, 10, 20]. Preformed malonaldehyde and malonaldehyde generated from precursors during the assay react with TBA to a defined chromogenic condensation product (MDA-TBA adduct) consisting of two molecules TBA and one molecule MDA. The unusual high absorption of the MDA-TBA adduct (molar absorption of 153000 at 532 nm) and its strong fluorescence at 553 nm makes the TBA assay extremely sensitive. One disadvantage is that a number of substances not related to lipid peroxidation can react with TBA to chromogens with absorbency around 530–535 nm; and it is this possibility of interferences which have caused severe doubts on the validity of this TBA test. Nevertheless, the TBA test is the favorite assay for most lipid peroxidation studies including relevant clinical investigations. Moreover, perhaps all important discoveries on pathological consequences of increased lipid peroxidation were made using the TBA test. In our opinion, the problem is not the test itself, but rather the numerous variations of the TBA assay, differing in sample pretreatment, acid concentration and type of acid, heating time and temperature, absence or presence of antioxidants, and/or catalytically active ferrous ions [12, 20]. Clearly, one cannot expect that tests, which are not standardized, yield comparable results. The only consensus reached so far regards terminology, that is to use the phrase TBARS (TBA reactive substances) instead of MDA. Since calibration of the TBA test is done with authentic MDA standards, concentration of TBARS are numerically equivalent to MDA concentrations.

Table 2 gives a survey of TBARS values, which were reported to be present in human plasma. It is evident that the values show, depending on the method of determination, an extreme wide variation from 0.0 to 47 nmol TBARS/mL plasma. The highest values were found in assays, where the whole plasma was boiled in a strong acidic TBA reagent and only the developed 532 nm absorbency was measured. It is reasonable to assume that under such drastic conditions most of the TBARS are artefactually formed during the assay itself.

Table 2. TBARS reported for normal human plasma. The values are means given in nmol MDA equivalent/mL plasma

Authors	TBARS	Reaction conditions
Largilliere et al. 1988 [29]	0.00	Deproteinized plasma was separated by HPLC and peak absorbance measured at 267 nm
Lee 1988 [30]	0.32	Plasma was reacted with TBA for 90 min at 60°C
Wong et al. 1987 [11]	0.60	Total plasma was reacted with phosphoric acid/TBA for 60 min at 100°C and determined by HPLC
Rabl et al. 1992 [31]	0.70	Total plasma was reacted with phosphoric acid /TBA for 60 min at 100°C and determined by HPLC
Suematsu et al. 1977 [32]	0.90	Phosphotungstic acid precipitate of serum was reacted with TBA/acetic acid for 60 min at 95°C
Ledwozyw et al. 1986 [33]	0.94	Plasma was reacted with TBA/HCL/TCA for 30 min at 100°C
Maseki et al. 1981 [34]	3.30	Phosphotungstic acid precipitate of serum was reacted with TBA/acetic acid for 60 min at 95°C
Satoh 1978 [35]	3.40	TCA precipitate of serum was reacted with TBA/ Na_2SO_4 for 30 min at 100°C
Yasaka et al. 1981 [36]	3.74	Phosphotungstic acid precipitate of serum was reacted with TBA/acetic acid for 60 min at 95°C
Hunter et al. 1986 [37]	3.80	TCA precipitate of plasma was reacted with TBA/Na_2SO_4 for 30 min at 100°C
Nishigaki et al. 1981 [38]	3.92	Phosphotungstic acid precipitate of serum was reacted with TBA/acetic acid for 60 min at 95°C
Santos et al. 1980 [39]	35.10	Plasma was reacted with TBA/HCL/TCA for 30 min at 100°C
Aznar et al. 1983 [40]	47.20	Plasma was reacted with TBA/HCL/TCA for 30 min at 100°C

In our opinion, one of the most reliable TBA assay is the one developed by Wong et al. [11]. In this assay, the whole TBA reaction mixture is separated by HPLC and the peak of the MDA-TBA adduct is quantified. This minimizes interferences with other compounds and therefore significantly increases the specificity. Wong et al. [11] found with this assay in human plasma 0.60 ± 0.13 nmol TBARS/mL ($n=41$). Using exactly the same protocol, we found [31] in healthy controls 0.70 ± 0.21 nmol TBARS/mL plasma (range 0.385 to 1.291 nmol/mL). The assay is easy to perform and exhibits an excellent reproducibility, and can be considered as a useful clinical chemical test for assessment, whether a certain pathological condition has led to an increase of plasma peroxides above the baseline level. Using this test, Rabl et al. [31] were able to demonstrate in human patients that plasma TBARS show a strong transient increase about 1 h after onset of reperfusion. In patients (n=9) receiving kidney allograft, plasma TBARS were 1 h after onset of reperfusion 2 fold above baseline. Figure 1 shows as example the plasma TBARS profile in 4 patients receiving kidney allograft. In patients (n=28) undergoing limb operation, plasma TBARS were 1 h after reperfusion 1.5 fold above baseline. Two hours after onset of reperfusion TBARS decreased in both groups of patients close to the preoperative level. These findings are in support of the assumption that oxygen radicals and lipid peroxidation mediated reperfusion injury occurs in a narrow time window within the earliest time after successful revascularization. Intravenous infusion of an antioxidant mix before onset of reperfusion prevented increase of TBARS [41].

Determination of HNE and other Aldehydes

Degradation of lipid hydroperoxides by β-cleavage reactions results in the formation of a great variety of aldehydes including alkanals, 2-alkenals, 2.4-

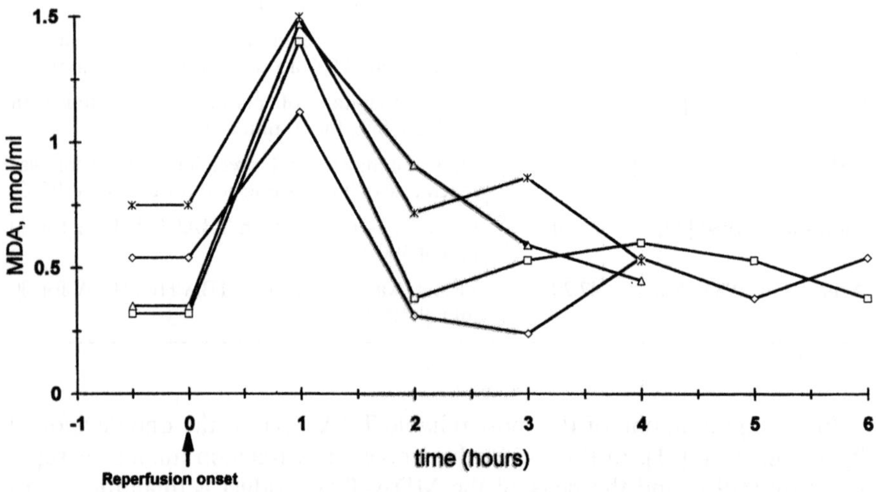

Fig. 1. Time profile of the change of plasma TBARS in four patients receiving kidney allograft. (From [31] with permission.)
A volume of 50 μL EDTA plasma obtained at the indicated time points before and after onset of reperfusion was mixed with 0.75 mL 0.44 M H_3PO_4, 0.25 mL aqueous 42 mM TBA and 0.45 mL H_2O (final volume 1.5 mL). The mixture was heated in a boiling waterbath for 60 min. After cooling, 1.5 mL alkaline methanol (50 mL methanol + 4.5 mL 1 N NaOH) was added. A volume of 20 μL of the neutralized mixture was then separated by HPLC on a RP-18 column with a mixture of 50 mM phosphate buffer pH 6.9 (600 mL) and methanol (450 mL). Detection was done fluorimetrically at 550 nm with 525 nm excitation. The detection limit for the assay was 0.3 picomol per 20 μL sample injected into the HPLC. This corresponds to 0.05 nmol TBARS/mL plasma

alkadienals and 4-hydroxyalkenals [12, 20]. In many instances, the major individual aldehydes are hexanal and 4-hydroxynonenal (HNE) produced by oxidation of omega-6 fatty acids. Aldehydes, in particular 4-hydroxynonenal possess cytotoxic, hepatotoxic, mutagenic and genotoxic properties, and it has been suggested that they act as a kind of "second toxic messengers" of oxygen radicals and lipid peroxidation [12]. The measurement of these compounds gains therefore increasing acceptance (Table 3), both as an index of the extent of lipid peroxidation and as an aid to elucidate the role of aldehydes as causative agents in certain pathological conditions [20]. The reported [20, 47, 49] values for HNE in plasma of healthy human subjects are in the range of about 0.08 to 0.70 nmol/mL. The carriers of HNE in plasma are most likely lipoproteins. Several experimental animal studies indicate that HNE levels significantly increase under conditions of oxidative stress or vitamin E deficiency [12]. For example, in dogs a 50 fold increase (<1 vs 45 nmol/mL) of plasma HNE was found after reperfusion following hypervolemic traumatic shock [50]. Many methods are now available to determine HNE in plasma (Table 3). Perhaps the most reliable and reproducible one is

Table 3. Methods for determination of HNE and other aldehydes in peroxidized biological samples

Authors	Derivatization reagent/ separation	Comments
Esterbauer et al. 1990 [20]	dinitrophenylhydrazine/HPLC	very frequently used, suited for HNE and other aldehydes, tedious, human plasma gives 0.28 ± 0.34 nmol HNE/mL [12]
Tomita et al. 1987 [42]	1,3-cyclohexanedione/HPLC	suited for HNE and other aldehydes, simple, rigorous controls necessary
Lang et al. 1985 [43]	Silylation/GC	suited only for HNE concentration above 10 μM
Tamura et al 1991 [44]	N-methylhydrazine + silylation/GC-MS	used for HNE and MDA
Oarada et al. 1986 [45]	N-dimethylhydrazine + silylation/GC-MS	used for HNE in oils
Van Kuijk et al. 1990 [46]	pentafluorobenzyloxime + silylation/GC-MS	very frequently used for HNE, human plasma contains 0.68 ± 0.41 nmol HNE/mL [47]
Norsten-Höög et al. 1990 [48]	hydroxylamine + silylation/GC-MS	used for HNE and other aldehydes
Kinter et al. 1992 [49]	hydroxylamine + silylation/GC-MS	perhaps the best method for HNE in plasma, 3-hydroxynonenal as internal standard, in reference serum 0.082 nmol/mL

that recently reported by Kinter et al. [49]. The advantage of this method is that it includes internal standardization with 3-hydroxynonenal.

Immunological Assays

An important development which will gain increasing attention in the future is the application of antisera and monoclonal antibodies recognizing proteins modified by lipid peroxidation products. Using such antibodies, it was recently shown with immunostaining that HNE- and MDA-conjugated proteins are present in atherosclerotic lesions of rabbits and humans [14, 17, 18] and that autoantibodies against such aldehyde-modified proteins occur in human plasma [19]. This is the first clear evidence that proteins modified by lipid peroxidation products do in fact occur *in vivo* and probably play a role in the pathogenesis of a human disease. Antibodies were also successfully used for immunocytochemical demonstration of HNE and MDA-modified proteins in fibroblasts in which lipid peroxidation was initiated by ascorbate/iron [16]. These highly sensitive and specific immunological techniques are very promising tools which will allow researchers in the future to study lipid peroxidation at the cellular level. Moreover, it should not be too difficult to develop ELISAs for routine quantification of proteins modified by HNE, MDA or other lipid peroxidation products in cells, tissue and human plasma.

Conclusion

Numerous methods have been developed to measure lipid peroxidation products and lipid peroxidation damage in tissue, cells and body fluids. The choice of which method is most appropriate depends on the specific interest of the investigator. In the routine clinical praxis, the determination of TBARS in serum or plasma by HPLC under strictly standardized conditions should be the first choice. If levels of TBARS are increased, other more sophisticated assays (e.g. exhaled pentane, ethane, levels of plasma antioxidants, fluorescent plasma proteins and lipids) should be included for verification. A very promising development are immunological assays, based on detection of peroxidatively damaged proteins in plasma by the ELISA technique.

Acknowledgements. The authors work has been supported by the Association for International Cancer Research (AICR) and by the Jubiläumsfonds der Österreichischen Nationalbank.

References

1. Sies H (ed) (1991) Oxidative stress: Oxidants and antioxidants. Academic Press, London
2. Esterbauer H (1993) Cytotoxicity and genotoxicity of lipid oxidation products. Am J Clin Nutr (in press)
3. Halliwell B, Gutteridge JMC (eds) (1989) Free radicals in biology and medicine, 2nd edn. Clarendon Press, Oxford
4. Slater TF (1987) Free radicals and tissue injury: Fact and fiction. Br J Cancer 55 (Suppl):5–10
5. Gutteridge JMC, Halliwell B (1990) The measurement and mechanism of lipid peroxidation in biological systems. Trends in Biochem Science 15:129–135
6. Steinberg D, Parthasarathy S, Carew TE, Khoo JC, Witztum JL (1989) Beyond cholesterol. Modifications of low-density lipoprotein that increases its atherogenicity. N Eng J Med 320:915–924
7. Esterbauer H, Gebicki J, Puhl H, Jürgens G (1992) The role of lipid peroxidation and antioxidants in oxidative modification of LDL. Free Rad Biol Med 13:341–390
8. Steinberg D, Berliner JA, Burton GW, et al (1992) Antioxidants in the prevention of human atherosclerosis. Circulation 85:2338–2344
9. Janero DR (1990) Malondialdehyde and thiobarbituric acid-reactivity as diagnostic indices of lipid peroxidation and peroxidative tissue injury. Free Rad Biol Med 9:515–540
10. Draper HH, Hadley M (1990) Malondialdehyde determination as index of lipid peroxidation. Meth Enzymol 186:421–431
11. Wong SHY, Knight JA, Hopfer SM, Zaharia O, Leach CN Jr, Sunderman FW (1987) Lipoperoxides in plasma as mesured by liquid-chromatographic separation of malondialdehyde-thiobarbituric acid adduct. Clin Chem 33:214–220
12. Esterbauer H, Schaur RJ, Zollner H (1991) Chemistry and biochemistry of 4-hydroxynonenal, malonaldehyde and related aldehydes. Free Rad Biol Med 11:81–128
13. Jeejeebhoy KN (1991) In vivo breath alkane as an index of lipid peroxidation. Free Rad Biol Med 10:191–193
14. Haberland ME, Fong D, Cheng L (1988) Malondialdehyde-altered protein occurs in atheroma of Watanabe heritable hyperlipidemic rabbits. Science 241:215–218
15. Kergonou JF, Pennacino I, Lafite C, Ducousso R (1988) Immunological relevance of malonic dialdehyde (MDA): III. Immunoenzymatic determination of human immunoglobulin binding to MDA-cross-linked proteins. Biochem Internat 16:845–852
16. Chojier M. Houglum K, Solis-Herruzo J, Brenner DA (1989) Stimulation of collagen gene expression by ascorbic acid in cultured human fibroblasts – A role for lipid peroxidation? J Biol Chem 264:16957–16962
17. Palinski W, Ylä-Herttuala S, Rosenfeld ME, et al (1990) Antisera and monoclonal antibodies specific for epitopes generated during oxidative modification of low density lipoprotein. Arteriosclerosis 10:325–335
18. Chen Q, Esterbauer H, Jürgens G (1992) Studies on epitopes on low-density lipoprotein modified by 4-hydroxynonenal. Biochem J 288:2249–2254
19. Salonen JT, Ylä-Herttuala S, Yamamoto R, et al (1992) Autoantibody against oxidized LDL and progession of carotid atherosclerosis. Lancet 339:883–887
20. Esterbauer H, Cheeseman KH (1990) Determination of aldehydic lipid peroxidation products: Malonaldehyde and 4-hydroxynonenal. Meth Enzymol 186:407–421
21. El-Saadani M, Esterbauer H, El-Sayed M, Goher M, Nasser AY, Jürgens G (1989) A spectrophotometric assay for lipid peroxides in serum lipoproteins using a commercially available reagent. J Lipid Res 30:627–630
22. Cramer GL, Miller JF, Pendleton RB, Lands WEM (1991) Iodometric measurement of lipid hydroperoxides in human plasma. Anal Biochem 193:204–211
23. Miyazawa T (1989) Determination of phospholipid hydroperoxides in human blood plasma by a chemiluminescence-HPLC assay. Free Rad Biol Med 7:209–217

24. Yamamoto Y, Ames BN (1987) Detection of lipid hydroperoxides and hydrogen peroxide at picomole levels by an HPLC and isoluminol chemiluminescence assay. Free Rad Biol Med 3:359–361
25. Kikugawa K, Beppu M (1987) Involvement of lipid oxidation products in the formation of fluorescent and cross-linked proteins. Chem Phys Lipids 44:277–296
26. Koller E, Quehenberger O, Jürgens G, Wolfbeis OS, Esterbauer H (1986) Investigation of human plasma low density lipoprotein by three-dimensional fluorescence spectroscopy. FEBS (Lett) 198:229–234
27. Van Kuijk FJGM, Thomas DW, Stephens RJ, Dratz EA (1990) Gas chromatography-mass spectrometry assays for lipid peroxides. Meth Enzymol 186:388–398
28. Cadenas E, Sies H (1984) Low-level chemiluminescence as an indicator of singlet molecular oxygen in biological systems. Meth Enzymol 105:221–231
29. Largilliere C, Melancon SB (1988) Free malondialdehyde determination in human-plasma by high-performance liquid-chromatography. Anal Biochem 170:123–126
30. Lee DM (1980) Malondialdehyde formation in stored plasma. Biochem Biophys Res Commun 95:1633–1672
31. Rabl H, Khoschsorur G, Colombo T, Tatzber F, Esterbauer H (1992) Human plasma lipid peroxide levels show a strong transient increase after successful revascularization operation. Free Rad Biol Med 13:281–288
32. Suematsu T, Kamada T, Abe H, Kikuchi S, Yagi K (1977) Serum lipoperoxide level in patients suffering from liver diseases. Clin Chim Acta 79:267–270
33. Ledwozyw A, Michalak J, Stepien A, Kadziolka A (1986) The relationship between plasma trilycerides, cholesterol, total lipid and lipid peroxidation products during human atherosclerosis. Clin Chim Acta 155:275–284
34. Maseki M, Nishigaki I, Hagihara M. Tomoda Y, Yagi K (1981) Lipid peroxide levels and lipid content of serum lipoprotein fractions of pregnant subjects with or without pre-eclampsia. Clin Chim Acta 115:155–161
35. Satoh K (1978) Serum lipid peroxide in cerebrovascular disorders determined by a new colorimetric method. Clin Chim Acta 90:37–43
36. Yasaka T, Ohya I, Matsumoto J, Shiramizu T, Sasaguri Y (1981) Acceleration of lipid peroxidation in human paraquat poisoning. Arch Intern Med 141:1169–1173
37. Hunter MIS, Mohamed JB (1986) Plasma antioxidants and lipid peroxidation products in Duchenne muscular dystrophy. Clin Chim Acta 155:123–132
38. Nishigaki I, Hagihara M, Tsunekawa H, Maseki M, Yagi K (1981) Lipid peroxide levels of serum lipoprotein fractions of diabetic patients. Biochem Med 25:373–378
39. Santos MT, Valles J, Aznar J, Vilches J (1980) Determination of plasma malondialdehyde-like material and its clinical application in stroke patients. J Clin Pathol 33:973–976
40. Aznar J, Santos MT, Valles J, Sala J (1983) Serum malondialdehyde-like material (MDA-LM) in acute myocardial infarction. J Clin Pathol 36:712–715
41. Rabl H, Khoschsorur G. Colombo T, et al (1993) A multivitamin infusion prevents lipid peroxidation and improves performance of transplanted kidneys in humans. Kidney Internat (in press)
42. Tomita I, Yoshino K, Sano M (1987) Formation of aliphatic aldehydes in the plasma and liver of vitamin E deficient rats. In: Hayaishi O, Mino M (eds) Clinical and nutritional aspects of vitamin E. Elsevier Science Publ, Amsterdam, pp 277–280
43. Lang J, Celotto C, Esterbauer H (1985) Quantitative determination of the lipid peroxidation product 4-hydroxynonenal by high-performance liquid chromatography. Anal Biochem 150:369–378
44. Tamura H, Shibamoto T (1991) Gas chromatographic analysis of malonaldehyde and 4-hydroxy-2-(E)-nonenal produced from arachidonic acid and linoleic acid in a lipid peroxidation model system. Lipids 26:170–173
45. Oarada M, Miyazawa T, Kaneda T (1986) Distribution of 14-C after oral administration of (U-14-C) labelled methyl linoleate hydroperoxides and their secondary oxidation products in rats. Lipids 21:150–154
46. Van Kuijk FJGM, Thomas DW, Stephens RJ, Dratz EA (1990) Gas chromatography-mass spectrometry of 4-hydroxy-nonenal in tissues. Meth Enzymol 186:399–406

47. Selley ML, Bartlett MR, McGuiness JA, Hapel A, Ardlie NG, Lacey MJ (1989) Determination of the lipid peroxidation product trans-4-hydroxy-2-nonenal in biological samples by high performance liquid chromatography and combined capillary gas chromatography/negative ion chemical ionization mass spectrometry. J Chromatography 488:329–340
48. Norsten-Höög C, Cronholm T (1990) Analysis of aldehydic lipid peroxidation products in rat liver and hepatocytes by gas chromatography and mass spectrometry of the oxime-t-butyl-dimethylsilyl derivatives. Anal Biochem 189:131–137
49. Kinter M, Sullivan S, Roberts RJ, Spitz D (1992) Trace quantitation of 4-hydroxy-2-nonenal in biological samples as its oxime-bis-tert-butyldimethylsilyl derivative using 3-hydroxynonenal as an internal standard. J Chromatography 578:9–16
50. Lieners C, Redl H, Molnar H, Fürst W, Hallström S, Schlag G (1989) Lipid peroxidation in a canine model of hypovolemic-traumatic shock. Progr Clin Biol Res 308:345–350

What Type of Metabolic Support?

Does Indirect Calorimetry Reflect Energy Expenditure in the Critically Ill Patient?

R. L. Chioléro, D. Bracco, and J. P. Revelly

Introduction

Energy processes intimately linked to life in all its manifestations. They are essential to perform such diverse functions as to adapt to changes in the environment, to grow, to move and to reproduce. This is also true in healthy humans and during acute illness, where reduced energy production may be related to the fatal autcome.

The discovery of "oxygène" during the 18th century as an elementary gas which generates carbonic gas and heat during combustion of organic substances, produced the physical basis for the development of the science of calorimetry. The theory of combustion coupled to metabolism was developed by Lavoisier who showed that *in vitro* (fire) and *in vivo* combustion (life) produced the same amount of heat per quantum of O_2 consumed and CO_2 produced [1]. He developed a direct ice calorimeter which enabled him to measure heat losses in small animals.

In most conditions, energy production is directly dependent on cellular oxidative processes. Energy expenditure (EE) and oxygen consumption ($\dot{V}O_2$) are therefore closely correlated physiologic parameters. In critically ill patients under various conditions, it has been repeatedly shown that decreased $\dot{V}O_2$ is associated with increased mortality, particularly in those with low cardiac output syndromes [2, 3]. Recent studies have given evidence that among acutely ill traumatized or septic subjects, those with supra-normal O_2 delivery and O_2 consumption had higher survival rate [4–6], although this point is yet controversial. EE is therefore an essential physiological parameter, which can be assessed at the bedside in the acutely ill patient, during various clinical conditions including mechanical ventilation.

In this chapter, we shall review the most relevant physiological aspects of EE, the methods of measurements as well as the pitfalls in the field of intensive medicine. The interrested reader, searching extensive technical information on the practice of indirect calorimetry is referred to a recent publication [7].

Energy Expenditure: Physiological Aspects

Enery is utilized in the cells to perform electrochemical, mechanical and synthetic work. In mammals, energy is released mainly from substrate oxidation. This process is coupled to high energy molecules synthesis (mostly ATP), while the cellular consuming energy reactions are coupled to ATP hydrolysis. All the chemical reactions release heat, which is therefore the end-product of energy utilization by the cells in resting condition. This is not true during exercise, where a part of energy is transformed into external work.

The fate of nutrients as energy source in the body is illustrated in Fig. 1. The energy content of nutrients is called gross energy and corresponds to their heat of combustion in a bomb calorimeter. Only a small part of energy ingested is lost in faeces and urine (mostly proteins end-products). Metabolizable energy, defined as gross energy minus the faecal and urinary losses, is that available to tissues during energy metabolism. *In vivo*, energy is gradually released along the chain of oxidative pathway of metabolism. At each step, a significant part of energy is transformed into heat. For example, during aerobic work, it has been calculated that 27% of metabolizable energy is transformed into mechanical work, while 73% of energy is released as heat. During ATP synthesis, 65% of energy is transferred to ATP, while 35% is released as heat. During the conversion of ATP energy to mechanical work, 40% of energy is transformed into mechanical work, while a further 60% is released as heat. The overall efficiency of aerobic was therefore calculated to be 27% (i.e. 65% × 40% = 27%) [8, 9]. This example illustrates clearly the relationship between energy production and heat generation during the oxidative processes.

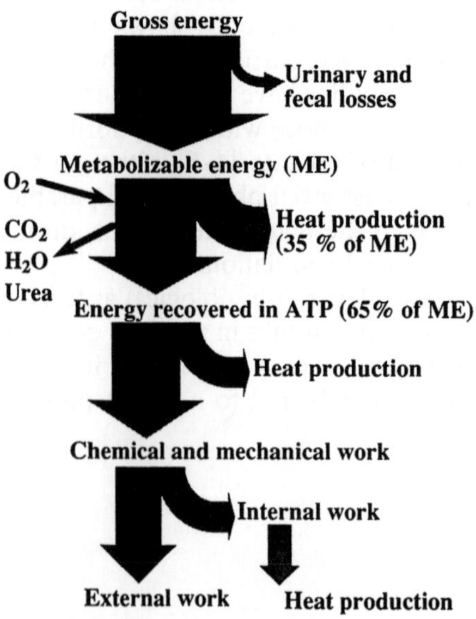

Fig. 1. Fate of energy during aerobic work. Except for urinary and fecal losses, all the energy is transformed into heat and external work. Measurement of O_2 consumption, CO_2 production and urinary N excretion represents the basis of indirect calorimetry. Direct measurement of heat losses represents the basis of direct calorimetry (From [9] with permission)

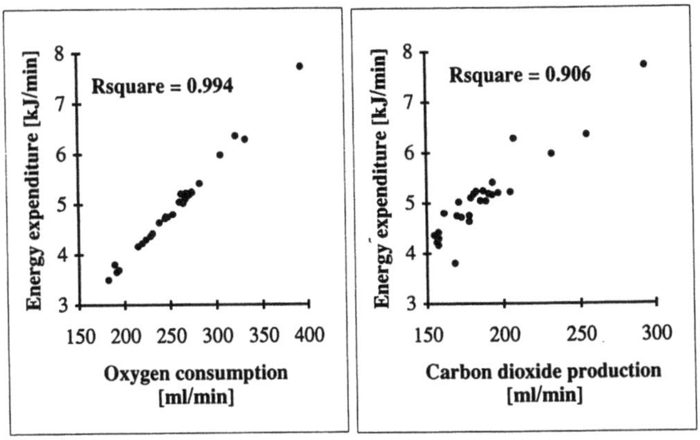

Fig. 2. Correlation between oxygen consumption, carbon dioxide production and energy expenditure in 10 postoperative cardiac surgery patients

Since energy is derived mainly from substrate oxidation, $\dot{V}O_2$ and EE are closely correlated. This is illustrated in Fig. 2, showing the relationship between resting EE and $\dot{V}O_2$ in cardiac surgery patients during the first postoperative hours. This relationship is usually expressed as the caloric equivalent of O_2, which corresponds to the number or Kcal (or KJ) released for each litre of O_2 consumed. The caloric equivalent of O_2 is influenced, although not much, by the type of substrate oxidized. It amounts to 4.69 kcal/L O_2 (STPD) during fat oxidation, 5.05 kcal/L O_2 during glucose, and 4.46 kcal/L O_2 for protein oxidation (Table 1). By contrast the energy released by gram of substrate oxidized is strongly influenced by the type of substrate.

Table 1. Oxygen and carbon dioxide equivalents of some foods and nutritional solutions. (From [24] with permission.)

Nutrients	Energy equivalent kJ/g	kcal/g	O_2 Equiv. kJ/l	CO_2 Equiv. kJ/l	RQ
Average carbohydrates	**17.5**	**4.18**	**21.12**	**21.12**	**1.00**
Glucose	15.56	3.719	20.84	20.84	1.00
Glycerol	18.00	4.305	21.16	21.16	1.00
Average lipids	**39.5**	**9.44**	**19.60**	**27.61**	**0.71**
Average parenteral lipids	37.1	8.87	19.62	27.13	0.723
Medium chain triglycerides	34.9	8.339	19.63	26.63	0.737
Human milk	39.32	9.398	19.58	27.58	0.710
Average proteins	**19.68**	**4.704**	**19.48**	**23.33**	**0.835**
Average TPN amino acid mixture	19.62	4.701	19.52	23.41	0.834
BCAA enriched aa mixture	25.98	6.209	19.57	26.52	0.738
Ethanol	29.67	7.091	20.33	30.50	0.67

The correlation between $\dot{V}CO_2$ and EE is weaker, since CO_2 production is markedly influenced by the type of nutrients oxidized (Fig. 2) [10–14]. The ratio of $\dot{V}CO_2$ to $\dot{V}O_2$ is defined as the respiratory quotient (RQ). In steady state condition, it is related to the nutrients that are oxidized by the body. The simultaneous measurement of $\dot{V}O_2$, $\dot{V}CO_2$ and urinary nitrogen excretion (Nu) allows to calculate the overall rate of oxidation of protein, carbohydrate and lipid of the body.

Methods to Assess Energy Expenditure

Assessment of energy production are based on calorimetric methods, i.e. aiming to quantify body heat production, or on methods based on other principles, i.e. the non-calorimetric methods.

Some of non-calorimetric methods rely on the relationship between EE and various physiological parameters, within an individual, such as heart rate [15], minute ventilation [16, 17] or electromyography [18]. Similar approaches have tried to correlate EE with indexes of physical activity (i.e. pedometer or accelorometer [19]). Other methods use isotopic tracers to assess EE, such as the doubly labelled water ($^2H_2{}^{18}O$) [20, 21], in which the rate of CO_2 production is determined from the difference in the turnover of deuterium and ^{18}O. It is doubtful that these methods will find a place in the intensive care unit, since they only measure $\dot{V}CO_2$ and do not allow to measure accurately EE at a given moment, but only to assess its changes over prolonged periods (i.e. days or weeks).

The calorimetric methods are presently the most accurate to asses EE. They include the direct and indirect calorimetry. In the former, the heat released by the body is directly measured, whereas in the latter the heat produced by the oxidative processes is calculated from $\dot{V}O_2$, $\dot{V}CO_2$ and urinary N excretion (Fig. 1) [10, 12].

The principle of direct calorimetry is simple, but the applicability of this method is difficult, since it implies to put the whole body in a tiny chamber or a suit [22]. It is therefore not usable at the bedside and obviously not practicable for acutely ill patients.

Indirect calorimetry relies on the principle that the heat released by the oxidative processes can be calculated from $\dot{V}O_2$, knowing the caloric equivalent of the O_2 consumed (Fig. 1 and Table 1). However, since the caloric equivalent of O_2 is influenced by the type of substrate oxidized, it is necessary to determine the proportion of the various substrates that are oxidized. This can be calculated from CO_2 production and urinary nitrogen excretion, simultaneously measured. When applying this principle, the energy produced by substrate or nutrient oxidation in the body is theoretically equal to the heat released by direct combustion in a bomb calorimeter. This is true for carbohydrate and lipid oxidation, which leave CO_2 and H_2O as end-products in addition to heat. This is not true for proteins, since urea and ammonia, the main end-products of protein oxidation are not totally oxidized and the energy released in the body is therefore lower than that produced in a bomb calorimeter. The caloric value of nitrogen by-products excreted in urine is equivalent in humans to 34.9 kJ/g (8.34 kcal/g) nitrogen oxidized or 5.61 kJ/g (1.34 kcal/g) protein oxidized.

Different physiological information are obtained by direct and indirect calorimetry. Any significant change in the rate or in the proportion of substrate oxidized will rapidly influence gas exchange and indirect calorimetry data, which therefore is appropriate to assess energy production in unstable conditions, such as exercise and critical illness. By contrast, the change in heat released is delayed. When heat production increases markedly, as during many infectious processes, a part of heat is stored in the body, producing a rise in body temperature. In such condition, the heat measured by direct calorimetry (i.e. the heat dissipated) will underestimate the heat truly produced by the tissues and therefore the energy expended.

In steady resting conditions, with no change of body heat content, similar EE values are found by direct and indirect calorimetry. This is illustrated in Fig. 3 showing the relation between EE assessed by both direct (H) and indirect (M) calorimetry in healthy women [23].

Indirect Calorimetry Technique: Energy Expenditure

As previously stated, the indirect calorimetry method calculates the metabolic rate from $\dot{V}O_2$, $\dot{V}CO_2$ and urinary nitrogen excretion, using one of the available equations. In our institution we use the following equation to calculate energy expenditure [24]:

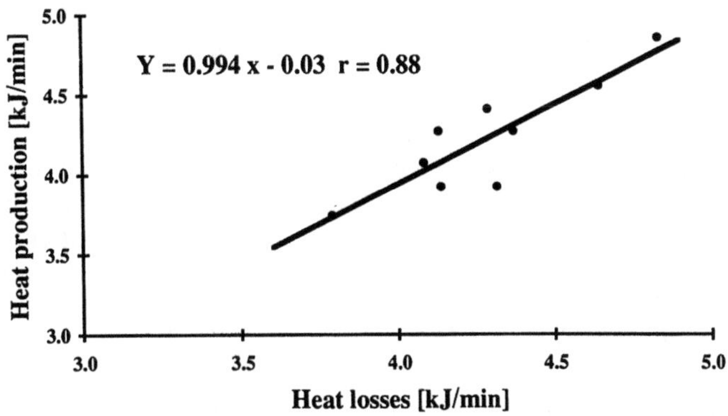

Fig. 3. Correlation between the energy dissipated (direct calorimetry) and energy produced (indirect calorimetry) in 10 healthy women (From [23] with permission)

$$\begin{aligned} EE\,(KJ/min) &= 15.90 \times \dot{V}O_2\,(L/min) \\ &\quad + 5.23 \times \dot{V}CO_2\,(L/min) - 9.33\,Nu\,(g/min). \\ EE\,(Kcal/min) &= 3.799 \times \dot{V}O_2\,(L/min) \\ &\quad + 1.249 \times \dot{V}CO_2\,(L/min) - 2.23\,Nu\,(g/min). \end{aligned} \tag{1}$$

It should be mentionned that this equation is applicable when the patient oxidized only the 3 usual substrates (i.e. proteins, lipids and carbohydrates). In addition, the equation shows that $\dot{V}O_2$ is the most important determinant of EE, whereas, $\dot{V}CO_2$ contributes less in the calculation of metabolic rate. A 5% error on $\dot{V}O_2$ will induce a 3.5% error on EE, whereas, a similar error on $\dot{V}CO_2$ will produce a 3 times lower error. The importance of Nu on EE determination is even less significant, since a 100% error on Nu will produce a 1% change in EE, a negligible error [7]. In 180 critically ill patients, Bursztein et al [25] noticed that the median Nu value was 18.25 g/day. Using this value for Nu to compute EE, they found that the mean error on EE was 1.8%. In the critically ill, as well as during exercise in normal subjects, it is a common practice to determine metabolic rate from $\dot{V}O_2$ only, while ignoring $\dot{V}CO_2$. Since RQ usually ranges between 0.80 and 0.95 in many critically ill patients receiving isocaloric nutrition, it should be possible to calculate EE with an error around 10%. However, this assumption has yet not been validated in ICU patients.

Indirect calorimetry can theoretically be achieved by two different techniques: first, by applying the reverse Fick equation to the pulmonary circulation; second, by the gas exchange method.

The reverse Fick equation is often used in the ICU to determine $\dot{V}O_2$, since pulmonary catheters are commonly inserted for monitoring, but the calculation of EE is rarely done. It consists in calculating body $\dot{V}O_2$ from cardiac output and from arterial and mixed venous O_2 contents, according to the equation:

$$\dot{V}O_2\,(mL/min) = 10 \times CO\,(L/min) \times (CaO_2\,(mL/dL) - C\bar{v}O_2\,(mL/dL)), \tag{2}$$

where CO is cardiac output, CaO_2 and $C\bar{v}O_2$ are arterial and venous O_2 contents. Discrepant results have been published concerning the value of the Fick method to determine $\dot{V}O_2$. In many studies, the Fick and the gas exchange methods were compared in critically ill patients: in some studies a biais was observed [26–30], whereas this was not the case in others [29, 31, 32]. In all, the limits of agreements were wide. In a recent study performed in cardiac surgery patients, we found a good agreement between $\dot{V}O_2$ measured by the Fick and the gas exchange methods, provided iced injectate was avoided for thermodilution and a meticulous technique was used [29]. However, the precision of the Fick method was lower than that of the gas exchange method.

Since arterial and venous CO_2 content determinations are hardly performed in clinical conditions, the use of the Fick method is limited and does not allow to determine $\dot{V}CO_2$. In a recent study performed in mechanically ventilated patients, it was shown that $\dot{V}CO_2$ determined by the Fick equation had an exceedingly weak correlation with $\dot{V}CO_2$ assessed by the gas exchange method ($r^2=0.26$) [28]. It is therefore clear that EE determined by the Fick principle relies on $\dot{V}O_2$ measurement only, whose precision is not high by this method.

The gas exchange method is the only one providing accurate measurement of EE, that is easily applicable in ICU patients during various clinical conditions, including mechanical ventilation. The indirect calorimeter continuously measures O_2 and CO_2 concentrations in the respiratory gases, as well as their flow rates.

$\dot{V}CO_2$ is calculated according to the following equation:

$$\dot{V}CO_{2STPD} = V_E \times F_ECO_2 - V_I \times F_ICO_2 \tag{3}$$

where V_I and V_E are the inspiratory and expiratory minute ventilation, F_ECO_2 and F_ICO_2 are the inspired and expired CO_2 concentration. Since inspired CO_2 concentration is usually assumed to be negligible ($\approx 0.03\%$), the following equation can be derived:

$$\dot{V}CO_{2STPD} = V_E \times F_ECO_2 \tag{4}$$

$\dot{V}O_2$ is determined, using the same principle:

$$\dot{V}O_{2STPD} = V_I \times F_IO_2 - V_E \times F_EO_2 \tag{5}$$

Inspiratory and expiratory gas flows are not identical, due to the differences in body $\dot{V}O_2$ and $\dot{V}CO_2$. Since it is technically difficult to measure both inspiratory and expiratory gas flow rates, more complex equations have been developed, based on two assumptions: first, there is no net N_2 exchange in the lung under steady conditions, and second, the inspired and expired gases are composed of O_2, CO_2 and N_2 only.

$$V_{ISTPD} \times F_IN_2 = V_{ESTPD} \times F_EN_2 \tag{6}$$

This allows to measure expiratory flow rate only and to calculate inspiratory flow rate.

$$V_{ISTPD} = \frac{1 - F_EO_2 - F_ECO_2}{1 - F_IO_2} \times V_{ESTPD} \tag{7}$$

$$\dot{V}O_{2STPD} = V_{ESTPD} \times \left(\frac{F_IO_2 \times (1 - F_ECO_2) - F_EO_2}{1 - F_IO_2} \right) \tag{8}$$

while

$$RQ = \frac{\dot{V}CO_{2STPD}}{\dot{V}O_{2STPD}} = \frac{(1 - F_IO_2) \times F_ECO_2}{F_IO_2 \times (1 - F_ECO_2) - F_EO_2} \tag{9}$$

This system of equation was originally developed by Haldane in 1920. A typical example is developed in appendix 1. Particular equations, taking into account the inspired CO_2 fraction or anesthetic gases are shown in appendix 2.

The use of nitrogen as a tracer gas shows the limitation of the Haldane's correction when the inspiratory O_2 fraction increases: the estimation of V_I is based on the expired/inspired nitrogen ratio. As nitrogen fractions are reduced, the precision of their ratio decreases. When there is no nitrogen (i.e. $F_IO_2 = 1.0$) in the respiratory gases, the calculation of $\dot{V}O_2$ by this method is not possible.

Accuracy and Precision of the Gas Exchange Method

In healthy resting subjects, both the accuracy and the precision of indirect calorimetry by the gas exchange method are excellent, averaging 1–4% and 2–3%, respectively [7, 33]. In critically ill patients, several factors have been shown to influence EE measurement with this method. In such clinical conditions, it is difficult to determine exactly the accuracy and the precision of indirect calorimetry, since there are no other validated method for EE assessment, which is easily applicable at the bedside and to which the former may be compared. *In vitro* studies, using the combustion of a gas such as butane or simulation tests performed by infusing known amounts of CO_2 and nitrogen in a bag, allow to assess the effect of these factors on the error of measurement of $\dot{V}O_2$.

F_IO_2 is a critical factor for both the accuracy and the precision of $\dot{V}O_2$ measurement. This is essentially due to the fact that $\dot{V}O_2$ is calculated by means of the Haldane correction with the gas exchange method. A mathematical analysis of error of $\dot{V}O_2$ determination as a function of F_IO_2 has been developed [25, 34]. *In vitro* studies have shown that the error on $\dot{V}O_2$ measurement increases significantly with F_IO_2, particularly for F_IO_2 exceeding 60–80%. The results of some of the recent *in vitro* studies performed with commercial calorimeters are shown in Fig. 4. From these data, it is clear that $\dot{V}O_2$ can be measured with a 5% accuracy, provided F_IO_2 is limited to a 60% level [35–40].

In patients receiving high F_IO_2, the gas exchange method must be avoided. This is unfortunate, since these patients are among the most desperately ill and may beneficiate of EE assessment for their management. In such conditions, the calculation of $\dot{V}O_2$ by the Fick method, which is not directly affected by the level of F_IO_2, remains the only useful tool to determine EE.

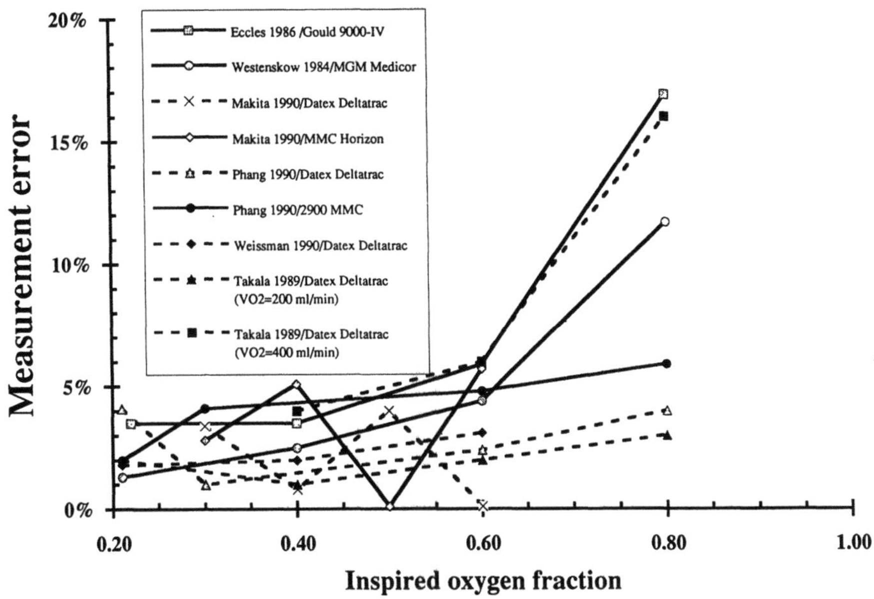

Fig. 4. In vitro testing of some commercially available calorimeters at increasing F_IO_2. Values are absolute errors and not biais

Stable minute ventilation, as well as steady CO_2 body stores (including the bicarbonate pool) are important for $\dot{V}CO_2$ measurement but less critical for adequate $\dot{V}O_2$ determination. The gas exchange method measures CO_2 release at the airway level. This reflects the tissue $\dot{V}CO_2$ provided steady state conditions are achieved. Since body CO_2 stores are large ($\approx$120 L), acute changes in alveolar ventilation may produce a state where tissue and respiratory CO_2 exchanges are unequal. The effect on $\dot{V}O_2$ is minimal due to the small size of body O_2 stores ($\approx$0.6 L O_2) and to its short time-constant (turnover of 42%/min in stable resting conditions). Fig. 5 shows the influence of a period of hyperventilation followed by a period of compensatory hypoventilation on gas exchanges in a healthy subject. In practice, the effect of unstable respiratory minute ventilation is not important for the assessment of metabolic rate, but critical during substrate oxidation calculations.

The duration of gas exchange measurement is another import factor to consider. Respiratory gas exchange is a discontinuous process over the respiratory cycle while tissue gas exchange is continuous. Due to this phenomenon, a sufficient period of measurement is required. The latter should be of 20–30 min, according to the conditions. In patients with fair stable conditions, a 15–20 min period is usually sufficient to achieve a good plateau in both $\dot{V}O_2$ and $\dot{V}CO_2$, whereas in less stable conditions it is recommended to prolong the measurements over 30 min [7, 33].

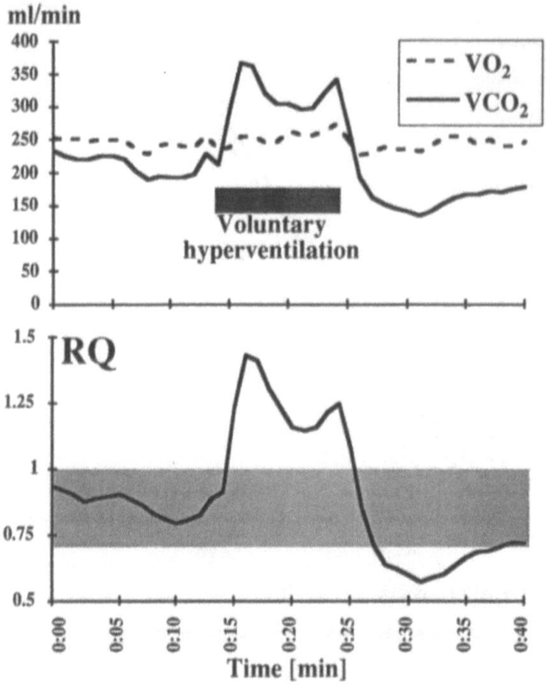

Fig. 5. Effect of transient voluntary hyperventilation and compensatory hypoventilation on oxygen consumption, carbon dioxide production and RQ, in a healthy subject

Conditions required for Accurate Energy Expenditure Measurement

Several conditions are required in healthy subjects to perform accurate and precise measurements of EE by the gas exchange method. In general, similar conditions are required in acutely ill patients breathing spontaneously:

1) There must be no leaks in the system collecting the respiratory gases and no pulmonary and pleural gas leaks, as can occur through chest tubes,
2) Minute ventilation must be stable, to provide stable body CO_2 stores,
3) A sufficient period of measurement must be provided to achieve steady $\dot{V}O_2$ and $\dot{V}CO_2$ levels. In stable conditions, a period of 20 min is recommended,
4) The calorimeter must be correctly calibrated, particularly the gas analyzers and the flow measurement system. At regular intervals, the instrument must be tested *in vitro*, using a gas infusion system or a combustion system,
5) The $\dot{V}O_2$ and $\dot{V}CO_2$ must be converted and expressed using constant gas conditions (usually STPD). This is important due to the significant effects of temperature, pressure and humidity on gas volumes, and

6) Steady hemodynamic, respiratory and metabolic states must be present to insure that respiratory gas exchange is equivalent to tissue gas exchange. The bicarbonate and urea pools must be constant. This is particularly important for basal and resting EE measurements, as well as for substrate oxidation assessment.

In acutely ill patients on mechanical ventilation, additional conditions have to be fullfilled:

7) There must be no gas leaks via or around the endotracheal tube and all the tubing connections of the ventilators,
8) F_IO_2 must be stable and below 60%. A high precision blender is mandatory, providing accurate inspiratory O_2 concentration over the whole range of inspiratory flow (Fig. 6),
9) A proper mixing of the expiratory gases must be achieved to measure stable expiratory gas concentrations,
10) There must be no decompensated failure of circulation, respiration and metabolism. Anaerobic metabolism must be excluded since in this condition, there is an energy expenditure which is not related to oxygen consumption,

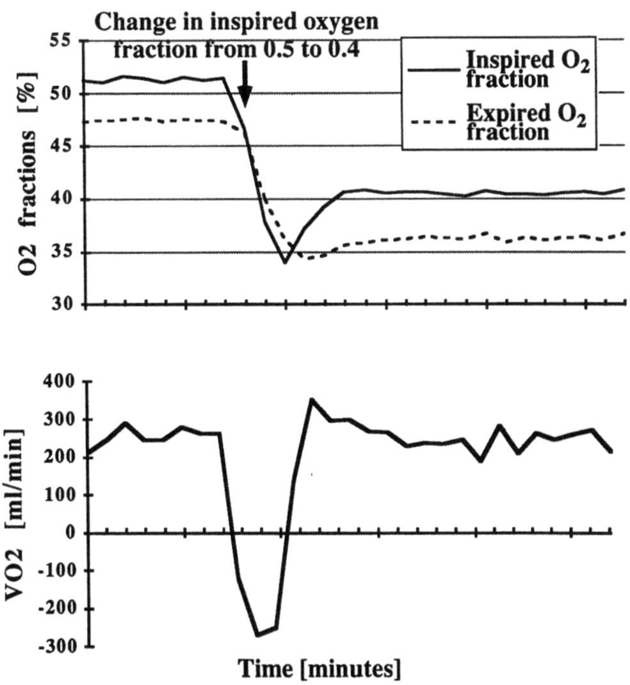

Fig. 6. Effect of acute F_IO_2 change on gas exchange measurements

11) A stable bicarbonate pool must be ascertained, in particular no renal or digestive losses and no alkali therapy must occur. Changing metabolic acid-base status (i.e. developing or resolving lactic or ketonic acidosis) must be excluded. Such conditions commonly occur in ICU patients, and should be ruled out to apply the indirect calorimetry method, and
12) No extra-corporeal CO_2 removal or oxygenation device may be used.

Measured Energy Expenditure and its Components

Indirect calorimetry gives a value of EE which is called measured EE or total EE. In clinical practice, it is important to consider the various components of total EE, particularly when aiming at determining the effect of acute illness on energy metabolism.

In the healthy adult subject, total EE can be divided into three main components: basal EE (also called basal metabolic rate), physical activity EE, and a third component due to the effects of various physiological and unphysiological causes. The latter include the thermogenic effect of food (also called diet induced thermogenesis), cold and physiological stimuli. The energy required for growth slightly increases the metabolic rate in children, whereas the metabolic effects of pregnancy has to be considered in pregnant women, particularly in the third trimester (Table 2). Basal EE corresponds to the energy measured in resting postabsorptive normothermic subjects under very standardized conditions. It is dependent upon the mass of active cells and has been shown to be highly correlated with fat-free mass. Although the vital organs contribute little to body weight, they are the most

Table 2. Conditions changing EE

	REE change, %
Healthy subjects	
Basal metabolic rate	–10
Nutrition	+3–+20
Sleeping	–5––10
Exercise – Light	+100–+200
Exercise – Moderate	+200–+500
Exercise – Heavy	+500–+1500
Pregnancy third trimester	+10–+20
Lactation	+10
Growth – Premature babies	+10–+15
Growth – Children	+5
Patients	
Sitting	+7.9
Standing	+17.4
Fever (per °C)	+10–+15
Critical illness	–20–+80

important contributor to basal EE: it has been estimated that liver, heart, brain and kidneys account for 60–70% of basal EE [41, 42].

In clinical conditions, particularly in ICU conditions, the patients even when resting are very rarely in basal conditions. One usually refers to resting EE, which can be defined as the rate of energy expended by resting healthy or ill subjects, who may not be in thermoneutral conditions, or may have fever, receive drugs, nutritional support or supportive treatments.

Exposure to a cold environment increases metabolic rate via two physiological mechanisms: non-shivering and shivering-thermogenesis. This is also true in ICU patients who not uncommonly are naked. Moreover, many severely traumatized or burned patients have a rise in the central temperature setpoint, which will further enhance cold induced thermogenesis, if not exposed at a proper temperature.

Physical activity produces the largest fluctuations in EE. Even a moderate physical activity largely overcomes the highest rise in EE due to the acute illness. This point is also relevant in the critically ill, who may be agitated or have seizures, postures or increased muscular tone.

It is important to realize that it is difficult to assess the effect of the acute illness or the supportive treatment on the metabolic rate, due to the number of confounding factors. The most important factors who may influence EE in the critically ill patient are summarized in Table 3. They are mainly related to the acute illness, the endocrine and metabolic responses as well as to the effect of supportive treatments. Adrenergic activity is markedly enhanced in the traumatized and burned patients. Various studies have evaluated the ef-

Table 3. Acute effects of therapeutics on energy expenditure on O_2 consumption

Intervention	Clinical situation	Effect on EE or VO_2	Ref.
1. Drugs			
Catecholamines	Circulatory failure	up to 32% increase ($\dot{V}O_2$)	[59]
Beta-blockers	Head injury	6% decrease (EE)	[60]
	Burn (adults)	7% decrease (EE)	[61]
	Burn (children)	16% decrease (EE)	[62]
Opiates	Analgesia during MV	9% decrease (EE)	[63]
Opiates	Postoperative shivering	59% decrease ($\dot{V}O_2$)	[64]
Sedation	Postoperative patients	20–55% decrease ($\dot{V}O_2$)	[43]
Barbiturates	Head injury	32% decrease (EE)	[44]
Muscular relaxants	Head injury	42% decrease (EE)	[45]
Opiates	Postoperative rewarming	26% decrease ($\dot{V}O_2$)	[65]
2. Mechanical ventilation	Acute respiratory failure/ weaning failure	25% decrease ($\dot{V}O_2$)	[56]
	Acute respiratory failure/ weaning failure	34% decrease ($\dot{V}O_2$)	[57]
3. Nutritional support	Burn	20% increase (EE)	[66]

MV = mechanical ventilation

fect of sympatho-adrenal hyperactivity on metabolic rate by administrating β-blockers. Other drugs such as opiates, muscular relaxants, and sedatives also lower the resting EE (Table 3). Sedatives produce a dose-dependent decrease in $\dot{V}O_2$, as shown in a recent study [43]. Barbiturates in head injured patient decrease markedly EE, below the normal prediction value [44]. A small or moderate physical activity may increase EE by 10 to 40%, whereas muscular relaxation may have the opposite effect [45]. Nutritional support may enhance resting EE by 20 to 30%, whereas undernutrition may diminish EE under the normal values [46–48]. The contribution of the respiratory muscles to resting EE is normally 3–5%, but can increase over 20% during acute respiratory failure. Mechanical ventilation may only marginally lower EE but may also decrease it significantly. All these examples illustrate clearly the difficulty to interpret the data of calorimetry, particularly to delineate the effect of the acute illness *per se* in critically ill patients. This difficulty is well illustrated by the data of the literature in patients with acute brain injury. The measured EE is often elevated in these patients, but can be normal or even decreased. The individual reported EE values range between 43 and 280% of the predicted values [49, 50]!

Indirect Calorimetry Technique: Substrate Oxidation

Conceivebly, the method of indirect calorimetry allows to calculate the overall amount of substrate that are oxidized in the body. For this purpose, N_u must be accurately measured in addition to gas exchange. This can be difficult in ICU conditions, particularly in patients with changing urea pool, such as in patients with varying renal function or receiving diuretics. The usual calculations are based on the assumption that only 3 groups of nutrients are oxidized: protein, carbohydrate, and lipid. This requires a system of three equations containing 3 parameters: $\dot{V}O_2$, $\dot{V}CO_2$ and N_u. The calculation is done in several steps:

1) Protein oxidation is calculated from the quantity of nitrogen eliminated in the urine;
2) This corresponds to a known amount of oxygen ($\dot{V}O_{2Prot}$) and carbon dioxide ($\dot{V}CO_{2Prot}$), allowing to compute the non-protein O_2 consumption ($\dot{V}O_{2Non\,Prot}$), the non-protein CO_2 production ($\dot{V}CO_{2Non\,Prot}$), as well as the non-protein respiratory quotient ($RQ_{NonProt}$); and
3) From NPRQ, the proportion of fat and carbohydrate oxidation and their energy equivalents are determined (see Appendix 3 for a complete mathematical development).

It should be pointed out that this assessment is strongly dependent on the accuracy and precision of both $\dot{V}O_2$ and $\dot{V}CO_2$ measurements. A 0.01 error on RQ induces a 3% error on the proportion of substrate oxidized; this produces a even larger error on the absolute value of substrate oxidation (Table 3).

This method has been validated in healthy subjects by simultaneous assessment of substrate oxidation using both the indirect calorimetry method and isotopic tracers. However the agreement between both methods was not very high, showing that indirect calorimetry provides only a crude estimation of substrate oxidation. In the acutely ill patient, it is even more problematic to rely on calorimetry to evaluate the rate of substrate utilization since its accuracy and precision are lower than in healthy subjects. There is yet no study validating this method in such condition.

It is important to point out that indirect calorimetry does not measure the true oxidation rates of carbohydrates, lipids and proteins but only their overall disappearance rates (Fig. 7) and therefore does not provide information on the intermediate metabolic processes [51]. Although under most circumstances, the disappearance of substrate from their respective metabolic pool is largely achieved by oxidation, there are frequent situations in which a substrate is not only oxidized but also converted or utilized for other purposes. This is the case for lipogenesis (conversion from carbohydrates to lipids) and neoglucogenesis (conversion of amino acids to glucose). In such conditions, the following equations are used:

$$\mathrm{CHO}_{\text{disappearance rate}} = \text{CHO oxidation} - \text{Neoglucogenesis} + \text{Lipogenesis} \quad (10)$$

$$\mathrm{Lipid}_{\text{disappearance rate}} = \text{Lipid oxidation} - \text{Lipogenesis} \quad (11)$$

$$\mathrm{Protein}_{\text{disappearance rate}} = \text{Protein oxidation} + \text{Neoglucogenesis} \quad (12)$$

The predicted RQ of neoglucogenesis from amino acids is close to 0.40. However, a perceptible drop in respiratory quotient is observed only when this process is highly activated and when the neoformed glucose is stored in the body or lost in urines and not completely oxidized to CO_2 and H_2O. However, in such conditions, the overall RQ will not drop substantially below 0.7, due to the fact that the process of neoglucogenesis contributes little

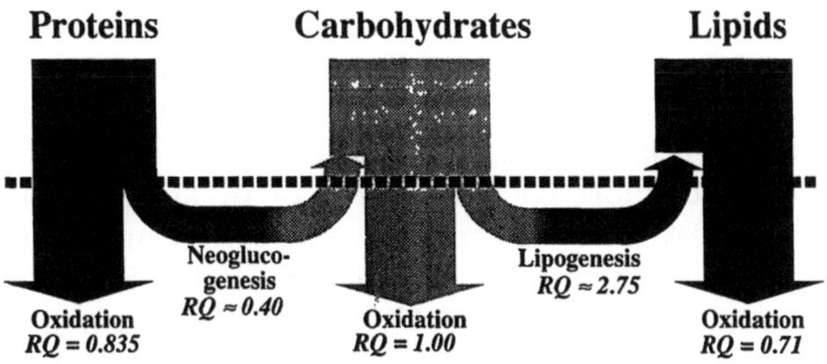

Fig. 7. Substrate flows assessement by the indirect calorimetry method. Indirect calorimetry measures only the overall disappearance rate (broken line) and not the true oxidation rate. For protein, the disappearance rate consists of the true oxidation rate plus the rate of neoglucogenesis. The same is true for carbohydrates (oxidation + lipogenesis – neoglucogenesis) and lipids (oxidation – lipogenesis)

to the overall metabolism. Indirect calorimetry thus allows to calculate overall substrate oxidation by the body, but not to determine the various intermediate metabolic processes.

It is also possible to use substrate labelled with stable isotopes in order to get an insight into the rate of substrate oxidation [52]. It should be noted that when a tracer is used (e.g. ^{13}C glucose) specific models must be developed. A simple model for assessing glucose oxidation in which all carbon atoms are ^{13}C labelled (U-^{13}C glucose) assumes that both the labelled and unlabelled glucose enter a single homogenous plasma glucose pool. From this pool, it can be either oxidized to CO_2, stored as glycogen, transformed into fat by lipogenesis or be used for non-essential amino acid synthesis. Glucose oxidation can be calculated from the $^{13}CO_2$ enrichment in expired air, $\dot{V}CO_2$ and ^{13}C enrichment of glucose administered. A correction factor for CO_2 retention in the bicarbonate pool must be also applied since the recovery is not equal to 100% but is generally 80% [53].

There are some problems related to the assessment of substrate oxidation by stable isotopes. They include:

1) the fact that the method is not completely independent from indirect calorimetry since $\dot{V}CO_2$ must be measured simultaneously, and
2) There may be a selective labelled CO_2 fixation by the body when, for example, the tracer is fixed or exchanged in the metabolism and the non-labelled tracer can be regenerated. In addition, CO_2 can be lost in bone bicarbonate which have a slow turnover but this will equally affect the calculation by indirect calorimetry and tracer studies.

Clinical Relevance in Intensive Care Medicine

EE is an important physiological parameter in critically ill patients. EE is highly correlated with $\dot{V}O_2$, due to the fact that it is directly dependent on cellular oxidative processes. When condidering the energy status of the body and the function of vital organs, these two parameters are physiologically equivalent. However, when the interest is directed to nutrition, to the utilization of nutrients and to their effects on the respiratory system, the indirect calorimetry method, which relies on the measurements of $\dot{V}O_2$, $\dot{V}CO_2$ and urinary N excretion, gives more information than the assessment of VO_2 only. No information on tissue or organ metabolism is provided by this method, which measures only whole body metabolic processes.

The first interest in using the gas exchange method in ICU patients is to accurately measure body $\dot{V}O_2$, while EE computation is often omitted. It is easily applied in patients breathing room air. By contrast, in acutelly ill mechanically ventilated patients, numerous conditions must be throughout satisfied to apply this technique, in order to avoid bias and inaccuracies. If this is the case, the accuracy and precision of $\dot{V}O_2$ measurement are superior to that achieved by the Fick method using a pulmonary artery catheter. One important limitation of the gas exchange method is related to the inspiratory O_2 fraction, which influences markedly the error on $\dot{V}O_2$ measurement. Above 60% F_IO_2, the error on $\dot{V}O_2$ increases dramatically, making this method inappropriate. In such condition, $\dot{V}O_2$ assessment relies on the Fick method only. Thus in the most severely ill patients whose survival is often critically dependent on the maintenance of $\dot{V}O_2$, the only valid method is the least accurate one.

Indirect calorimetry in severely ill patients is also used to assess EE, in order to provide an adequate nutritional support and adequate amounts of energy supply. For this purpose, the method is appropriate, provided carefull measurement conditions are satisfied, including a sufficient number of measurements of adequate duration. In healthy subjects, indirect calorimetry allows to assess the proportion of protein, carbohydrate, and fat oxidized. This require highly accurate determination of gas exchange and urinary N excretion. Such demanding measurements cannot be insured in critically ill patients in whom this method provides, at best, a crude estimation of nutrient utilization.

In patients with prolonged weaning from mechanical ventilation, indirect calorimetry provides several important information. Resting EE is difficult to predict in these patients, in whom adequate nutritional support is mandatory [54, 55]. The increase in $\dot{V}O_2$ due to the discontinuation of respiratory mechanical support (O_2 cost of breathing) is related to the outcome of weaning [56, 57]. $\dot{V}CO_2$ is dependent on energy supply and the type of nutrients administered. These two factors influence directly the level of alveolar ventilation required to achieve a given level of $PaCO_2$, and thus work of breathing [54, 58].

Appendix 1: Practical Example: Calculating Energy Expenditure and Substrate Oxidation

Part 1: Calculating $\dot{V}O_2$, $\dot{V}CO_2$, RQ and EE in a Patient on Mechanical Ventilation with the Following Parameters

$V_{E STPD} = 5$ L/min $\quad F_IO_2 = 50\%$

$F_ECO_2 = 4\%$ $\quad F_EO_2 = 45.5\%$

Calculations of oxygen consumption and carbon dioxide production

$$\dot{V}CO_{2STPD} = 5 \text{ L/min} \times 0.04 = 200 \text{ mL/min} \tag{A-1}$$

$$V_{ISTPD} = \frac{1-0.455-0.04}{1-0.5} \times 5 \text{ L/min} = 5.05 \text{ L/min} \tag{A-2}$$

$$\dot{V}O_{2STPD} = 5 \text{ L/min} \times \left(\frac{0.5 \times (1-0.04) - 0.455}{1-0.5}\right) = 250 \text{ mL/min} \tag{A-3}$$

$$RQ = \frac{\dot{V}CO_{2STPD}}{\dot{V}O_{2STPD}} = \frac{200\ mL/min}{225\ mL/min} = 0.80 \qquad (A\text{-}4)$$

$$EE = 15.90 \times 0.225 + 5.23 \times 0.2 - 9.33 \times 0.0013 = 4.6\ kJ/min = 1.1\ kcal/min \qquad (A\text{-}5)$$

If the Haldane correction is omitted (i.e. assuming $V_I = V_E$), oxygen consumption and RQ can be rewritten:

$$\dot{V}O_{2STPD} = V_{In} \times F_IO_2 - V_E \times F_EO_2 = 5\ L/min \times 0.5 - 5\ L/min \times 0.455 = 225\ mL/min$$

$$RQ = \frac{\dot{V}CO_{2STPD}}{\dot{V}O_{2STPD}} = \frac{200\ mL/min}{250\ mL/min} = 0.89 \qquad (A\text{-}6)$$

In this example, the Haldane correction on flow measurement is 1% and leads to a 10% error on $\dot{V}O_2$ and a 30% error or RQ (assuming a 0.7–1 range).

Part 2: Calculations of Substrate Oxidations

To calculate the substrate oxidation rates, we need an additional parameter: nitrogen excretion which averaged 18 g/24 h (0.0013 g/min) in this example. As developed in appendix 3, measured oxygen consumption and carbon dioxide production is the sum of the partial contribution of each substrate. Using the constants for average protein, lipids and carbohydrates proposed by Elia and Livesey [24] (Table 1), and assuming 6.25 g prot/g N, the equations A-7 to A-9 can be rewritten:

$$CHO_{Oxidation} = -2.956 \times + 4.164 \times \dot{V}CO_2 - 3.286 \times Urin\ N_{Excr} \qquad (A\text{-}7)$$

$$Lipids_{Oxidation} = 1.711 \times \dot{V}O_2 - 1.711 \times \dot{V}CO_2 - 1.783 \times Urin\ N_{Excr} \qquad (A\text{-}8)$$

$$Prot_{Oxidation} = 6.25 \times Urin\ N_{Excr} \qquad (A\text{-}9)$$

Including Haldane correction:

$CHO_{oxidation}$ = 0.05 g/min = 0.92 kJ/min = 18% of EE

$Lipids_{Oxidation}$ = 0.06 g/min = 2.51 kJ/min = 50% of EE

$Prot_{Oxidation}$ = 0.08 g/min = 1.55 kJ/min = 31% of EE

Without Haldane correction:

$CHO_{Oxidation}$ = 0.13 g/min = 2.22 kJ/min = 48% of EE

$Lipids_{Oxidation}$ = 0.02 g/min = 0.79 kJ/min = 18% of EE

$Prot_{Oxidation}$ = 0.08 g/min = 1.55 kJ/min = 34% of EE

Appendix 2: Sets of Equations Used to Determine $\dot{V}O_2$, $\dot{V}CO_2$ and RQ in Particular Conditions

A) If inspired carbon dioxide fraction has to be taken into account:

$$\dot{V}CO_{2STPD} = V_{ESTPD} \times \left(\frac{F_ECO_2 \times (1 - F_IO_2) - F_ICO_2 \times (1 - F_EO_2)}{1 - F_IO_2 - F_ICO_2} \right) \qquad (A\text{-}10)$$

$$\dot{V}O_{2STPD} = V_{ESTPD} \times \left(\frac{F_IO_2 \times (1 - F_ECO_2) - F_EO_2 \times (1 - F_ICO_2)}{1 - F_IO_2 - F_ICO_2} \right) \quad \text{(A-11)}$$

$$RQ = \frac{F_ECO_2 \times (1 - F_IO_2) - F_ICO_2 \times (1 - F_EO_2)}{F_IO_2 \times (1 - F_ECO_2) - F_EO_2 \times (1 - F_ICO_2)} \quad \text{(A-12)}$$

B) If other gases are used, or water partial pressure have to be taken into account, calculate the inspired (F_IG) and expired (F_EG) fraction of all the gas:

$$\dot{V}CO_{2STPD} = V_{ESTPD} \left(\frac{F_ECO_2 \times (1 - F_IO_2 - F_IG) - F_ICO_2 \times (1 - F_EO_2 - F_EG)}{1 - F_IO_2 - F_ICO_2 - F_IG} \right) \quad \text{(A-13)}$$

$$\dot{V}O_{2STPD} = V_{ESTPD} \left(\frac{F_IO_2 \times (1 - F_ECO_2 - F_EG) - F_EO_2 \times (1 - F_ICO_2 - F_IG)}{1 - F_IO_2 - F_ICO_2 - F_IG} \right) \quad \text{(A-14)}$$

$$RQ = \left(\frac{F_ECO_2 \times (1 - F_IO_2 - F_IG) - F_ICO_2 \times (1 - F_EO_2 - F_EG)}{F_IO_2 \times (1 - F_ECO_2 - F_EG) - F_EO_2 \times (1 - F_ICO_2 - F_IG)} \right) \quad \text{(A-15)}$$

Appendix 3: Substrate Disappearance Rates and Energy Expenditure: Mathematical Development of Equations

Part 1: Proteins, carbohydrates, and lipids

The concept is based upon the fact that total oxygen consumption and carbon dioxide production measured are the sum of the contribution of each of the three substrates:

$$\dot{V}O_2 = \dot{V}O_{2Prot} + \dot{V}O_{2Lipids} + \dot{V}O_{2CHO} \quad \text{(A-16)}$$

$$\dot{V}CO_2 = \dot{V}CO_{2Prot} + \dot{V}CO_{2Lipids} + \dot{V}CO_{2CHO} \quad \text{(A-17)}$$

$$\text{Protein oxidation} = \text{N urinary} \times \text{Constant} \quad \text{(A-18)}$$

Where $\dot{V}O_{2Prot}$, $\dot{V}O_{2Lipids}$ and $\dot{V}O_{2CHO}$ represent the oxygen consumption attributable to each substrate, which can be calculated according to the following equations:

$$\dot{V}O_{2Lipids}[\text{mL/min}] = \frac{\text{Energy equiv. [kJ/g]}}{\text{Oxygen equivalent [kJ/mL } O_2]} \times \text{Lipid ox [g/min]} \quad \text{(A-19)}$$

$$\dot{V}CO_{2Lipids}[\text{mL/min}] = \frac{\text{Energy equiv. [kJ/g]} \times QR_{Lipids}}{\text{Oxygen equiv. [kJ/mL } O_2]} \times \text{Lipid ox [g/min]} \quad \text{(A-20)}$$

etc. ...

By solving these equations in terms of carbohydrates, lipids, and protein oxidations:

$$CHO_{Oxidation} = \dot{V}O_2 \times \frac{RQ_{Lipids} \times O_2Equiv_{CHO}}{Energy_{CHO} \times (RQ_{Lipids} - RQ_{CHO})} + \dot{V}CO_2 \times \frac{O_2Equiv_{CHO}}{Energy_{CHO} \times (RQ_{CHO} - RQ_{Lipids})}$$

$$+\text{Urinary } N_{Excr}\times N_{constant} \times \frac{\text{Energy}_{Prot}\times O_2\text{Equiv}_{CHO}\times(RQ_{Prot}-RQ_{Lipids})}{O_2\text{Equiv}_{Prot}\times \text{Energy}_{CHO}\times(RQ_{Lipids}-RQ_{CHO})} \qquad \text{(A-21)}$$

$$\text{Lipid oxidation}=\dot{V}O_2\times\frac{RQ_{CHO}\times O_2\text{Equiv}_{Lipids}}{\text{Energy}_{Lipids}\times(RQ_{CHO}-RQ_{Lipids})}$$

$$+\dot{V}CO_2\times\frac{O_2\text{Equiv}_{Lipids}}{\text{Energy}_{Lipids}\times(RQ_{Lipids}-RQ_{CHO})}$$

$$+\text{Urin. } N_{Excr}\times N_{constant} \times\frac{(\text{Energy}_{Prot}\times O_2\text{Equiv}_{Lipids}\times(RQ_{Prot}-RQ_{CHO}))}{(O_2\text{Equiv}_{Prot}\times\text{Energy}_{Lipids}\times(RQ_{CHO}-RQ_{Lipids}))} \qquad \text{(A-22)}$$

$$\text{Protein oxidation}=\text{Urin. } N_{Excr}\times N_{constant}$$

$\dot{V}O_2$ and $\dot{V}CO_2$ are in mL/min, whereas Energy equivalents are in kJ/g, and oxygen equivalents in kJ/mL O_2. Urinary nitrogen excretion is expressed in g/min. Substrate oxidation is calculated as g/min.

EE is calculated as the sum of the EEs due to each substrate:

$$EE=EE_{Prot}+EE_{Lipids}+EE_{CHO} \qquad \text{(A-23)}$$

$$EE=(\text{Protein oxidation}\times\text{Energy equiv}_{Prot}) +(\text{Lipid}_{Oxidation}\times\text{Energy equiv}_{Lipids}) +(\text{CHO}_{Oxidation}\times\text{Energy equiv}_{CHO}) \qquad \text{(A-24)}$$

$$EE=\dot{V}O_2\times\frac{(O_2\text{Equiv}_{Lipids}\times RQ_{CHO})-(O_2\text{Equiv}_{CHO}\times RQ_{Lipids})}{RQ_{CHO}-RQ_{Lipids}}$$

$$+\dot{V}CO_2\times\frac{O_2\text{Equiv}_{CHO}-O_2\text{Equiv}_{Lipids}}{RQ_{CHO}-RQ_{Lipids}}$$

$$+\text{Urin. } N_{Excr}\times N_{constant}\times\text{Energy}_{Prot} \times\left(1-\frac{O_2\text{Equiv}_{CHO}\times(RQ_{Prot}-RQ_{Lipids})+O_2\text{Equiv}_{Lipids}\times(RQ_{CHO}-RQ_{Prot})}{O_2\text{Equiv}_{Prot}\times(RQ_{CHO}-RQ_{Lipids})}\right) \qquad \text{(A-25)}$$

This system of equations is applicable in any situation where these three substrates are used and allows the calculation of oxidations. It requires to determine the energy content, the oxygen equivalent (also called heat equivalent) and the respiratory quotient of proteins, carbohydrates, and lipids. It also necessitates to define the protein equivalent of nitrogen, which is usually set at 6.25 g of protein oxidized per gram nitrogen excreted.

Part 2: Calculation principles when oxidizing a fourth substrate (ethanol, acetate, etc. ...)

When dealing with 4 substrates, we have to measure the disappearance rate of the fourth substrate by an independent method: It is mathematically impossible to resolve a system including 3 equations with 4 unknown variables. This is usually achieved by estimating the distribution volume of the substrate and measuring blood clearance rate. For example, measurement of ethanol in expired air is a non-invasive way to assess its blood level with a negligible loss. Equations A-16 and A-17 have to take this fourth substrate into account:

$$\dot{V}O_2 = \dot{V}O_{2Prot} + \dot{V}O_{2Lipids} + \dot{V}O_{2CHO} + \dot{V}O_{2\,4^{th}Substrate} \quad \text{(A-26)}$$

$$\dot{V}CO_2 = \dot{V}CO_{2Prot} + \dot{V}CO_{2Lipids} + \dot{V}CO_{2CHO} + \dot{V}CO_{2\,4^{th}Substrate} \quad \text{(A-27)}$$

Step by step process to solve theses equations:

1) Measure the 4th substrate disappearance rate by an independent method;
2) Calculate the oxygen consumption and the carbon dioxide production due to this substrate

$$(\dot{V}O_{2\,4^{th}Substrate}, \dot{V}CO_{2\,4^{th}Substrate});$$

3) Deduce these values from the total $\dot{V}O_2$ and $\dot{V}CO_2$ measured to assess the oxygen consumption due to protein, lipids, and CHO;
4) Process as developed here above in equations A-16 to A-23, to calculate protein, lipid, and CHO oxidation rates;
5) Include the contribution of the 4th substrate to the total EE:

$$EE = EE_{Prot} + EE_{Lipids} + EE_{CHO} + EE_{4^{th}Substrate} \quad \text{(A-28)}$$

It is important to note that equations (1) and (2) do not apply in such conditions (as well as all other related equations).

References

1. Kleiber M (1975) The fire of life: An introduction to animal energetics. RE Kreiger Inc:pp 116
2. Bland R, Shoemaker W (1985) Common physiologic pattern in general surgical patients: Hemodynamic and oxygen transport changes during and after operation in patients with and without associated medical problems. Surg Clin North Am 65:793–809
3. Wilson R, Christensen C, LeBlanc L (1972) Oxygen consumption in critically ill surgical patients. Ann Surg 176:801–804
4. Shoemaker W, Kram H, Appel P, Flemming A (1990) The efficacy of central venous and pulmonary artery catheters and therapy based upon them in reducing mortality and morbidity. Arch Surg 125:1332–1338
5. Edwards J (1989) Optimal levels of oxygen transport in critically ill patients. In: Vincent JL (ed) Update in intensive care and emergency medicine, Vol 8. Springer Verlag, Berlin, Heidelberg, New York. pp 205–214
6. Shoemaker W, Appel P, Kram H, Waxman K, Lee T (1988) Prospective trial of supranormal values of survivors as therapeutic goals in high-risk surgical patients. Chest 94:1176–1186
7. Bursztein S, Elwyn DH, Askanazi J, Kinney JM (1989) Energy metabolism, indirect calorimetry, and nurtrition. Williams & Wilkins, Baltimore
8. Pahud P, Ravussin E, Jéquier E (1980) Energy expended during deficit period of submaximal exercise in man. J Appl Physiol 48:770–775
9. Jéquier E, Flatt J (1986) Recent advances in human energetics. News Physiol Sciences 1:112–114
10. Ferrannini E (1988) The theoretical bases of indirect calorimetry. A review. Metabolism 37:287–301

11. Jéquier E, Schutz Y (1983) Long-term measurements of energy expenditure in human using a respiration chamber. Am J Clin Nutr 38:989–998
12. Jéquier E, Felber J (1987) Indirect calorimetry. Baillière's Clin Endocr Metab 1:911–935
13. Jéquier E, Acheson K, Schutz Y (1987) Assessment of energy expenditure and fuel utilization in man. Ann Rev Nutr 7:187–208
14. Jéquier E (1984) Energy expenditure in obesity. Clin Endocr Metab 13:563–580
15. Spurr G, Prentice A, Murgatroyd P, Goldberg G, Reina J, Christman N (1988) Energy expenditure from minute heart rate recording: Comparison with indirect calorimetry. Am J Clin Nutr 48:552–559
16. Durnin J, Edward R (1955) Pulmonary ventilation as an index of energy expenditure. Quart J Expt Physiol 40:370–377
17. Ford A, Hellerstein A (1959) Estimation of energy expenditure from pulmonary ventilation. J Appl Physiol 14:981–984
18. Harding R, Sen R (1970) Evaluation of total muscular activity by quantification of electro-myograms, through a summing amplifier. Med Biol Erg 8:343–356
19. Stunkard A (1960) A method of studying physical activity in man. Am J Clin Nutr 8:595–601
20. Coward W, Prentice A (1985) Isotope method for the measurement of carbon dioxide production in man. Am J Clin Nutr 41:659–661
21. Schoeller D, van Stanten E (1982) Measurement of energy expenditure in man by doubly-labelled water method. J Appl Physiol 53:955–959
22. Spinnler G, Jéquier E, Favre R, Dolivo M, Vanotti A (1973) Human calorimeter with a new type of gradient layer. J Appl Physiol 35:159–165
23. Frascarolo P, Schutz Y, Jéquier E (1990) Decreased thermal conductance during the lutheal phase of the menstrual cycle in women. J Appl Physiol 69:2029–2033
24. Livesey G, Elia M (1988) Estimation of energy expenditure, net carbohydrate utilization, and net fat oxidation and synthesis by indirect calorimetry: Evaluation of errors with special reference to the detailed composition of foods. Am J Clin Nutr 47:608–628
25. Bursztein S, Saphar P, Singer P, Elwyn D (1989) A mathematical analysis of indirect calorimetry measurements in acutely ill patients. Am J Clin Nutr 50:227–230
26. Behrends W, Weiland C, Giani J (1987) Continuous measurement of oxygen uptake: Evaluation of the Enström metabolic computer and clinical experiences. Acta Anaesthesiol Scand 31:10–14
27. Bizouarn P, Soulard D, Blanloeil Y, Guillet A, Goarin Y (1992) Oxygen consumption after cardiac surgery: A comparison between calculation by Fick's principle and measurement by indirect calorimetry. Intensive Care Med 18:206–209
28. Brandi L, Grana M, Mazzanti T, Giunta F, Natali A, Ferrannini E (1992) Energy expenditure and gas exchange measurements in postoperative patients: Thermodilution versus indirect calorimetry. Crit Care Med 20:1273–1283
29. Chioléro R, Mavrocordatos P, Bracco D, Schutz Y, Cayeux C, Revelly J (1993) Cold iced injectate should not be used to assess O_2 consumption in acutelly ill patients (submitted)
30. Myburgh J, Webb R, Worthley L (1992) Ventilation/perfusion indices do not correlate with the difference between oxygen consumption measured by the Fick principle and metabolic monitoring systems in critically ill patients. Crit Care Med 20:479–482
31. Vermeij C, Feenstra B, Bruining H (1990) Oxygen delivery and oxygen uptake in postoperative and septic patients. Chest 98:415–420
32. Ronco J, Phang T, Walley K, Wiggs B, Fenwick J, Russel J (1991) Oxygen consumption is independent of changes in oxygen delivery in severe adult respiratory distress syndrome. Am Rev Respir Dis 143:1267–1273
33. Damask M, Schwarz Y, Weissman C (1987) Energy measurements and requirements of critically ill patients. Crit Care Clin 3:71–96
34. Ultman J, Bursztein S (1981) Analysis of error in the determination of respiratory gas exchange at varying FiO_2. J Appl Physiol 50:210–216

35. Eccles R, Swinamer D, Jones R, King G (1986) Validation of a compact system for measuring gas exchange. Crit Care Med 64:807–811
36. Westenskow D, Cutler C, Wallace W (1984) Instrumentation for monitoring gas exchange and metabolic rate in critically ill patients. Crit Care Med 12:183–187
37. Makita K, Nunn J, Royston B (1990) Evaluation of metabolic measuring instruments for use in critically ill patients. Crit Care Med 18:638–644
38. Phang P, Rich T, Ronco J (1990) A validation and comparison study of two metabolic monitors. JPEN 14:259–261
39. Weissman C, Sardar A, Kemper M (1990) Techniques, materials, and devices. JPEN 14:216–221
40. Takala J, Keinänen O, Väisänen P, Karl A (1989) Measurement of gas exchange in intensive care: Laboratory and clinical validation of a new device. Crit Care Med 17:1041–1047
41. Weinsier RL, Schutz Y, Bracco D (1992) Reexamination of the relationship of resting metabolic rate to fat-free mass and to the metabolically active components of fat-free mass in human. Am J Clin Nutr 55:790–794
42. Grande F, Keys A (1980) Body weight, body composition, and calorie status. In: Goodhart R, Shils M (eds) Modern nutrition in health and disease, 6 edn. Lea and Febiger, Philadelphia, PA, pp 3–34
43. Boyd O, Grounds M, Bennett D (1992) The dependency of oxygen consumption on oxygen delivery in critically ill postoperative patients is mimicked by variations in sedation. Chest 101:1619–1624
44. Dempsey D, Guenter P, Mullen J, et al (1985) Energy expenditure in acute trauma to the head with and without barbiturate therapy. Surg Gynecol Obstet 16:128–134
45. Clifton G, Robertson C, Choi S (1986) Assessment of nutritional requirements of head-injured patients. J Neurosurg 64:895–901
46. Vaisman N, Rossi MF, Goldberg E, Dibden L, Wykes LJ, Pencharz PB (1988) Energy expenditure and body composition in patients with anorexia nervosa. J Pediatr 113:919–924
47. Casper R, Schoeller D, Kuschner R, Hnilicka J, Gold S (1991) Total daily energy expenditure and activity level in anorexia nervosa. Am J Clin Nutr 53:1143–1150
48. Melchior J, Rigaud D, Rozen R, Malon D, Apfelbaum M (1989) Energy expenditure economy induced by decrease in lean body mass in anorexia nervosa. Eur J Clin Nutr 43:793–799
49. Chioléro R, Lemarchand T (1992) Modifications hormonales après traumatisme crânien sévère. In: Boles JJ (ed) Conséquences endocriniennes des états d'agression aiguë. Arnette, Paris pp 79–90
50. Chioléro R, Schutz Y, Lemarchand T, et al (1989) Hormonal and metabolic changes following severe head injury or noncranial injury. JPEN 13:5–12
51. Simonson DC, DeFronzo RA (1990) Indirect calorimetry: Methodological and interpretative problems. Am J Physiol 258:E399–E412
52. Rosenblatt J, Wolfe R (1988) Calculation of substrate flux using stable isotopes. Am J Physiol 254:E526–E531
53. Irwing C, Wong W, Shulman R, O'Brian Smith E, Klein P (1983) 13C bicarbonate kinetics in human: Intra-vs interindividual variations. Am J Physiol 245:R190–R202
54. Weissmann C, Hyman A (1987) Nutritional care of the critically ill patient with respiratory failure. Crit Care Clin 3:185–202
55. Wilson D, Rogers R, Hoffman R (1985) Nutrition and chronic lung disease. Am Rev Respir Dis 132:1347–1365
56. Lewis W, Chwals W, Benotti P, et al (1988) Bedside assessment of the work of breathing. Crit Care Med 16:117–122
57. Shikora S, Bistrian B, Borlase B, Blackburne G, Stone M, Benotti P (1990) Work of breathing: Reliable predictor of weaning and extubation. Crit Care Med 18:157–162
58. Talpers S, Romberger D, Bunce S, Pingleton S (1992) Nutritionally associated increased carbon dioxide production. Excess total calories vs high proportion of carbohydrate calories. Chest 102:551–555

59. Chioléro RL, Revelly JP, Jéquier E (1991) Effects of catecholamines on oxygen consumption and oxygen delivery in critically ill patients. Chest 100:1676–1684
60. Chioléro R, Breitenstein E, Thorin D, et al (1989) Effects of propranolol on resting metabolic rate after severe head injury. Crit Care Med 17:328–344
61. Breitenstein E, Chioléro R, Jéquier E, Dayer P, Krupp S, Schutz Y (1990) Effects of beta-blockade on energy metabolism following burns. Burns 16:259–269
62. Wolfe R, Herndon DN, Jahoor F, Miyosi H, Wolfe M (1987) Effect of severe burn injury on substrate cycling by glucose and fatty acids. N Engl J Med 317:403–408
63. Swinamer D, Phang P, Jones R, Grace M, King E (1988) Effect of routine administration of analgesia on energy expenditure in critically ill patients. Chest 92:4–10
64. Macintyre P, Pavlin E, Dwersteg J (1987) Effect of meperidine on oxygen consumption, carbon dioxide production and respiratory gas exchange in postanaesthesia shivering. Anesth Analg 66:751–755
65. Rodriguez J, Weissman C, Damask M, Askanazi J, Hyman A, Kinney J (1983) Morphine and postoperative rewarming in critically ill patients. Circulation 68:1238–1246
66. Allard JP, Pichard C, Hoshino E, et al (1990) Validation of a new formula for calculating the energy requirements of burn patients. JPEN 14:115–118

Are We Giving Unbalanced Amino Acid Solutions?

– From Protein Hydrolysates to Tailored Solutions –

P. Fürst and P. Stehle

Introduction

Ideal Composition? Ideal Amounts? Disease-specific Solutions?

It has been known for more than 50 years that a severe traumatic injury gives rise to striking changes in metabolism. In particular, there is a marked increase in nitrogen (N) excretion indicating net protein catabolism and an enhanced oxygen utilization, demonstrating increased oxidation of energy substrates [1]. Recent developments in nutritional support of such patients have enabled body mass to be preserved while healing occurs [2]. Today consensus has been reached that amino acid nutrition beneficially affects net nitrogen balance during episodes of trauma, injury or infection [3–6]. Negative N-balance after severe trauma or injury can therefore be minimized if large amounts of amino acid N together with energy substrates are provided by the intravenous route [5, 7].

Although such nutritional therapy has concentrated upon giving, often IV, large amounts of both organic N and energy substrates, it is by no means clear what is the ideal composition of the diet of these patients. An additional fundamental question might be, whether a unique composition of nutrients is required for certain special disorders. It even has been questioned whether provision of N is beneficial during the early period of increased protein loss [8]. Accordingly, in some studies, increase in dietary input in the immediate posttrauma period has not led to the expected improvement of clinical outcome.

As an explanation, the hypothesis has been brought forward that either the proportions in presently available solutions are not suitable, or it was postulated that these solutions are incomplete, since important amino acids such as glutamine, tyrosine and cystine are not included [9]. These amino acids are either poorly soluble or unstable during heat sterilization.

In the present chapter, relevant historical aspects of parenteral amino acid substrates will receive brief comments. Current nutritional implications will be evaluated in the face of known metabolic alterations as affected by provision of various amino acid solutions. Finally, future aspects and prospects will be elaborated in the hope that these ideas will focus attention and research upon the need to correlate nutrition more directly with cellular biochemistry.

Amino Acid Nutrition: A Remarkable Evolution [10, 11]

The idea of intravenously infusion protein hydrolysates and amino acids arose simultaneously with the realization that ingested proteins are hydrolyzed in the gastrointestinal tract: the resulting low-molecular "building blocks" being subsequently absorbed and transported via the portal venous system to the liver. For the first time, Neumeister reported in 1889 that a mild alkaline hydrolysate of casein could be intravenously administered to experimental animals without producing signs of toxicity. In 1904, Friedrich infused nitrogen in form of a peptone solution together with fat, glucose, and salt. In the same year, Abderhalden and Rona injected enzymatic hydrolysates of casein which contains a mixture of amino acids and peptides. About 10 years later, Henriques and Andersen reported what is generally considered the first successful achievement of positive N balance by the continuous IV infusion of an enzymatic hydrolysate of meat, glucose and salt into a goat for 16 days.

The therapeutic implication of this experiment did not follow until 24 years later when Elman published the first of his many outstanding papers and classic monographs dealing with the experimental and clinical use of IV protein hydrolysates and amino acids. Elman could achieve positive N balance by infusion of a protein hydrolysate together with glucose. Subsequently, intensive studies performed by Wretlind led to the industrial production of enzymatic hydrolysate of casein containing up to 65% free amino acids and 35% low-molecular peptides. Until the 1960s, such preparations have been widely used in clinical practice for enteral and parenteral protein nutrition.

A milestone in clinical protein nutrition was the development of relatively inexpensive synthesis procedures for the large scale production of amino acids by Japanese scientists. The availability of crystalline amino acids opens the possibility to formulate and create a great variety of aqueous preparations for parenteral use. The composition of the first generation amino acid solutions were based on the so called "Rose-pattern": these preparations contained all essential L-amino acids according to the "safe intake" defined by William Rose and, in addition, glycine as non-specific nitrogen source as well as arginine and histidine. Several alternative approaches have been used to further optimize amino acid preparations, e.g. mixtures which are close to the amino acid composition of a protein with high biological value like potato-egg pattern. The plasma-/transfer-adapted solutions are based on the hypothesis that the plasma transfer rate of a selected amino acid determines its requirement. The clinical implication of these amino acid solutions, though based upon various theoretical approaches, generally reveals very similar effects upon pertinent-clinical chemical variables. Obvious differences in these formulations are only related to the number of amino acids included. Whether these differences in the concentrations of single essential and/or nonessential amino acids have any significance in clinical setting is still to be determined.

At the present time, many investigators are proceeding on the assumption that "tailored" solutions will increase the benefits of IV nutrition for specific patient groups [9, 11]. We have already seen the development of amino acid mixtures for the treatment of renal and liver disease. Other investigators are working on solutions to optimize the growth of young infants. Still other investigators hope for the use of solutions enriched in branched-chain amino acids. The postulated anabolic role of these amino acids on protein synthesis is highly controversial [9, 11].

Interpretation of Cellular Amino Acid Imbalance: The Intracellular Amino Acid Concept

Clinical observation has confirmed that practically every condition which is associated with weight loss is also associated with muscle wasting. The accelerated muscle protein breakdown in catabolic patients suggests an alteration of the cytoplasmic amino acid profile in muscle, which could affect protein synthesis at the cellular level in the ribosomes. Analysis of skeletal muscle tissue may provide the best estimation of the average intracellular composition in the whole organism, since skeletal muscle is by far the most abundant cellular tissue in the body and relatively uniform as to cellular composition [12].

The Unique Intracellular Pattern of Catabolism: The Effect of Nutrition

Free amino acid patterns in muscle have been measured in healthy man and in various catabolic conditions [13]. One important finding is that the concentrations of free amino acids in muscle change in response to changes in diet and physiological and pathological states. Each catabolic condition appears to have its own unique and reproducible intracellular pattern. Valine, like the other branched-chain amino acids (BCAA), increases in trauma and during starvation but is unchanged in diabetes. Glutamine, by contrast, decreases considerably in trauma and starvation but is unchanged in uremia and diabetes. In chronic uremia, selective decreases in valine and threonine are consistent findings. Changes in plasma free amino acid concentrations may parallel those in muscle, but frequently differ either quantitatively or qualitatively (Fig. 1). These results indicate that the intracellular free amino acid pattern of muscle is characterized by a "unique pattern of catabolism" distinctive for the disease or condition studied.

Interestingly, the unique pattern of trauma was apparently little influenced by parenteral nutrition. Alterations in the individual amino acid concentrations appeared not to be affected by the total amounts or mixtures of amino acids given. Surprisingly, the high amounts of amino acids given were not reflected in an increased amino acid pool in muscle, and the sustained decrease in muscle glutamine concentration persisted irrespective of nutritional efforts. Infusion of various amino acid solutions was accompanied by an increase of intracellular concentration of BCAA, especially those of valine and leucine [13]. The combined results suggest that the observed changes as well as the depleted pools of certain amino acids are due to imbalanced composition of the amino acids infused rather than the total amount given. Antagonism of structurally related amino acids such as leucine, isoleucine and valine have been reported earlier. Excess of any of these amino acids results in depression of growth which can be relieved by addition of the other two amino acids. Excessive intake of leucine depressed the isoleucine and valine levels in plasma and skeletal muscle; the decreased values are easily corrected by administration of isoleucine and valine [14]. There is evidence that amino acid imbalances and/or antagonisms result in a decrease in the pool of amino acids which is already limiting for protein synthesis and consequently stimulate amino acid catabolism and thereby cause increased requirement [14].

Intracellular glutamine depletion is a typical feature of the response of malnutrition, trauma and infection, irrespective of dietary regimen or the extent of injury. None of the solutions employed influenced the low intracellular glutamine concentration in the immediate post-injury state [13]. This finding is certainly due to the fact that none of the commercially available amino acid solutions contain glutamine (Vide infra).

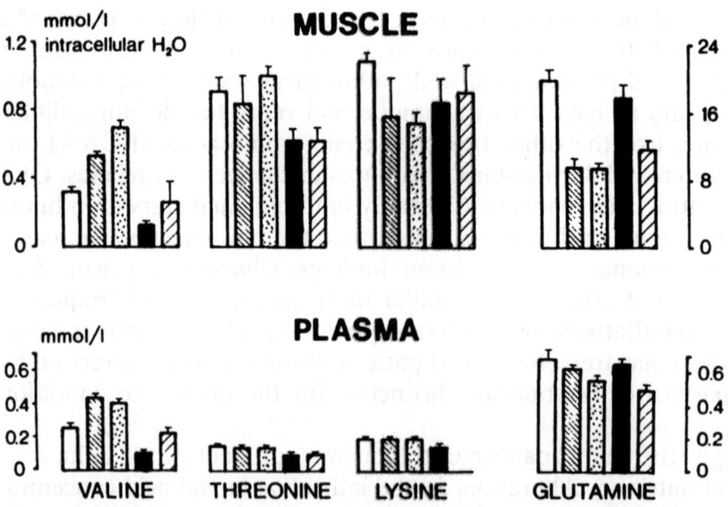

Fig. 1. Selected free amino acids in different catabolic states □ normal, ■ uremia-untreated, ▨ 11 day fast, ▨ diabetes-untreated, ▦ after total HIP replacement

Interpretation of Amino Acid Patterns

Successful normalization or partial correction of an abnormal plasma amino acid pattern is often taken as a guarantee of adequate amino acid utilization. However, the limitations inherent to methodology and to data interpretation are sadly often neglected. There are many factors which influence amino acid concentrations [13, 15]. Diurnal variation, previous nutrition, physical activity and technical errors should be considered. Age and sex are two further important factors affecting amino acid concentrations [15]. Measurements of free amino acids are usually made at a single point in time and an adequately controlled data base is of the utmost importance in deciding whether a subject manifests normal or abnormal amino acid metabolism.

An essential question is how to identify a pathological amino acid profile and whether the therapeutic intention should be to normalize, by whatever means, the pathological pattern. According to our opinion, it is worth striving to achieve a normal pattern if the high or low values are due to an amino acid imbalance or antagonism. Intracellular depletion of amino acids is always a sign of deficiency and thus might be corrected. Increase in the amino acid concentrations, without obvious presence of a concomitant imbalance, is, however, difficult to interpret and further investigations are therefore warranted.

We believe that direct measurements of muscle intracellular amino acid patterns in different catabolic situations may provide a better understanding of post-injury intracellular metabolism and assist in the development of guidelines to improve timing and composition of nutritional support.

The Concept of Conditionally Indispensable Amino Acids

One of the affected areas, clearly applicable to the practice of clinical nutrition, is of “tailor-made solutions” [9, 11]. Although many of the above nutrition formulae are now available, they have been designed to improve tolerance of nitrogen load in presence of illness, malnutrition or organ dysfunction rather than to provide specific nutrients for individual organs or tissues [16].

The present direction considers individual amino acids in single nutrients an important alternative approach. Certain diseases accompanied by deficiencies, antagonisms or imbalances in a particular compartment or in various organ tissues might selectively require one or more amino acids which are appropriate for use just in that given condition to support the attenuated tissue [9, 17]. In this situation, some classical “non-essential” amino acids have to be reconsidered to yield as “conditionally indispensable” substrates. Administration of required substrates might thus greatly facilitate an anabolic response to a life-threatening disease [18]. The major questions are: which particular amino acids should be considered, and in what amount should they be administered?

In the following, some potentially indispensable amino acids will be listed and their clinical implication scrutinized. The direct aims of these evaluations are to determine which amino acids in what particular clinical conditions are to be included in future parenteral solutions. Indeed, the final goal is to develop amino acid preparation with suitable composition for the treatment of the critically ill and/or special disorders.

Histidine

In infants, the evidence for a dietary histidine requirement was an early observation [19], whereas in adults, histidine was considered a dispensable amino acid. Recent studies in normal men, however, showed that long-term histidine-deficient diet (1–8 weeks) led to a significant fall in plasma histidine levels [20]. This observation seriously raised the question whether during long term TPN a supplementation with histidine might be beneficial.

In the early 1970s, Fürst and Bergström [21] could provide first evidence that histidine might be an indispensable amino acid in uremia. Accordingly, supplementation of tailored IV diets given to uremic patients with histidine resulted in a considerably improved, even positive N balance [22].

Serine

In healthy adults, serine can be readily synthesized from glycine and activated formaldehyde. Indeed, serine is the only non-essential amino acid which has been shown to stimulate protein synthesis *in vitro* [23]. In all clinical situations with impaired kidney function, endogenous synthesis might not cover serine requirements resulting in low extra- and intracellular serine concentrations [24]. These findings suggest that serine may be indispensable for uremic patients on maintenance hemodialysis, and that serine depletion may be another limiting factor for protein synthesis, thereby contributing to the increased protein requirements in these patients.

Arginine

Arginine as intermittant metabolite of the urea cycle significantly reduces blood ammonia and, thus, can counteract a high ammonia load administered with protein hydrolysates/amino acid solutions [25]. Currently, arginine receives new attention in the critically ill because of its potential role in immunomodulation [26]. It is hypothesized that arginine enhances the depressed immune response of individuals suffering from injury, surgical trauma, malnutrition, or sepsis. In experimental animals as well as in human studies, supplementation with arginine resulted in an improved cellular response, a decrease in trauma-induced reduction in the T-cell function, and a higher phagocytosis rate [27]. Moreover, daily supply of 30–35 g of arginine is claimed to retard tumor growth and to diminish tumor metastasis [36, 37]. When dealing with the parenteral supply of arginine, it is important to note that arginine has a specific drawback in its competition with lysine for tubular reabsorption (Fig. 2) [28]. Thus, parenteral administration of excessive amounts of arginine may result in lysine deprivation.

Taurine

Taurine (2-aminoethane sulfonic acid) is the most abundant free amine in the intracellular compartment [29]. Low muscle intracellular taurine concentrations are a typical feature in patients with chronic renal failure [30]. Intracellular taurine depletion might be associated with the well-known muscle fatigue in uremia. Additional functions of intracellular taurine like stabilization of the membrane potential and promotion of the calcium transport may render this amine as a positive ionotropic and antiarrhythmic agent.

There is some evidence that taurine might be indispensable during parenteral nutrition. Low taurine concentrations in plasma, platelet, and urine have been described in infants and children, but also in adult trauma patients undergoing taurine free long-term parenteral nutrition including methionine

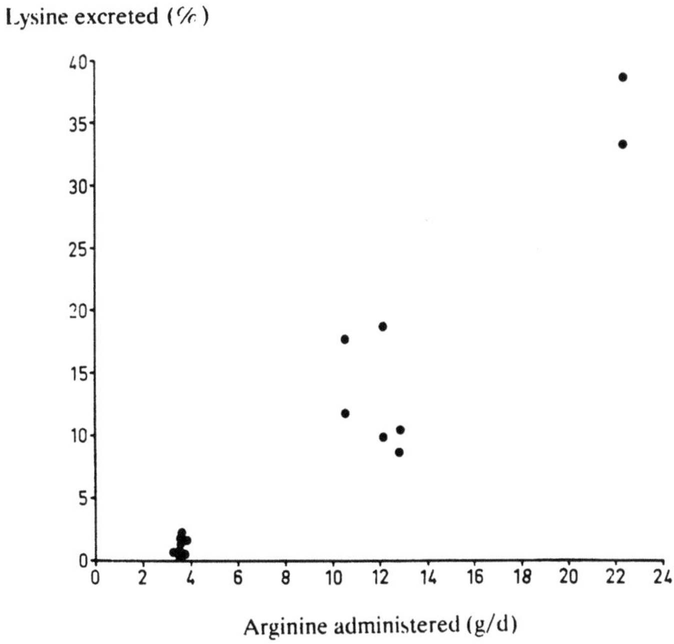

Fig. 2. Lysine excreted in human urine (expressed as % of amount infused, 2.6 g) plotted against the quantity of arginine simultaneously infused (From [28] with permission)

[31, 32]. Since these patients did not receive cysteine, which is a metabolic precursor of taurine, it could not be excluded that an inadequate conversion of methionine could contribute to low taurine levels. Plasma taurine deficiency after intensive chemotherapy and/or radiation was more severe in those patients receiving taurine free parenteral nutrition than in orally fed patients [33]. In pediatric TPN patients, low plasma taurine was accompanied by abnormal electroretinograms; addition of taurine (1.5–2.25 g/d) to the IV solutions restored plasma levels and normalized electroretinograms [31]. Kopple et al. [34] reported that 10 mg taurine/kg BW/d IV normalized plasma and blood cell taurine concentrations in long-term TPN patients.

Cyst(e)ine

In healthy adults, the sulfur-containing amino acid cysteine can be synthesized from methionine via the liver-specific transsulfuration pathway. In liver tissue of fetuses, preterm and term infants, the activity of cystathionase, key enzyme in the transsulfuration pathway, has been found to be low or undetectable [35]. In liver disease, cysteine requirements of the body cannot be covered due to diminished transsulfuration capacity. In all these particular conditions, cyst(e)ine should be exogenously administered [36].

Interestingly, the route of nutrient administration seems also to influence the rate of hepatic cysteine synthesis by altering the delivery of cysteine precursors to the liver. Stegink et al. [37] could demonstrate in healthy men that IV infusion of solutions containing methionine but no cysteine resulted in depressed levels of all three forms of circulating cysteine (free cysteine, free and protein-bound cystine). This result may suggest that parenteral solutions should not only contain sufficient methionine but additional amounts of cysteine. Presumably, such a supplementation with cysteine may be also beneficial with respect to taurine requirements during long-term TPN. Addition of cysteine to TPN solutions is however problematic. At neutral or slightly alkaline pH, cysteine rapidly oxidizes during heat sterilization and storage to yield the dimer cystine which itself is very poorly soluble and, thus, precipitates in the solution. Acidic conditions may lead to a reduction of the SH-group and the formation of H_2S.

Tyrosine

The aromatic amino acid tyrosine has been traditionally considered a nonessential amino acid for adult humans. Tyrosine is synthesized exclusively from phenylalanine by hydroxylation; inclusion of tyrosine in the diet exerts a sparing effect on the dietary phenylalanine requirement. However, under certain pathological conditions like classic phenylketonuria, liver and kidney diseases, and also in premature infants, tyrosine has to be considered a conditionally indispensable amino acid. The essentiality of tyrosine is attributed to lacking or diminished activity of liver phenylalanine hydroxylase or is due to reduced oxidation of tyrosine from phenylalanine resulting from a partial inhibition of this enzyme. In particular cases, a reduced endogenous tyrosine synthesis may also occur in full-term infants [38].

Rudman et al. [36, 39] reported that cirrhotic patients receiving a standard TPN exhibited hypotyrosinemia, hypocystinemia and hypotaurinemia. They suggested that these patients may have impaired liver capacity to synthesize these amino acids due to pathological alterations in liver tissue.

Due to its low solubility in aqueous solutions, the concentration of tyrosine in amino acid preparations does not exceed 0.4–0.5 g/L, an amount which might be insufficient to cover tyrosine requirements in the above mentioned situations.

Glutamine

Glutamine is the most prevalent free proteic amino acid in the human body. In skeletal muscle, glutamine constitutes more than 60% (>19.5 mM ICW) of the total free amino acid pool [29]. Glutamine acts not only as a precursor for protein synthesis but is an important intermediate in a large number of metabolic pathways. As the highest concentrated amino acid in the blood stream, glutamine serves as nitrogen transporter between various tissues.

It is well known that glutamine represents an important metabolic fuel for the cells of the GI tract (enterocytes, colonocytes) [40, 41]. Recently, overwhelming evidence have been brought forward that all rapidly proliferating cells, mainly those of the immune system, strictly depend on the availability of glutamine as energy (carbon, nitrogen) source [42]. Hypercatabolic and hypermetabolic situations are accompanied by a strong glutamine deprivation. After elective operations, major injury, burns, infections, and pancreatitis, intramuscular glutamine concentrations are decreased; the depletion being independent from nutritional efforts [9, 13].

Two recent observations suggest that glutamine is involved in the regulation of muscle protein balance: the striking direct correlation between muscle glutamine and the rate of protein synthesis, and the positive effect of maintaining intracellular glutamine content on protein anabolic processes *in vitro* [43, 44]. If maintenance of intracellular glutamine pool promotes conservation of muscle protein, there is a theoretical case for glutamine supplements in the parenteral nutrition of stressed and malnourished patients.

The inclusion of free glutamine in commercially available amino acid preparations is hampered by the quantitative decomposition of aqueous glutamine to the cyclic product pyroglutamic acid associated with ammonia liberation (Fig. 3) [45], and because of its limited solubility in water (2–3 g/100 mL). Glutamine-containing TPN solutions have to be freshly prepared under strict aseptic conditions and stored at 4°C (max. 2 days) as recommended by Khan and colleagues [46]. To diminish the risk of precipitation, the glutamine concentrations in such solutions should not exceed 1–1.5%. Consequent-

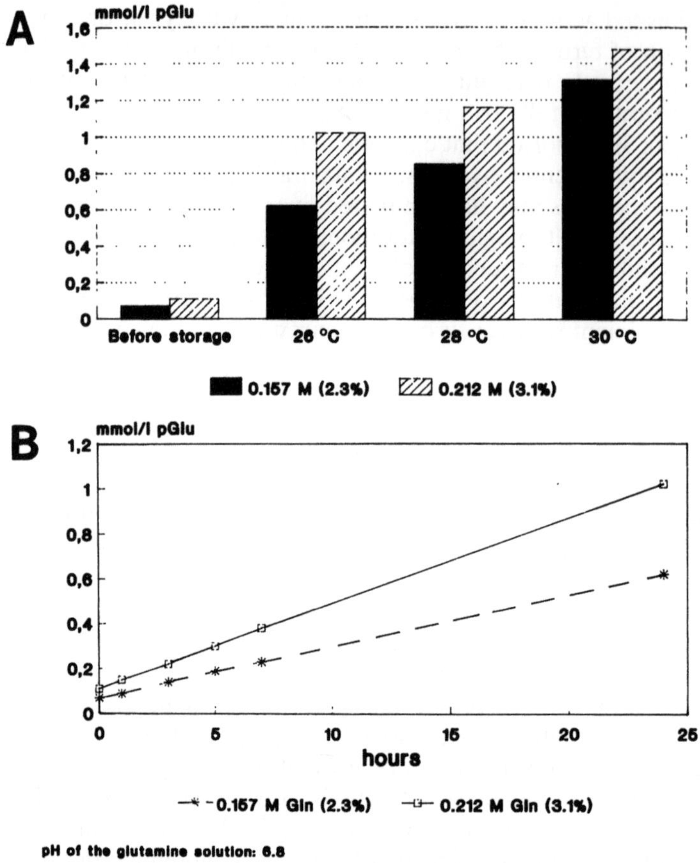

Fig. 3. Stability of glutamine during storage. Influence of temperature (A) and duration of storage (B) on pyroglutamic acid (pGlu) liberation

ly, provision of adequate amounts of glutamine to injured or critically ill patients with such a low concentrated solution represents a severe burden, especially in volume-restricted situations. Thus, the parenteral use of free glutamine is reserved for controlled and well-conducted clinical trials.

Pharmacokinetics and clinical/metabolic effects of IV administration of free glutamine have been investigated in healthy humans [47] as well as in selected patient population [48, 49]. Hammarqvist et al. [48] evaluated N balance, plasma and intracellular muscle amino acids in patients following elective cholecystectomy receiving glutamine-supplemented TPN. In the glutamine group, the postoperative decrease in the intracellular glutamine concentration as well as the cumulative N loss was less pronounced than in the control group. In patients undergoing allogenic bone marrow transplantation (BMT), glutamine enriched TPN (0.57 g glutamine/kg/d) resulted in an improved N balance and a significant reduced 3-methylhistidine/creatinine excretion ratio compared to controls receiving isocaloric and isonitrogenous TPN [49]. More importantly, post-BMT morbidity was diminished with glutamine supplementation: the incidence of clinical infection, total and site-specific microbial colonization, and the length of hospital stay were reduced compared with controls.

New Substrates in Protein Nutrition: The Dipeptide Concept

As mentioned, tyrosine and cysteine are poorly soluble, and glutamine is too unstable for addition to existing preparation in their native form. This drawback can be overcome by use of synthetic short-chain peptides. Undoubtedly, this new approach has introduced a new dimension, though the explosion of new information about peptide assimilation is only a prelude, prior to IV use of peptides in common clinical practice. The dipeptides are highly soluble in water and sufficiently stable during sterilization procedures to be approved by the authorities as constituents of parenteral solutions.

Basic studies with various synthetic glutamine-, tyrosine- and cysteine-containing short-chain peptides provide convincing evidence that these new substrates are rapidly cleared from plasma after parenteral administration without being accumulated in tissues and with inconsequential losses in urine. Considerable hydrolase activity in extra-/intracellular tissue compartments [50] ensures a quantitative peptide hydrolysis, the liberated amino acids being available for protein synthesis and/or generation of energy. Following a bolus injection or under conditions of continuous TPN, these peptides provide tyrosine, cystine, and glutamine, respectively, for maintenance of their intra- and/or extracellular pools. Parenteral dipeptide nutrition promotes growth and nitrogen retention [50–55]. Interestingly, IV provision of L-alanyl-L-glutamine (Ala-Gln) reduces muscle loss of glutamine during stress [56] and prevents intestinal mucosal atrophy in parenterally fed rats [57].

Human studies in healthy volunteers demonstrated that Ala-Gln [58], glycyl-L-tyrosine (Gly-Tyr) [58], and L-alanyl-L-tyrosine (Ala-Tyr) [59] are readily hydrolyzed after their bolus injection; the elimination half-time ranging between 3.3 and 5.8 min. Continuous infusion of a commercial amino acid solution supplemented with Ala-Gln and Gly-Tyr was not accompanied by any side effects and no complaints were reported [60].

In patients undergoing major elective surgery, infusion of Ala-Gln supplemented TPN over 5 days resulted in an improvement of the N balance on each postoperative day compared with controls receiving isonitrogenous and isoenergetic TPN without the peptides (Fig. 4) [61]. The improved net N balance was associated with maintenance of the intracellular glutamine pool, whereas in patients receiving the control solution, glutamine levels were markedly decreased compared to preoperative values (Fig. 5). The infusion of the solutions was free of any side effects, and postoperative recovery was normal for each patient.

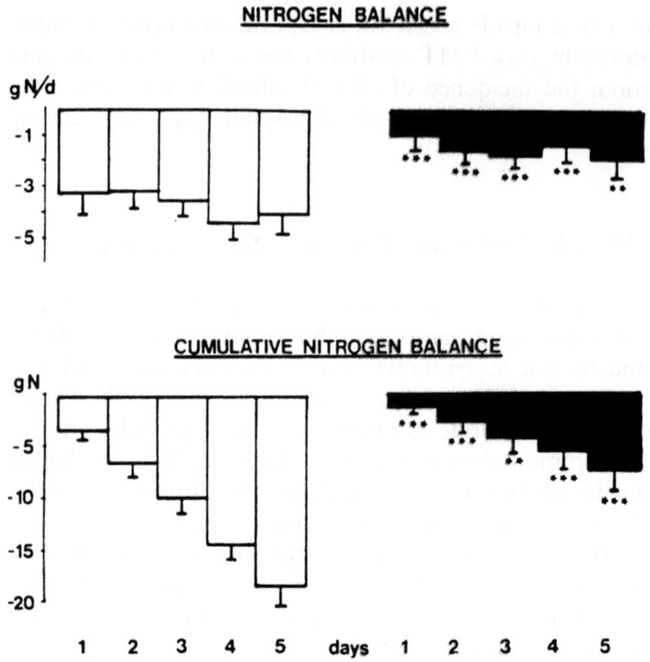

Fig. 4. Day-to-day and cumulative nitrogen balance (mean ± SEM, n = 6) in patients after major elective surgery receiving Ala-Gln (280 mg/kg BW per day) supplemented (*black columns*) or conventional TPN (*open columns*) ***p < 0.001; **p < 0.01

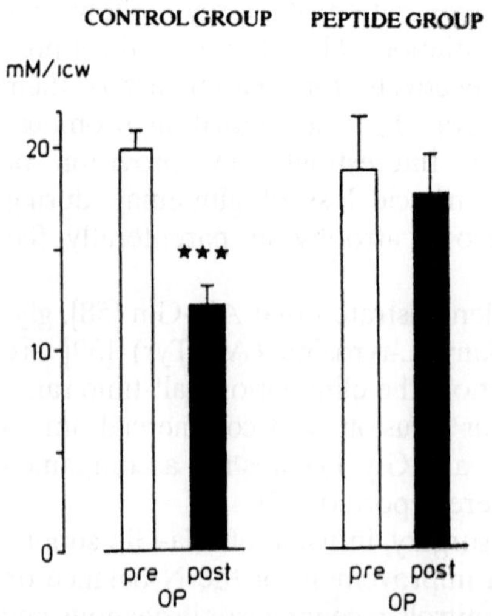

Fig. 5. Intracellular muscle glutamine concentration (mean ± SEM, n = 6) in control patients and in patients receiving Ala-Gln (280 mg/kg BW per day) supplemented TPN (peptide group).
icw, intracellular water; ***p < 0.001

In good agreement with these results, IV supply of Ala-Gln following cholecystectomy preserved the intracellular glutamine pool (91% of preoperative value), and the characteristic postoperative change in muscle ribosome profile was abolished [62]. Beneficial effects of short-term infusion of Ala-Gln on muscle protein synthesis assessed by [^{13}C]leucine incorporation were reported by Barua et al. [63] in post-surgical patients receiving glutamine free parenteral nutrition. Most importantly, current results of Tremel et al. [64] indicate that Ala-Gln supplemented parenteral nutrition may avoid TPN related intestinal atrophic response in ICU patients.

N-Acetylated Amino Acids

Early studies in experimental rats undergoing long-term TPN clearly have shown that highly soluble and stable N-acetylated amino acids, acetylcysteine, acetyltyrosine and acetylglutamine, are rapidly taken up and are subsequently hydrolyzed by acylases after their parenteral administration in dogs. However, poor utilization of parenterally supplied acetylglutamine was associated with a large urinary excretion (38% of the amount infused). Among the organs studied, only kidney cleared acetylglutamine in a measurable extent [9, 17].

Studies in healthy volunteers brought strong evidence forward that acetylated amino acids are only poorly metabolized in humans. Continuous infusion of acetylglutamine [65], acetyltyrosine, or acetylcysteine [66] resulted in an accumulation of the respective compound in plasma whereas no or minor effects on plasma levels could be observed (Fig. 6). The urinary excretion rate of the acetylated amino acids approached 40–50% of the amount given. After bolus injection of acetyltyrosine, Druml et al. [59] observed little if any hydrolysis of the acetylated amino acids.

In the light of these results, it is to be concluded that N-acetylated amino acids are poorly utilized in humans due to restricted acylase capacities.

Conclusion

Administration of required substrates might greatly facilitate an anabolic response to a life-threatening disease [18].

The present direction of clinical nutrition considers two main approaches. Provision of tailor-made solutions is an approach assuming increased benefits for specific patient groups like children, renal and liver diseases. Indeed, the presently available nutrition formulae have been designed to improve tolerance of nitrogen load rather than to provide an appropriate composition for individual organs or tissues. Consequently, an important alternative proposal is the consideration of individual amino acids as tissue/organ specific single nutrients. Accordingly, some "classic non-essential amino acids" like histidine, serine, arginine, tyrosine, cystine, taurine and glutamine have to be reconsidered as "conditionally indispensable" substrates. In order to overcome the problems associated with poor solubility (tyrosine and cystine) and instability (glutamine and cysteine) the dipeptide concept has been developed. By using modern biotechnological methods, stable and highly soluble glutamine, cystine and tyrosine containing dipeptides have been synthetized.

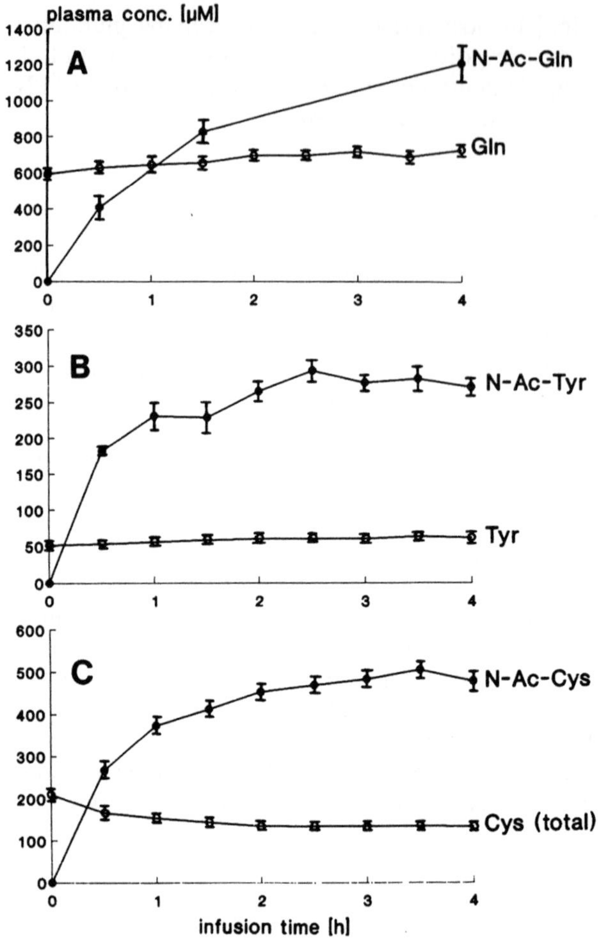

Fig. 6. Human plasma concentrations of acetylglutamine (Ac-Gln), acetyltyrosine (Ac-Tyr) and acetylcysteine (Ac-Cys) before and during intravenous infusion of Ac-Gln, Ac-Tyr and Ac-Cys, respectively (From [65, 66] with permission)

The dipeptides are efficiently and safely utilized in various clinical conditions.

Efficient protein metabolism requires the simultaneous presence of each proteic amino acid in appropriate proportions. The intracellular concentration of amino acids would then represent the balance between the rate of production (entry of amino acids into the intracellular pool) and the rate of the utilization of amino acids from this pool. Low intracellular amino acid concentrations may thus be due to either a decreased uptake from the extracellular compartment, or a reduction in protein catabolism, or an increased utilization.

An altered cellular amino acid pattern may affect ribosomal protein synthesis. The tissue pool size of the first limiting amino acid influences polysome aggregation [67]. It is known that the rate of polysome aggregation and the activity of amino acid activating enzymes regulate cellular protein syn-

Table 1. Are we giving imbalanced amino acid solutions?

Too much	Too little
Glycine	Valine
Phenylalanine	Serine
Leucine	Lysine[a]
Threonine?	Histidine?
Lacking (must be added)	
Glutamine (glutamine-peptide)	20–25 g/L
Tyrosine peptide	3 g/L
Cyst(e)ine-peptide	1–3 g/L
Taurine	1–2 g/L

[a] especially in association with high arginine nutrition?

thesis [68, 69]. In case of amino acid imbalance, the mechanism for protein synthesis would be presented with an amino acid substrate complex, not only low in concentration, but also of unsuitable composition. Therefore, regardless of its initial cause, the imbalance of cellular amino acids catabolic stress may be one of the fundamental inadequacies in cell nutrition adversely affecting protein synthesis.

Direct measurements of cellular amino acids indicate that proportion and requirements based on data from healthy subjects cannot be applied in catabolic patients. It appears that intravenous provision of glycine, phenylalanine, leucine and probably threonine is too excessive, while too little amounts of valine, serine and presumably lysine and histidine are administered. Glutamine, tyrosine, cystine and taurine are not included in presently available solutions. To develop suitable preparations for the treatment of critically ill patients these lacking amino acids (amine) must be incorporated in future solutions (Table 1).

References

1. Cuthbertson DP (1932) Observations of the disturbances of metabolism produced by injury to the limbs. Q J Med 1:223–230
2. Davies JWL, et al (1977) The nutrition of patients with burns. In: Richards JR, Kinney JM (eds) Nutritional aspects of care in the critically ill. Churchill Livingstone, London, pp 595–612
3. Van Way CW, Meng HC, Sandstead HH (1975) Nitrogen balance in postoperative patients receiving parenteral nutrition. Ann Surg 110:272–276
4. Fürst P, Bergström J, Kinney JM, Vinnars E (1977) Nutrition in post-operative catabolism. In: Richards JR, Kinney JM (eds) Nutritional aspects of care of the critically ill. Churchill Livingstone, Edinburgh, pp 389–410
5. Shenkin A, Neuhäuser M, Bergström J, et al (1980) Biochemical changes associated with severe trauma. Am J Clin Nutr 33:2119–2127

6. Iapichino G, Gattinoni L, Solca M, et al (1982) Protein sparing and protein replacement in acutely injured patients during TPN with and without amino acid supply. Intensive Care Med 8:25–31
7. Kinney JM, Elwyn DH (1983) Protein metabolism and injury. Annu Rev Nutr 3:433–466
8. Moore FD, Brennan MR (1975) Intravenous amino acids. N Engl J Med 293:194–195
9. Fürst P, Stehle P (1992) New substrates for protein nutrition. In: Schlierf G (ed) Recent advances in clinical nutrition. Smith-Gordon, London, pp 213–229
10. Levenson SM; Hopkins BS, Waldron M, Canham JE, Seifter E (1984) Early history of parenteral nutrition. Fed Proc 43:1391–1406
11. Fürst P, Stehle P (1990) Künstliche Ernährung – gestern, heute, morgen. Infusionsther Klin Ern 17:237–244
12. Fürst P (1985) Regulation of intracellular metabolism of amino acids. In: Bozetti F, Dionigi R (eds) Nutrition in trauma and cancer sepsis. Karger, Basel, pp 21–53
13. Fürst P (1983) Intracellular muscle free amino acids – their measurement and function. Proc Nutr Soc 42:451–462
14. Harper AE (1964) Amino acid toxicities and imbalances. In: Munro HN, Allison JB (eds) Mammalian protein metabolism. Academic Press, New York, pp 87–134
15. Fürst P (1983) Criteria underlying the formulation of amino acid regimens: Established and new approaches. In: Kleinberger G, Deutsch E (eds) New aspects of clinical nutrition. Karger, Basel, New York, pp 361–376
16. O'Dwyer ST, Smith RJ, Kripke SA, Settle RG, Rombeau JL (1990) New fuels for the gut. In: Rombeau JL, Caldwell MD (eds) Clinical nutrition: Enteral and tube feeding. WB Saunders Co, Philadelphia, pp 540–555
17. Fürst P, Stehle P (1993) The potential use of parenteral dipeptides in clinical nutrition. Nutr in Pract 8 (in press)
18. Wilmore DW (1989) The practice of clinical nutrition: How to prepare for the future. JPEN 13:337–343
19. Snyderman SE (1970) The protein and amino acid requirements of the premature infant. In: Jonxis JHP, Visser HKA, Troelstra JA (eds) Metabolic processes in the foetus and newborn infant. Stenfert Kroese, Leiden, pp 128–141
20. Anderson HL, Cho ES, Wixom RL (1986) Effects of long-term, low histidine diet on men. In: Fürst P, Kluthe R (eds) Histidine III. Wissenschaftliche Verlagsgesellschaft, Stuttgart, pp 2–25
21. Fürst P (1972) 15N-studies in severe renal failure. II. Evidence for the essentiallity of histidine. Scand J Clin Lab Invest 30:307–312
22. Fürst P (1989) Amino acid metabolism in uremia. J Am Coll Nutr 8:310–323
23. Galbraith RA, Buse MG (1981) Effects of serine on protein synthesis and insulin receptors. Am J Physiol 241:C167–C171
24. Bergström J, Alvestrand A, Fürst P (1990) Plasma and muscle free amino acids in maintenance hemodialysis patients without protein malnutrition. Kidney Int 38:108–114
25. Najarian N, Harper AE (1956) A clinical study of the effect of arginine on blood ammonia. Am J Med 21:832–842
26. Kirk SJ, Barbul A (1990) Role of arginine in trauma, sepsis, and immunity. JPEN 14:226S–229S
27. Daly JM, Reynolds J, Thom A (1988) Immune and metabolic effects of arginine in the surgical patients. Ann Surg 208:512–523
28. Vinnars E, Fürst P, Hallgren B, Hermansson IL, Josephson B (1970) The nutritive effect in man of non-essential acids infused intravenously (together with the essential ones). I. Individual non-essential amino acids. Acta Anaesth Scand 14:147–172
29. Bergström J, Fürst P, Noree LO, Vinnars E (1974) Intracellular free amino acid concentration in human muscle tissue. J Appl Physiol 36:693–697
30. Bergström J, Alvestrand A, Fürst P, Lindholm B (1989) Sulphur amino acids in plasma and muscle in patients with chronic renal failure. Evidence for taurine depletion. J Int Med 226:189–194

31. Geggel HS, Ament ME, Heckenlively JR, Martin DA, Kopple BS, Kopple JD (1985) Nutritional requirement for taurine in patients receiving long-term parenteral nutrition. N Engl J Med 312:142–146
32. Zelikovic I, Chesney RW, Friedman AL, Ahlfors CE (1990) Taurine depletion in very low birth weight infants receiving prolonged total parenteral nutrition: Role of renal immaturity. J Pediatr 116:301–306
33. Desai TK, Maliakkal J, Kinzie JL, Ehrinpreis MN (1992) Taurine deficiency after intensive chemotherapy and/or radiation. Am J Clin Nutr 55:708–711
34. Kopple JD, Vinton NE, Laidlaw SA, Ament ME (1990) Effect of intravenous taurine supplementation on plasma, blood cell, and urine taurine concentrations in adults undergoing long-term parenteral nutrition. Am J Clin Nutr. 52:846–853
35. Sturman JA, Gaull G, Räihä NCR (1970) Absence of cystathionase in human fetal liver. Is cystine essential? Science 169:74–75
36. Chawla RK, Lewis FW, Kutner M, Bate DM, Roy RGB, Rudman D (1984) Plasma cysteine, cystine, and glutathione in cirrhosis. Gastroenterology 87:770–776
37. Stegink LD, Den Besten L (1972) Synthesis of cysteine from methionine in normal adult subjects: Effect of route of alimentation. Science 178:514–516
38. Räihä NCR (1973) Phenylalanine hydroxylase in human liver during development. Pediat Res 7:1–4
39. Rudman D, Williams PJ (1985) Nutrient deficiencies during total parenteral nutrition. Nutr Rev 43:1–13
40. Windmueller HG, Spaeth AE (1974) Uptake and metabolism of plasma glutamine by the small intestine. J Biol Chem 249:5070–5079
41. Souba WW (1991) Glutamine: A key substrate for the splanchnic bed. Annu Rev Nutr 11:285–308
42. Newsholme EA, Newsholme P, Curi R, Challoner E, Ardawi MSM (1988) A role for muscle in the immune system and its importance in surgery, trauma, sepsis and burns. Nutrition 4:261–268
43. Jepson MM, Bates PC, Broadbent P, Pell JM, Millward DJ (1988) Relationship between glutamine concentration and protein synthesis in rat skeletal muscle. Am J Physiol 255:E166–E172
44. MacLennan PA, Brown RA, Rennie MJ (1987) A positive relationship between protein synthetic rate and intracellular glutamine concentration in perfused rat skeletal muscle. FEBS (Lett) 215:187–191
45. Fürst P, Albers S, Stehle P (1990) Glutamine-containing dipeptides in parenteral nutrition. JPEN 14:118S–124S
46. Khan K, Hardy G, McElroy B, Elia M (1991) The stability of L-glutamine in total parenteral nutrition solutions. Clin Nutr 10:193–198
47. Lowe DK, Benfell K, Smith RJ, et al (1990) Safety of glutamine-enriched parenteral nutrient solutions in humans. Am J Clin Nutr 52:1101–1106
48. Hammarqvist F, Wernerman J, Ali R, Von der Decken A, Vinnars E (1989) Addition of glutamine to total parenteral nutrition after elective abdominal surgery spares free glutamine in muscle, counteracts the fall in muscle protein synthesis, and improves nitrogen balance. Ann Surg 209:455–461
49. Ziegler TR, Young LS, Benfell K, et al (1992) Clinical and metabolic efficacy of glutamine-supplemented parenteral nutrition after bone marrow transplantation. A randomized, double-blind, controlled study. Ann Intern Med 116:821–828
50. Fürst P (1991) Peptides in clinical nutrition. Clin Nutr 10:519–524
51. Daabees TT, Stegink LD (1978) L-alanyl-L-tyrosine as a tyrosine source during intravenous nutrition of the rat. J Nutr 108:1104–1113
52. Neuhäuser M (1985) Utilization of glycyl-L-tyrosine during long-term parenteral nutrition in the growing rat. Clin Nutr 4 (Suppl):124–130
53. Stehle P, Ratz I, Fürst P (1989) In vivo utilization of intravenously supplied L-alanyl-L-glutamine in various tissues of the rat. Nutrition 5:411–415
54. Stehle P, Ratz I, Fürst P (1991) Whole-body autoradiography in the rat after intravenous bolus injection of L-alanyl-L-[U-^{14}C]glutamine. Ann Nutr Metab 35:213–220

55. Stehle P, Albers S, Pollack L, Fürst P (1988) In vivo utilization of cystine-containing synthetic short chain peptides after intravenous bolus injection in the rat. J Nutr 118:1470–1474
56. Roth E, Karner J, Ollenschläger G, Simmel A, Fürst P, Funovics J (1988) Alanylglutamine reduces muscle loss of alanine and glutamine in postoperative anaesthetized dogs. Clin Sci 75:641–648
57. Tamada H, Nezu R, Imamura I, et al (1992) The dipeptide alanyl-glutamine prevents intestinal mucosal atrophy in parenterally fed rats. JPEN 16:110–116
58. Albers S, Wernerman J, Stehle P, Vinnars E, Fürst P (1988) Availability of amino acids supplied intravenously in healthy man as synthetic dipeptides: Kinetic evaluation of L-alanyl-L-glutamine and glycyl-L-tyrosine. Clin Sci 75:463–468
59. Druml W, Lochs H, Roth E, Hübl W, Balcke P, Lenz K (1991) Utilization of tyrosine dipeptides and acetyltyrosine in normal and uremic humans. Am J Physiol 260:E280–E285
60. Albers S, Wernerman J, Stehle P, Vinnars E, Fürst P (1989) Availability of amino acids supplied by constant intravenous infusion of synthetic dipeptides in healthy man. Clin Sci 76:643–648
61. Stehle P, Zander J, Mertes N, et al (1989) Effect of parenteral glutamine peptide supplements on muscle glutamine loss and nitrogen balance after major surgery. Lancet 1:231–233
62. Hammarqvist F, Wernerman J, Von der Decken A, Vinnars E (1990) Alanyl-glutamine counteracts the depletion of free glutamine and the postoperative decline in protein synthesis in skeletal muscle. Ann Surg 212:637–644
63. Barua JM, Wilson E, Downie S, Weryk B, Cuschieri A, Rennie MJ (1992) The effect of alanyl-glutamine peptide supplementation on muscle protein synthesis in post-surgical patients receiving glutamine-free amino acids intravenously. Proc Nutr Soc 51:104A
64. Tremel H, Kienle B, Weilemann LS, et al (1992) Glutamine dipeptide supplemented TPN maintains intestinal function in critically ill. Clin Nutr 11:25 (Abst)
65. Magnusson I, Kihlberg R, Alvestrand A, Wernerman J, Ekman L, Wahren J (1989) Utilization of intravenously administered N-acetyl-L-glutamine in humans. Metabolism 38 (Suppl 1):82–88
66. Magnusson I, Ekman L, Wangdahl M, Wahren J (1989) N-acetyl-L-tyrosine and N-acetyl-L-cysteine as tyrosine and cysteine precursors during intravenous infusion in humans. Metabolism 38:957–961
67. Clement CY, Harper AE (1974) Liver polysome profile and protein synthesis in rats fed a threonine-imbalanced diet. J Nutr 104:252–260
68. Gaetani S, Paulucci AM, Spadoni MA, Tomassi G (1964) Activity of amino acid activating enzymes in tissues from protein depleted rats. J Nutr 84:173–181
69. Noda K, Taniguchi H, Kitasaka R (1975) Effect of amino acid imbalance on protein synthesis of skeletal muscle and liver in rats. Nutr Rep Inter 11:129–134

Anabolic Drive in Critically Ill Patients: Pros and Cons a Prevailing Glucose System

G. Iapichino and D. Radrizzani

Introduction

In view of the influence of different calorie substrates on protein metabolism, we need to consider the interactions between substrate disposal and hormonal control of body metabolism that constitute the so called "anabolic drive" [1]. Moreover, we know that amino acids have a dominant role in regulating protein synthesis. The role of amino acids exceeds that of calories and is in part independent from their property to induce the production of insulin and other hormones involved in protein metabolism [1–6].

There is also a body of evidence that nutrient assumption induces metabolic processes like absorption, interconversion, oxidative disposal or storage and ultimately changes in body composition and weight [7]. These metabolic effects differ from nutrient to nutrient, and could variably affect protein and thus energy metabolism [8].

Hitherto, the best way to study the protein sparing properties of different calorie substrates is to minimize the anabolic effect of amino acids by reducing the protein supply, and possibly not to overcome the measured or presumed calorie needs to avoid important increases in energy metabolism. Moreover, if the treatment supports enough energy and nitrogen (N), it is quite unlikely to see any difference in N retention in non-catabolic and non-malnourished subjects because of the inability of normally nourished, non-catabolic individuals to increase their body cell mass (BCM), i.e. to develop a positive N balance [9]. Many authors directly addressed this topic comparing glucose and lipid system, and the extensive literature is controversial, probably due to the above methodological considerations. Further information comes from several available studies on N retention (protein metabolism) conducted with different calorie systems but not primarily addressed to explore the role of glucose and lipids. Moreover, the relationship between calorie system, insulin plasma levels, and the resulting protein balance could be explored for further insights.

The aim of this chapter is to review, as widely as possible, the literature on these topics, also taking into account the potential confounding factors like methodological differences (experimental design, sample size and matching of control groups, time span of the study, quality and amount of both energy and amino acids utilized, insulin supply and sensitivity of the methods adopted to measure the experimental response), clinical characteristics, and metabolic environment (age, disease process, nutritional status, degree and stability of the stress reaction during the study and clinical course: complicate or uneventful) of studied subjects. The majority of the studies deal with IV nutritional support.

Glucose vs Glucose-Fat Mixed System

Normal Man

In normal adults, glucose is the substrate with the strongest action on the protein metabolism [10, 11]. Lipids have a minor effect by their glycerol content [12]. Nevertheless a full energy dose of fats, associated with amino acids, can minimize a negative N balance [13].

Two recent reports seem at variance. Parenteral repletion after 10 days of starvation in volunteers [14] reduced the whole body protein breakdown, eventually reaching a net N retention regardless of the calories' source (glucose vs 50% mixed system). However, the N supply, a far more important regulator of protein synthesis [1, 5, 6], was so large (0.29 g of N/kg in spite of fasting urinary N loss of 0.10 g/kg) and the non-protein energy load so high (35 kcal/kg/day) that, even in the lipid subset, glucose plus glycerol intake (18 kcal) exactly coped with the fasting REE of these subjects.

A 14-day study period in volunteers [8] fed with diet yielding 37 kcal and 1 g protein/kg maintained N balance irrespectively of the substrate composition (fat/glucides 1/1 or 1/2). Again, the high fat diet supplied glucides and glycerol in an amount, able to exactly cope the measured REE (21 kcal/kg) so that nutritional allowance of the subjects were widely met with both diets. Hence, it is not surprising that no difference was found.

Malnourished Patients Marginally or not Stressed

Eleven comparisons are available (Table 1). 5 were in favor of glucose, 1 of a 60% fat system [15], and 5 found no difference. A critical review of the studies strenghtens the influence of glucose. The 4 studies performed with a not so large N intake (0.16–0.22) as to obscure the influence of calorie substrate [9, 16–18], resulted in a better protein sparing action of the glucose system. In the 5th study [19] the glucose system resulted in a greater increase of BCM even if the treatment yielded less nonprotein kcal (35 vs 42 kcal/kg) and N (0.19 vs 0.27 gN/kg) than 70% lipid system.

At variance, a study planned with high N intake resulted in a better body protein accretion with the 60% lipid system [15]. However, the assessment of protein balance was performed with neutron activation analysis, a method that lacks sufficient sensitivity for short-term treatment [20, 21]. Moreover, a study with the same design and method of assessment of protein balance, carried out later in the same institution [22], failed to show any difference

Table 1. Glucose vs mixed system in malnourished patients

Authors	Ref.	No of Pts	No of days of TPN	Non-protein kcal/kg	Glucose %	gN_i/kg	N Bal g/kg
Tulikoura and	[16]	9	12	48	100	0.18	+0.06
Huikuri (1981)		8	12	54	44	0.18	+0.05[b]
Iapichino	[17]	8	8	47	100	0.22	+0.019
et al. (1987)		8	8	48	66	0.22	−0.020[b]
Jeejeebhoy	[18]	24	7	40	100	0.16	+0.058
et al. (1976)			7	40	17	0.16	+0.044[b]
Shizgal and	[9]	55[a]	14	44	98	0.20	36 kcal
Forse (1980)		29[a]	14	52	53	0.22	55 kcal[b,c]
Shizgal and	[19]	23[a]	15	35	99	0.19	+0.062
Forse (1981)		23[a]	15	42	32	0.27	+0.014[b]
Macfie	[15]	16	14	49	100	0.31	TBN=
et al. (1981)		16	14	51	41	0.32	TBN↓
Almond	[22]	12	14	41	100	0.28	TBN=, TBK↑
et al. (1989)		12	14	40	42	0.28	TBN=
Nordenstrom	[23]	5	7	31	100	0.40	+0.092
et al. (1983)			7	32	50	0.40	+0.088
Gazzaniga	[24]	18	16	6–35	100	0.15–0.20	[d]
et al. (1975)			15	4–38	20	0.13–0.19	
Shaw and	[25]	15	5 h	24±10	100	0	−0.39[e]
Holdaway (1988)		11	5 h	29±27	0	0	−0.31[e]
		9	5 h	id	100	0	−0.18[e]
		8	5 h	id	0	0	−0.13[e]

[a] many patients underwent > one study; [b] significant difference; [c] np kcal needed to maintain BCM; [d] NS difference in the number of positive N Bal days; [e] net protein catabolism.

between the two systems. This study recorded a significant increase of TBK^+ only with the glucose system. Even though this is controversial, TBK^+ increase is generally related to an increase in BCM [21].

The other 4 comparisons (no differences) include a study planned with a huge N supply [23] as to obscure the calorie effect, a study in which the nutrient intake was very variable [24], and a sophisticated isotopic study performed with glucose and pure lipids without amino acids supply [25]. Forty-three of the 80 patients were malnourished patients with gastrointestinal cancer divided according the upper and lower location of the cancer. The experimental protocol raises some questions, i.e. the clinical meaning of only 5 h of substrate infusion (particularly fat) with a calorie infusion rate presented for the whole patient population. When it was recalculated, it showed a huge variability especially for the lipid regimen.

Catabolic Patients

These are patients studied just after surgery [23, 26–30], trauma [23, 29, 31, 32], burn [30, 31] or medical illness [32]; many are infected [23, 29, 30, 32]. The increase in REE and N loss ranges from a minimum increase in elective surgery to a maximum in septic or burned patients.

Nutritional status was clearly defined in the majority of studies. The studies that enrolled only postoperative surgical patients [26–28] were quite satisfactory with respect to the patients homogeneity. All the others included patients with a variable degree of stress and nutritional status. Anyway, 8 comparisons are available (Table 2), 4 are in favor of glucose, 1 in favor of a 50% mixed system, and 3 did not find any difference. Going into details, the glucose system was further strenghened.

Among the studies in favor of glucose, 2 were conducted with low N intake [26, 31], 1 with and without N intake [30], and 1 had a variable clinical TPN protocol [29].

The study supporting a mixed system [32] included a mix of septic, ventilated patients. Notwithstanding the moderate-low N intake, both groups resulted in a positive N balance (protein turnover and N determination) as it was expected in an overall malnourished population. Indeed, this population had received an inadequate calorie and protein intake for a mean of 2.2 weeks prior to the study. Moreover, the lipid group included much older and significantly more depleted patients than the glucose group. In view

Table 2. Glucose vs mixed system in stressed-catabolic patients

Authors	Ref.	No of Pts	No of days of TPN	Non-protein kcal/kg	Glucose %	gN_i/kg	N Bal g/kg
Henneberg	[26]	10	10	35	91	0.16	+0.004
et al. (1985)		10	10	35	20	0.16	−0.05[a]
Woolfson	[31]	8	3	34	100	0.13	0.12
et al. (1979)			3	34	58	0.13	0.14[a]
Gazzaniga	[29]	8	8	33	100	0.27	+0.047
et al. (1985)		9	7	29	0	0.27	−0.027[a]
		10	8	34	25	0.23	−0.012
Long	[30]	5	3–12	[b]	[b]	[b]	UPR↓[a]
et al. (1977)							
Roulet	[32]	5	4	26	100	0.21	+0.003
et al. (1983)		6	4	29	50	0.19	+0.09[a]
Nordenstrom	[23]	8	4	29	100	0.28	+0.004
et al. (1983)		11	4	31	55	0.29	−0.02
Dworkin	[28]	17	7	440	100	0.19	−18[c]
et al. (1983)		11	7	550	0	0.19	−28[c]
Bark	[27]	4	6	50	100	0.3	−0.025
et al. (1976)		5	6	50	30	0.3	−0.01

[a] significant difference; [b] variable amount; [c] cumulative N Bal g.

of these flaws in group matching, the results should be interpreted cautiously.

Among the 3 studies showing no difference between calorie systems, two were conducted with a consistent N load in gastroresected [27] and in catabolic injured or infected patients [23]. Notwithstanding the large N load, the latter study showed an evident trend in favor of the glucose system. The 3rd study (hypocaloric, normo N supply in cystectomized patients) [28], showed a non-significant trend in favor of the glucose system.

Studies with Major Heterogeneity in Design

Four studies planned to compare glucose and fats did not find any difference between the two protocols (Table 3). Several flaws in experimental design could have influenced these results.

The first study [33] included 25 patients with a variety of illnesses: 13 had benign GI diseases, 2 were receiving chemotherapy, 3 had carcinoma resected, 4 sepsis and 3 had severe burns. All patients studied except the septic patients had lost more than 10% of their BW prior to the institution of TPN. The calorie intake ranged 18–85 kcal/kg and the N intake 0.08–0.24 gN.

The second study [34] included 20 critically ill mechanically ventilated patients with a wide variety of illnesses, and entered the 14-day study one week after ICU admission. However, when compared to the predicted value, the measured fasting REE was identical in 6, higher in 8, and lower in 6 patients. Moreover, the patients BW ranged from 59 to 168% of their ideal BW. Six patients were in the range of +10 to +20% and 6 patients were over +20%. Nevertheless, substrate supply was based on actual BW and the results were normalized for it.

Table 3. Glucose vs mixed system in miscellanea patients (The treatment resulted in no difference)

Authors	Ref.	No of Pts	No of days of TPN	non-protein kcal/kg	Glucose %	gN_i/kg
Bocking	[33]	13	14–21	18–25	100	0.08–0.24
et al. (1980)		12	14–21	22–43	40	
Baker	[34]		4–7	40	100	0.16
et al. (1984)		20[a]	4–7	40	75	0.16
			4–7	40	25	0.16
Glynn	[35]	6	5	20–32	100	0.16–0.25
et al. (1987)			5		30	
Shaw and	[25]	14	5 h	24±10	100	0
Holdaway (1988)		24	5 h	29±27	0	0

[a] many patients underwent > one study.

The third study [35] included 6 gastroenterological patients in stable conditions who had no recent surgery. Four patients were depleted, at least 2 were septic from the beginning, and 1 became septic during the 5 day glucose crossover period. Moreover, N intake ranged from 0.16 to 0.25 gN/kg and calorie intake ranged from 20 to 32 kcal/kg.

Finally, the fourth comparison (between pure glucose and pure fat, no N regimen) [25] is presented in the previously mentioned study including malnoursihed patients; 38 of the 81 patients were affected by sepsis and/or trauma. In addition to the methodological question discussed before about malnourished patients no information was available about age, nutritional status, severity of trauma and time of the study in relation to the phase of injury and stress.

In conclusion, the analysis of the glucose vs fat studies demonstrate that:

- a mixed system does probably not show a better protein sparing of fat than a glucose system;
- a glucose system results in a better protein sparing of fat when the studies are planned with appropriate methodology. This applies to normal subjects as well as patients. Nine of 23 comparisons performed on patients favored a glucose system;
- Many of the studies conducted in healthy as well as in patients (12/23) that showed no difference were conducted with a methodological design that was probably unable to find any effects. Nevertheless, 3 of these comparisons in patients still show a trend in favor of a glucose system.

Analysis of Clinical Studies

The available studies on metabolic nutritional support were stratified according to clinical results, i.e. the degree of protein replacement. We separated the studies performed on malnourished, catabolic marginally or not stressed patients, from the studies on catabolic patients.

Malnourished Patients

We found 27 groups of patients treated within a range of 0.16–0.40 gN/kg and 27–56 nonprotein kcal/kg/day (Table 4). An insufficient clinical result (negative net protein balance or steady BCM), was obtained in 5 groups: 3 were treated with a 44% [17], 50% [36], and 60% [22] lipid system, respectively, and 2 with a glucose system [15, 22]. One of these groups [22] showed an increase of TBK^+.

Twenty-two of 27 study groups showed the possibility to reach an accrual of body protein stores in malnourished patients. Seven of 22 groups were treated with 50–80% lipid system [9, 15, 16, 18, 19, 23, 36]. The others 15/22 groups received a 95–100% glucose system.

Table 4. Clinical studies in malnourished patients

Authors	Ref.	No of Pts	No of days of TPN	non-protein kcal/kg	Glucose %	gN_i/kg
Negative results						
Almond et al. (1989)	[22]	12	14	40	42	0.28[e]
Shaw (1988)	[36]	8[a]	7	40	50	0.27
Iapichino et al. (1987)	[17]	8	8	48	66	0.22
Macfie et al. (1981)	[15]	16	14	49	100	0.31
Almond et al. (1989)	[22]	12	14	41	100	0.28[f]
Positive Results						
Shaw (1988)	[36]	4[b]	7	40	50	0.27
Macfie et al. (1981)	[15]	16	14	51	41	0.32
Jeejeebhoy et al. (1976)	[18]	24[c]	7	40	17	0.16
Tulikoura and Huikuri (1981)	[16]	8	12	54	44	0.18
Nordenstrom et al. (1983)	[23]	5[c]	7	32	50	0.40
Shizgal and Forse (1980)	[9]	29[d]	14	52	53	0.22
Shizgal and Forse (1981)	[19]	35	15	42	32	0.27
Tulikoura and Huikuri (1981)	[16]	9	12	48	100	0.18
Nordenstrom et al. (1983)	[23]	5[c]	7	31	100	0.40
Burt et al. (1984)	[61]	11[a]	14	36	100	0.26
Iapichino et al. (1987)	[17]	8	8	47	100	0.22
Robin et al. (1989)	[40]	8	6	29	100	0.29
Shizgal and Posner (1989)	[21]	51[d]	15	49	94	0.24
		39[d]	15	43	95	0.20
Forse et al. (1990)	[60]	12[c]	8	27	93	0.50
Loder et al. (1990)	[99]	9[c]	3	28	100	0.20
			3	42	100	0.30
			3	56	100	0.40
Jeejeebhoy et al. (1976)	[18]	24[c]	7	40	100	0.16
Shizgal and Forse (1980)	[9]	55[d]	14	44	98	0.20
		50[d]	14	44	94	0.38
Shizgal and Forse (1981)	[19]	23[d]	15	35	99	0.19

[a] cancer patients; [b] no cancer patients; [c] crossover study; [d] many patients underwent > one study; [e] TBN and TBK do not vary; [f] TBK increases.

Better nutritional state and higher stress level can inversely affect the efficacy of the metabolic treatment [9, 19, 36]. Even though patients from all these studies have a different metabolic environment, studies should guarantee a roughly casual distribution of depleted and stressed patients between the 2 treatment groups. In conclusion, 15 of 17 glucose systems resulted in positive protein balance (and another in positive TBK^+ balance), and 7 of 10 with mixed systems.

Stressed Patients with Variable Degree of Malnutrition

To reduce the variability of this kind of patients and to better compare different studies, the stress reaction was considered as moderate or severe, according to the REE and/or N losses [37, 38].

Moderately stressed patients. Patients with a REE < 25 kcal/kg/day [23, 32, 39–41], or with urinary N loss < 15 g/day [26, 27, 29, 38, 42, 43]. This resulted in 21 groups of patients, some of which including also severely stressed patients, as reported or judged by the variability of the fasting REE [23, 29, 40, 41], or the N output [38, 43]. Malnutrition was also present, particularly in the studies by Greig et al. [41] and Roulet et al. [32]. A criteria for inclusion was a treatment with at least 18 non protein kcal/kg and 0.16 gN/kg/day (Table 5). A negative N balance was obtained in 8 of 21 groups; including 6 with a mixed system (50–100% fat) [23, 26, 27, 29, 41], and 2 with a glucose system [27, 42]. A zero or marginally positive N balance was reached in 13 of 21

Table 5. Clinical studies in moderately stressed catabolic patients

Authors	Ref.	No of Pts	No of days of TPN	non-protein kcal/kg	Glucose %	gN_i/kg
Marginally negative results						
Henneberg et al. (1985)	[26]	10	10	35	20	0.16
Greig et al. (1987)	[41]	6[a]	6	29	50	0.19
Nordenstrom et al. (1983)	[23]	8	4	31	55	0.29
Gazzaniga et al. (1985)	[29]	9	7	29	0	0.27
		10	8	34	25	0.23
Bark et al. (1976)	[27]	5	6	50	30	0.3
Tulikoura et al. (1988)	[42]	14	3	34	100	0.19
Bark et al. (1976)	[27]	4	6	50	100	0.3
Positive results						
Brandi et al. (1990)	[39]	7	2	27	63	0.19
Greig et al. (1987)	[41]	6[a]	6	23	50	0.37
		6	4	29	50	0.19
Roulet et al. (1983)	[32]	5	4	26	100	0.21
Robin et al. (1989)	[40]	5	6	29	100	0.29
Henneberg et al. (1985)	[26]	10	10	35	91	0.16
Nordenstrom et al. (1983)	[23]	11	4	29	100	0.28
Cerra et al. (1987)	[38]	53	7	18	100	0.16
		8	5	31	100	0.34
Iapichino et al. (1988)	[43]	8	5	32	100	0.35
Tulikoura (1988)	[42]	14	3	27	100	0.49
Iapichino et al. (1982)	[37]	4	5	31	100	0.23
Gazzaniga et al. (1985)	[29]	8	8	33	100	0.27

[a] crossover study.

groups, including 3 with a mixed system (40–50% fat) [32, 39, 41], and 10 with a glucose system [23, 26, 29, 32, 38, 40, 42–44].

In conclusion, 10 of 12 glucose systems and 3 of 9 mixed systems reached a positive clinical result.

Severely stressed patients. Patients who had a REE higher than 25 kcal/kg [36, 37, 45–48] or a daily fasting urinary N loss exceeding 15 gN [43, 49–54]. This resulted in 19 study groups (Table 6) in which the treatment generally spanned from 2 to 7 days in the early acute flow phase of stress reaction. Two studies on septic patients lasted 10 [52] and 14 [53] days, respectively, and could have included different metabolic phases during stress reaction. One study [52] is difficult to evaluate because of major patient heterogeneity (nutritional status, degree of organs failure, N input related to renal failure, and clinical course during the 10-day TPN study) and method used in the estimation of protein balance: i.e. neutron activation analysis.

The criteria for selecting these studies was a calorie intake superior to the patient's need and in any case 0.20 gN/kg.

Hence, they were ranked according to the results in protein balance:

- weak anticatabolic effect (>10 gN net loss/day): 3 groups all with a 50% mixed system [36, 46, 52];

Table 6. Clinical studies in severely stressed catabolic patients

Authors	Ref.	No of Pts	No of days of TPN	non-protein kcal/kg	Glucose %	gN_i/kg
Weak results (>10 gN net loss)						
Streat et al. (1987)	[52]	8	10	34	50	0.29
Shaw and Wolfe (1989)	[46]	49	7	32	50	0.27
Shaw (1988)	[36]	18	7	40	50	0.27
Marginally negative results (3–10 gN net loss)						
Shaw et al. (1987)	[45]	22	8	42	50	0.24/0.35
Shaw (1988)	[36]	16	7	40	50	0.27
Larsson et al. (1990)	[51]	30	7	47	50	0.2/0.25/0.30
Pitkanen et al. (1991)	[48]	30	2	30	50	0.20/0.26
Shenkin et al. (1980)	[55]	7	7	40	50	0.32
Iapichino et al. (1990)	[50]	10	2	30	100	0.30
Iapichino et al. (1988)	[43]	20	5	30	100	0.24
Jeevanandam et al. (1990)	[47]	8	5	31	100	0.26
Marginally positive results (±2 gN net loss)						
Shizgal and Martin (1988)	[53]	86[a]	14	41	90	0.22
Iapichino et al. (1982)	[37]	8	5	38	100	0.26
Clowes et al. (1980)	[54]	6	3	45	100	0.34
Iapichino et al. (1985)	[49]	14	5	31	100	0.35

[a] many patients underwent > one study.

- marginally negative protein balance (3–10 gN net loss/day): 12 groups. Nine of these were conducted with 50% mixed system [36, 45, 48, 51, 55] and 3 with glucose [43, 47, 50]; and
- near balance (2 gN net loss or gain/day): 4 groups all conducted with 90–100% glucose [37, 49, 53, 54].

Nevertheless, if the marginally negative balance is accepted as a valuable clinical result in the acute phase after severe injury, 9 of 12 mixed systems and 7 of 7 glucose systems can be considered as acceptable. Moreover, considering all the 40 study groups in catabolic patients, a clinical satisfactory result was reached in 12 of 21 mixed systems and in 17 of 19 glucose systems.

Optimal Rate of N Intake in Stressed Patients

Another interesting indirect information can also be achieved considering the controversial results on the optimal rate of N intake in stressed patients. In fact, according to well designed studies, this figure does not exceed 0.24 gN intake/kg/day [41, 45, 51, 56]. In other studies, even though protein store accretion (positive balance) is not the main goal in the acute injury phase and is also unlikely to reach, the optimal N intake ranged between 0.28–0.35 gN/kg/day [37, 38, 42, 43, 50, 54, 57–59]. The discrepancy between these studies might be explained by N needs equal or exceeding 0.24 g/kg. Nevertheless, the studies supporting a lower N figure were all conducted with a mixed regimen, all the others with a glucose system. This suggests a different anabolic drive and a net protein utilization elicited by different calorie systems.

Insulin Response to Substrate

The degree of insulin response to the infused calorie and amino acids could explain the better protein sparing capacity of a prevalent glucose amino acids regimen.

Malnourished Patients

This is clearly stated by Forse et al. [60] while comparing an hypocaloric to normocaloric system, and by Burt et al. [61] who, in cancer patients (radiation therapy), found the largest rate of whole body protein synthesis associated with a net increase in plasma insulin level of about 40–120 mU/L spontaneously reached with TPN (Table 7).

A comparable insulin level and a better N balance was found by Jeejeebhoy et al. [18] only in the glucose group. A further indirect evidence of this

Table 7. Glucose supply (kcal/kg) and plasma insulin level (mU/L) when submaximal or maximal protein sparing (PS) effect is obtained

		Submaximal PS		Maximal PS	
		Glucose	Insulin	Glucose	Insulin
Malnourished patients					
Burt et al. (1984)	[61]	36	8–30	36	48–130
Forse et al. (1990)	[60]	7	25	25	53[a]
Jeejeebhoy et al. (1976)	[18]	7	13	40	53[a]
Warnold et al. (1988)	[62]	11	19	18	43[a]
Catabolic patients					
Long et al. (1977)	[30]	<25	15–30	>25	35–80[a]
Woolfson et al. (1979)	[31]	20	29	34	47[a]
Chiarelli et al. (1990)	[63]	<20	34	>20	104[a]
Enzi et al. (1990)	[64]	<20	18	>20	50[a]

[a] plasma level significantly different vs submaximal PS group.

physiological relationship [1] was suggested by the Warnold et al. study [62]. This study on depleted cancer patients suggested "the inefficiency to stimulate protein synthesis of 6 h TPN", supplied with 120% of the fasting REE as a 50% mixed system, and 0.2 gN/kg resulting in 19 mU/L insulin. On the contrary, the "inefficiency" becomes an "efficiency" when increasing the N supply and doubling the energy supply. The latter regimen yielded exactly the fasting REE in glucose and doubles insulin plasma level (43 mU/L). Moreover, the result in protein gain was predictable only by the N and glucose load regardless of the lipid load [21, 44, 60].

Hence, the maximal protein sparing effect seems associated, in these reports [18, 60–62], with a plasma insulin level ranging from 43 to 130 mU/L i.e. 3 to several fold higher than the one (8 to 30 mU/L) reached by the groups with less efficient protein sparing effect. Other authors obtained a higher plasma insulin level (either significant: 5 vs 18 and 3 vs 18 mU/L [25], 8 vs 17 mU/L [23] or as a trend 8 vs 28 mU/L [35]) with a glucose system. However, it does not result in a better protein sparing activity than the mixed one. Interestingly enough, the plasma insulin level spontaneously reached with a glucose system in these studies, was below the suggested optimal range.

Catabolic Patients

In the studies showing a different effect on body catabolism of IV calorie sources [30, 31] and early enteral or a IV conventional approach (burns) [63, 64], better results were again associated with a higher insulin – glucose mediated – plasma levels (range 50–104 vs 15–35) (Table 7). The same insulin behavior (51 vs 29 mU/L) was also reported by a study [23] that found only a better N balance trend for glucose. On the contrary, when the better protein sparing effect resulted with the mixed system [32], positive N balance was reached also with a glucose system. Nevertheless, the achieved plasma insulin levels were not significantly different, and were both in the range associated with the optimal influence on protein metabolism.

In conclusion, also in patients, the anabolic drive elicited by nutritional intake seems to be mediated by endogenous insulin secretion in a dose dependent manner. The optimal insulin level seems to depend on patient's metabolic environment, particularly nutritional status and stress state. In any case, the nutrient mix that results in the more efficient increase in insulin production rate (and probably other anabolic factors) is constituted by amino acids and a prevalent glucose system.

Effect of Insulin Supply

The hypothesis that the best anabolic drive could be elicited by an optimal plasma insulin level supports the reasonable attempt to reach such a plasma level by supplying insulin as an anabolic drug.

Nine papers deal with the metabolic manipulation in patients that can tolerate the glucose load with and without insulin supply (Table 8). Three case reports [30, 65, 66] and 3 prospective studies [21, 31, 66] could demonstrate a positive effect of insulin supply on protein metabolism in patients with various degrees of stress and nutritional status. Homogeneity of the patient population [30, 65–67] and careful experiment design [21, 31] support the credibility of such results [68]. The addition of insulin (20–200 mU/m^2·min) to nutritional fluids reduced the rate of urea production (UPR) by 23 to 50% [30, 31, 66, 67], enhanced protein synthesis by 34% [65], and the rate at

Table 8. Effects of insulin (I) supply (mU/m^2·min) on I plasma level (mU/L) and protein metabolism

		I supply	Insulinemia no I	Insulinemia Yes I	Results	
Hinton et al. (1971)	[66]	77–230	–	–	UPR	40–50%
Long et al. (1977)	[30]	variable	15–30[a]	35–80	UPR	50%
Woolfson et al. (1979)	[31]	19–190	65[a]	210	UPR	23–34%
Burke et al. (1979)	[65]	variable	60[a]	72	P Synt	34%
Inculet et al. (1986)	[67]	50	40[a]	75	UPR	25%
					AA efl.	59%
					3-MHu	19%
Shizgal and Forse (1986)	[21]	variable	59[a]	100	BCM	35%

[a] significant difference vs insulin addition.

UPR = rate of urea production; P Synt = Protein synthesis; AA = amino acids; BCM = body cell mass; 3-MHu = urinary 3-methylhistidine.

which BCM was increased by 35% in malnourished patients [21]. The protein sparing effect was proportional to the catabolic rate [31] and to the degree of malnutrition [21].

Three papers in malnourished patients did not confirm these results: Macfie et al. [69] in 2 matched groups of gastroenterologic patients, failed to detect any increase of total body N with insulin (neutron activation analysis). To the contrary, a significant increase in TBK^+ was found. Moreover, changes in TBK^+ are consistent with BCM changes reported by Shizgal and Posner [21]. In Powell-Tuck's studies on postoperative [70] or non-surgical [71] malnourished patients, the insulin supply (insulin plasma levels increased significantly only for postoperative patients) was not associated with changes in UPR, 3-methylhistidine excretion or whole-body protein turnover rates. However, patient's age, nutritional status, nutrient (31–78 and 25–65 kcal/kg/day; 0.16–0.39 and 0.23–0,39 gN/kg/day) and insulin (20–50 mU/$m^2 \cdot$min) supply were quite heterogeneous in the small sample size [68].

Further insights come from a study performed in malnourished patients varying both insulin and glucose load, while maintaining constant energy supply. This resulted in 2 isocaloric groups: a 100% glucose (30 mU/$m^2 \cdot$min insulin) and a 67% glucose (16 mU/$m^2 \cdot$min insulin) system.

The better N retention found in the 100% glucose group was related to higher insulin plasma levels (>130 vs 70–30 mU/L), supporting the concept that insulin supply might be the anabolic trigger for the optimal protein sparing activity [17].

Another possibility for studying insulin action in severely stressed patient who cannot receive glucose without insulin, is to test different glucose and insulin loads. A supply of 30 kcal/kg/day glucose, insulin (1U/6g) and N reduced fasting net leg N output by 60%. The N efflux was about 20% lesser than with a supply of 15 kcal/kg/day [50].

Criticism of the Use of Glucose

Many studies performed in volunteers as well as in malnourished and catabolic patients suggest a powerful action of amino acids and endogenous or exogenous insulin on the anabolic drive. Nevertheless, while the controversies regarding the role of amino acids in anabolic drive are of relatively minor importance, those on the use of a prevalent or exclusive glucose system with insulin (a problem practically limited to the IV approach) are more important. In fact, strong criticisms to the use of a prevalent glucose system [57, 72–74] has been based on the inability to oxidize the glucose load. Despite, this defect seems to be overemphasized even in less favorable conditions [39, 75–78].

Other criticisms arise from the effects of glucose on lungs, liver and brain. Ventilatory insufficiency with hypercapnia is a feared complication of glucose loading. Gas exchange largely reflects the composition of the burned fuels. Oxygen consumption is minimal burning carbohydrates and increases with lipid (7%) and protein (16%) oxidation. On the other hand CO_2 production is maximal with carbohydrates and decreases with protein (7%) and fat (24%) oxidation. Moreover, the supply of substrate at a rate exceeding energy demand results in storage as fat.

Liposynthesis from carbohydrates has high energy cost (12% of the stocked energy) and yields a large amount of CO_2. Fat storage from fats hardly consumes any O_2 or produces CO_2. Theoretically, shifting from fasting (fat oxidation) to a carbohydrate regimen will result in an increase in O_2 consumption and CO_2 production by the induced thermogenesis of the diet (DIT). However, the increase in O_2 consumption is damped by a lesser oxidation of body fat and protein (reduced neoglucogenesis and protein sparing action).

Shifting from fasting to a fat regimen should minimally influence gas exchange because of a minor effect on body protein oxidation and a weaker DIT. Protein supply tends to increase gas exchange because of the higher DIT (35%) and because of a consistent increase in UPR.

However, providing that the energy intake (as a prevalent 80–100% glucose system) remains within the measured fasting expenditure and includes about 0.25–0.3 g/kgN, the variation in O_2 consumption and CO_2 production is minimal [79–80]. Moreover, it would be clinically relevant in only small fraction of patients.

Fat store replacement, when needed, can be accomplished by an additional amount of fat with a lesser impact on the cardiocirculatory system [39, 42, 76–83].

On the other hand, the fatty liver syndrome was also shown to be directly related to the severity of illness, and not to the nature of nutritional support [84]. Fat liver content, in an animal sepsis model [85], as well as in stressed patients [86], depends mainly on peripheral free fatty acid release, hepatic clearance, reesterification, and trapping for the impaired Apo-B protein synthesis which is necessary for the formation of the VLDL-TG complex prior to secretion. From this point of view, the reduction of free fatty acid release induced by glucose and insulin can be seen as therapeutic [85, 87]. In head injured patients [46, 57, 72–74], cerebral damage associated with hyperglycemia has not been yet clearly demonstrated [88].

Furthermore, glucose is claimed to cause wide variations in the planned energy input, making the feeding of critically ill patients very unpredictable [52, 89]. From this point of view, a mixed system is certainly advantageous, but these practical difficulties can be overcome simply by adding insulin in a dose-titrated fashion (ranging from 1 U/2–18 g glucose) to glucose load and to stress level. This approach is better than to treat hyperglycemia only when it occurs [41, 52].

Other reasons against the fixed use of insulin have been put forward:

- this therapy adds to the complication of parenteral feeding [90, 91];
- insulin could block amino acids mobilization and as a consequence might adversely affect the outcome [57]; and
- the ability of insulin to suppress proteolysis wanes after prolonged infusion.

The reply to the first objection is trivial. The degree of professionality reached by intensive care teams in the use of drugs (steroids, catecholamines, heparin, thrombolytics, antisera, etc. ...), is a strong guarantee. The second question is indeed very valid. It stems from the hypothesis [92] that the mobilization of the amino acids from the periphery to deliver N to the viscera is beneficial and that glucose and insulin could spare muscle but starve central tissue. This was exactly the phenomenon we addressed [50, 93], pointing out the need of matching the quantitative and qualitative amino acids allowance of viscera in the setting of stress, possibly by using new tissue-specific nutrients.

The latter remark is based on the observation by the De Fronzo's group that in volunteers endogenous leucine flux, acutely inhibited by insulin, returned to the pre-insulin basal rate, following 24 h of hyperinsulinemia. They postulate a reduction in the plasma and intracellular concentrations of leucine, an important inhibitor of proteolysis [1–3], in response to insulin infusion. This in turn may cause an up regulation of protein turnover [AS Petrides 1992, personal communication]. Nevertheless, in injured patients, we demonstrated that the suppression of proteolysis was again present after 5 days of treatment while stopping glucose and insulin infusion for 24 h (UPR up to the basal value [37]) or TPN for 6 h (significantly reduced amino acids leg efflux back to pre-treatment values [94]).

Conclusion

The established agreement, mainly based on studies conducted with a mixed system, is that injured and septic patients are not prevented from consistent protein loss even if they are not aggressively supported. Otherwise, even if they are not malnourished and in the early days of unjury (2–3 days for elective operation to weeks or month for severe sepsis or burn), the protein loss of injured patients can be reduced to a minimum ($\sim$5 gN or less/day) adopting a N supply titrated on fasting N loss coupled with prevalent glucose system ($\geq$80%) that permits an "optimal" plasma insulin level. This is reached by a spontaneous increase of insulin secretion or by a planned supply to overcome resistance. The positive effect of increasing energy intake (particularly with carbohydrates) on protein metabolism has been established in normal volunteers [5, 10], in stable malnourished patients [21, 44, 60], and in catabolic, but not malnourished patients [53, 58]. Nevertheless, for the implications of calorie supply on gas exchange, the assessment of the minimum energy supply that allows the maximum anabolic drive could be particularly important. A 3–4 mg/kg·min glucose infusion for few hours (i.e. roughly the energy requirement on a 24 h basis) results in a plasma insulin level of 33-38 mU/L and permits a half maximal whole body and muscle protein breakdown in volunteers [95, 96].

A glucose load just in range of the energy requirements can achieve an "optimal" anabolic insulin plasma level in stable, malnourished patients (Table 7). Moreover, when energy intake as glucose reaches the balance, the plateau of N loss is also achieved [37]. The same calorie supply/requirement ratio was needed by stressed patients to spontaneously obtain the "optimal" insulin level (Table 7) and to plateau the N loss when 1 U insulin/4–7 g glucose was added [37].

In conclusion, today, a prevalent glucose system ($\geq 80\%$) yelding the overall measured or expected energy requirement, coupled with insulin supply to maintain normoglycemia, reaches an "optimal" anabolic insulin level that, with protein supply, seems to be the most efficient tool to optimize protein metabolism. This IV approach is very similar in composition to the balanced enteral diet which in any case should be administrated as soon as possible.

The treatment supplied to less catabolic and/or malnourished patients is also able to replace the depleted protein stores.

Whether or not the best anabolic drive could make the difference in the treatment of critically ill patients remains unsettled, but this possibility offered by metabolic support must be considered. The intensivist will select the kind of patients and the right time during the course of the illness in which the best anabolic drive is desirable.

The increasing interest in nutrient requirements of specific organs or tissues (glutamine and short-chain fatty acids for the gut), the availability of the conditionally essential amino acids (tyrosine, cystine, taurine) to better improve protein synthesis, the possibility to nutritionally manipulate the immunological response (arginine and omega-3 fatty acids), together with the administration of the next available growth factors and the possibility to alter the stress response [57, 97, 98] certainly will increase the effectiveness on nutritional support.

References

1. Millward DJ (1990) The hormonal control of protein turnover. Clinical Nutrition 9:115–126
2. Bennett WM, Connacher AA, Scrimgeour CM, Smith K, Rennie MJ (1989) Increase in anterior tibialis muscle protein synthesis in healthy man during mixed amino acid infusion: Studies of incorporation of [1–13C] leucine. Clin Sci 76:447–454
3. Tessari P, Inchiostro S, Biolo G, et al (1987) Differential effects of hyperinsulinemia and hyperaminoacidemia of leucine-carbon metabolism in vivo. J Clin Invest 79:1062–1069
4. Barbul A (1986) Arginine: Biochemistry, physiology, and therapeutic implications. JPEN 10:227–238
5. Young VR (1987) Kinetics of human amino acid metabolism: Nutritional implications and some lessons. Am J Clin Nutr 46:709–725
6. Pellett PL (1990) Protein requirements in humans. Am J Clin Nutr 51:723–737
7. Garrow JS (1978) Energy balance and obesity in man. 2nd ed. Elsevier North-Holland
8. McCargar LJ, Clandinin MT, Belcastro AN, Walker K (1989) Dietary carbohydrate-to-fat ratio: Influence on whole-body nitrogen retention, substrate utilization, and hormone response in healthy male subjects. Am J Clin Nutr 49:1169–1178

9. Shizgal HM, Forse RA (1980) Protein and calorie requirements with total parenteral nutrition. Ann Surg 192:562–568
10. Moore FD (1980) Energy and the maintenance of the body cell mass. JPEN 4:228–260
11. Vasquez JA, Morse EL, Adibi SA (1985) Effect of dietary fat, carbohydrate, and protein on branched-chain amino acid catabolism during caloric restriction. J Clin Invest 76:737–743
12. Brennan MF, Fitzpatrick GF, Cohen KH, Moore FD (1975) Glycerol: Major contribution to the short term protein sparing effect of fat emulsion in normal man. Ann Surg 182:386–394
13. Wolfe BM. Culebras JM, Sim AJW, Ball MR, Moore FD (1977) Substrate interaction in intravenous feeding. Comparative effects of carbohydrate and fat on amino acid utilization in fasting man. Ann Surg 186:518–540
14. Tracey KJ, Legaspi A, Albert JD et al (1988) Protein and substrate metabolism during starvation and parenteral refeeding. Clin Sci 74:123–132
15. Macfie J, Smith RC, Hill GL (1981) Glucose or fat as a nonprotein energy source? A controlled clinical trial in gastroenterological patients requiring intravenous nutrition. Gastroenterology 80:103–107
16. Tulikoura I, Huikuri K (1981) Changes in nitrogen metabolism in catabolic patients given three different parenteral nutrition regimens. Acta Chir Scand 147:519–524
17. Iapichino G, Radrizzani D, Leoni L, et al (1987) A comparison of mixed and glucose systems in the total parenteral nutrition of malnourished patients. Clinical Nutrition 6:1–4
18. Jeejeebhoy KN, Anderson GH, Nakhooda AF, Greenberg GR, Sanderson I, Marliss EB (1976) Metabolic studies in total parenteral nutrition with lipid in man. Comparison with glucose. J Clin Invest 57:125–136
19. Shizgal HM, Forse RA (1981) Total parenteral nutrition with vamin and intralipid. JPEN 5:391–396
20. King RFJH, MacMahon MJ, Burkinshaw L, et al (1988) A comparison of changes in body nitrogen measured by in vivo neutron activation analysis and urinary nitrogen balance. Clinical Nutrition 7:231–236
21. Shizgal HM, Posner B (1989) Insulin and the efficacy of total parenteral nutrition. Am J Clin Nutr 50:1355–1363
22. Almond DJ, King RFGJ, Burkinshaw L, Laughland A, MacMahon MJ (1989) Influence of energy source upon body composition in patients receiving intravenous nutrition. JPEN 13:471–477
23. Nordenström J, Askanazi J, Elwyn DH et al (1983) Nitrogen balance during total parenteral nutrition. Ann Surg 197:27–33
24. Gazzaniga AB, Bartlett RH, Shobe JB (1975) Nitrogen balance in patients receiving either fat or carbohydrate for total intravenous nutrition. Ann Surg 182:163–168
25. Shaw JHF, Holdaway CM (1988) Protein-sparing effect of substrate infusion in surgical patients is governed by the clinical state, and not by the individual substrate infused. JPEN 12:433–440
26. Henneberg S, Eklund A, Stjernström H, Hellsing K, Sjölin J, Wiklund L (1985) Postoperative substrate utilization and gas exchange using two different TPN-systems: Glucose versus fat. Clinical Nutrition 4:235–242
27. Bark S, Holm I, Hâkansson I, Wretlind A (1976) Nitrogen-sparing effect of fat emulsion compared with glucose in the postoperative period. Acta Chir Scand 142:423–427
28. Dworkin B, Daly J, Massar E, Alcock N, Dudrick SJ, Copeland III EM (1983) Intravenously administered amino acids with either dextrose or lipid as nutritional support in surgical patients. Surg Gynecol Obstet 156:577–581
29. Gazzaniga AB, Day AT, Sankary H (1985) The efficacy of a 20 per cent fat emulsion as a peripherally administered substrate. Surg Gynecol Obstet 160:387–392
30. Long III JM, Wilmore DW, Mason AD, Pruitt BA (1977) Effect of carbohydrate and fat intake on nitrogen excretion during total intravenous feeding. Ann Surg 185:417–422

31. Woolfson AMJ, Heathley RV, Allison SP (1979) Insulin to inhibit protein catabolism after injury. N Engl J Med 300:14–17
32. Roulet M, Detsky AS, Marliss EB, et al (1983) A controlled trial of the effects of parenteral nutritional support on patients with respiratory failure and sepsis. Clinical Nutrition 2:97–105
33. Bocking JK, Holliday RL, Reid B, Mustard R, Duff JH (1980) Total exchangeable potassium in patients receiving total parenteral nutrition. Surgery 88:551–555
34. Baker JP, Detsky AS, Stewart S, Whitwell J, Marliss EB, Jeejeebhoy KN (1984) Randomized trial of total parenteral nutrition in ciritically ill patients: Metabolic effects of varying glucose-lipid ratios as the energy source. Gastroenterology 87:53–59
35. Glynn MJ, Metzner S, Halliday D, Powell-Tuck J (1987) Whole body protein metabolism in parenterally fed patients: Glucose versus fat as the predominant energy source. Clinical Nutrition 6:91–96
36. Shaw JHF (1988) Influence of stress, depletion, and/or malignant disease on the responsiveness of surgical patients to total parenteral nutrition. Am J Clin Nutr 48:144–147
37. Iapichino G, Gattinoni L, Solca M, et al (1982) Protein sparing and protein replacement in acutely injured patients during TPN with and without amino acid supply. Intensive Care Med 8:25–31
38. Cerra F, Hirsch J, Mullen K, Blackburn G, Luther W (1987) The effect of stress level, amino acid formula, and nitrogen dose on nitrogen retention in traumatic and septic stress. Ann Surg 205:282–287
39. Brandi LS, Frediani M, Oleggini M, et al (1990) Insulin resistance after surgery: Normalization by insulin treatment. Clin Sci 79:443–450
40. Robin AP, Elwyn DH, Nordenström J, Carpentier YA, Askanazi J, Kinney JM (1989) Fatty acid kinetics in man during chronic and acute illness. J Surg Res 47:65–73
41. Greig PD, Elwyn DH, Askanazi J, Kinney JM (1987) Parenteral nutrition in septic patients: Effect of increasing nitrogen intake. Am J Clin Nutr 46:1040–1047
42. Tulikoura I (1988) Maintenance of visceral protein levels in serum during postoperative parenteral nutrition. JPEN 12:597–601
43. Iapichino G, Radrizzani D, Scherini A, et al (1988) Essential and non-essential amino acid requirement in injured patients receiving total parenteral nutrition. Intensive Care Med 14:399–405
44. Radrizzani D, Iapichino G, Scherini A, et al (1986) Main nitrogen balance determinants in malnourished patients. Intensive Care Med 12:308–311
45. Shaw JHF, Wildbore M, Wolfe RR (1987) Whole body protein kinetics in severely septic patients. Ann Surg 205:288–294
46. Shaw JHF, Wolfe RR (1989) An integrated analysis of glucose, fat, and protein metabolism in severely traumatized patients. Ann Surg 209:63–72
47. Jeevanandam M, Young DH, Schiller WR (1990) Influence of parenteral nutrition on rates of net substrate oxidation in severe trauma patients. Crit Care Med 18:467–473
48. Pitkänen O, Takala J, Poyhonen M, Kari A, Miettinen P, Alhava E (1991) Nitrogen and energy balance in depleted patients undergoing major gastrointestinal surgery: Response to TPN. Clinical Nutrition 10:36–42
49. Iapichino G, Radrizzani D, Solca M, Bonetti G, Leoni L, Ferro A (1985) Influence of total parenteral nutrition on protein metabolism following acute injury: Assessment by urinary 3-methylhistidine excretion and nitrogen balance. JPEN 9:42–46
50. Iapichino G, Radrizzani D, Bonetti G, et al (1990) Influence of parenteral nutrition on leg nitrogen exchange in injured patients. Crit Care Med 18:1367–1373
51. Larsson J, Lennmarken C, Martensson J, Sandstedt S, Vinnars E (1990) Nitrogen requirements in severely injured patients. Br J Surg 77:413–416
52. Streat SJ, Beddoe AH, Hill GL (1987) Aggressive nutritional support does not prevent protein loss despite fat gain in septic intensive care patients. J Trauma 27:262–266
53. Shizgal HM, Martin MF (1988) Caloric requirement of the critically ill septic patient. Crit Care Med 16:312–317
54. Clowes Jr GHA, Heideman M, Lindberg D, et al (1980) Effect of parenteral alimentation on amino acid metabolism in septic patients. Surgery 88:531–543

55. Shenkin A, Neuhäuser M, Bergström J, et al (1980) Biochemical changes associated with severe trauma. Am J Clin Nutr 33:2119–2127
56. Wolfe RR, Goodenough RD, Burke JF, Wolfe MH (1983) Response of protein and urea kinetics in burn patients to different levels of protein intake. Ann Surg 197:163–171
57. Cerra FB (1990) How nutrition intervention changes what getting sick means. JPEN 14:164s–169s
58. Iapichino G, Radrizzani D, Solca M, et al (1984) The main determinants of nitrogen balance during total parenteral nutrition in critically ill injured patients. Intensive Care Med 10:251–254
59. Humberstone DA, Koea J, Shaw JHF (1989) Relative importance of amino acid infusion as a means of sparing protein in surgical patients. JPEN 13:223–227
60. Forse RA, Elwyn DH, Askanazi J, Iles M, Schwarz Y, Kinney JM (1990) Effects of glucose on nitrogen balance during high nitrogen intake in malnourished patients. Clin Sci 78:273–281
61. Burt ME, Stein TP, Schwade JG, Brennan MF (1984) Whole-body protein metabolism in cancer-bearing patients. Effect of total parenteral nutrition and associated serum insulin response. Cancer 53:1246–1252
62. Warnold I, Edén E, Lundholm K (1988) The inefficiency of total parenteral nutrition to stimulate protein synthesis in moderately malnourished patients. Ann Surg 208:143–149
63. Chiarelli A, Enzi G, Casadei A, Baggio B, Valerio A, Mazzoleni F (1990) Very early nutrition supplementation in burned patients. Am J Clin Nutr 51:1035–1039
64. Enzi G, Casadei A, Sergi G, Chiarelli A, Zurlo F, Mazzoleni F (1990) Metabolic and hormonal effects of early nutritional supplementation after surgery in burn patients. Crit Care Med 18:719–721
65. Burke JF, Wolfe RR, Mullany CJ, Mathews DE, Bier DM (1979) Parameters of optimal glucose infusion and possible hepatic and respiratory abnormalities following excessive glucose intake. Ann Surg 190:274–283
66. Hinton P, Allison SP, Littlejohn S, Lloyd J (1971) Insulin and glucose to reduce catabolic response to injury in burned patients. The Lancet 1:767–769
67. Inculet RI, Finley RJ, Duff JH, et al (1986) Insulin decreases muscle protein loss after operative trauma in man. Surgery 99:752–758
68. Shizgal HM (1990) Reply to Powell-Tuck and Glynn. Am J Clin Nutr 52:579–580
69. Macfie J, Yule AG, Hill GL (1981) Effects of added insulin on body composition of gastroenterologic patients receiving intravenous nutrition – A controlled clinical trial. Gastroenterology 81:285–289
70. Powell-Tuck J, Fern EB, Garlick PJ, Waterlow JC (1984) The effect of surgical trauma and insulin on whole-body protein turnover in parenterally-fed undernourished patients. Human Nutrition: Clin Nutr 38C:11–22
71. Powell-Tuck J, Glynn MJ (1985) The effect of insulin infusion on whole-body protein metabolism in patients with gastrointestinal disease fed parenterally. Human Nutrition: Clin Nutr 39C:181–191
72. Berger R, Adams L (1989) Nutritional support in the critical care setting (Part 1). Chest 96:139–150
73. Meguid MM, Campos AC, Hammond WG (1990) Nutritional support in surgical practice: Part I. Am J Surg 159:345–358
74. Weissman C (1990) The metabolic response to stress: An overview and update. Anesthesiology 73:308–327
75. Shangraw RE, Jahnoor F, Miyoshi H, et al (1989) Differentiation between septic and postburn insulin resistance. Metabolism 38:983–989
76. Long CL (1987) Fuel preferences in the septic patients: Glucose or lipid? JPEN 11:333–335
77. Iapichino G, Radrizzani D (1988) Metabolic support and energy supply for critically ill patients: A pathophysiological approach. Intensive Care World 5:48–51
78. Radrizzani D, Iapichino G (1990) Gas exchange and substrate oxidation during energy supply. In: Hull SM, Behr SR, Fugate CP (eds) The role of nutrition in pulmonary disease, Abbott Park, Illinois, pp 46–51

79. Iapichino G, Radrizzani D (1991) Nutritional strategy during acute respiratory failure. J Drug Dev 4:82–85
80. Talpers SS, Romberger DJ, Bunce SB, Pingleton SK (1992) Nutritionally associated increased carbon dioxide production. Excess total calories vs high proportion of carbohydrate calories: Chest 102:551–555
81. Goodenough RD, Wolfe RR (1984) Effect of total parenteral nutrition on free fatty acid metabolism in burned patients. JPEN 8:357–360
82. Askanazi J, Carpentier YA, Elwyn DH, et al (1980) Influence of total parenteral nutrition on fuel utilizations in injury and sepsis. Ann Surg 191:40–46
83. Iapichino G (1989) Nutrition in respiratory failure. Intensive Care Med 15:483–485
84. Wolfe BM, Walker BK, Shaul DB, Wong L, Ruebner BH (1988) Effect of total parenteral nutrition on hepatic histology. Arch Surg 123:1084–1090
85. Wolfe RR, Shaw JHF, Durkot MJ (1985) Effects of sepsis on VLDL kinetics: Responses in basal state and during glucose infusion. Am J Physiol 248:E732–E740
86. Klein S, Peters EJ, Shangraw RE, Wolfe RR (1991) Lypolitic response to metabolic stress in critically ill patients. Crit Care Med 19:776–779
87. Wolfe RR, Janhoor F, Shaw JHS (1990) Metabolic response of critically ill patients. Riv Ital Nutr Par Ent 8:63–69
88. Robertson CS, Goodman JC, Narayan RK, Contant CF, Grossman RG (1991) The effect of glucose administration on carbohydrate metabolism after head injury. J Neurosurg 74:43–50
89. Stoner HB, Little RA, Frayn KN, Elebute AE, Tresedern J, Gross E (1983) The effect of sepsis on the oxidation of carbohydrate and fat. Br J Surg 70:32–35
90. Herndon DN, Barrow RE, Kunkel KR, Broemeling L, Rutan RL (1990) Effects of recombinant human growth hormone on donor-site healing in severely burned children. Ann Surg 212:424–429
91. Powell-Tuck J, Glynn MJ (1990) Insulin supplementation during total parenteral nutrition. Am J Clin Nutr 52:578–579
92. Hasselgren PO, Pedersen P, Sax HC, Warner W, Fischer JE (1988) Current consepts of protein turnover and amino acid transport in liver and skeletal muscle during sepsis. Arch Surg 123:992–999
93. Radrizzani D, Iapichino G, Cambisano M, Bonetti G, Ronzoni G, Colombo A (1988) Peripheral, visceral and body nitrogen balance of catabolic patients, without and with parenteral nutrition. Intensive Care Med 14:212–216
94. Iapichino G, Radrizzani D, Bonetti G, et al (1985) Parenteral nutrition of injured patients. Effect of manipulation of aminoacid infusion (increasing branched chain while decreasing aromatic and sulphurated aminoacids). Clinical Nutrition 4:121–128
95. Tessari P, Trevisan R, Inchiostro S, et al (1986) Dose-response curves of effects of insulin on leucine kinetics in humans. Am J Physiol 251:E334–E342
96. Shangraw RE, Stuart CA, Prince MJ, Peters EJ, Wolfe RR (1988) Insulin responsiveness of protein metabolism in vivo following bedrest in humans. Am J Physiol 255:E548–E558
97. Wilmore DW (1991) Catabolic illness: Strategies for enhancing recovery. N Engl J Med 325:695–702
98. Long CL, Lowry SF (1990) Hormonal regulation of protein metabolism. JPEN 14:555–562
99. Loder PD, Smith RC, Kee AJ, et al (1990) What rate of infusion of intravenous nutrition solution is required to stimulate uptake of amino acids by peripheral tissues in depleted patients? Ann Surg 211:360–368

Are Present Fat Emulsions Appropriate?

Y. A. Carpentier

Introduction

Lipid emulsions used in parenteral nutrition are administered to supply both energy and essential fatty acids to different tissues. Traditionally, these emulsions have been prepared using long-chain triglycerides (LCT) derived from soybean oil and phospholipids derived from egg yolk [1]. They have been marketed as 10% and 20% preparations, differing in the phospholipid/triglyceride ratio since the same amount of phospholipids (1.2 g/dL) was used in both types of preparations. Including these emulsions in the parenteral regimen of critically ill patients was shown to have beneficial effects, with respect to:

1. providing efficiently utilized energy substrates;
2. reducing the carbohydrate load and the associated respiratory and hepatic complications; and
3. avoiding or correcting essential fatty acid deficiency syndromes.

However, the high phospholipid content of some 10% emulsions was shown to alter plasma lipid and lipoprotein pattern. In addition, the fatty acid composition of soy triglycerides has been suggested to induce side-effects, such as enhancement of inflammatory reactions, depression of immune defenses, and increased production of free radicals.

Recently, new preparations have been developed with a modified pattern of trigylceride fatty acids obtained by mixing different oils or by producing synthetic triglyceride molecules, or else by reducing the phospholipid content.

The purpose of this chapter is to review recent advances in lipoprotein and fatty acid metabolism in order to critically assess which modifications are particularly relevant to optimally answer the specific requirements of the critically ill patient.

Structure and Metabolism of Lipid Emulsions

Emulsion particles have been designed on the model of the endogenous triglyceride-rich chylomicrons and serve as vehicles for transport of the water-insoluble triglyceride molecules [2]. This triglyceride core is stabilized by a phospholipid surface. However, phospholipids are present in greater amounts in lipid emulsions than in chylomicrons and the surplus of phospholipids can be isolated by ultracentrifugation as a separate fraction of vesicular or liposomal particles [3].

Metabolism of Triglyceride-rich Particles

Hydrolysis of triglycerides present in the core of emulsion particles can take place either at the endothelial site of extra-hepatic tissues under the action of lipoprotein lipase (LPL), or in the liver under the action of hepatic lipase (HL). Immediately after their infusion into the circulation, emulsion particles acquire different apolipoproteins (apo's) transferred from the high density lipoprotein (HDL) pool (Fig. 1). Apo C-II plays an essential role in the recognition of emulsion particles by the receptor site of lipoprotein lipase (LPL) and activation of its hydrolytic site [4]. Transfer of apo C-II is very efficient [5] and only small amounts are required for activating LPL; thus, except for extreme conditions of altered protein synthesis or massive losses, apo C-II deficiency is unlikely to be rate-limiting for extra-hepatic lipolysis. Hydrolysis of exogenous triglycerides is regulated by endogenous factors (such as the availability of active lipoprotein lipase and its distribution between various tissues), as well as by the lipid composition of the emulsion. Indeed, in order to become accessible to the hydrolytic action of the lipase, triglyceride molecules have to partition from particle core into the phospholipid surface. The amount of triglycerides that can be dissolved into a phospholipid layer is largely dependent on the chain length and degree of unsaturation of triglyceride fatty acids, but also on phospholipid composition. For example, medium-chain triglycerides (MCT) are 4 to 5 times more soluble into the same phospholipid layer than soybean-derived LCT [6]. This factor probably plays an important role in the faster hydrolysis by LPL of MCT vs LCT and explains why MCT dissapear more rapidly than LCT from a particle containing a mixture of both types of triglycerides. In normal post-prandial conditions, fatty acids (FA) resulting from triglyceride hydrolysis by LPL are largely taken up by adjacent tissues and only a small fraction is released into the circulation to increase the plasma pool of free or non-esterified fatty acids (Nefas) largely associated to albumin. The situation can be quite different in parenteral nutrition since lipid emulsions are sometimes infused at a fast rate. The immediate effect of triglyceride hydrolysis by LPL is to release large amounts of FA at the site of the endothelial wall. If they are not efficiently assimilated by the adjacent tissues, FA accumulate and exert a feedback inhibition on LPL activity [7]; this effect is more pronounced for long-chain than medium-chain FA. In addition, locally high concentrations of FA can detach LPL from the endothelium and release it into the circulation. LPL was recently suggested to promote the binding to their receptors of TG-rich remnants [8] and other lipoproteins [9]. It is reasonable to speculate a similar role for LPL towards emulsion remnants. Thus, the

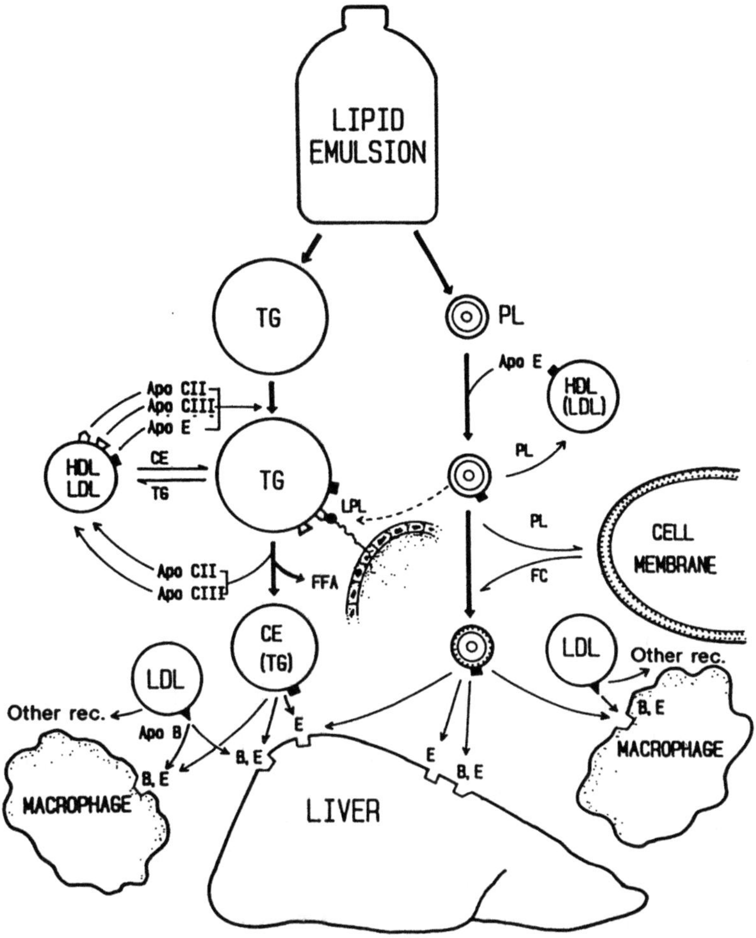

Fig. 1. Intravascular metabolism of both (triglyceride (TG)-rich and phospholipid (PL)-rich particles present in a lipid emulsion. The four key steps previously outlined for the metabolism of endogenous chylomicrons are represented for the triglyceride-rich emulsion particles. On the right side, the formation of phospholipid-free cholesterol complexes having acquired apoprotein (apo) E is represented, as is the competitive effect of liposomes for lipoprotein lipase (LPL). In the lower part, we have speculated on the potential competition of exogenous remnants between themselves and with endogenous lipoproteins for binding to the low-density lipoprotein (LDL) B, E receptor and the chylomicron remnant E receptor, at the site of different tissues. HDL = high-density lipoprotein; FFA = free fatty acids.

infusion rate together with the capacity of extra-hepatic tissues for assimilating FA released from TG hydrolysis may largely influence, not only the release of Nefas and LPL in the plasma, but also the amount of TG remaining in the particles to be delivered to the liver. Recent work from Sniderman and his associates [10] strongly suggests that assimilation of FA by peripheral tissues (and namely adipose tissues) is regulated by an acylation stimulating protein (ASP) which acts separately from insulin to promote re-esterification of FA into triglycerides. Impaired activity of this protein would lead to an increased content of triglycerides in remnant particles, together with a higher release of Nefas into the circulation. Although LPL is capable of hydrolyzing various lipid components contained in different lipoproteins, the enzyme appears to interact preferentially with large-sized particles such as chylomicrons and very low density lipoproteins (VLDL) and its activity on phospholipids represents only a few percent of that directed on trigylcerides. In addition, the enzyme shows a specifity for cleaving preferentially FA with a chain length not longer than 18 carbon atoms from the sn-1 and the sn-3 positions of triglyceride molecules. It was recently suggested that the hepatic lipase (HL) could have a complementary role by hydrolyzing from the particle surface residual lipids which have not been properly attacked by LPL [11]. These successive actions of LPL and HL lead to a preferential channelling of some FA to extra-hepatic tissues, while others are mainly delivered to the liver.

Exchange of core components between triglyceride-rich particles and cholesterol-rich lipoproteins represents another important step in the intravascular metabolism of lipid emulsions. This process is mediated by the cholesteryl ester transfer protein (CETP) which is present in man and in only some animal species [12]. These exchanges are regulated by the amount (and the composition) of triglyceride-rich particles present into the circulation, but also by the concentration of phospholipids and Nefas. Transfer of triglycerides to LDL (and HDL), in exchange of cholesteryl esters, results in a substantial core remodelling, which can effect particle recognition by specific receptors [13]. At the same time, emulsion particles loose triglycerides (both by hydrolysis and transfer) and acquire cholesteryl esters to form remnants which may play a substantial role in the reverse transport of cholesterol from peripheral tissues to the liver.

Uptake of these remnants is the last, but crucial step in the intravascular metabolism of emulsion triglyceride-rich particles. Indeed, in relation to their lipid content, remnant disposal may represent a substantial supply of fatty acids, cholesterol and phospholipids to the liver. In case of impaired hepatic uptake, remnants are diverted to other tissues (i.e. macrophages) by the so-called scavenger pathway(s). It was known for long that remnant removal could proceed not only through the B, E receptors, but also through a receptor recognizing only apo E. More recently, it was shown that infusion of recombinant apo E in rabbits largely accelerates the elimination of cholesteryl esters contained in remnants [14, 15]. Evidence is developing that the recently isolated low density receptor related protein (LRP) could be the long sought chylomicron remnant (or apo E) receptor [16]. Confirmation that LRP is this putative receptor would be extremely relevant for the care of patients, since:

1. LRP has been isolated not only in hepatocytes, but also in other tissues such as bone marrow; and
2. LRP also binds some proteins, such as α-2 macroglobulin and plasminogen activator inhibitor (PAI-1). If there was a competition between these proteins and remnants for the same receptor sites, this could not only delay the catabolism of TNF (and other cytokines linked with α-2 macroglobulin), but also enhance the tendency to thrombosis by reducing the fibrinolytic process.

Although some aspects of this integrated view on the intravascular metabolism of triglyceride-rich particles are still speculative, the concept that emulsion FA partitioning between peripheral tissues and the liver may be affected by triglyceride composition and by different mediators, is gaining support. Progresses in this area may be particularly relevant to the care of critically ill patients who tend to have high plasma levels of triglyceride-rich lipoproteins and Nefas.

Uptake of fatty acids by tissues can be realized by different mechanisms, as shown by the following examples:

- immediate uptake of FA released at the endothelial site by hydrolysis of trigylcerides certainly represents a major pathway for LPL rich extra-hepatic tissues, such as adipose tissues and muscles, but also the lungs; evidence for the presence of high LPL concentrations (and efficient uptake of triglyceride FA) in several areas of the central nervous system (CNS) [17] should lead to a re-evaluation of fat metabolism in the brain;
- endocytosis of remnants derived from triglyceride-rich particles followed by intracellular hydrolysis of triglycerides takes place in liver and potentially in bone marrow and macrophages;
- many circulating cells and macrophages bear on their outer membrane a lipase similar to LPL; in addition, platelets have a lipase cleaving FA from monoglycerides; and
- Nefas circulating in plasma in association with albumin are available for most or all tissues.

Metabolism of Phospholipid-rich Particles

The proportion of phospholipids present in the liposomal fraction is much larger in the classical 10% emulsions with a phospholipid/triglyceride (wt/wt) ratio of 0.12 than in the 20% emulsions with a phospholipid/triglyceride ratio of 0.06 [18]. Since their plasma elimination is relatively slow, infusion at high rate of phospholipid-rich emulsions induces a prolonged accumulation of liposomal particles [19, 20]. In the circulation, these particles may interfere with other lipoproteins and emulsion particles at several steps of their metabolism (Fig. 1). For example, they compete with triglyceride-rich particles for binding to LPL, which may impede peripheral hydrolysis of triglycerides [3]. They acquire apoproteins (e.g. apo E) from the HDL reservoir and are capable of competing with other particles for binding to apo E and B, E receptors [21]. In addition, liposomal phospholipids can substantially modify the composition of cell membranes by attracting free cholesterol, as demonstrated for erythrocytes [22]. Phospholipid-free cholesterol complexes bind to albumin and form particles similar to lipoprotein X (LpX) which was primarily isolated from the plasma of cholestatic patients. LpX is expected to be eliminated in the liver; hepatic accumulation of phospholipids has been reported to occur in patients on long-term TPN with lipids [23].

Because of these effects at several steps of lipid metabolism, attention has recently been paid to reduce the liposomal content of lipid emulsions. In addition to the 20% preparations, phospholipid-reduced 10% emulsions as well as 30% emulsions (with a phospholipid/triglyceride ratio of 0.06 and 0.04, respectively) have now become available. Of interest, not only the amount of phospholipids, but also their composition, may affect emulsion metabolism. For instance, we found differences of triglyceride elimination and FA release into the circulation between 2 apparently similar preparations to be associated to a different phosphatidylcholine/phosphatidylethanolamine ratio in egg phospholipids.

Lipid and Lipoprotein Metabolism in ICU Patients

Changes of lipid metabolism in critically ill patients result from a marked modification of the hormonal milieu, as well as from the production of inflammatory mediators. The increased release of counterregulatory hormones (catecholamines, cortisol and glucagon) largely counteracts the effect of insulin and stimulates the activity of hormone-sensitive lipase in adipose (and probably muscular) tissues. This results in an increased hydrolysis of triglycerides and release of glycerol and FA. A substantial proportion of fatty acids are re-esterified in the liver and repackaged into nascent VLDL. In addition, cytokines such as TNF enhance *de novo* FA synthesis in the liver while they possibly inhibit LPL activity in adipose tissue. Thus, the increased hepatic lipogenesis and triglyceride secretion is not matched by a rise of removal, which leads to an elevated plasma level of triglyceride-rich particles. It has recently been suggested that these triglyceride-rich particles could have a beneficial effect in trapping and inactivating endotoxins [24]. In most hypermetabolic conditions, oxidation of FA is enhanced by comparison to carbohydrates, which leads to a relatively lower carbon dioxide production and reduced minute ventilation. Cholesterol concentration is markedly reduced, particularly in HDL. Indeed, HDL possess anti-inflammatory properties and are "consumed" in some immune processes [25]. HDL are known to decrease degranulation of neutrophil leukocytes [26] and to inhibit cytolytic activity of complement's complex C5b-9 [27, 28]. HDL are also actively catabolyzed by activated and proliferating lymphocytes [29] and reticuloendothelial cells [30], as a result of increased cellular demand for lipids and aminoacids [31]. These specific functions of HDL may partially explain the major hypoalphalipoproteinemia encountered in critically ill patients. This increased HDL uptake is associated with an increased catabolism of apo A-1 which may be further enhanced by the parenteral nutrition with LCT emulsions [32]. Since apo A-1 rich HDL are known to have a potent effect in stabilizing prostacyclin (PGI_2) [33], this could further accentuate the thrombotic tendency encountered in these patients.

Inflammatory mediators stimulate the production of several acute-phase proteins, including apo SAA, which is found mainly in HDL but also in other lipoproteins [34]. The role of this apoprotein is not well-known, but the hypothesis may be raised that it would promote the delivery of cholesterol and phospholipids to certain types of rapidly dividing cells [35].

Development of New Lipid Emulsions

Triglycerides derived from soybean are particularly rich in essential polyunsaturated FA with a carbon chain length of 18 carbon atoms, since they contain an average of 54% linoleic (C18:2 n-6) and 8% α-linolenic (C18:3 n-3) acids. While being efficient oxidative substrates, these FA also compete between each other for the formation of other essential FA with a longer carbon chain and a higher degree of desaturation, through a common elongase-

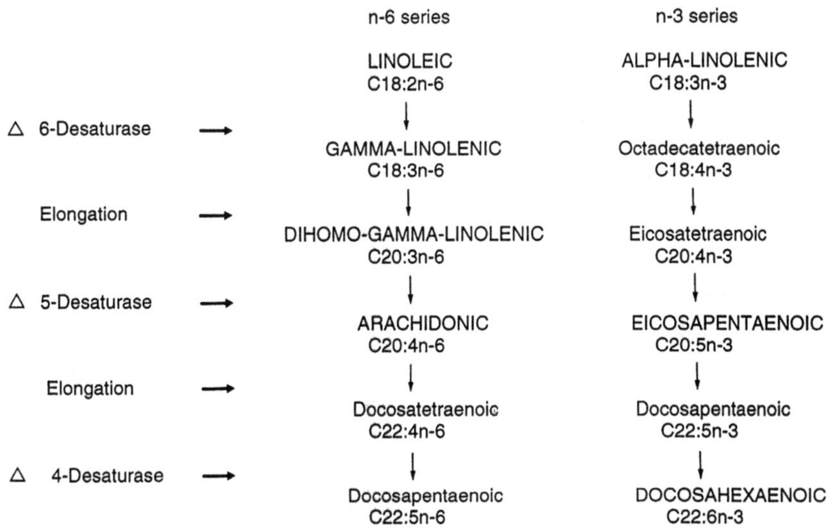

Fig. 2. Desaturase-Elongase pathways for n-6 and n-3 essential fatty acids. The same enzymatic pathway is used for elongation and desaturation of C18 n-6 and n-3 fatty acids. Fatty acids playing a major role in humans (at the exception of those involved in brain metabolism) are presented in capital letters.

desaturase pathway (Fig. 2). The major FA derived from linoleic acid (n-6 series) are γ-linolenic (C18:3 n-6), di-homo γ linolenic (C20:3 n-6), and arachidonic (C20:4 n-6) acids; and those derived from α-linolenic acid (n-3 series) are eicosapentanoic (C20:5 n-3; EPA) and docosahexanoic (C22:6 n-3; DHA) acids, the latter being found in high concentration in fish oils.

Essential FA are important components of plasma and cell membrane phospholipids. Their relative concentration in cell membranes (and in intracellular organelles) can affect the physical properties, but also the activity of membrane receptors and enzymes. In addition, essential FA with 20 carbon atoms are the precursors of various eicosanoids (Fig. 3). Except for PGI_2, eicosanoids derived from arachidonic acid (dienoic prostaglandins and thromboxane, and tetraenoic leukotrienes) tend generally to be more pro-coagulant and pro-inflammatory than the corresponding mediators (trienoic prostaglandins and thromboxane, and pentaenoic leukotrienes) derived from eicosapentanoic acid. In addition, supply of n-3 long-chain FA to normal subjects decreases the production of inflammatory cytokines (IL-1 and TNF) by immune cells [36] and reduces the sensitivity of tissue receptors to these mediators [37].

Infusion of soy emulsions has also been associated with the formation of products derived from the action of free radicals on polyunsaturated FA, and

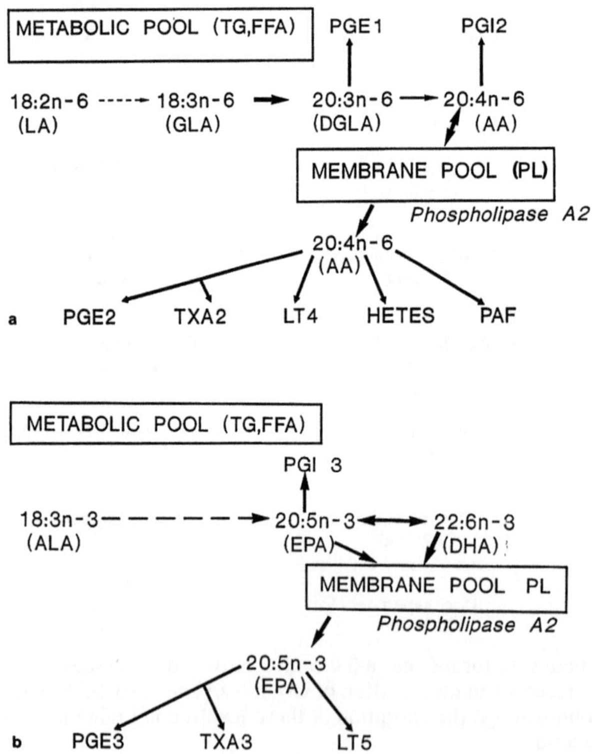

Fig. 3a, b. Formation of major eicosanoids from n-6 **(a)** and n-3 **(b)** essential fatty acids. TG: triglycerides; FFA: free fatty acids; LA: linoleic acid; GLA: gamma-linolenic acid; DGLA: di-homo gamma-linolenic acid; AA: arachidonic acid; ALA: alpha-linolenic acid; EPA: eicosapentanoic acid; DHA: docosahexanoic acid; PG: prostaglandin; TX: thromboxane; LT: leukotrienes; HETES: hydroxy-eicosatetraenoic acids; PAF: platelet aggregating factor.

the consumption of plasma anti-oxidants such as vitamin E [38–40]. The general view is that the amount of α-tocopherol contained in soy oil is insufficient to prevent peroxidative attacks and that anti-oxidant supply should be raised. Of course, this holds true for preparations containing other polyunsaturated, such as long-chain n-3 FA. We have recently provided evidence that enriching soy emulsions with α-tocopherol could restore plasma and lipoprotein levels [41]. Increasing plasma anti-oxidant capacity may be particularly relevant in most neonatal and adult ICU patients, whether they are supplied or not with parenteral nutrition and lipid emulsions.

Attempts have recently been made for reducing the total intake of n-6 polyunsaturated FA contained in soy emulsions or for changing the balance between n-6 and n-3 compounds. This can be achieved by replacing a proportion of soy oil by medium-chain triglycerides (or olive oil), or by adding triglycerides derived from fish oil. At the same time, new types of structured triglycerides are developed, which contain in the same molecule specific FA with different chain length, put in a pre-determined position or assembled at random.

Considering lipid emulsions not only as a means of providing energy, but also of modifying cell membrane composition and regulating the production (and action) of several mediators represents a new and exciting approach which currently stimulates extensive research, as assessed by the rapidly growing literature. Taking into consideration the numerous implications of lipid compounds in metabolic reactions, it is understandable that a study can (and should) address only a limited number of aspects. Therefore, caution is needed in order to avoid overinterpretation of the data.

Influence of Triglyceride FA Composition on the Metabolism of Lipid Emulsions

Emulsions containing Medium-Chain Triglycerides

In this part, we propose to summarize recent data evaluating the effect of replacing half the amount of soy triglycerides by MCT on different steps of the intravascular metabolism of lipid emulsions. These studies have been conducted in normal subjects, using the hypertriglyceridemic clamp model developed in our unit [42]. This model allows to measure key parameters in a system which largely reproduces conditions of patients receiving parenteral nutrition with lipids. Indeed, an infusion of glucose and amino acids is started prior to and continued throughout lipid administration at rates of 0.25 and 0.16 $g \cdot kg^{-1} \cdot h^{-1}$, respectively. In addition, this combined infusion of glucose and amino acids minimizes the contribution of endogenous fat stores to plasma Nefas (and ketones) and lipid oxidation, and induces a stabilization of substrate and hormone levels within 3 h [43].

After an initial infusion of lipid emulsions at a rate of 1 $g \cdot kg^{-1} \cdot h^{-1}$ during 18 min, plasma triglyceride concentration has been stabilized at 6 mmol/L to comparatively study the metabolism of a MCT/LCT (50%/50% wt/wt) mixture vs a pure soy-derived LCT emulsion in normal subjects [44]. We have observed:

- a higher elimination rate of infused triglycerides for the MCT/LCT emulsion; indeed, MCT/LCT infusion had to be raised to a rate of $0.24 \pm 0.04\ g \cdot kg^{-1} \cdot h^{-1}$ while that of LCT was decreased to $0.12 \pm 0.02\ g \cdot kg^{-1} \cdot h^{-1}$. Analysis of FA composition in plasma triglycerides showed that the difference between both emulsions was primarily due to a much faster hydrolysis of MCT while that of LCT remained unaffected by the presence of MCT;
- a higher rise of plasma Nefas during MCT/LCT (from 0.05 to 1.52 mmol/L) than during LCT (from 0.11 to 0.53 mmol/L) infusion; analysis of FA pattern in plasma Nefas showed a much larger contribution of medium-chain than long-chain FA in this increase;
- a much lower enrichment of cholesteryl esters in the TG-rich particles (isolated in the $d < 1.006$ g/mL fraction) during MCT/LCT than LCT infusion; this is in agreement with *in vitro* data showing that the relatively high concentration of MCT in the phospholipid surface inhibits acquisition of cholesteryl esters;
- a lower increase of plasma phospholipid level with MCT/LCT, in spite of a much higher rate of infusion, suggesting a much faster phospholipid elimination from this emulsion.

In addition, the faster hydrolysis of emulsion triglycerides was not associated with a higher, but to the contrary with a lower accumulation of remnants derived from MCT/LCT than LCT. As previously mentioned, this latter observation may reflect an important aspect if it was confirmed that the hepatic removal of remnants interferes with the catabolism of α-2 macroglobulin.

Additional studies comparing the same emulsions, included for 3 months in the regimen of patients on long-term HPN (in a cross-over design), showed advantages for the MCT/LCT mixture with respect to:

- a lower (and practically no) incidence of liver test alterations [45];
- the maintenance of a balanced FA pattern in RBC phospholipids, versus a marked accumulation of linoleate observed with the LCT emulsion [46]; and
- the maintenance of a normal HDL/LDL cholesterol ratio, versus a substantial decrease observed with the LCT preparation.

However, it is difficult to determine whether these advantages resulted from the reduced intake of soy-derived FA, or from the infusion of MCT. Also, indirect calorimetry measurements performed in normal subjects did not show a substantially greater rate of total body fat oxidation with MCT/LCT versus LCT, suggesting that the higher rate of MCT oxidation reported from isotopic studies may be at the expense of LCT oxidation. In addition, we could demonstrate that the metabolism of medium-chain FA is not totally independent from carnitine [47].

Emulsions Enriched with Fish Oil Triglycerides

Although the potential interest of n-3 FA in inflammatory conditions is well-recognized, their application in clinical nutrition is related to some important questions:

- What is the effect of fish oil supplementation on triglyceride hydrolysis by LPL and remnant formation?
- What is the rate of incorporation of n-3 FA into cellular membrane of different tissues?
- How to antagonize the peroxidative susceptibility of these very unsaturated FA?

In vitro data have shown that addition of more than 10% fish oil (i.e. ~5% n-3 FA) to a soy emulsion exerted a marked inhibitory effect on LPL activity [48]. Hence, we have used the hypertriglyceridemic clamp stabilized over 5 h at 6 mmol/L to study the effect of supplementing a regular soybean emulsion with 10% fish oil triglycerides on the intravascular metabolism of exogenous lipids in normal subjects. EPA and DHA accounted for respectively 1.8 and 1.7% of triglyceride FA in the fish oil enriched emulsion and were not present in the control triglycerides. However, the phospholipid emulsifier also contained 0.5% EPA and 2.9% DHA.

Although the infusion rate required to maintain plasma triglyceride concentration at a level of 6 mmol/L had to be temporarily decreased more with the fish oil enriched emulsion, the total amount of trigylcerides infused over the 285 min period following the priming was the same with both preparations (46 ± 6 g fish oil enriched triglycerides vs 47 ± 4 g of control soy emulsion). Plasma Nefa concentration rose from 0.02 ± 0.01 to 0.31 ± 0.04 mmol/L with the fish oil enriched, and from 0.02 ± 0.01 to 0.39 ± 0.04 mmol/L with the control soy emulsion. This difference was not statistically significant.

Similar changes in the lipid composition of endogenous lipoproteins and of exogenous particles were observed with both emulsions. This suggests that neutral lipid transfer between emulsion TG-rich particles and cholesterol-rich LDL and HDL were not affected by fish oil supplementation. In addition, no differences in the amount of triglycerides and cholesterol present in remnant particles at the end of lipid infusion were observed between both emulsions.

Thus, enrichment of a soy-derived emulsion with 10% of a fish oil-derived preparation has no significant influence on the major parameters characterizing the intravascular metabolism of lipid emulsions during one single infusion in man.

The incorporation of exogenous FA into different tissue lipids was studied in 2 groups of 4 Beagle dogs (age 13±1 month; weight 14.7±1.1 kg) randomized to receive TPN with a pure soy-derived emulsion, or the same preparation enriched with 10% fish oil. Lipid intake was 5 g TG/kg·day and contributed to 60% of non-protein calories. Biopsies of different tissues were taken 2 weeks before starting and again on the day following TPN. It was interesting to observe that EPA and DHA could not be detected in adipose tissue trigylcerides while significant enrichment with 18:2 n-6 and 18:3 n-3 was observed [49]. In the liver, 18:2 n-6 content was markedly increased, both into triglycerides and phospholipids. A slight enrichment of EPA and DHA was observed in liver triglycerides of ¾ animals infused with the fish oil enriched emulsion. In contrast, a marked enrichment with DHA, and to a minor extent with EPA, was present in liver phospholipids. Thus, long-chain n-3 FA do not accumulate into storage lipids, but are efficiently incorporated into tissue phospholipids, with substantial interorgan differences.

Recent data suggest that n-3 FA can be incorporated into pulmonary macrophages within only a few days of enteral supplementation [50]. In 2 studies where infusions of either a fish oil derived or a soy derived emulsion were started prior to an endotoxin challenge in animals, fish oil appeared to reduce the level of lactic acidosis (by enhancing hepatic clearance of lactate) and to maintain a better tissue perfusion, particularly in the intestine [51, 52]. However, it is difficult to determine whether the positive effects resulted from a reduction of n-6 FA intake, or from the supply of n-3 FA.

In the past years, experimental data have been reported on the use of structured triglycerides in parenteral nutrition. In a first series of experiments in animal models of burns and cancer, beneficial effects were observed with respect to protein-sparing and reduced tumor growth [53, 54). However, these studies were comparing triglycerides made of fish oil and medium-chain FA to a regular soy emulsion. Hence, it was not possible to separate the effect of FA composition from that of triglyceride structure. In a recent paper, the same group [55] compared structured triglycerides made of an isomolar mixture of MCT and soy LCT to blended oils with the same FA composition, and to a pure soy emulsion in a model of burned rats. No difference was observed between the 3 substrates with respect to their nitrogen sparing effect. These investigations were performed with structured triglycerides prepared by allowing long and medium-chain FA to re-esterify at random on the glycerol backbone. However, Redgrave et al. [56] have emphasized the role of FA in triglyceride sn-2 position on peripheral hydrolysis by lipoprotein lipase, and mainly in hepatic uptake of remnants. In collaboration with R. J. Deckelbaum and Th. Olivecrona, we noticed marked differences between different types of well-defined structured triglycerides (e.g. LML and MLM) with respect to *in vitro* hydrolysis by LPL and neutral lipid exchange [57, 58]. This suggests the potential for triglycerides with a different structure to have a specific behavior at several steps of intravascular metabolism.

Acknowledgements. The studies summarized in the present review have been performed with the support of grants nr 3.4568.91 and 3.4632.92 from the Belgian "Fonds de la Recherche Scientifique Médicale". The emulsions were kindly provided by Fresenius AG (Bad Homburg, Germany) and by B. Braun (Melsungen, Germany).

References

1. Wretlind A (1981) Development of fat emulsions. JPEN 5:230–235
2. Carpentier YA, Van Gossum A, Dubois DY, Deckelbaum RJ (1993) Lipid Metabolism. In: JL Rombeau, MD Caldwell (eds): "Clinical Nutrition: Parenteral Nutrition, 2nd edition". WB Saunders Philadelphia, USA, pp:35–74
3. Haumont D, Deckelbaum RJ, Richelle M, et al (1989) Plasma lipid and plasma lipoprotein concentrations in low birth weight infants given parenteral nutrition with twenty or ten percent lipid emulsion. J Pediatr 115:787–793
4. Olivecrona T, Bengtsson-Olivecrona G (1990) Lipases involved in lipoprotein metabolism. Curr Opin Lipidol 1:116–121
5. Tonouchi H, Iriyama K, Carpentier YA (1990) Transfer of apolipoproteins between plasma lipoproteins and exogenous lipid particles after repeated bolus injections or during a continuous infusion of fat emulsion. JPEN 14:381–385
6. Deckelbaum RJ, Hamilton JA, Moser A, et al (1990) Medium-chain versus long-chain triacylglycerol emulsion hydrolysis by lipoprotein lipase and hepatic lipase: Implications for the mechanisms of lipase action. Biochemistry 29:1136–1142
7. Peterson J, Bihain BE, Bengtsson-Olivecrona G, Deckelbaum RJ, Carpentier YA, Olivecrona T (1990) Fatty acid control of lipoprotein lipase. A link between energy metabolism and lipid transport. Proc Natl Acad Sci 87:909–913
8. Beisigel U, Weber W, Bengtsson-Olivecrona G (1991) Lipoprotein lipase enhances the binding of chylomicrons to low density lipoprotein receptor-related protein. Proc Natl Acad Sci USA 88:8342–8346
9. Rumsey SC, Obunike JC, Arad Y, Deckelbaum RJ, Goldberg IJ (1992) Lipoprotein lipase-mediated uptake and degradation of low density lipoproteins by fibroblasts and macrophages. J Clin Invest 90:1504–1512
10. Sniderman A, Baldo A, Cianflone K (1992) The potential role of acylation stimulating protein as a determinant of plasma trigylceride clearance and intracellular triglyceride synthesis. Curr Opin Lipidol 3:202–207
11. Melin T, Qi C, Bengtsson-Olivecrona G, Akesson A, Nilsson A (1991) Hydrolysis of chylomicron polyenoic fatty acid esters with lipoprotein lipase and hepatic lipase. Biochim Biophys Acta 1075:259–266
12. Tall AR (1986) Plasma lipid transfer protein. J Lipid Res 27:361–368
13. Packard CJ, Munro A, Lorimer AR, Gotto AM, Sheperd J (1984) Metabolism of apolipoprotein B in large triglyceride-rich hypertriglyceridemic subjects. J Clin Invest 74:2178–2192
14. Mahley RW, Weisgraber KH, Hussain MM, et al (1989) Intravenous infusion of apolipoprotein E accelerates clearance of plasma lipoproteins in rabbits. J Clin Invest 83:2125–2130
15. Yamada N, Shimano H, Mokuno H, et al (1989) Increased clearance of plasma cholesterol after injection of apolipoprotein E into Watanabe heritable hyperlipidemic rabbitts. Proc Natl Acad Sci 86:665–669
16. Brown MS, Herz J, Kowal RC, Goldstein JL (1991) The low-density lipoprotein receptor-related protein: Double agent or decoy? Curr Opin Lipidol 2:65–72
17. Bessesen DH, Richards CL, Etienne J, Goers JW, Eckel RH (1993) Spinal cord of the rat contains more lipoprotein lipase than other brain regions. J Lipid Res 34:229–238

18. Haumont D, Richelle M, Deckelbaum RJ, Coussaert E, Carpentier YA (1992) Effect of liposomal content of lipid emulsions on plasma lipids in low birth weight infants receiving parenteral nutrition. J Pediatrics 121:759–763
19. Griffin E, Breckenridge WC, Kuksis A, Bryan MH, Angel A (1979) Appearance and characterization of lipoprotein X during continuous Intralipid infusions in the neonate. J Clin Invest 64:1703–1712
20. Untracht S (1982) Alterations of serum lipoproteins resulting from total parenteral nutrition with Intralipid. Biochim Biophys Acta 711:176–192
21. Williams KJ, Scanu AM (1986) Uptake of endogenous cholesterol by a synthetic liopoprotein. Biochim Biophys Acta 875:183–194
22. Dahlan W, Richelle M, Kulapongse S, Deckelbaum RJ, Carpentier YA (1992) Modification of erythrocyte membrane lipid composition induced by a single intravenous infusion of phospholipid-triacylglycerol emulsions in man. Clin Nutr 11:255–261
23. Degott C, Messing B, Moreau D, et al (1988) Liver phospholipidosis induced by parenteral nutrition: Histologic, histochemical, and ultrastructural investigations. Gastroenterology 95:183–191
24. Harris HW, Grunfeld C, Feingold KR, Rapp JH (1990) Human very low density lipoproteins and chylomicrons can protect against endotoxin-induced death in mice. J Clin Invest 86:696–702
25. Dubois DY (1993) Contribution à l'étude du métabolisme des HDL chez l'être humain. Mise en évidence de fonctions spécifiques des HDL en dehors du Reverse Cholesterol Transport. PhD Thesis, Université Libre de Bruxelles, Brussels
26. Blackburn WD, Dohlman JG, Venkachalapathi YV, et al (1991) Apolipoprotein A-I decreases neutrophil degranulation and superoxide production. J Lipid Res 32:1911–1918
27. Packman CH, Rosenfeld SI, Leddy JP (1985) High-density lipoproteins and its apolipoproteins inhibit cytolytic activity of complement. Studies on the nature of the inhibitory moieties. Biochim Biophys Acta 812:107–115
28. Jordan-Stack TC, Witte DP, Aronow BJ, Harmony JAK (1992) Apolipoprotein J: A membrane policeman? Curr Opin Lipidol 3:75–85
29. Cuthbert JA, Lipsky PE (1987) Provision of cholesterol to lymphocytes by high density and low density lipoproteins. Requirement for low density lipoprotein receptors. J Biol Chem 262:7808–7818
30. Ginsberg H, Grabowski GH, Gibson JC, et al (1984) Reduced plasma concentrations of total, low density lipoprotein and high density lipoprotein cholesterol in patients with Gaucher type I disease. Clin Genetics 26:109–116
31. Malmendier CL, Lontie J-F, Dubois DY (1991) Mechanisms of hypocholesterolemia. Adv Exp Med Biol 285:173–182
32. Hajri T, Ferezou J, Steinmetz P, Lutton C (1993) Total parenteral nutrition and plasma lipoproteins in the rat: Evidence for accelerated clearance of apo-A-I-rich HDL. Biochim Biophys Acta 1166:84–91
33. Yui Y, Aoyama T, Morishita H, Takahashi M, Takatsu Y, Kawai C (1988) Serum prostacyclin stabilizing factor is identical to apolipoprotein A-I (Apo A-I). A novel function of Apo A-I. J Clin Invest 82:803–807
34. Bekaert ED, Dole E, Dubois DY, et al (1992) Alterations in lipoprotein density classes in infantile visceral Leishmaniasis: Presence of apolipoprotein SAA. Eur J Clin Invest 22:190–199
35. Dubois DY, personal communication
36. Endres S, Ghorbani R, Kelley VE, et al (1989) The effect of dietary supplementation with n-3 polyunsaturated fatty acids on the synthesis of interleukin-1 and tumor necrosis factor by mononuclear cells. N Engl J Med 320:265–271
37. Tisdale MJ, Beck SA (1991) Inhibition of tumor-induced lipolysis in vitro and cachexia and tumour growth in vivo by eicosapentaenoic acid. Biochem Pharmacol 41:103–107
38. Lemoyne M, Van Gossum A, Kurian R, Jeejeebhoy KN (1988) Plasma vitamin E and selenium and breath pentane in home parenteral nutrition patients. Am J Clin Nutr 48:1310–1315

39. Van Gossum A, Lemoyne M, Sharriff R, Kurian A, Jeejeebhoy KN (1988) Increased lipid peroxidation after lipid emulsion as measured by breath pentane output. Am J Clin Nutr 48:1394–1399
40. Pitkanen O, Hallmann M, Andersson S (1991) Generation of free radicals in lipid emulsion used in parenteral nutrition. Pediatr Res 29:56–59
41. Traber MG, Carpentier YA, Kayden HJ, Richelle M, Galeano N, Deckelbaum RJ (1993) Alterations in the distribution of alpha- and gamma-tocopherols in human lipoproteins in response to intravenous infusion of triglyceride-rich emulsions. Metabolism (in press)
42. Carpentier YA, Kinney JM, Siderova VS, et al (1990) Hypertriglyceridaemia clamp: A new model for studying lipid metabolism. Clin Nutr 9 (Suppl):1
43. Carpentier YA, Bihain B, Rubin M, et al (1990) Stabilization of plasma substrate concentrations: A model for conducting metabolic studies. Clin Nutr 9:313–318
44. Richelle M (1992) Influence of intravenous lipid emulsions on cholesterol homeostasis. Clin Nutr 11:49–52
45. Carpentier YA, Richelle M, Haumont D, Deckelbaum RJ (1990) New developments in fat emulsions. Proc Nutr Soc 49:375–380
46. Dahlan W, Richelle M, Rössle C, Deckelbaum RJ, Carpentier YA (1992) Effects of essential fatty acid contents of lipid emulsions on erythrocyte polyunsaturated fatty acid composition in patients on long-term parenteral nutrition. Clin Nutr 11:262–268
47. Rössle C, Carpentier YA, Richelle M, et al (1990) Medium chain triglycerides induce alterations in carnitine metabolism. Am J Physiol 258:E944–E947
48. Oliviera T, Carpentier YA, Hansen I, Deckelbaum RJ (1992) Triglyceride hydrolysis of soy vs fish oil LCT emulsions. Clin Nutr 11 (suppl):44
49. Rössle C (1993) Intravascular metabolism of a fish oil-supplemented lipid emulsion in an experimental dog model: Effects on plasma and liver lipids, lipoproteins and incorporation of long-chain n3 fatty acids into plasma lipids. Clin Nutr (in press)
50. Palombo J, Lydon E, Bistrian B, Forse A (1993) Rapid modulation of rat alveolar macrophage and lung phospholipid fatty acids (PLFA) by continuous enteral feeding with fish oil. JPEN 17:27S
51. Pomposelli JJ, Flores E, Hirschberg Y, et al (1990) Short-term TPN containing n-3 fatty acids ameliorate lactic acidosis induced by endotoxin in guinea pigs. Am J Clin Nutr 52:548–552
52. Pscheidl EM, Wan JM, Blackburn GL, Bistrian BR, Istfan NW (1992) Influence of w-3 fatty acids on splanchnic blood flow and lactate metabolism in an endotoxemic rat model. Metabolism 41:698–705
53. Mok KT, Maiz A, Yamazaki K, et al (1984) Structured medium-chain and long-chain trigylceride emulsions are superior to physical mixtures in sparing body protein in the burned rat. Metabolism 33:910
54. Ling PR, Istfan NW, Lopes SM, et al (1991) Structured lipid made from fish oil and medium-chain triglycerides alters tumor and host metabolism in Yoshida-sarcoma-bearing rats. Am J Clin Nutr 53:1177
55. Gollaher CJ, Swenson ES, Mascioli EA, Babayan VK, Blackburn GL, Bistrain BR (1992) Dietary fat level as determinant of protein-sparing actions of structured triglycerides. Nutrition 8:348–353
56. Redgrave TG, Kodali DR, Small DM (1988) The effect of triacyl-sn-glycerol structure on the metabolism of chylomicrons and triacylglycerol-rich emulsions in the rat. J Biol Chem 263:5118–5123
57. Olivecrona T, Bengtsson-Olivecrona G, Carpentier YA, Deckelbaum RJ, Hansen T, Frokjaer S (1990) Lipolysis of emulsions containing structured triglycerides with medium and long chain fatty acids. Clin Nutr 9 (Suppl):10
58. Richelle M, Deckelbaum RJ, Olivecrona T, Hansen T, Frokjaer S, Carpentier YA (1990) Triglyceride structure determines cholesterol transport by lipid emulsions. Clin Nutr 9 (Suppl):32

Organ Specific Nutrients and Associated Therapy

Effects of Enteral Nutrients on the Critically Ill Gut

J. I. Lew and J. L. Rombeau

Introduction

Traditional teachings state that the gut is quiescent in the critically ill patient. These teachings, however, are undergoing rigorous scientific scrutiny. It is now known that the gut is both physiologically and metabolically active despite the presence of critical illness. Moreover, recent investigations have shown that enteral nutrients, and in some instances the provision of enterocyte and colonocyte fuels, enhance structure and function of the intestine during stress and disease. This chapter reviews the structure and function of the normal intestinal epithelium and the adverse effects of critical illness on the gut. In addition, the role of enteral nutrients in preventing and treating these adverse effects is discussed. This information in part has been reviewed in a previous report from our laboratory (Lew JI and Rombeau JL, unpublished data).

Normal Intestinal Epithelium

Cellular Proliferation and Differentiation

Intestinal epithelial cells have one of the most rapid turnover rates of any tissue in the human body. Turnover of the intestinal epithelium involves the proliferation, migration, differentiation, maturation and eventual exfoliation of its component cells. Intestinal epithelial cell renewal depends on the continual division of proliferating stem cells deep within mucosal crypts. DNA synthesis associated with proliferation occurs in these stem cells of the small intestine and colon. New epithelial cells migrate from the lower half of crypts to the mucosal surface where they are, by this time, mature and eventually lost to the lumen. Under normal conditions, proliferation is balanced by exfoliation so that epithelial cell populations are preserved at a steady state [1].

Cell proliferation, and consequently DNA synthesis, is initiated when certain changes in metabolic activity occur. Precursor nucleic acid enzymes required in DNA synthesis, such as thymidine kinase and thymidylate synthetase, increase in activity as cell proliferation begins in the bases of the intestinal crypts. After proliferation, intestinal epithelial cells move into differentiative and maturative phases of the cell cycle. Differentiation, which occurs after proliferation, is associated with a decrease in important cell constituents necessary for DNA synthesis. While protein and other syntheses still occur in differentiating cells, their ability to proliferate decreases and eventually ceases. Thus, DNA synthesis occurs before cell differentiation which indicates a mutually exclusive relationship between cell proliferation and differentiation [2].

Specialized structures characteristic of intestinal epithelial cells are associated with the later stages of cell differentiation and maturation. For example, mature villous columnar cells of the small intestine are highly polarized and possess well developed brush borders. Additionally, hydrolases commonly found in these brush borders further characterize differentiated and matured cells. Thus, changes in precursor nucleic acid enzyme activity, enzyme variability and template stability are associated with cell differentiation and have a role in regulating the cessation of DNA synthesis before this phase [2]. Furthermore, structural specializations characteristic of certain cells serve as markers for cell maturation (Lew JI and Rombeau JL, 1993).

Small intestine. The epithelial cells of the small intestine (enterocytes) form an important lumenal interface with the outside environment. Absorption is greatly enhanced in the small bowel by mucosal projections called villi which extend into its lumen. The surface which covers the villi is comprised mainly of three enterocyte types: villous columnar cells, goblet cells, and enteroendocrine cells. These cells are bound together by tight junctions which maintain an impermeable barrier between the lumenal contents and intestinal submucosa [3]. The cells of small bowel crypts differ from the covering villi. The crypts contain 4 types of enterocytes: crypt base columnar cells, immature goblet cells, Paneth cells, and enteroendocrine cells.

The crypt base columnar cells of the small intestine are stem cells which differentiate into other constituent enterocyte types as they migrate up to the villi. Most of the enterocytes from crypt base to villi are absorptive columnar cells that transcend from crypt cell columnar cells to become differentiated villous columnar cells. In humans, the time involved for columnar cells to reach the lumen is 5 to 6 days in most of the small bowel, and 3 days in the ileum [2].

The two kinds of mucus cells in the small intestine are immature goblet cells, found exclusively in the crypts, and mature mucus secreting goblet cells located in the upper crypts and villi. These cells begin as immature goblet cells that migrate with columnar cells to the villous tips where they mature to become mucus secreting goblet cells. Additionally, Paneth cells do not divide and originate higher in crypts of the small intestine where they eventually degenerate and descend into the crypt base to be phagocytosed by macrophages. Renewal of these cells takes place after several weeks. Finally, enteroendocrine cells also migrate toward the villous tips, taking about 4 days to reach the surface. As these cells mature, they acquire an increased number of cytoplasmic granules and lose the ability to divide [2].

Large intestine. In contrast to the small intestine, the human large intestine (colon) has no villi. The absorptive epithelium is planar and consists of straight tubular crypts which extend into the lamina propria. The colonic epithelial cells or colonocytes consist of 3 types: absorptive columnar cells, mucus secreting goblet cells, and enteroendocrine cells [4].

The colonic crypts consist primarily of mucus releasing goblet cells with occasional enteroendocrine cells. The colonic surface is comprised mainly of absorptive columnar cells which have microvilli on their lumenal surfaces found less abundantly than those in the small intestine. At colonic base crypts, there are stem cells that differentiate into the different colonocyte types. The stem cells of the ascending colon are small columnar cells while those of the descending colon and rectum called vacuolated cells contain secretory vesicles. Before they reach the lumenal surface, these vacuolated cells lose their vesicles and mature into typical columnar cells with a brush border. The columnar, mucous and enteroendocrine cells proliferate in the lower two thirds of colonic crypts. Migration of these cells to the lumenal surface takes about 3 to 8 days in humans [2, 5].

Intestinal Barrier

The normal intestinal epithelium allows for selective passage of nutrients into blood and lymph circulation, while serving as a protective physical barrier against the absorption of intralumenal bacteria and their toxins. The epithelial cell membranes prevent transcellular migration of such antigens, and the tight junctions between these cells hinder particle movement through paracellular channels. Furthermore, mucus cell secretions prevent the adherence and invasion of enteric bacteria and toxins.

The intestinal barrier is characterized by several immunologic components. The mucosa and submucosa are replete with lymphocytes, macrophages, neutrophils and Peyer's patches which are lymphoid aggregates to the terminal ileum. Found abundantly in bile and intestinal secretions, IgA binds and mediates the recognition of such antigens as bacteria and their toxins. Furthermore, hepatic Kupffer cells are in a key position to collect and detoxify antigens that penetrate beyond the intestinal wall and regional lymphatic tissue. The epithelium and its immunologic constituents are the major components of intestinal barrier function, although cell mediated immunity may play a supportive role to the mucosa [6].

Nutrients and Intestinal Growth and Function

As mentioned, enterocyte and colonocyte renewal is dependent on the continued division of proliferating stem cells located deep within mucosal crypts. Mucosal growth is determined by the rates of epithelial cell proliferation and exfoliation. Normal mucosa is maintained at a steady state when cell proliferation is balanced by surface epithelial cell exfoliation. For mucosal growth to occur, the rate of cell production must be greater than the rate of cell loss. Growth may occur when the rate of cell proliferation increases and cell loss remains constant or when cell production remains the same and cell exfoliation decreases. Furthermore, mucosal atrophy or hypoplasia occurs when cell proliferation is insufficient or exfoliation increases. In contrast, mucosal hyperplasia results when cell production increases or cell life is prolonged. Thus, the rate of intestinal cell turnover determines mucosal growth, and any alteration in these processes will result in physiologic changes [1].

Since epithelial cell metabolic activity consumes most of the nutrient requirements of normal intestine, the most important stimulus for mucosal growth and function is the presence of lumenal (enteral) nutrients. Enteral nutrition (EN), the direct provision of nutrients into the intestinal lumen, mediates mucosal trophism by several mechanisms, namely, physical contact, stimulation of trophic gastrointestinal (GI) hormones, enhancement of intestinal blood flow and incitement of the autonomic nervous system.

Physical Contact of Nutrients

The stimulatory effects of nutrients on mucosal growth is a result of two processes; namely by enteral nutrients, and by dietary induced trophic factors independent of nutritional value. Enteral nutrients in the form of digestible or indigestible material in the intestinal lumen directly stimulate mucosal growth by physical contact.

Several studies have demonstrated the importance of EN in the maintenance of intestinal mucosal growth, especially in intestinal adaptation after surgical resection (Lew JI and Rombeau JL, 1993). EN maintains cell proliferation consistently in the small intestinal mucosa after bypass surgery. Additionally, nonspecific esterase and α-glucosidase activity is elevated in villous columnar cells compared to control values [7]. Enteral contents in the form of a fiber-free diet with poorly fermentable pure cellulose are capable of maintaining colonic mucosal growth. Cellulose causes a marked increase in crypt column height and may play a regulatory role on mucosal growth [8].

Certain enteral nutrients stimulate mucosal growth when converted into trophic factors by the action of digestive enzymes or bacteria within the intestinal lumen. Recent studies indicate that dietary fiber may belong in this category. Although dietary fiber is not digested by small intestinal secretions, there is significant fiber degradation in the ascending colon by bacterial fermentation [9]. The extent of fermentation is determined by the type of fiber and bacterial flora. Numerous species of colonic bacteria have necessary enzymes required to digest or ferment dietary fiber. Metabolism of these fibers nourishes the colonic microflora and produces the major end-products of fermentation, namely, volatile short-chain fatty acids (SCFA) which primarily include acetate, propionate, and n-butyrate in humans [10, 11].

Studies with [3H] thymidine clearly show that animals on fiber supplemented diets have increased crypt cell turnover rates and faster cell migration to the villous columns in the small intestine [12]. Rats fed pectin and guar gum supplemented diets demonstrated faster rates of enterocyte turnover than those fed with oat bran and fiber free diets [13]. In the jejunum, pectin stimulated cell proliferation more than guar gum. Similar effects were noted in the ileum. No significant effects were found in the duodenum.

Other studies have shown that fiber ingestion is important in the maintenance and growth of the colonic epithelium. Low fiber diets produce atrophy as noted by mucosal hypoplasia and a decreased rate of colonocyte renewal [14]. Although other dietary components such as cellulose may be important in sustaining colonic mucosal integrity [8], it is generally believed that the trophic effects in the colon are mediated by the fermentation products from dietary fiber and undigested starch [15].

Enterotrophic Gastrointestinal Hormones

The role of nutrient-induced GI hormones in the regulation of intestinal mucosal growth has not been fully elucidated. Nevertheless, some studies reveal that gastrin and enteroglucagon have trophic effects in the small intestine and colon.

Gastrin, a peptide, is trophic for certain types of normal intestinal mucosa. This hormone stimulates cell proliferation and increases levels of DNA, RNA and protein content in duodenal, ileal and proximal colonic mucosa [1]. Additionally, removal of the antrum with G cells that synthesize gastrin decreases DNA content in the colon [16]. In an *in vitro* study with normal human colonic epithelial cells, pentagastrin caused a fivefold increase in cell number compared to a threefold increase in cells treated with saline [17]. The extent of the effects of gastrin in intestinal growth, however, are still not entirely clear. While studies clearly demonstrate that gastrin stimulates gastric cell proliferation, similar effects in the small intestine and colon have been contradictory [18, 19].

Enteroendocrine cells in the ileum and colon produce enteroglucagon. Although there is a strong correlation between increased enteroglucagon levels and intestinal mucosal growth, to our knowledge, no studies have clearly demonstrated that enteroglucagon stimulates this growth (Lew JI and Rombeau JL, 1993). While glucagon has a small effect on colonocyte proliferation, enteroglucagon plays a larger role in enterocyte proliferation [20]. Enteroglucagon was thought to stimulate cell proliferation in the small intestine after discovery of intestinal hypertrophy in a patient with an enteroglucagon secreting tumor. After tumor resection, the small bowel hypertrophy in this patient disappeared [21]. Finally, other studies suggest intestinal resection and glucose perfusion increase intestinal cell proliferation and plasma levels of enteroglucagon (Lew JI and Rombeau JL, 1993).

Intestinal Blood Flow

While reports on the effects of enteral nutrients on intestinal blood flow have been scarce, some studies suggest that SCFA have a trophic effect on colonic mucosa by increasing blood flow to this organ [22, 23]. Intralumenal placement of SCFA at postprandial concentrations increases colonic blood flow or hyperemia in dogs, suggesting these substances directly dilate colonic vasculature [22]. Acetate appears to produce a greater increase of blood flow than propionate and n-butyrate [22, 24].

In an *in vitro* study with resected human colons, SCFA, and not glutamine, individually and in combination caused concentration-dependent dilation of resistance arteries. This *in vitro* effect suggests SCFA may improve colonic microcirculation thereby providing a partial explanation for their trophic effect on colonic mucosa. Furthermore, such results might explain how modest doses of parenterally delivered SCFA produce trophic effects on rat intestinal mucosa [25–27].

Autonomic Nervous System

Studies on the effects of the autonomic nervous system (ANS) on the GI tract have been limited, except for the small intestine. Several studies suggest the ANS influences enterocyte proliferation. Sympathectomy inhibits DNA synthesis in intestinal crypts and decreases normal circadian rhythm in mitotic activity of undifferentiated enterocytes (Lew JI and Rombeau JL, 1993). In small bowel mucosa, β-adrenergic stimulation with isoproterenol decreases enterocyte proliferation, and consequently, cell turnover [28]. Noradrenergic fibers originate in the crypt base and rise into the villous tips [29]. At the crypt base, these fibers make direct contact between epithelial cells and nerve terminals [30, 31]. Recent work from our laboratory suggests that the ANS is important in the mediation of enterotrophic effects of cecally produced SCFA [32]. Rats with denervated ceca had significantly less SCFA mediated enterotrophism when compared to animals with normal cecal innervation. When considered together, these findings strongly suggest that there are autonomic receptors which play an important role in nutrient-induced regulation and proliferation of epithelial cells in the small intestinal mucosa.

Growth Factors

Several growth factors help regulate mucosal growth in the small intestine and colon. Although some of their effects are tissue specific, alteration of cell proliferation is a common mechanism shared by all growth factors. Growth factors affecting cell proliferation in the intestinal mucosa include growth hormone, insulin like growth factor I, epidermal growth factor, neurotensin and transforming growth factors α and β. An extensive review of this topic is included in chapter by Young et al.

Alteration of the Intestinal Barrier in Critical Illness

The intestinal tract is one of several main target organs that are compromised in the critically ill patient. Stresses such as cardiogenic shock, hypovolemia, sepsis and thermal injury can produce necrotic lesions in the intestinal mucosa. These conditions, with low mesenteric blood flow, disrupt the integrity of the intestinal barrier [33]. In addition to these stresses, malnutrition, starvation and altered intestinal flora, caused by broad spectrum antibiotics, further impair intestinal absorption. Stress-induced lesions of the intestinal mucosa begin at the apices of the villi and progress downward to separate the epithelium from the lamina propria in some instances. If such lesions continue, destruction of the lamina propria, ulceration and transmural necrosis of the intestinal barrier may occur. Such disruption of mucosal integrity allows for invasion by intralumenal constituents such as bacteria and endotoxin into the portal circulation [33]. Thus, the eroded mucosa becomes an ineffective barrier which allows disease processes to occur.

Hypoxia, associated with low blood flow, is an important cause of intestinal mucosal lesions during stress [34]. Exfoliation of intestinal epithelial cells, decreased mucus production and increased mucosal permeability to intralumenal particles occur with hermorrhagic shock. Furthermore, in such states of shock, lysosomal rupture renders the intestinal mucosa more susceptible to digestion by released enzymes. The lumenal presence of pancreatic enzymes such as elastase and trypsin also plays an important role in the pathogenesis of barrier dysfunction in intestinal ischemia. Accordingly, preservation of blood flow and perfusion of the intestinal lumen with nutrients and oxygen may protect the mucosa from damage in the ischemic gut [33].

Although intestinal ischemia is a major cause of mucosal barrier lesions, past studies suggest reperfusion of such ischemic tissue promotes oxygen-free (superoxide) radical formation which causes further barrier damage and eventual organ destruction. Generated by xanthine oxidase, superoxide radicals are eliminated by endogenous oxygen radical scavengers such as superoxide dismutase, catalase and glutathione [33, 35]. Glutathione, a tripeptide and major antioxidant, consists of glutamate derived from glutamine, cysteine and glycine. Recent studies suggest prophylactic administration of glutamine after intestinal shock, and ischemia-reperfusion preserves glutathione stores which may enhance antioxidant protection [36, 37].

Bacterial Translocation

Bacterial translocation is defined as the process by which bacteria migrate across the intestinal mucosal barrier to invade the liver, spleen and mesenteric lymph nodes. Any combination of three conditions often found in critically ill patients will promote bacterial translocation. These conditions are physical disruption of mucosal barrier (i.e. hermorrhagic shock, sepsis), microflora imbalance resulting in bacterial overgrowth of enteric bacilli (i.e. broad spectrum antibiotic therapy), and impaired host immune system (i.e. immunosuppressive drugs, protein deficiency) [6, 38].

Intestinal barrier failure and bacterial translocation is not an all or none phenomenon [35]. Disintegration of any one component of the intestinal barrier facilitates translocation of bacteria to the mesenteric lymph nodes, liver and spleen. However, in the healthy host, translocated bacteria do not multiply and spread systemically. Microorganisms are localized in the afore mentioned organs and eventually eliminated by tissue macrophages. In conditions of severe or complete intestinal barrier failure, translocating bacteria invade mesenteric lymph nodes, systemic organs and the circulatory system. The majority of animal models with this condition usually survive. However, those animals with thermal injury or protein deficiency receiving nonlethal doses of endotoxin frequently die from the translocation of bacteria [35].

Although a physical mucosal barrier and host immune system are necessary for effective barrier function, an intact epithelial barrier will preclude bacterial translocation despite impaired cell-mediated immunity. Thus, the intestinal mucosal barrier may play a primary role in preventing bacterial translocation while host immune defenses may serve a secondary role in intestinal barrier function [35]. An extensive review of this topic is included in chapter by MP Fink.

Endotoxemia

Bacterial endotoxins may also cross an impaired intestinal barrier. Normally, endotoxins enter the portal system in small amounts and are detoxified rapidly by hepatic Kupffer cells. Intestinal ischemia markedly potentiates the systemic effect of endotoxemia. If the superior mesenteric artery is temporarily occluded in rabbits, fatal endotoxemia can occur. Interestingly, when the intestinal microflora of these animals is removed, fatal endotoxemia does not occur when the same artery is occluded [39]. In mice, endotoxin enhances bacterial translocation from the intestinal lumen to the mesenteric lymph nodes in a dose dependent fashion. Lethal doses of bacterial toxins disrupt intercellular tight junctions, increasing permeability to bacteria and maintaining or amplifying endotoxemia [40].

Endotoxemia occurs in critically ill patients with low blood flow (i.e. cardiogenic or hypovolemic shock). A large percentage of trauma patients in shock have endotoxemia without evidence of visceral perforations. Of those with systolic blood pressures less than 80 mmHg at hospital admission, 56% patients have endotoxemia. Furthermore, of those with systolic blood pressures greater than 80 mmHg at admission, endotoxemia occurs in 9% of these patients [41]. Thus, severe hypotension leads to marked increases in endotoxemia.

Multiple Organ Failure Syndrome

Multiple organ failure (MOF) syndrome is a significant cause of morbidity and mortality in critically ill patients. Initially, MOF was thought to be exclusively due to sepsis [35, 42]. However, recent evidence suggests it can occur in the absence of infection [43, 44]. Enteric bacteremia is found in some critically ill patients dying of MOF and, in such cases, no septic focus can be found either clinically or by autopsy. Consequently, increasing attention has been directed to the investigation of gut derived bacteria as translocating pathogens responsible for initiating sepsis and perpetuating MOF.

In the gut origin hypothesis of MOF, translocated enteric bacteria and endotoxin travel to organs and tissues causing sepsis, macrophage cytokine secretion, neutrophil protease stimulation, oxidant production, proinflammatory endothelial cell promotion, and complement and coagulation system activation. These processes are thought to be self-sustaining and responsible for initiating MOF [42, 45].

There is no definitive evidence currently to support gut origin sepsis as a major cause of MOF. In fact, evidence for this hypothesis rests primarily on laboratory experiments with animal models. In the opinion of one of the authors (JL Rombeau), gut induced MOF occurs only in a very small percentage of malnourished, critically ill patients who are severely septic and immunosuppressed with significantly compromised gut barrier function.

Enteral Nutrients in Critical Illness

Since most critically ill patients are unable to eat voluntarily, nutrients must be administered either enterally or parenterally. Although total parenteral nutrition (TPN) has contributed significantly to the management of critically ill patients, enteral nutrition (EN) may be equally, if not more, beneficial to these patients. With improved methods of delivery, EN enhances intestinal structure and function. Although TPN may be used to maintain patients unable to receive EN, prolonged TPN administration leads to intestinal mucosal atrophy, enterocyte hypoplasia and decreased intestinal enzyme activity. These combined effects may in turn contribute to intestinal barrier disruption, hypermetabolism and other detrimental sequelae. Essential nutrients required for normal mucosal growth are usually not found in prolonged administrations of TPN used for treatment of critical illness. In fact, TPN is often associated with iatrogenic bowel malnutrition that impairs intestinal epithelial cell proliferation and mucosal repair [6].

The intestinal tract in critical illness has traditionally been considered to be inactive as a consequence of primary disease, infection, injury or medicinal side effects. Paralytic ileus usually occurs at some point in the course of treating critically ill patients. Different components of the intestinal tract are not equally susceptible to paralytic ileus. The small intestine is somewhat resistant to ileus development, and impaired absorption and dysmotility usually resolve within the first 24 h following insult. The colon and stomach, however, may take more than 3 days to regain normal motility after injury [46]. Consequently, early postoperative EN, which bypasses the stomach and delivers nutrients directly into the small bowel, is often used in critically ill patients [47, 48].

Paralytic ileus also promotes enteric bacterial overgrowth. Thus, in addition to rapid repair or prevention of intestinal muscosal injury, control of microfloral overgrowth and mediation of the host immune system against translocating bacteria and endotoxins may be efficacious in treatment of critically ill patients. Accumulating evidence suggests early administration of EN preserves intestinal barrier function by maintaining mucosal mass, preventing disruption of normal microflora balance and modulating host immune defenses [49].

In a recent comparative study, EN and TPN altered immunologic and metabolic response to endotoxemic injury in normal human volunteers [50]. These subjects received either isocaloric, isonitrogenous EN or TPN for 7 days and were then given IV injections of *E. Coli* endotoxin. TPN significantly worsened systemic manifestations of endotoxemia when compared to EN. Parenterally fed subjects demonstrated increased arterial and hepatic versus cachectin production consistent with activated reticuloendothelial cell response (Fig. 1). Furthermore, TPN subjects showed greater adverse effects of endotoxemic injury as indicated by increased peripheral lactate production and peripheral amino acid release. This study suggests TPN or the lack

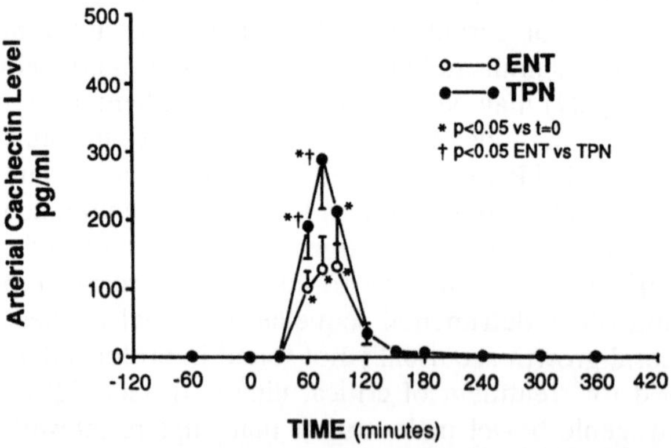

Fig. 1. Comparison of arterial cachectin levels before and after endotoxin injection in enteral vs parenteral feeding in normal human subjects. EN = enteral nutrition. TPN = total parenteral nutrition (From [50] with permission)

of enteral nutrients impairs intestinal barrier function and increases hepatic and splanchnic host exposure to bacteria and endotoxin. These events may amplify cytokine response by increasing splanchnic and reticuloendothelial cell activation to subsequent injury. Cytokines produced and secreted by hepatic Kupffer cells and splanchnic lymphocytes also enhance production of counterregulatory hormones which may transiently down regulate cytokine production, increase output of hepatic produced acute phase proteins and reduce gluconeogenesis [49]. Thus, antecedent route of nutritional support may influence immunologic and metabolic responses in critically ill patients to subsequent insults. An extensive review of this topic is included in Chapter by S Lowry.

Clinical Trials

Recent controlled clinical trials have shown that EN improves clinical outcome, especially decreased sepsis, in critically ill postoperative trauma patients.

In one trial, administration of enteral protein and rate of sepsis was studied in patients with blunt multiple trauma [51]. One reference group received more enteral protein (0.61 g/kg·day) and less IV protein (0.47 g/kg·day) while another group received no enteral protein and all IV protein (1.82 g/kg·day) for a 6 to 21 day period. The two groups began at the same degree of sepsis and differed after 21 days of study. Patients with no enteral protein intake had significantly more sepsis by all criteria than those receiving enteral protein. Furthermore, the larger amounts of protein given intravenously to the patients with no enteral protein did not compensate for the increased

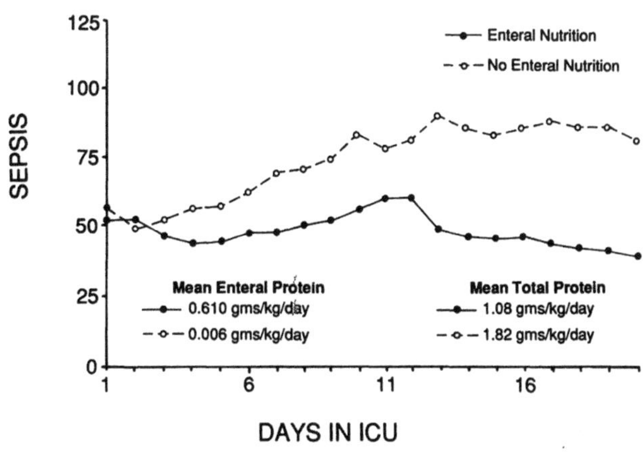

Fig. 2. Rate of sepsis in critically ill patients after 21 days of enteral protein vs intravenous protein. Enteral Nutrition = enteral protein. No enteral Nutrition = intravenous protein (From [51] with permission)

rate of sepsis (Fig. 2). Thus, absence of enteral protein intake increased rate of sepsis in patients with blunt multiple trauma.

In another study, EN was compared to TPN following postoperative infection in patients with abdominal trauma index above 15 [52]. Patients were randomly assigned to receive EN and TPN within 12 h after surgery. Infections developed in 17% of the EN patients contrasted to 37% of the TPN group. Furthermore, incidence of major septic morbidity was 3% in the EN group compared to 20% in those patients given TPN. Thus, EN compared to TPN improved resistance to infection in postoperative patients with severe abdominal trauma.

Finally, in a prospective trial, septic complications were studied in abdominal trauma patients who were randomly assigned to either early EN and TPN [53]. When randomized patients received either enteral or parenteral feeding within 24 h of injury, the enteral group developed fewer pneumonias, intra-abdominal abscess and line sepsis than the parenteral group (Fig. 3). Significantly fewer infections were found in enterally fed patients with an injury severity score above 20 or an abdominal trauma index above 24. In a subpopulation of the patients with an abdominal trauma index above 40 needing more than 20 units of blood or requiring more surgery within 72 h, there were significantly fewer infected patients and infections per infected patient in the enterally fed group. Thus, enterally fed trauma patients had significantly lower septic complications than parenterally fed trauma patients, with most of the significant changes found in the more severely injured.

In summary, these clinical trials illustrate that EN is well tolerated in severely injured patients. Furthermore, early enteral feeding reduces septic complications in these critically ill patients.

Metabolic Intestinal Fuels

Metabolic fuels of the intestinal tract have trophic effects on mucosal growth and the small intestine and colon differ in fuel preference. Glutamine and

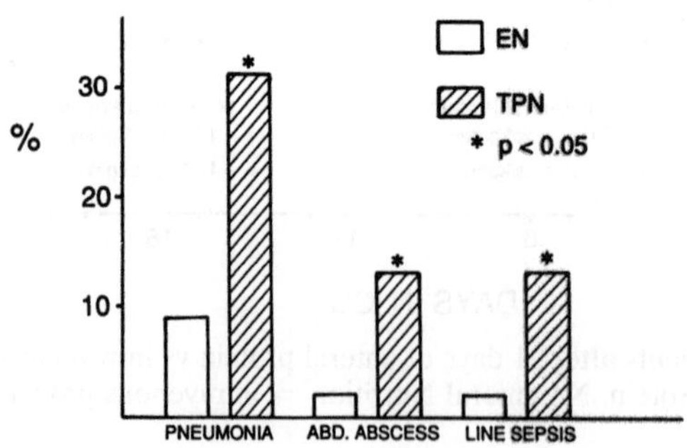

Fig. 3. Comparison of the effects of enteral vs parenteral nutrition on septic complications in postoperative patients with abdominal trauma. EN = enteral nutrition. TPN = total parenteral nutrition (From [53] with permission)

butyrate are the preferred metabolic fuels respectively for rapidly proliferating enterocytes and colonocytes. When EN is ineffective and TPN is required in the critically ill, such nutritional support generally fails to provide these two essential intestinal nutrients. In fact, glutamine is absent in all currently available formulations of TPN in the United States. Furthermore, butyrate is not enterally administered to the colon in critically ill patients, and concomitant antibiotic therapy suppresses colonic microflora that produce butyrate from dietary fiber and undigested starch. Thus, at a time when the gut might conceivably benefit from appropriate feeding, the prescribed nutritional therapy paradoxically starves the intestinal tract and leads to mucosal atrophy. Current studies suggest that EN supplemented with intestinal specific metabolic fuels such as glutamine and butyrate may be more efficacious in critically ill patients with intestinal dysfunction when compared to providing formulations without these fuels.

Glutamine

Glutamine is a non-essential amino acid that plays a major role in the maintenance of intestinal metabolism, structure and function. A principal fuel for enterocytes, glutamine may be especially important in critical illness when the intestinal barrier appears to be vulnerable [54, 55]. In the jejunum, enterocytes possess very active glutaminases which hydrolyze glutamine to glutamate and ammonia. Enterocytes use glutamine from the circulation as a metabolic fuel, and the majority of its nitrogen end-products appear in ammonia, alanine and citrulline. Moreover, such nitrogen end-products are released into the portal circulation after enteral glutamine administration, and are collected by the liver before reaching the systemic circulation. Thus, glutamine is metabolized when it enters enterocytes either across the lumenal brush border or through the basolateral membrane from the systemic circulation [54, 55].

In critically ill patients, increased protein catabolism provides amino acids for other systemic organs. Skeletal muscle, a source of body protein, is the primary organ of glutamine synthesis and storage. Accordingly, the concentration of this amino acid is 30 times higher in skeletal muscle than in the circulation [55]. Although glutamine release from skeletal muscle markedly increases during critical illness, circulating concentrations of this amino acid are decreased, indicating its increased uptake by other tissues [6, 55]. In patients with multisystem trauma, increased and selective uptake of glutamine occurs in the intestinal tract [56]. In stressed conditions, glutamine depletion surpasses that of all other amino acids and endures during recovery after all other amino acids have returned to normal levels [57].

Although included in some current EN formulations, these provisions of glutamine are probably administered in insufficient amounts to support intestinal mucosal growth. Furthermore, current TPN formulae do not contain glutamine which may explain the intestinal mucosal atrophy found in patients receiving prolonged parenteral feeding. Although such mucosal disruption may be the result of decreased nutrient contact or insufficient production of enterotrophic GI hormones, the lack of glutamine in parenteral formulae may also cause such atrophy. Elevated plasma glutamine levels above control values cause trophic effects on rat intestinal mucosa [58]. Additionally, TPN with glutamine diminishes gut atrophy and stimulates small bowel dissaccharidase activity [59]. Similar results occur when glutamine is administered enterally [60, 61]. Finally, both enteral and parenteral infusions significantly increase mucosal mass of intestinal grafts in rats receiving heterotopic small bowel isografts compared to non-glutamine controls [62, 63].

Current TPN formulae without glutamine promote bacterial translocation in rats. Bacterial translocation is reduced in rats fed glutamine orally, while it does not occur in those animals fed regular chow diets [64]. Furthermore, EN and TPN glutamine enriched formulae increase intestinal glutaminase activity and glutamine uptake. Accordingly, glutamine supplemented TPN maintains immune cellularity better than standard formulations [65, 66]. Glutamine supplemented TPN maintains IgA at normal physiologic levels which, in turn, prevent bacterial adherence to enterocytes. Thus, glutamine supplementation decreases bacterial translocation and preserves intestinal immune function during TPN.

Several studies suggest glutamine enhanced EN and TPN benefit animals with intestinal mucosal injury due to chemotherapy. Glutamine enriched EN preserves intestinal mass and improves survival of rats with methotrexate-induced enterocolitis [67]. Similar results were found in rats on glutamine enriched TPN after receiving 5-fluorouracil (5-FU). Increased villous height and mucosal DNA content were found in these rats. When the supplemented TPN was given before 5-FU administration, there was further increased mucosal cellularity and significantly lower mortality compared to controls [68].

As mentioned, glutathione (GSH) is a major antioxidant consisting of glutamate derived from glutamine. GSH protects normal tissue from oxidant injury and improves resistance to chemotherapy and radiation related injury in tumor tissue. Oral glutamine supplementation may restore depleted GSH to normal levels in cancer patients thereby providing the intestinal tract and other organs a form of acquired resistance to oxygen free radicals generated by chemotherapy and radiation therapy. Thus, enteral glutamine supplementation may enhance the selectivity of antitumor drugs by protecting normal tissue and sensitizing tumor cells to chemotherapy related injury [57] (Rouse K et al., personal communication).

In a recent double-blind, randomized, controlled clinical trial, patients given glutamine supplemented TPN after bone marrow transplantation demonstrated improved nitrogen balance, reduced infection, lower rates of microfloral overgrowth and shortened hospital stay compared to patients receiving standard TPN [69]. Although nutrient intake was similar in both groups, nitrogen balance improved in glutamine supplemented TPN patients compared to controls (-1.4 ± 0.5 vs -4.2 ± 1.2 g/d; $P = 0.002$). Furthermore, fewer experimental patients (13%) developed clinical infections in contrast to controls (43%). Finally, patients receiving glutamine had significantly lower incidences of microfloral colonization and shortened hospitalizations (29 ± 1 vs 36 ± 2 days; $P = 0.017$).

Although enteral diets supplemented with glutamine alone maintain intestinal mucosal integrity, the addition of epidermal growth factor has a synergistic effect on mucosal growth in the small intestine [70]. Additionally, glucocorticoid hormones may enhance intestinal glutamine utilization by increasing glutaminase expression, thereby providing more energy for enterocytes in stress related states [71]. Thus, growth factors and hormones may act as trophic factors in conjunction with glutamine to maintain the integrity of the intestinal mucosa.

Butyrate

Short chain fatty acids (SCFA), the most important of which include acetate, n-butyrate and propionate, are fermentation end-products of enzymatic breakdown of dietary fiber and undigested starch by the colonic microflora. SCFA are essential for the metabolic welfare of colonocytes and are important regulators of the colonic milieu. SCFA increase colonocyte proliferation, stimulate mucosal growth, enhance blood flow and improve energy metabolism. Numerous studies indicate increased mitotic indices and labelling index scores in crypts of colonic mucosa infused with SCFA (Lew JI and Rombeau JL, 1993). Acetate, n-butyrate and propionate account for the majority of SCFA produced in the human colon. Of these, butyrate is preferentially oxidized by normal colonocytes when compared to such common fuels as glucose, glutamine and ketone bodies [15, 72, 73]. Butyrate has a sparing effect on glucose and glutamine oxidation. Accordingly, glucose or glutamine does not decrease the entry of butyrate carbons in the Krebs cycle (Roediger WEW, 1993, personal communication).

Normal colonocytes depend on fatty acid oxidation (β-oxidation) for energy production, and SCFA availability strongly affects this oxidation process (Roediger WEW, 1993). When starved of SCFA, colonocytes oxidize butyrate at a significantly diminished rate with decreased ketogenesis. Since butyrate is not synthesized by mammalian tissue, the colonic mucosa can only obtain it from bacterial fermentation of polysaccharides predominantly found in dietary fiber and undigested starch. In normal colonocytes, preferred activation of butyrate to its CoA derivatives by short chain CoA synthetases leads to production of ATP and acetyl CoA essential for cellular metabolism. Thus, butyrate deprivation, and consequently diminished β-oxidation, can cause severe functional consequences for colonocytes. Butyrate deficiency may lead to decreased absorption, diminished lipid synthesis, reduced mucus production and impaired detoxification mechanisms in the colon. These conditions, in turn, may lead to colonocyte barrier breakdown and other detrimental sequelae (Roediger WEW, 1993).

Past studies demonstrate that butyrate is the most important SCFA in eliciting colonocyte proliferation [15, 74]. Experiments *in vivo* demonstrate a dose-dependent stimulatory effect of SCFA on crypt cell production rate in the order of effectiveness: n-butyrate, propionate, and acetate in rats [15, 72]. Furthermore, intralumenal perfusion of butyrate concentrations of 20, 40, and 150 mM into cecectomized rat colon increase segmental DNA by 100, 100, and 50%, respectively. Infusion of 20 mM butyrate stimulates colonic mucosal growth similarly to physiologic concentrations of acetate, butyrate and propionate. Moreover, butyrate concentrations 7.5 times the normal colonic concentration (20 mM) do not significantly increase colonocyte proliferation and mucosal growth. Thus, butyrate is the primary fuel for colonocytes, and normal colonic concentrations of this fatty alone is optimal for colonocyte proliferation [73, 75].

In a clinical study, 7 patients with diversion colitis received SCFA irrigations (butyrate 40 mmol/L, propionate 30 mmol/L, and acetate 60 mmol/L) twice daily for 2 to 6 weeks. Endoscopic appearance of colonic mucosa of patients treated with SCFA improved after 2 weeks, and progressively after 4 to 6 weeks when compared to saline controls. Histologic degree of colonic inflammation decreased dramatically [76]. In another study, butyrate enemas (100 mmol/L) given twice daily to 10 patients with distal ulcerative colitis for 2 weeks returned colonocyte production to normal values and expanded proliferative zones within the mucosa. Stool frequency and rectal bleeding regressed in patients receiving butyrate enemas. Furthermore, endoscopic appearance of colonic mucosa improved considerably and histologic findings of inflammation decreased significantly [77].

Butyrate studies *in vitro* demonstrate paradoxical results to the *in vivo* studies. While some experiments demonstrate that butyrate stimulates colonic epithelial cell proliferation in 25 and 60 mM concentrations *in vitro*, other cell studies show that butyrate concentrations of 2 to 8 mM have no effect or decrease cell proliferation [78–80]. If these *in vitro* studies receive further confirmation, the possibility that butyrate acts via an intermediary found only in intact colonic mucosa appears likely. The paradoxical effects of butyrate *in vitro* merit further investigation.

In critically ill patients unable to eat voluntarily, prolonged TPN administration does not provide butyrate to the starving colon. Such fasting conditions decrease β-oxidation in colonocytes without compensation from other metabolic mechanisms. In past experimental models, when butyrate has been withheld from the colon, mucosal absorption of sodium and water is significantly reduced (Roediger WEW, 1993). Severe starvation of the colon may lead to mucosal alterations known as colitis which is seen under famine conditions. Some detrimental effects of colonocyte starvation are reversed by SCFA infusions (i.e. butyrate) as demonstrated in dog colonic loops and human colon affected by diversion colitis [76, 81]. Orally administered butyrate is quickly and completely absorbed in the jejunum and does not reach the colon. Since a slow release form of butyrate has not been developed, it is presently administered therapeutically by rectal irrigation (Scheppach W, Bartram P, Richter F, 1993).

In summary, there is conclusive evidence that butyrate metabolism is essential for normal colonocyte function. Colonocyte β-oxidation of butyrate is involved in such processes as ATP production, lipogenesis, sodium absorption, histone acetylation and detoxification (Roediger WEW, 1993). Since butyrate is not synthesized in mammalian tissue, lack of enteral nutrients or suppressed colonic microflora due to antibiotic therapy may starve colonocytes and cause mucosal barrier breakdown. Theoretically, butyrate may prevent such functional and structural alterations within the colon in critical illness. While initial clinical trials are encouraging, more extended human studies with butyrate are needed.

Future Directions

Although recent studies have shown that the provision of enteral nutrients benefit the structure and function of the intestinal tract in critically patients, the mechanism by which this occurs is still not entirely known. Nutritional research has only begun to provide new information as to the vital role of enteral nutrition on the intestinal epithelium. Such information has broadened our understanding of the importance of nutrition not as a separate entity *per se*, but as an integral part of the maintenance and welfare of multiple organ systems. Indeed, the field of nutrition encompasses all fields of basic science and clinical medicine. Current research in enteral feeding has expanded into immunology, molecular biology and cellular physiology to further elucidate its prophylactic and therapeutic indications.

New immunoregulatory components in enteral nutrition such as omega-3 fatty acids (fish oils), RNA nucleotides and arginine may stimulate the gut immune system and maintain intestinal barrier integrity [82]. Immunonutrition refers to the effects of EN and TPN on the immune system. Since they may modulate immune function, the dietary presence of these immunonutrients in various levels may be utilized to alter host immune and accessory cell response. This is of particular interest because such nutrients added to enteral formulations or special therapeutic diets may benefit critically ill patients.

Omega-3 fatty acids of fish oil alter inflammatory reactions by down-regulating eicosanoid production. Increased levels of eicosanoids elevate PGE_2 production which results in severe host immunosuppression. Excess PGE_2 has been associated with postoperative infection, trauma and sepsis. Following severe trauma or surgery, increased PGE_2 production by host macrophages and monocytes causes diminished T cell function, reduced T cell proliferative response and increased suppressor T cell activity [83]. These changes may contribute in part to high infection rates in critically ill patients. Recent studies suggest omega-3 fatty acids ameliorate the condition of these immunosuppressed patients by depressing eicosanoid production and action.

In one study, high levels of dietary omega-3 fatty acids reduced PGE_2 synthesis in rat spleen and thymus following immune challenge [84]. Additionally, intravenously fed fish oil emulsions markedly improved survival in guinea pigs administered single doses of endotoxin [85]. In rats administered fish oil derived fatty acids for 50 days, decreased PGE_2 production during the chronic phase of inflammation occurred after antigenic challenge [86]. Thus, omega-3 fatty acid supplemented enteral diets may down-regulate eicosanoid production in critically ill patients with severe sepsis.

Dietary nucleotides stimulate growth and function of intestinal epithelial cells, lymphocytes and macrophages. In particular, RNA nucleotides have an immunostimulatory effect by increasing expression of mature T lymphocytes [82]. In a study to assess dietary nucleotide effects against infection, mice fed RNA or uracil supplemented diets demonstrated significantly increased resistance to IV *S. aureus* challenge compared to mice fed adenine-supplemented or nucleotide-free diets [87]. Nucleotide-free diets decrease host restistance to infection, impair cellular immune function and decrease rate of allograft rejection [88]. Additionally, absence of dietary nucleotides may inhibit enterocyte and colonocyte production and function, thereby disrupting the intestinal mucosa. Thus, manipulation of nucleotide content in therapeutic enteral diets may bolster intestinal immunity and maintain intestinal barrier function.

Arginine has many immunomodulatory effects that are not entirely understood. This dibasic amino acid has a thymotrophic effect that increase production and release of natural killer and helper T cells. Arginine also promotes release of IL-2 which is partially responsible for metabolic response to stress. Furthermore, IL-2 itself plays a key role in host antitumor activity, transplant rejection, blood transfusion crossreactivity and humoral response reaction [82]. In a study with injured rats, arginine supplemented enteral and parenteral diets reduced post-traumatic weight loss, increased collagen deposition and accelerated wound healing [89]. In a randomized, prospective trial, arginine supplemented enteral diets fed to cancer patients prevented postoperative reduction in blastogenic response to the mitogens con A and PHA [90]. This effect of arginine on the immune system may benefit critically ill patients at risk of infection. Furthermore, arginine is an important substrate precursor for nitric oxide (NO) production. NO synthase converts arginine in the presence of cofactors, NADPH and oxygen to citrulline and NO [91]. NO is yet another agent which has been implicated in a wide range of immunologic functions that may prove therapeutic to critically ill patients.

Recent studies suggest endogenous NO preserves the integrity of intestinal mucosa and microvasculature following severe endotoxemia. In humans, NO is derived from endothelium of arteries and veins and mediates or regulates cell function in several normal physiologic and disease states. In animal models, NO interacts with superoxide anions to form less toxic species, and inhibits neutrophil adhesion and emigration [92]. This evidence suggests NO may reduce oxygen radical damage caused by endotoxin and may protect the intestine by restricting the damaging effects of endotoxin activated neutrophils. Further research is required to clearly define the role of arginine supplementation and NO mediation in intestinal inflammation where tissue damage involving superoxides, neutrophils or vasoactive mediators may occur. Such information may explain the pathogenesis of such intestinal inflammatory diseases such as ulcerative or Crohn's colitis. Furthermore, NO used clinically with nutritional support may have a synergistic effect in treating critically ill patients with compromised intestinal barrier function.

The relationship between nutrition and the intestinal tract not only involves the presence of lumenal nutrients, but also the direct or indirect effects of nutrients on production of gut hormones, growth factors, immunologic gut components, blood flow and neural activity in the regulation of the intestinal milieu. Since there are countless possible nutrient admixtures and many homeostatic mechanisms, it will be some time before we fully know how the intestinal tract ably responds to its ever changing environment.

Conclusion

The most important stimulus for intestinal growth and function is the presence of enteral nutrients within the gut lumen. The small bowel and colonic epithelium preferentially utilize glutamine and butyrate respectively as respiratory fuels. Increasing evidence demonstrates that the gut is metabolically active during critical illness. Most critically ill patients do not receive enteral nutrients or intestinal fuels. Recent investigations in animals and humans document reduced sepsis due to the provision of enteral nutrients during critical illness. The mechanism(s) for this effect remain to be fully elucidated. Nevertheless, they appear to be due in part to maintenance of intestinal barrier integrity. Further studies are needed to identify the role of specific nutrients in mediating and enhancing these enterotrophic responses.

References

1. Johnson LR (1987) Regulation of gastrointestinal growth. In: Johnson LR (ed) Physiology of the gastrointestinal tract. 2nd edn. Raven Press, New York, pp 301–333
2. Lipkin M (1987) Proliferation and differentiation of normal and diseased gastrointestinal cells. In: Johnson LR (ed) Physiology of the gastrointestinal tract, 2nd edn., Raven Press, New York, pp 255–284
3. Madara JL, Tries JS (1987) Functional morphology of the mucosa of the small intestine. In: Johnson LR (ed) Physiology of the gastrointestinal tract. 2nd edn., Raven Press, New York, pp 1209–1249
4. Shamsuddin AM, Phelps PC, Trump BF (1982) Human large intestinal epithelium: Light microscopy, biochemistry, and ultrastructure. Hum Path 13:790–803
5. Colony PC (1989) The identification of cell types in the normal adult colon. In: Augenlicht LH (ed) Cell and molecular biology of colon cancer, CRC Press Inc., Boca Raton, Florida, pp 2–21
6. Wilmore DW, Smith RJ, O'Dwyer ST, Jacobs DO, Ziegler TR, Wang XD (1988) The gut: A central organ after surgical stress. Surgery 104:917–923

7. Rijike RPC, Plaisier HM, DeRuiter H, Galjaard H (1977) Influence of experimental bypass on cellular kinetics and maturation of small intestinal epithelium in the rat. Gastroenterology 72:896–901
8. Cameron IL, Ord VA, Hunter KE, Van Nguyen M, Padilla GM, Heitman DW (1990) Quantitative contribution of factors regulating rat colonic crypt epithelium: Role of parenteral and enteral feeding, caloric intake, dietary cellulose level and the colon carcinogen DMH. Cell Tissue Kinet 23:227–235
9. Cummings JH, Branch WJ (1986) Fermentation and the production of short chain fatty acids in the human large intestine. In: Vahouny GV, Kritchevsky D (eds) Basic and medical aspects of dietary fiber, Plenum Press, New York, pp 131–149
10. Cummings JH (1984) Colonic absorption: The importance of short chain fatty acids in man. Scand J Gastroenterol 19:90–99
11. Vahouny GV (1987) Effects of dietary fiber on digestion and absorption. In: Johnson LR (ed) Physiology of the gastrointestinal tract. 2nd edn. Raven Press, New York, pp 1623–1648
12. Vahouny GV, Cassidy MM (1986) Dietary fiber and intestinal adaptation. In: Vahouny GV, Kritchevsky D (eds) Basic and medical aspects of dietary fiber. Plenum Press, New York, pp 181–209
13. Jacobs LR (1989) Dietary fiber and the intestinal mucosa. In: Cummings JH (ed) The role of dietary fiber in enteral nutrition, Abbott International, Abbott Park, Illinois, pp 24–35
14. Bristol JB, Williamson CN (1984) Large bowel growth. Scand J Gastroent 19:25–34
15. Sakata T (1987) Stimulatory effect of short chain fatty acids on epithelial cell proliferation in the rat intestine: A possible explanation for trophic effects of fermentable fibre, gut microbes and luminal trophic factors. Br J Nutr 58:95–103
16. Dembinski AB, Johnson LR (1979) Growth of pancreas and gastrointestinal mucosa in antrectoma and gastrin treated rats. Endocrinology 105:769–773
17. Sirinek KR, Levine BA, Moyer MP (1985) Pentagastrin stimulates in vitro growth of normal and malignant human colon epithelial cells. Am J Surg 149:35–39
18. Johnson LR (1979) Regulation of gastrointestinal mucosal growth. J Surg 3:477–487
19. Ryberg B, Axelson J, Hakanson R, Sundler F, Mattsson H (1990) Trophic effects of continuous infusion of [Leu15]-gastrin-17 in the rat. Gastroenterology 98:33–38
20. Goodlad RA, Al Mukhtar MYT, Ghatei MA, Bloom SR, Wright NA (1983) Cell proliferation plasma enteroglucagon and plasma gastrin levels in starved and refed rats. Virchows Arch Cell Pathol 43:55–62
21. Gleeson MM, Bloom SR, Polak JK, et al (1971) Endocrine tumor in kidney affecting small bowel structure, mobility and absorptive function. Gut 122:773–782
22. Kvietys PR, Granger ND (1981) Effect of volatile fatty acids on blood flow and oxygen uptake by the dog colon. Gastroenterology 80:962–969
23. Demigné C, Remesy C (1985) Stimulation of absorption of volatile fatty acids and minerals in the cecum of rats adapted to a very high fiber diet. J Nutr 115:53–60
24. Cummings JH, Pomare EW, Branch WJ, Naylor CPE, MacFarlane GT (1987) Short chain fatty acids in human large intestine, portal, hepatic and venous blood. Gut 28:1221–1227
25. Sakata T (1986) Effects of indigestible dietary fibre bulk and short-chain fatty acids on tissue and weight and epithelial proliferation rate of the digestive tract in rats. J Nutr Sci Vitaminol 32:355–362
26. Mortensen FV, Nielsen H, Mulvany MJ, Hessov I (1990) Short chain fatty acids dilate isolated human colonic resistance arteries. Gut 31:1391–1394
27. Karlstad MD, Killeffer JA, Bailey JW, DeMichele SJ (1992) Parenteral nutrition with short-and long-chain triglycerides: Triacetin reduces atrophy of small and large bowel mucosa and improves protein metabolism in burned rats. Am J Clin Nutr 55:1005–1011
28. Tutton PJM, Helme RD (1974) The influence of adrenoceptor activity on crypt cell proliferation in the rat jejunum. Cell Tissue Kinet 7:125–136
29. Thomas EM, Templeton D (1981) Noradrenergic innervation of the villi of rat jejunum. J Auton Nerv Syst 3:25–29

30. Jacobowitz D (1965) Histochemical studies of the autonomic innervation of the gut. J Pharmacol Exp Ther 149:358–364
31. Newson B, Ahlman H, Dahlström Å, Das Gupta TK, Nyhus LM (1979) On the innervation of the ileal mucosa in the rat – a synapse. Acta Physiol Scand 105:387–389
32. Frankel WL, Zhang W, Singh A, et al (1992) Stimulation of autonomic nervous system mediates SCFA induced jejunal trophism. Surgical Forum 43:24–26
33. Saadia R, Schein M, MacFarlane C, Boffard KD (1990) Gut barrier function and the surgeon. Br J Surg 77:487–492
34. Jones WG, Minei JP, Barber AE, Fahey TJ, Shires III GT, Shires GT (1991) Splanchnic vasoconstriction and bacterial translocation after thermal injury. Am J Physio 261:H1190–H1196
35. Deitch EA (1990) Bacterial translocation of the gut flora. J Trauma 30:S184–S189
36. Hong RW, Rounds JD, Helton WS, Robinson MK, Wilmore DW (1992) Glutamine preserves liver glutathione after lethal hepatic injury. Ann Surg 215:114–119
37. Robinson MK, Rounds JD, Hong RW, Jacobs DO, Wilmore DW (1992) Glutathione deficiency increases organ dysfunction after hemorrhagic shock. Surgery 112:140–149
38. Berg RD (1983) Translocation of indigenous bacteria from the intestinal tract lumen. In: Hentges DJ (ed) Intestinal microflora in health and discase, Academic Press, New York, pp 333–352
39. Hammer-Hodges D, Woodruff P, Cuevas P, Kaufmann A, Fine J (1974) Role of intraintestinal gram-negative bacterial flora in response to major injury. Surg Gynecol Obstet 138:599–603
40. Deitch EA, Berg R, Specian R (1987) Endotoxin promotes the translocation of bacteria from the gut. Arch Surg 122:185–190
41. Rush BF, Sori AJ, Murphy TF, Smith S, Flanagan JJ, Machiedo GW (1988) Endotoxemia and bacteremia during hemorrhagic shock: The link between trauma and sepsis? Ann Surg 207:549–554
42. Deitch EA (1992) Multiple organ failure: Pathophysiology and potential future therapy. Ann Surg 216:117–134
43. Goris RJA, Boekholtz WKF, van Bebber IPT, Nuytinck JKS, Schillings PHM (1986) Multiple organ failure and sepsis without bacteria: An experimental model. Arch Surg 121:897–901
44. Border JR (1992) Multiple systems organ failure. Ann Surg 216:111–116
45. Zhi-Yong S, Yuan-Lin D, Xiao-Hong W (1992) Bacterial translocation and multiple system organ failure in bowel ischemia and reperfusion. J Trauma 32:148–153
46. Rolandelli RH, Rombeau JL (1989) Enteral nutrition in critically ill patients. Perspectives in Critical Care 2:1–16
47. Ryan JA (1983) Jejunal feeding. In: Fischer JE (ed) Surgical Nutrition, 1st edn. Little, Brown and Company, Boston, pp 757–777
48. Muggia-Sullam M, Bower RH, Murphy RF, Joffe SN, Fischer JE (1985) Postoperative enteral versus parenteral nutritional support in gastrointestinal surgery. Am J Surg 149:106–112
49. Lowry SF (1990) The route of feeding influences injury responses. J Trauma 30:S10–S15
50. Fong Y, Marano MA, Barber A, et al (1989) Total parenteral nutrition and bowel rest modify the metabolic response to endotoxin in humans. Ann Surg 210:449–457
51. Border JR, Hassett J, LaDuca J, et al (1987) The gut origin septic states in blunt multiple trauma (ISS = 40) in the ICU. Ann Surg 206:427–448
52. Moore FA, Moore EE, Jones TN, McCroskey BL, Peterson VM (1989) TEN versus TPN following major abdominal trauma-reduced septic morbidity. J Trauma 29:916–923
53. Kudsk KA, Croce MA, Fabian TC, et al (1992) Enteral versus parenteral feeding. Ann Surg 215:503–513
54. Windmueller HG (1982) Glutamine utilization by the small intestine. Adv Enzymol 53:201–237
55. Souba WW, Herskowitz K, Austgen TR, Chen MK, Salloum RM (1990) Glutamine nutrition: Theoretical considerations and therapeutic impact. JPEN 14:237S–243S

56. McAnena OJ, Moore FA, Moore EE, Jones TN, Parsons P (1991) Selective uptake of glutamine in the gastrointestinal tract: Confirmation in a human study. Br J Surg 78:480–482
57. Herskowitz K, Souba WW (1990) Intestinal glutamine metabolism during critical illness: A surgical perspective. Nutrition 6:199–206
58. O'Dwyer ST, Smith RJ, Hwang TL, Wilmore DW (1989) Maintenance of small bowel mucosa with glutamine-enriched parenteral nutrition. JPEN 13:579–585
59. Grant J, Snyder PJ (1988) Use of L-glutamine in total parenteral nutrition. J Surg Res 44:506–513
60. Jacobs DO, Evans A, O'Dwyer ST, et al (1987) Disparate effects of 5-fluorouracil on the ileum and colon of enterally fed rats with protection by dietary glutamine. Surg Forum 38:45–49
61. Smith RJ, O'Dwyer ST, Wang XD, et al (1988) The gastrointestinal response to injury, starvation and enteral nutrition. Report of the Eighth Ross Conference of Medical Research. Columbus, Ohio
62. Schroeder P, Schweizer E, Blömer A, Deltz E (1992) Glutamine prevents mucosal injury after small bowel transplantation. Transplantation Proc 24:1104
63. Frankel WL, Zhang W, Afonso J, et al (1993) Glutamine enhancement of structure and function in the transplanted small intestine in the rat. JPEN 17:47–55
64. Alverdy JC, Aoys E, Moss G (1988) Total parenteral nutrition promotes bacterial translocation from the gut. Surgery 104:185–190
65. Burke D, Alverdy JC, Aoys E, Moss G (1989) Glutamine supplemented TPN improves gut immune function. Arch Surg 124:1396–1399
66. Alverdy JC, Aoys E, Weiss-Carrington P, Burke D (1992) The effect of glutamine-enriched TPN on gut immune cellularity. J Surg Res 52:34–38
67. Fox AD, Kripke SA, DePaula J, Berman JM, Settle RG, Rombeau JL (1988) Effect of a glutamine-supplemented enteral diet on methotrexate-induced enterocolitis. JPEN 12:325–331
68. O'Dwyer ST, Scott T, Smith RJ, et al (1987) 5-fluorouracil toxicity on small intestinal mucosa but not white blood cells is decreased by glutamine. Clin Res 35:369a (Abst)
69. Ziegler TR, Young LS, Benfell K, et al (1992) Clinical and metabolic efficacy of glutamine-supplemented parenteral nutrition after bone marrow transplantation. Ann Intern Med 116:821–828
70. Jacobs DO, Evans DA, Mealy K, O'Dwyer ST, Smith RJ, Wilmore DW (1988) Combined effects of glutamine and epidermal growth factor (EGF) on GI mucosal cellularity. Surgery 104:358–364
71. Sarantos, P, Abouhamze A, Souba WW (1992) Glucocorticoids regulate intestinal glutaminase expression. Surgery 112:278–283
72. Roediger WEW (1982) Utilization of nutrients by isolated epithelial cells of the rat colon. Gastroenterology 83:424–429
73. Kripke SA, Fox AD, Berman JM, Settle RG, Rombeau JL (1989) Stimulation of intestinal mucosal growth with intracolonic infusion of short chain fatty acids. JPEN 13:109–116
74. Sakata T, Yajima T (1984) Influence of short chain fatty acids on the epithelial cell division of digestive tract. Quart J Exp Physio 69:639–648
75. Rombeau JL, Kripke SA, Settle RG (1990) Short-chain fatty acids: Production, absorption, metabolism and intestinal effects. In: Kritchevsky D, Bonfield C, Anderson JW (eds) Dietary fiber: chemistry, physiology and health effects. Plenum Press, New York, pp 317–337
76. Harig JM, Soergel KH, Komorowski RA, Wood CM (1989) Treatment of diversion colitis with short chain fatty acid irrigation. New Engl J Med 320:23–28
77. Scheppach WM, Sommer H, Kirchner T, et al (1992) Effect of butyrate enemas on the colonic mucosa in distal ulcerative colitis. Gastroenterology 103:51–56
78. Friedman E, Lightdale C, Winawer S (1988) Effects of psyllium fiber and short-chain organic acids derived from fiber breakdown on colonic epithelial cells from high risk patients. Cancer (Letters) 43:121–124

79. Young GP, Gibson PR (1991) Contrasting effects of butyrate on proliferation and differentiation of normal and neoplastic cells. In: Short-chain fatty acids: metabolism and clinical importance. Ross Laboratories, Columbus, OH, pp 50–55
80. Scheppach WM (1991) Short-chain fatty acids are a trophic factor for the human colonic mucosa in vitro. In: Short-chain fatty acids: metabolism and clinical importance. Ross Laboratories, Columbus, OH, pp 90–93
81. Roediger WEW, Rae DA (1982) Trophic effect of SCFAs on mucosal handling of ions by the defunctioned colon. Br J Surg 69:23–25
82. McClave SA, Lowen CC, Snider HL (1992) Immunonutrition and enteral hyperalimentation of critically ill patients. Dig Dis Sci 37:1153–1161
83. Kinsella JE, Lokesh B, Broughton S, Whelan J (1990) Dietary polyunsaturated fatty acids and eicosanoids: Potential effects on the modulation of inflammatory and immune cells; An overview. Nutrition 6:24–44
84. Marshall LA, Johnston PV (1982) α-Linolenic and linoleic acids and the immune response. Prog Lipid Res 20:731–734
85. Mascioli E, Leader L, Flores E, Trimbo S, Bistrian B, Blackburn G (1988) Enhanced survival to endotoxin in guinea pig fed IV fish oil emulsions. Lipids 23:623–625
86. Yoshino S, Ellis EF (1987) Effect of a fish-oil-supplemented diet on inflammation and immunological processes in rats. Intern Arch Allergy Appl Immun 84:233–240
87. Kulkarni AD, Fanslow WC, Randolph FB, Van Buren CT (1987) Modulation of delayed hypersensitivity in mice by dietary nucleotide restriction. Transplantation 44:847–849
88. Randolph FB, Kulkarni AD, Fauslow WC, Pizzini RP, Kumar S, Van Buren CT (1990) Role of RNA as a dietary source of pyrimidines and purine in immune function. Nutrition 6:45–52
89. Seifter E, Rettura G, Barbul A, Levenson SM (1978) Arginine: An essential amino acid for injured rats. Surgery 84:224–230
90. Daly JM, Reynolds J, Thom A, et al (1988) Immune and metabolic effects of arginine in the surgical patient. Ann Surg 208:512–523
91. Stamler JS, Singel DJ, Loscalzo J (1992) Biochemistry of nitric oxide and its redox-activated forms. Science 258:1898–1902
92. Stark ME, Szurszewski JH (1992) Role of nitric oxide in gastrointestinal and hepatic function and disease. Gastroenterology 103:1928–1949

Nutrition of some Cells of the Immune System and its Importance in the Response to Trauma

E. A. Newsholme

Introduction

Lymphocytes and macrophages play an important role in the immune response during which these cells undergo increased rates of production and recruitment, and alterations in function. It was for this reason that these cells were investigated in relation to their nutrition. Mature lymphocytes recirculate through lymphoid tissues via blood and lymph in a relatively quiescent state until stimulated to proliferate during, for example, a bacterial or viral infection. By contrast, macrophages are terminally differentiated end-cells in which the ability to proliferate is gradually lost.

Despite the undoubted importance of these cells, it was surprising that, until the recent work from the author's laboratory, relatively little was known about their metabolism: the fuels they require to carry out their functions, the rates of utilization and fates of these fuels, and whether any differences in metabolism or nutrition can be related to their specific cell biology as part of the immune system. Furthermore, and of considerable clinical importance, if these cells have unique nutritional requirements, does this have specific consequences for the animal as a whole especially in conditions of injury, etc. ...?

Lymphocytes are small round cells with characteristic large nuclei and a thin rim of cytoplasm. Cells of similar morphology are found in the spleen, bone marrow, lymph nodes, thymus, and other areas, such as Peyer's patches and tonsils. Lymphocytes in the tissue are in dynamic equilibrium with circulating blood. They may be categorized according to their surface markers, reactions to stimuli, migratory patterns, and life span. Of possible particular importance to their nutrition is the fact that, in their various locations within the body, the number of lymphocytes is very large: perhaps as many as 1500 g in the average man, but most of these reside within the lymphoid tissue; only a small proportion are in the circulation at any one time. Differentiated lymphocytes originate from primitive stem cells, which in mammals reside in the bone marrow. Further differentiation leads to the development of lymphoid stem cells that are directed to specific sites of the body for further differentiation. For example in the thymus, these cells acquire certain characteristics by which they become known as T-lymphocytes, that is, thymus-derived lymphocytes; these cells take part in cell-mediated immune reactions. B-lymphocytes mature in the bone marrow, and they are the precursors of antibody-forming cells. T-cells do not synthesize detectable amounts of immunoglobulin, but function as regulators of the immune response. This is achieved via interactions between various T-cell subsets (helper, suppressor, or cytotoxic T-cells) and macrophages during the operation of the cell-mediated immune response. Possible differences in nutrition and metabolism between T-cell subsets have not been studied; it is considered that any differences will be minor, but this area awaits further investigation.

In normal animals not subjected to a serious immune challenge, most of the lymphocytes will be in a quiescent state – known as resting lymphocytes. This has been taken to mean that such lymphocytes are also metabolically inactive. However, the role of these cells in the immune system means that they must be able at any time to respond rapidly and effectively to an immune challenge. Some of these requirements have been analysed by metabolic-control logic [1, 2]. Such adaptations and their basis in the nutritional requirements of these cells permit new interpretations for some of the responses to injury, trauma, sepsis and burns to be made. These are discussed below.

Macrophages are mononuclear cells that are formed from the monocytes. They are terminally differentiated end-cells in which the ability to proliferate is gradually lost. Mature resident macrophages are found to be more widely distributed in hematopoietic, lymphoid, and other tissues, where they exist as biosynthetically active cells. After an inflammatory or immunological stimulus, newly recruited macrophages with markedly different secretory and endocytic properties can accumulate in large numbers at specific sites. In spite of this functional heterogeneity, macrophages overall are characterized as motile, highly phagocytic cells that display marked plasma-membrane activity. Their versatile secretory activities, which include enzymes, hormone-like mediators of inflammation, and toxic oxygen products, can be altered by stimuli such as phagocytic particles, microbial products, and lymphokines acting on various macrophage plasma membrane receptors. The cell-biological function of these cells within the immune system would, therefore, appear to be quite distinct. It would not *a priori* be expected that their nutritional requirements and fuel metabolism, at least those that relate to cell function, would be similar. However the evidence is that they are similar [3–7].

It has been demonstrated in the author's laboratory that arginine, branched chain amino acids (leucine, isoleucine and valine), glutamine, glucose and saturated fatty acids (FA) are oxidized at high rates by lymphocytes and macrophages but the oxidation is only partial. It is considered that this partial oxidation of some, if not all, fuels has a specific role in these immune and other cells which is essential for maintenance of normal function of these cells. Polyunsaturated FA are less readily oxidized than saturated ones by these cells, but are more readily incorporated into the phospholipids of membranes, where they may cause changes in the fluidity.

This work provided, for the first time, evidence that these cells can use glutamine and/or long-chain FA for energy formation and, indeed, that these fuels could be quantitatively more important than glucose. Until this work, it had been considered that glucose was the major, if not the only, fuel to be used by lymphocytes. It has been shown, surprisingly, that the oxidation of all these fuels was only partial: for example glutamine is converted largely to glutamate, aspartate and alanine; glucose is converted to lactate; arginine is converted to ornithine and citrulline; FA may be converted largely to acetate or ketone bodies. The cells also use branched chain amino acid but their fate is not known. The need for high rates of partial oxidation of these fuels by these cells has been analysed theoretically by metabolic-control-logic. This approach suggests that these fuels may be utilized at high rates not only to provide energy but to provide optimal conditions for proliferation and to provide very specific signals for proliferation [4–9].

Glucose, Glutamine, Fatty Acid and Arginine Metabolism in Immune Cells

Branched-point Sensitivity and Precision in Control

Much of metabolism is branched and although this may be necessary as an essential part of the diversity of reactions in the body, it is considered that branched-points may also have been adapted for precision in regulation, as described below.

The increased sensitivity in control provided by the branched-point mechanism is similar in principle to that achieved in the substrate cycle; a continuous high flux in one branch of a pathway provides optimal conditions for the precise regulation of the (much smaller) flux in the other branch. Thus the increased sensitivity in the arm which has the smaller flux depends upon the ratio of fluxes in the two branches. This is equivalent to the sensitivity improvement in cycling which is provided by the ratio of cycling rate to the overall flux [2].

Glycolysis and glutaminolysis are examples of branched pathways since they provide intermediates that are precursors for biosynthetic pathway, but the fluxes through the biosynthetic pathways are normally very small (Fig. 1). However, these fluxes will increase considerably during the synthesis of DNA, RNA and protein, and also during synthesis of phospholipid for new cell membranes. The high rates of glycolysis and glutaminolysis in lymphocytes and macrophages are, therefore, considered to provide branch-point sensitivity, that is precision in control, to enable cell division to occur rapidly, effectively and with minimal cell death [8, 9]. The "inefficient" failure to oxidize these fuels in terms of energy provision is the "cost" that has to be paid for this precision in control.

A high rate of glutamine utilization can only be maintained if it is provided by muscle, and this may account for the somewhat surprising response to injury: loss of body nitrogen and mobilisation of FA that is resistant to insulin.

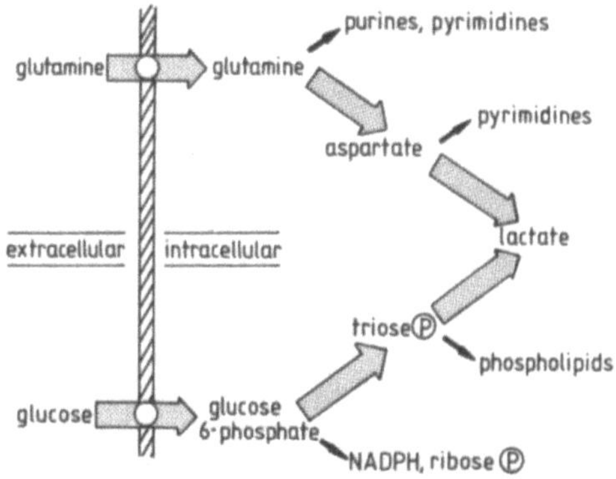

Fig. 1. The branch-points in the processes of glycolysis and glutamine utilization in the oxidative and biosynthetic branches of the lymphocytes and in macrophages. For glutaminolysis, glutamine provides nitrogen for both the purine and pyrimidine rings, and aspartate provides both nitrogen and carbon for the pyrimidine ring. For glycolysis, glucose 6-phosphate is the substrate for the pentose phosphate pathway which provides both ribose and NADPH, and triose phosphate provides glycerol 3-phosphate which is a component of phospholipids in membranes. (From [1] with permission)

The Intracellular and Extracellular Trigylceride/Fatty Acid Cycle as an Example of Branched-point Sensitivity

The reactions involved in the intracellular (Fig. 2) and extracellular cycles play a role in man [10]. The triglyceride/FA substrate cycle can be considered as a branch-point which occurs between the processes of esterification (cycling) and β-oxidation (Fig. 3). Both brown adipose tissue and red skeletal muscle have a high capacity for FA oxidation but, since this capacity will only be used infrequently, it is possible that cycling provides a branch-point in the pathway which might enable the process of β-oxidation to retain maximum possible sensitivity to its regulator(s) in these tissues. It is speculated that this may also be the case for lymphocytes and macrophages.

The high sensitivity will be achieved if the rates of lipolysis and esterification are high (that is, the cycling rate is high) and greater than that of β-oxidation. Under these conditions, an increased rate of FA oxidation to provide energy for the tissue will result in only a small decrease in the FA level

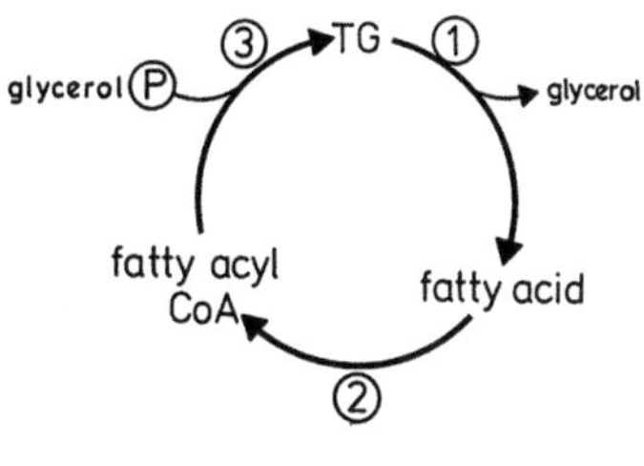

Fig. 2. The intracellular triacylglycerol-fatty acid substrate cycle. Reaction 1 is lipolysis, reaction 2 is fatty acid activation, and reaction 3 is the esterification process

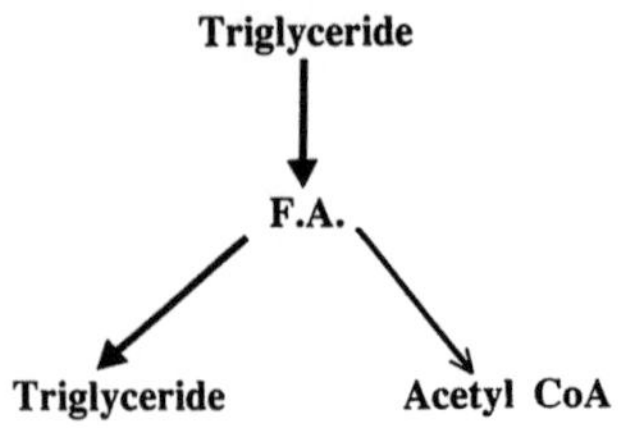

Fig. 3. The triacylglycerol-fatty acid substrate cycle and fatty acid oxidation interpreted as a branch-point pathway. The cycle represents the high-flux system, and oxidation represents the low-flux system

since it is "protected" by the lipolytic process. The triglyceride/FA substrate cycle can therefore be seen as a dynamic buffer system since a small decrease in the concentration of FA will not cause any marked opposition to the increased rate of oxidation. It will be of interest to determine the rate of such cycling in lymphocytes and macrophages, and whether this rate can be increased by cytokines that are released in injury, sepsis, etc. for reasons given below.

Fatty Acid Oxidation as a Branched Pathway to provide for Control in the Immune System

The rate of conversion of [1-^{14}C]-oleate into $^{14}CO_2$ by lymphocytes accounts for about 1% of the total oleate utilized by the cells. However, addition of oleate to isolated lymphocytes increases O_2 consumption to an extent that suggests that the FA contributes more than 30% to O_2 consumption of the isolated lymphocytes, in comparison with that of glucose and glutamine [11]. The apparent low rate of oxidation as indicated by conversion of [1-^{14}C]-oleate into $^{14}CO_2$, may be due to failure of acetyl CoA to be oxidized by the Krebs cycle.

There is evidence that lymphocytes possess the specific enzymes for producing acetoacetate (HMG-CoA synthase and lyase) and that incubated lymphocytes do in fact produce ketone bodies [12]. What is the role of ketogenesis in lymphocytes? It is possible that the primary role of this process is to maintain a high flux through a pathway in which acetyl CoA is an intermediate: such a high flux will act to "buffer" the concentration of acetyl CoA against any change in its rate of utilization in other pathways. Thus during cell division, acetyl CoA may be required for several essential processes as follows:

a) synthesis of FA and cholesterol for cell membranes;
b) formation of malonyl CoA for chain extension of FA for production of specific chain length FA (e. g. conversion of C18 to C20 or C22); and
c) the use of acetyl CoA as an acetylation agent in covalent modification of regulatory proteins (Fig. 4).

The ketogenic pathway would provide a further example of the mechanism of "branch-point sensitivity" in control of the rate of precursor utilization

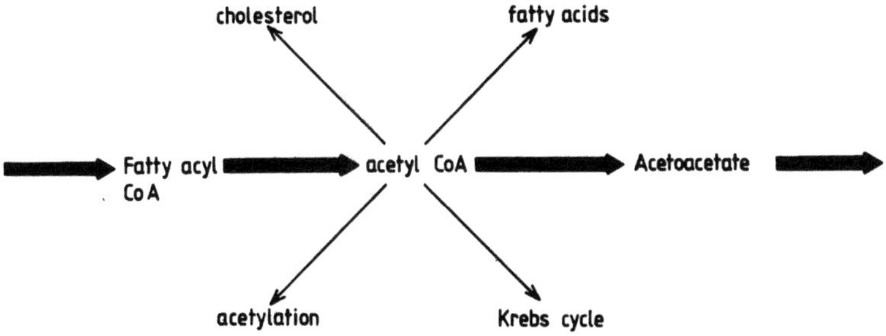

Fig. 4. Branch-point sensitivity for the ketogenic pathway in lymphocytes. Lymphocytes have a rate of formation of acetoacetate from endogenous substrate that is presumed to be fatty acids. The role of this pathway in lymphocytes is considered to be the maintenance of a constant concentration of acetyl-CoA despite marked variations in its rate of utilization by these cells for synthesis of specific fatty acids for chain extension of fatty acids for cholesterol synthesis, and for acetylation of proteins (e.g. histones). It may also allow extra ATP via the Krebs cycle at a specific time during the cell cycle

during the cell cycle. The buffering effect of the large flux into ketone bodies means that any increases in the rate of utilization of acetyl CoA in these pathways will not cause a major decrease in the concentration of acetyl CoA; and this will mean that these processes can change their rate dramatically without suffering any limitation due to changes in acetyl CoA concentration. This role is consistent with the finding that FA may be utilized and oxidized close to the maximal rate by lymphocytes and macrophages even in the fed state. This suggests that FA are taken up by the lymphocytes and macrophages not only to provide energy, but to provide acetyl CoA for important functions in the cells that are involved in immune function.

The Glucose/Fatty Acid Cycle

FA are mobilized from adipose tissue in conditions of trauma, surgery, burns, and sepsis. These are transported bound to albumin in the plasma, and their plasma concentration, in part, plays a role in control of the rate of oxidation of FA in muscle. However, FA not only play a role as a fuel but also as a regulator of glucose utilization and oxidation (Fig. 5). And this may be important for the immune system.

The concept of the glucose/FA cycle was put forward to explain the reciprocal relationship between the rates of oxidation of glucose and FA by muscle. Although some features of the cycle have been modified since that time, there is now considerable evidence to support the important proposal that, under conditions of "carbohydrate stress" (defined as when the glycogen store in the liver is depleted) FA are mobilized from adipose tissue so that their rate of oxidation by muscle increases and this, in turn, decreases the rate of glucose utilization [1]. Conversely, when the carbohydrate stress is

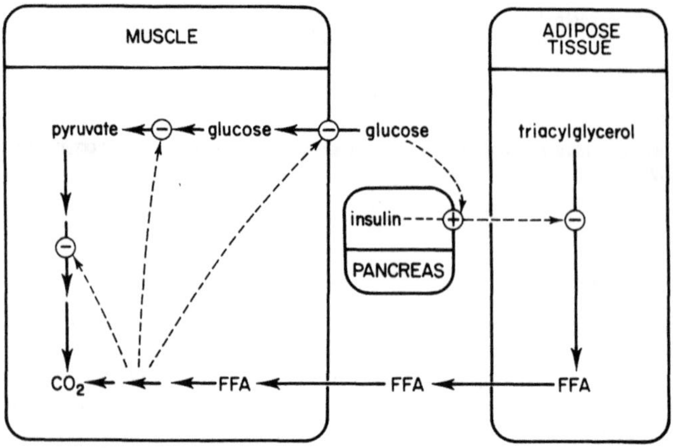

Fig. 5. The glucose/fatty acid cycle. Note that a change in the peripheral blood glucose concentration is less important than changes in the glucose concentration in hepatic portal blood in eliciting insulin release form the pancreas, since glucose absorption form the intestine is accompanied by secretion of duodenal hormones which increase the sensitivity of the β-cells to the stimulatory effect of glucose. (From [1] with permission)

removed (e.g. by refeeding a starved subject), the rate of FA release by adipose tissue is reduced, decreasing their rate of oxidation, so that the rate of glucose utilization by the muscle increases. These responses serve to stabilize the blood glucose concentration. The regulatory effect of FA on glucose utilization can be seen as a logical necessity when the small reserves of carbohydrate are taken into account together with the facts that some tissues have an obligatory requirement for glucose. The reason for this marked preference for lipid as a reserve fuel, which is not unique to man but is found in most animals, is that it is approximately nine times more efficient than carbohydrate as a storage fuel.

Although the role of this cycle has been considered to be particularly important in starvation, it may be even more important in injury, sepsis, burns, etc. ...

The Cycle in Trauma, Surgery, Sepsis, and Burns

Trauma, whether accidental or as a result of the surgeon's knife, sepsis or burns all result in an increased rate of mobilization of FA from adipose tissue and elevated FA plasma levels. Hence, the glucose/FA cycle operates under these conditions. It is generally assumed that the importance of this is to conserve glucose for the brain, since injury, etc. ... may restrict food intake, and in primitive man would have prevented hunting or gathering! However, from knowledge of the immune system, it is possible to propose that high rates of glucose utilization are required for some if not all the cells of the immune system, for fibroblasts and for phagocytic cells involved in repair [4, 7]. The enhanced rate of FA mobilization from adipose tissue may be caused by the effects of catecholamines, insulin and glucocorticoids on adipose tissue, but it is possible that cytokines may also be involved. It is also possible that the increased plasma triacylglycerol level under these conditions may provide a substrate for lipoprotein lipase released by macrophages at sites of injury or infection, for use not only by macrophages but all other cells involved in defense and repair functions.

The Possible Role of Polyunsaturated Fatty Acids as Immunosuppressive Agents

More than one half of the FA in the human diet are unsaturated and, although desaturation can be achieved by enzymes in the liver, certain polyunsaturated FA (PUFA), which are required by the body, cannot be made in this way and must be provided in the diet: these are termed essential FA. There are two major families of essential FA; the n-6 family derived from cis-linoleic acid, and the n-3 family derived from α-linoleic acid. Linoleate and α-linolenate are transformed in the body to arachidonate and eicosapentaenoate, respectively. Both of these FA are precursors for specific compounds that are known to play local messenger roles within and between cells: these are the prostaglandins, thromboxanes, prostacyclins, and leukotrienes.

It has been suggested that PUFA have several roles in the health of an individual, and one of these is an effect on the immune system. In particular, it has been suggested that PUFA possess immunosuppressive properties.

A systematic investigation of the effects of a wide range of FA on thymidine incorporation into concanavalin-A (Con-A)-stimulated rat lymph node lymphocytes has been carried out. The effects of saturated (myristate, palmitate, stearate), monounsaturated (oleate), omega-6 polyunsaturated (linoleate, arachidonate) and omega-3 polyunsaturated (linolenate, eicosapentaenoate, docosahexaenoate) FA were studied. The concentrations of FA used were physiological (30–500 μM) and the FA were added to the cell culture medium as preformed complexes with bovine serum albumin. All the FA tested had the ability to inhibit thymidine incorporation into lymph node lymphocytes. However, the extent of inhibition depended upon the particular FA, the FA concentration, the time during culture of FA addition, and the duration of exposure of the cells to FA. Generally, unsaturated FA were more inhibitory than saturated FA; the greatest inhibition of proliferation was caused by eicosapentaenoate and arachidonate, and the least inhibition was caused by myristate and palmitate. The mechanism for this inhibition may be caused by changes in membrane fluidity which then interferes with production of important cytokines and/or expression of key receptors on the plasma membrane. This lymphocyte proliferation is supported by the production of IL-2 by activated T-cells and the appearance on the cell surface of receptors for IL-2 and transferrin. It has been shown that unsaturated FA inhibit the production of IL-2 by concanavalin-A-stimulated lymphocytes isolated from the rat lymph node and human peripheral blood. FA did not affect expression of the IL-2 receptor, but they suppressed transferrin receptor expression by up to 50% [13–16].

Macrophage Functions and Fatty Acids

Macrophage adhesion is important in *in vivo* interactions such as binding to endothelial cells and migration into tissues. Using a sensitive method to measure adhesion of macrophages to different surfaces, it was found that saturated FA enrichment enhanced macrophage adhesion compared with enrichment in PUFA, which tended to decrease adhesion.

Phagocytosis is a major membrane-associated event in which particles are bound to membrane receptors and then are surrounded by the cell membrane, forming phagocytic vesicles, which are subsequently internalized and the contents digested. Macrophages enriched with saturated FA showed decreased rates of phagocytic uptake of unopsonised zymosan (boiled yeast cell walls) whilst those enriched with PUFA displayed increased phagocytic activity [17]. This suggests that membrane fluidity is an important determinant of phagocytic activity; indeed macrophage phagocytic activity was highly correlated with parameters of membrane fluidity determined from the phospholipid FA composition. Macrophages enriched with the fish oil-derived FA showed lower phagocytic activity than expected on the basis of the expected change in membrane fluidity of these cells. These findings raise the question of the composition of lipid that should be given to patients after injury, surgery, sepsis, or burns. It is possible that the normal lipolytic response to these conditions is to provide the correct "fatty acid" mixture for maintenance of the activity of the immune cells and repair processes. Any interference with this mobilization or modification of the plasma lipid profile may interfere with this precise but subtle role of FA.

The author has elsewhere questioned whether insulin normally plays a quantitatively important role in regulation of the blood glucose level suggesting that this may be achieved via changes in the concentration of IGF-I and possibly IGF-2 [18]. What then is the role of insulin? It is tempting to suggest it is the precise regulation of FA mobilization for various adipose tissue depots to provide the correct balance of FA to activate immune cells etc. ... In this case, insulin can really be considered as a cytokine!

Plasma Fatty Acid, Free Tryptophan and Branched-chain Amino Acid Concentrations and Fatigue

There is some evidence to support the view that, if the concentration of a neurotransmitter in the brain is decreased, this may limit the rate of neuronal firing in some parts of the brain, especially if the rate of neuronal firing is high. This inability of one part of the brain to function satisfactorily owing to a decrease in neurotransmitter concentration can result in changes in behavior. For example, in some parts of the brain, a decrease in the concentration of the monoamine neurotransmitters (norepinephrine, dopamine and/or 5-HT) can result in depression. In addition, there is evidence to support the view that an increase in the level of 5-HT in the brain can result in tiredness and sleep. It is therefore suggested, as a working hypothesis, that an increase in the concentration of this neurotransmitter in certain areas of the brain might ensure a high rate of neuronal firing in a specific part of the brain which then increases the sensitivity to fatigue. This would be described as central fatigue.

The logic underlying the hypothesis is as follows [19–21]:

1. Tryptophan is converted in the brain to a neurotransmitter known as 5-hydroxytryptamine (5-HT). This neurotransmitter may be involved in control of tiredness and sleep.
2. Branched-chain amino acids (leucine, isoleucine and valine) are not taken up by liver but by muscle and their rate of uptake is increased during exercise. Both branched-chain amino acids and tryptophan enter the brain upon the same amino acid carrier, so that competition between the two types of amino acids for entry into brain can occur.
3. An increased level of tryptophan in the brain will increase the rate of formation of 5-HT and hence increase the level of this neurotransmitter in the brain. This could result in increased firing of some 5-HT neurones and this "might" result in central fatigue: that is, it increases the mental effort necessary to maintain the pace of running, or the level of activity of the exercise.
4. Tryptophan is unique amongst the amino acids in that it is bound to plasma albumin, so that it exists as a bound and a free form, which are in equilibrium; this equilibrium is changed in favor of free tryptophan when the plasma FA level is raised above about 1 mM. This is probably caused by the binding of FA to albumin.

Although much of the discussion has focused attention on fatigue in relation to performance in athletes, this should not conceal the potential clinical importance of these ideas. Fatigue is a factor that can decrease the rate of recovery and increase the length of stay in hospital of patients after surgery, injury and infection. And, of considerable importance, the cause of chronic fatigue syndrome is still unknown. The concept that plasma amino acid concentration changes may play a role in fatigue opens up a new line of investigation and suggests a new role for administration of solutions containing branched-chain amino acids, overcoming fatigue in patients during recovery from injury, surgery, sepsis, and burns.

Glutamine: A Link between Muscle and the Immune System

Glutamine is used at a very high rate by some cells of the immune system. Why? The role of partial oxidation of glutamine (glutaminolysis) in rapidly-dividing cells has been considered previously to be the provision of energy and/or the provision of both nitrogen and carbon for precursors for synthesis of macromolecules (e.g. purine and pyrimidine nucleotides for DNA and RNA). However, there are problems with both explanations. Quantitative information, provided by the work from the author's laboratory with lymphocytes, shows that the rate of glutaminolysis is markedly in excess of that of the precursor requirements: the rate of glutamine utilization is at least 30-fold greater than the maximum capacity for pyrimidine nucleotide synthesis [22].

On the basis of metabolic control logic, it has been suggested that the high rates of glutaminolysis (and glycolysis) provide optimal conditions for the precise and sensitive control of the rate of use of the intermediates of these pathways for biosynthesis precisely at the time required by the synthetic processes during the cell cycle (e.g. glutamine for purine and pyrimidine nucleotide synthesis).

Both liver and muscle can produce and release glutamine into the bloodstream. But muscle may be quantitatively the most important tissue. Since the cells of the intestine have a large capacity to utilize glutamine, most of the glutamine that enters the body via the diet is utilized by the intestine. Hence glutamine production and release by muscle becomes of considerable physiological and immunological importance. Glutamine release by muscle is increased under conditions when it is required in greater rate by the immune system. Therefore, factors that increase the rate of release of glutamine may be beneficial in conditions of surgery, sepsis, and burns. Such factors are known to affect the immune system. These include glucocorticoids, growth hormone and thyroxine [23–25].

Growth Hormone and Glutamine in Relation to Wound Healing

It has recently been shown that administration of human growth hormone (GH) to the rat for 3 or 10 days increased the concentration of glutamine release from incubated soleus muscle isolated from rats treated with GH for 3 days. Since it is known that GH increases the rates of amino acid uptake by and protein synthesis in muscle, it has been generally assumed that this hormone would have similar effects on the rates of amino acid release. However, it is often overlooked that changes in the rates of release of amino acids from muscle are not directly related to rates of amino acid uptake, and may not reflect changes in protein metabolism. This is particularly important for glutamine, which is stored in muscle at a high concentration (approximately 20 mM in man) and makes only a small contribution (approximately 3%) to protein synthesis. For example, the rate of glutamine release from muscle may be decreased in certain conditions associated with an increase in the rate of net protein degradation.

The beneficial effect of GH supplementation on rates of wound healing could be explained, at least in part, by changes in the plasma concentration of glutamine. Thus, GH increased the rate of glutamine release from muscle which may, in turn, explain the GH-mediated increase in the plasma concentration of glutamine. Consequently, the concentration of glutamine at the site of wound healing may be maintained, which is essential for the normal functioning of immune cells and other rapidly dividing cells. This hypothesis suggests that GH administration increases the wound healing post-surgery via changes in glutamine metabolism by skeletal muscle. Further clinical work is required to confirm and extend these experimental findings.

Hence, it is now possible to propose a common mechanism by which GH could increase the rate of wound healing and improve nitrogen balance: it could increase the rate of protein synthesis in skeletal muscle, at least in part, by an increase in the concentration of glutamine in muscle; and GH therapy may enhance the rate of wound healing, at least in part, by increasing the rate of glutamine release from muscle, which in turn may increase the plasma glutamine concentration [24].

Glutamine and Overtraining

The overtraining syndrome in athletes is characterized by a number of signs and symptoms, including poor performance, fatigue, depression and an impairment of immune function; these may persist unless the athlete rests. The immunosuppression is characterized by a higher incidence of infectious diseases and slower wound healing. In addition to these effects of overtraining, there is evidence that a single bout of exercise can decrease the ability of cells of the immune system to respond to mitogenic stimulation. It is suggested that one cause of this impairment of immune function after a single bout of exercise or during the overtraining syndrome could be related to changes in plasma glutamine levels, since glutamine is utilized at a very high rate by cells of the immune system and is considered to be an important fuel for these cells and that it may have specific immunostimulatory properties [26].

The concentration of glutamine was decreased in plasma from overtrained athletes and from runners following a marathon race; the decrease in resting overtrained athletes was 9% and that after the marathon was 16%. Although these are small changes, it is possible that in overtrained athletes after prolonged exercise, the decrease in plasma glutamine levels may be considerably greater, and it is possible that the decrease in glutamine level may be greater in other areas of the body more prone to infection (e.g. buccal cavity, bronchi, skin).

The mechanism responsible for the decrease in plasma glutamine concentration in overtrained athletes and after long-term exercise is now known.

However, it is possible that these conditions may decrease the rate of glutamine release from muscle and thus could be responsible for the decrease. In support of this, the rate of glutamine release from skeletal muscle of the rat *in vitro* is decreased after prolonged exercise, and physical training decreases the maximum activity of glutamine synthetase in muscle.

It has been shown that overtraining is without effect on the plasma levels of IL-1 and -6 or on the kinetics of lymphocyte proliferation *in vitro*. Thus, the ability of lymphocytes to proliferate appears to be normal, at least when it is assessed *in vitro*, in controlled and defined medium containing physiological concentrations of glutamine. However in the overtrained athlete, the *in vitro* concentration of glutamine is below normal physiological levels which are known to be required for maximal rates of lymphocyte proliferation and macrophage phagocytosis: at least in culture *in vitro*. Thus, it is hypothesized that such a decrease in plasma glutamine concentration in overtraining or following long-term exercise may contribute to the impairment of immune function observed in these conditions *in vivo*. This hypothesis is supported by the observation that the overtraining syndrome is rarely seen in sprinters or power athletes, but affects endurance athletes, suggesting that repeated prolonged exercise is an important predisposing factor.

It is of course possible that changes in the concentration of other metabolites, hormones or cytokines may play a role in the immunosuppression in overtraining. For example, the plasma concentration of cortisol is elevated in overtrained athletes, although it is unclear whether a small increase in cortisol levels would impair the immune response [23].

Plasma Levels of Glutamine after Surgery

Surgery is known to impair the immune response. Although the mechanism underlying this impairment is not understood, the net effect is an increased risk of the development of postoperative sepsis. In an attempt to elucidate a possible mechanism for postoperative immunosuppression, our study has been carried out to examine the relationship between cytokine elaboration and glutamine metabolism.

It is known that surgery increases the rate of utilization of glutamine by the small intestine, and it would be expected to increase the rate of utilization by cells involved in the immune response to surgery. Consequently, it was considered important to study the sequential change in plasma glutamine and other amino acid levels in response to surgical operations of different severity.

A particular problem is that the plasma level of glutamine is routinely measured by automated amino acid analysis which may be unsatisfactory because glutamine is unstable in the acidic conditions used in this technique. It has now been shown that plasma level of glutamine rapidly decreased after the incision (2.5 h) and remained markedly lower than preoperative values for approx. 7 days following major surgery [27]. Larger decreases (51 to

58%) in the plasma glutamine level have been reported following major burns and in patients suffering from acute pancreatitis and multiple organ failure. It is likely that the decrease observed following major surgery is due to increased rates of glutamine utilization by cells of the immune system and intestinal cells, because under such conditions, it has been reported that the rate of release of glutamine by muscle is increased.

Given the proposed role of glutamine for cells of the immune system and the experimental evidence that suggests that normal plasma levels of this amino acid are essential for a response of these cells to an immune challenge, it is suggested that this large and prolonged decrease in the plasma glutamine level may be one factor that causes immunosuppression after major surgery. The hypothesis that maintenance of an adequate supply of glutamine to the small intestine prevents malfunction of this organ and enhances survival following injury has recently been successfully tested. Nutritional or pharmacological regimens that enhance the supply of glutamine to cells of the immune system after surgery may improve clinical outcome by maintenance or stimulation of the body's defense and repair mechanisms [27, 28]. Such regimens require further evaluation in the clinical setting.

A Putative Glutamine Nitrogen Cycle in the Body

The principal tissue for lactate utilization is liver. Most of the lactate that is removed by the liver is converted to glucose or glycogen, via gluconeogenesis. The conversion of lactate to glucose in the liver and the continuous formation of lactate from glucose in the other tissues of the body represents a cyclic flow of carbon that has been termed the Cori cycle (after Carl Cori, who originally put forward the idea). It may have greater physiological significance than just that of a carbon link between peripheral tissues and the liver. By maintaining a high flux through the Cori cycle, a dynamic buffer of key metabolic intermediates is provided, both in the tissues and in the bloodstream, so that they can be used by tissues when required [18]. If the rate of utilization of the intermediates is low, compared to the flux through the Cori cycle, this may provide for precision in regulation as described and defined elsewhere. This may be one reason for increased Cori cycle flux during injury, sepsis, post-surgery, and burns, when, although there is generalized resistance to insulin, muscle may have a higher rate of conversion of glucose to lactate although much less glucose is oxidized [29]. Alternatively or in addition, in these conditions, there will be increased utilization of glucose by cells of the immune system and repair cells, and the end-product of this metabolism is lactate. Hence, increased Cori cycle activity may stem from activity of the white cells and repair cells as well as muscle. The increased cycling may function to converse glucose for these cells whose role in repair and recovery would be jeopardized if the blood glucose level decreased. It is possible to speculate that the function of the increased muscle protein degradation that occurs in conditions of injury, sepsis, surgery, etc. ... is to provide nitrogen for glutamine synthesis because of the very high sensitivity provided by the branched-point system in immune and other cells. Since this latter system results in the formation of glutamine, aspartate and alanine as end-products, the question arises why there is not a cycle in nitrogen metabolism equivalent to the Cori cycle in glucose metabolism? Thus, the end-products of glutamine could be "disbanded" by the body for synthesis of glutamine with a corresponding saving in body protein degradation. Is there a metabolic "principle" in nitrogen metabolism that prevents such a cycle from operating satisfactorily? Alternatively, have the changes in diet of Western man over the past several hundred years caused changes which prevent the normal operation of this putative nitrogen cycle?

Conclusion

Glutamine and glucose are used at very high rates by some cells of the immune system. These high rates may provide ideal conditions for the precise and sensitive control of the rate of use of the intermediates of these pathways for biosynthesis, precisely at the time required by the biosynthetic process during the cell cycle. High rates can thus be seen as part of a mechanism of control to permit synthesis of macromolecules when required, without any need for complex regulatory mechanism or extracellular signals to make more glucose or glutamine available for the rapidly dividing cells. The process is known as branched-point sensitivity. Branch-points may provide precision in regulation if one of the fluxes at the branch is low compared with the other flux. Consequently, any decrease in the flux through this glutamine pathway – even if small – could impair the functioning of the immune system. Fat oxidation provides a fuel for many tissues and it provides an important signal to decrease glucose utilization and oxidation in muscle and so conserve glucose for essential organs such as the brain. The control of fatty acid oxidation is achieved in part through its plasma concentrations, which may be precisely controlled by the triacylglycerol-fatty acid substrate cycle, which can also, if oxidation is taken into account, be viewed as a branch-point in this important pathway. Both branch-points and substrate cycles are energetically expensive and may account for some of the increases in energy expenditure in conditions of injury, burns, and sepsis, and in the postexercise condition. Fatty acids, through effects on plasma free tryptophan concentrations and hence 5-hydroxytryptamine concentrations in the brain, may play a role in central fatigue. Polyunsaturated fatty acids are claimed to have immunosuppressive properties. Insulin may have an important role in regulating the plasma concentration of fatty acids to influence some of these functions.

References

1. Newsholme EA, Leech AR (1983) Biochemistry for the Medical Sciences, John Wiley and Sons, Chichester
2. Crabtree B, Newsholme EA (1985) A quantitative approach to metabolic control. Curr Top Cell Regul 25:21–76
3. Ardawi MSM, Newsholme EA (1983) Glutamine metabolism in lymphocytes of the rat. Biochem J 212:835–842
4. Ardawi MSM, Newsholme EA (1985) Metabolism in lymphocytes and its importance to the immune response. Essays Biochem 21:1–44
5. Newsholme P, Gordon S, Newsholme EA (1987) Rates of utilization and fates of glucose, glutamine, pyruvate, fatty acids and ketone bodies by mouse macrophages. Biochem J 242:631–636
6. Newsholme EA, Newsholme P, Curi R, Challoner E, Ardawi MSM (1988) A role for muscle in the immune system and its importance in surgery, trauma, sepsis, and burns. Nutrition 4:261–268
7. Newsholme P, Newsholme EA (1989) Rates of utilization of glucose, glutamine and oleate and formation of end products by mouse peritoneal macrophages in culture. Biochem J 261:211–218
8. Newsholme EA, Crabtree B, Ardawi MSM (1985) The role of high rates of glycolysis and glutamine utilization in rapidly-dividing cells. Biosci Rep 4:393-400
9. Newsholme EA, Crabtree B, Ardawi MSM (1985) Glutamine metabolism in lymphocytes, its biochemical, physiological and clinical importance. Q J Exp Physiol 70:473–489
10. Newsholme EA, Parry-Billings M (1992) Some evidence for the existence of substrate cycles and their utility *in vivo*. Biochem J 285:339–344
11. Ardawi MSM, Newsholme EA (1984) Metabolism of ketone bodies, oleate and glucose in lymphocytes of the rat. Biochem J 221:255–260
12. Curi R, Williams JF, Newsholme EA (1989) Formation of ketone bodies by resting lymphocytes. Int J Biochem 21:1133–1136
13. Calder PC, Bond JA, Bevan SJ, Hunt SV, Newsholme EA (1991) Effects of fatty acids on proliferation of concanavalin-A stimulated rat lymph node lymphocytes. Int J Biochem 23:579-588
14. Calder PC, Bevan SJ, Newsholme EA (1992) The inhibition of T-lymphocyte proliferation by fatty acids is an eicosanoid-independent mechanism. Immunology 75:108–115
15. Calder PC, Newsholme EA (1992) Polyunsaturated fatty acids suppress human peripheral blood lymphocyte proliferation and interleukin-2 production. Clin Sci 82:695–700
16. Calder PC, Newsholme EA (1992) Unsaturated fatty acids suppress interleukin-2 production and transferrin receptor expression by concanavalin A-stimulated rat lymphocytes. Mediat Inflamm 1:107–115
17. Calder PC, Bond J, Harvey DJ, Gordon S, Newsholme EA (1990) Uptake and incorporation of saturated and unsaturated fatty acids into macrophage lipids and their effect upon macrophage adhesion and phagocytosis. Biochem J 269:807–814
18. Newsholme EA, Bevan SJ, Dimitriadis GP, Kelly RP (1992) In: Ashcroft P, Ashcroft S (eds) Insulin action. Blackwell Scientific Publications, Oxford, pp 155–193
19. Blomstrand E, Celsing F, Newsholme EA (1988) Changes in plasma concentrations of aromatic and branched chain aminoacids during sustained exercise in man and their possible role in fatigue. Acta Physiol Scand 133:115–123
20. Blomstrand E, Hassen P, Ekblom B, Newsholme EA (1991) Administration of branched chain amino acids during sustained exercise: Effects on performance and on plasma concentrations of some amino acids. Eur J Appl Physiol 63:83–88
21. Newsholme EA, Blomstrand E, Ekblom B (1992) Physical and mental fatigue: Metabolic mechanisms and importance of plasma amino acids. Brit Med Bull 48:477–495

22. Szondy Z, Newsholme EA (1989) The effect of glutamine concentration on the activity of carbarnoyl-phosphate synthase II and on the incorporation of [^{3}H] thymidine into DNA in rat mesenteric lymphocytes stimulated by phytohemagglutinin. Biochem J 261:979–983
23. Parry-Billings M, Leighton B, Dimitriadis G, Bond J, Newsholme EA (1990) Effects of physiological and pathological levels of glutocorticoids on skeletal muscle glutamine metabolism in the rat. Biochem Pharmacol 40:1145–1148
24. Parry-Billings M, Dimitriadis GD, Leighton B, Dunger D, Newsholme EA (1993) The effects of growth hormone on skeletal muscle glutamine metabolism of the rat: A possible mechanism to explain the clinical benefits of growth hormone administration post-injury. Arch Surg (in press)
25. Parry-Billings M, Dimitriadis GD, Leighton B, et al (1990) Effects of hyperthyroidism and hypothyroidism on glutamine metabolism by skeletal muscle of the rat. Biochem J 272:319–322
26. Parry-Billings M, Budgett R, Koutedakis Y, et al (1992) Plasma aminoacid concentrations in the overtraining syndrome: Possible effects on the immune system. Med Sci Sports Exerc 24:1353–1358
27. Scheltinga MR, Young LS, Benfell K, et al (1991) Glutamine-enriched intravenous feedings attenuate extracellular fluid expansion after a standard stress. Ann Surg 214:385–392
28. Hammarqvist F, Wernerman J, van der Decken A, Vinnars E (1990) Alanyl-glutamine counteracts the depletion of free glutamine and the postoperative decline in protein synthesis in skeletal muscle. Ann Surg 212:637–642
29. Leighton B, Dimitriadis GD, Parry-Billings M, et al (1989) Effects of insulin on glucose metabolism in skeletal muscle from septic and endotoxemic rats. Clin Sci 77:61–67

The Impact of Nutrition on Muscle Tissue in Critical Illness

J. Wernerman, P. Garlick, and E. Vinnars

Introduction

In man, muscle tissue serves as a protein reservoir, which is mobilized to meet the specific metabolic needs associated with critical illness. Muscle proteins are then degraded into the constituent amino acids, which are exported to other tissues where they serve as substrates for oxidative processes, protein synthesis, gluconeogenesis, ureagenesis, nucleic acid synthesis, etc. ... Although muscle proteins serve important functions such contraction, enzymatic transformation of energy substrates into work and with vital functions such as breathing, they are sacrified in situations when a need of higher priority emerges. As long as skeletal muscle can provide amino acid precursors for these substrates, the critically ill subject will be able to support other vital organs metabolically, but terminally in disease as well as in malnutrition/ starvation, there is a depletion of skeletal muscle and then also of cardiac muscle proteins leading to cardiac failure and death. Modern metabolic and nutritional therapy can provide the necessary substrates for other tissues, but in spite of conventional nutritional therapy, the processes leading to protein depletion in muscle continue and they are only marginally attenuated or not influenced at all. It is therefore a great challenge to develop a nutritional therapy which can, among other things, also preserve muscle proteins during critical illness in order to facilitate mobilization and shorten convalescence.

The necessary background to develop such a metabolic and nutritional strategy is to describe the pathophysiology of critical illness at the tissue level. Skeletal muscle protein and amino acid metabolism had been addressed with the use of a number of different approaches. Although sampling of muscle tissue by biopsy is comparatively easy, the principles underlying the regulation of muscle protein metabolism are still only partially known. Furthermore, it is only very recently that quantitative estimates of the protein turnover rate in human skeletal muscle have become possible. Moreover, the lack of a gold standard among the different techniques used to study muscle protein metabolism in man calls for the use of several techniques in parallel to reflect the changes that occur. Hence this overview of muscle tissue in the context of nutritional therapy of the critically ill will first describe the available techniques of investigation, and thereafter develop the present state of knowledge concerning the physiology and pathophysiology of muscle protein metabolism. Finally, an overlook at new therapeutical strategies will be given.

Techniques of Investigation

Ribosome Analysis

The ribosomes are the intracellular particles on which the translation process takes place. One ribosome is made up of 2 subunits and the complete particle can ride along the mRNA molecule, reading the genetic message and translating it into a polypeptide chain. Several ribosomes can attach to the same mRNA simultaneously, thus making up a polyribosome complex. The ribosome particle is released from the mRNA after termination of translation, and eventually it is reutilized to translate another mRNA molecule. This is the polyribosome-subunit cycle in which ribosome particles are used over and over again. The total amount of ribosome particles in a tissues reflects the machinery for protein synthesis or the capacity for protein synthesis. Ribosome parameters therefore give a qualitative estimate of tissue protein synthesis. The relative proportion of polyribosomes to total ribosomes on the other hand reflects the activity of protein synthesis. The concentration and size distribution of ribosomes can be determined in biopsy samples of approximately 50 mg from human skeletal muscle [1]. The amount of ribonucleic protein is most easily quantified as the optical density at 260 nm, and the concentration of ribosomes is best related to the wet weight or the tissue content of DNA. Since such an analysis can be performed in a 50 mg tissue specimen, multiple sequential samples can be taken over time in the same subject to follow the course of the ribosome particles as a reflection of protein synthesis [2]. This allows for comparison of paired samples, which gives most information when longitudinal changes are studied. Also the problems with the sometimes large interindividual scatter is minimized when paired samples are used for comparison. Ribosome analysis is perhaps most informative when the rapid changes are studied in paired samples (Fig. 1), such as the effect of short-term starvation [1], refeeding [3], elective surgery [4], hemodialysis [5], and stress hormone infusion [6]. In addition, the effects of postoperative nutritional support, including amino acid solutions of different composition, have been elucidated [7–11]. In such studies, patiens have been randomized in different groups, and the changes in ribosome parameters have been compared. The use of paired samples has made such comparisons possible also in small groups of patients, provided the groups are homogeneous. Ribosome analysis is a direct measurement of an *in vivo* phenomenon. The ribonucleoprotein content of the tissue can be measured with a high precision and reproducibility within the same series of samples [12]. Between series, however, the variation is considerably larger which makes it desirable that all samples from one patient are analysed together.

Although ribosome measurement is preferable in situations with rapid changes in protein metabolism, the changes in ribosome configuration do not occur with such a high speed so that the result obtained is just an unrepresentative snap-shot. On the contrary, if the ribosome content changes

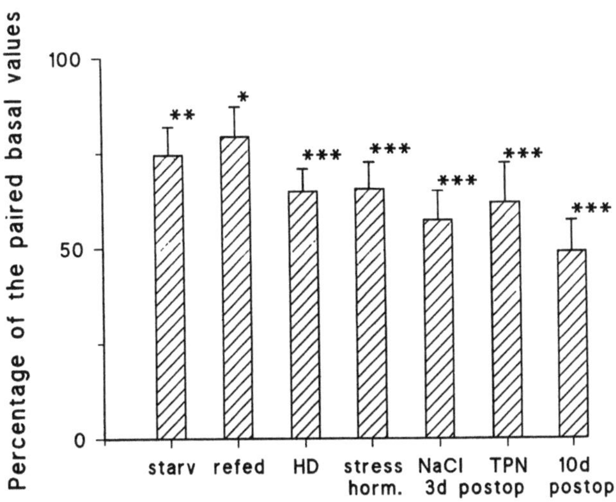

Fig. 1. The concentration of polyribosomes in skeletal muscle given as percentage of the paired basal values. The ribosomal changes in response to 3 days of starvation, 2 days of refeeding after 3 days of starvation, hemodialysis in patients with chronic renal failure, a 6 h stress hormone infusion in healthy volunteers, elective surgery on the 3rd postoperative day, with or without TPN, and finally on the 10th postoperative day. *, **, *** denotes significantly different from the paired basal values, *$p<0.05$, **$p<0.01$, and ***$p<0.001$, respectively. (From [1–6] with permission)

over hours, it is associated with rather dramatic situations such as hemodialysis [5] or stress hormone infusions [6]. Physiological changes in the nutritional intake, on the other hand, do not influence the ribosome configuration on a short-term basis. For example, food intake during the day does not cause any alternation of the ribosome parameters [13], and 36 h of starvation also leaves the ribosomes unaffected [1]. This means that changes recorded in ribosome content represent alternations that are real and consistent. The obvious shortcoming inherent to this technique is the qualitative character of the assay. Although the ribosomes can be quantified accurately, this is not synonymous with similar changes in protein synthesis. The direction of the changes is obviously indicative, but the changes in protein synthesis cannot be elucidated in quantitative terms. The value of the technique is the comparatively easy sampling procedure and its independence from the underlying assumptions that are required by isotopic labelling techniques. This makes ribosome analysis a preferable technique to use in conjunction with other techniques, when several different independent methodologies are needed in parallel to study changes in protein synthesis, especially when information concerning the level of regulation is desirable.

Determination of Specific Messengers

The development of modern molecular biology also opens the possibility to determine gene expression also in muscle tissue. So far only a small number of studies has been performed in human subjects. The high content of ribonucleases in muscle constitute a special problem in comparison with other tissues. When structural proteins such as actin and myosin are studied, quantitative estimates of the transcription are wanted. However, until now the dot-blot and nothern-blot techniques used, do not allow for more than semiquantitative estimates [14]. Nevertheless, it has been shown that the gene expression of myosin is influenced by work [15], hormones [16], and starvation [14, 17]. In the future, however, when probes corresponding to a large number of different messengers become available, finger prints of the gene expression can be obtained. Although not strictly quantitative in character, such information will be very valuable as a supplement when the quality of protein synthesis should be elucidated.

Free Amino Acids

The first technique to become available observing the *in vivo* situation in human skeletal muscle was measurement of the concentrations of the free amino acids [18]. The intracellular free amino acid pattern is distinctly different from that in plasma. The first and most important difference is the total concentration, 2.5 mmol/L in plasma versus approximately 50 mmol/L intracellular water (ICW) in muscle. The 20-fold difference in concentration is to a large extent due to taurine and glutamine, as these 2 amino acids maintain a concentration of around 20 mmol/L in ICW. Taurine has a very low concentration in plasma and is not present as an amino acid constituent of proteins. Taurine emanates from the metabolism of the sulphur containing amino acids methionine and cysteine, but the rationale for the very high concentration in human skeletal muscle is not understood at present. Glutamine on the other hand is also the most abundant amino acid in plasma, with a concentration of 0.6–0.8 mmol/L. This gives a gradient of approximately 30 between the intracellular and extracellular space. In proteins, though, glutamine constitutes only about 6% of the amino acid residuces, compared with 25–30% in plasma, and 40% in muscle. Glutamate and alanine also appear in high concentrations intracellularly, in the range of 2–5 mmol/L. For alanine, this is a 5–10 fold concentration gradient relative the extracellular space, while for glutamate the gradient is around 200. In contrast, the essential amino acids have less pronounced concentration differences. The pattern of free amino acids in muscle tissue differs considerably between species [19]. Therefore, the relevance of animal data to the amino acid metabolism of human muscle is questionable. In rat muscle, for example, the glycine concentration is very high.

The pattern of free amino acids in muscle is characteristically altered by a variety of metabolic states, such as surgical trauma [20], sepsis [21], pancreatitis [22], critical illness [23], immobilization [24], starvation [25], malnutrition [21, 26], uremia [28], hemodialysis [5], stress hormone infusion [29], etc. ... In several of these states, the changes are fairly uniform with decreases of glutamine and the basic amino acids (lysine, histidine and arginine) and concomitant elevations of the branched-chain (valine, isoleucine and leucine) and aromatic amino acids (tyrosine and phenylalanine). In summary, this means a decrease of the total free amino acid concentration which is completely accounted for by the decrease of the non-essential amino acids. The sum of essentials on the other hand is unaltered, as the decrease of lysine is compensated by the increase in the branched-chain and aromatic amino acids. This pattern is most marked in the critically ill, septic and pancreatitis patients [20–23], while subjects undergoing elective surgery or short-term starvation exhibit similar changes but of a more moderate degree [20, 25]. By contrast early after surgical trauma and during a short-term stress hormone infusion, the amino acid pattern appears different [29, 30]. In these circumstances, alanine is elevated while all the essentials and glutamate are decreased and glutamine is unaltered. This "early" pattern is then gradually transformed into the characteristic pattern of muscle protein catabolism. However, the changes in muscle amino acids are restored to normal very slowly [31], and glutamine is the last amino acid to regain the basal level after elective surgery [32]. This period of restitution is very variable inbetween individuals, ranging from 15 to more than 30 days. During refeeding after short-term starvation on the other hand (Fig. 2), the restitution is complete already after a few days [25].

The interpretation of the altered amino acid pattern in muscle is controversial. The statistical covariation between the glutamine level and muscle protein synthesis is of course very suggestive [33, 34]. On the other hand, this correlation does not indicate any causal connection. Furthermore, the parallel nature of changes in glutamine and protein synthesis is not absolute. Early during stress hormone infusion and during hemodialyses, the ribosome content decreases, while the glutamine level remains unaffected [5, 6, 29]. In the period immediately following elective surgery, the incorporation of [^{13}C] leucine or [d5]-phenylalanine drops dramatically by 20–30% without any alteration in muscle glutamine [30, 35, 36]. In critical illness, on the other hand, glutamine is reduced by 70–80% of normal values, while muscle protein synthesis rate, as estimated by the incorporation of [d5]-phenylalanine into muscle protein, decreases, by only about 20% [23, 37]. Overall, the muscle glutamine level seems to reflect, in a qualitative way, the combined effects of changes in muscle protein synthesis and degradation. The glutamine content does not change very rapidly over time, so the values obtained at analysis represent actual levels corresponding to the actual state of the individual. The reproducibility of the changes in muscle glutamine and the relative slowness with which changes occur make glutamine a valuable indicator of the alterations in amino acid

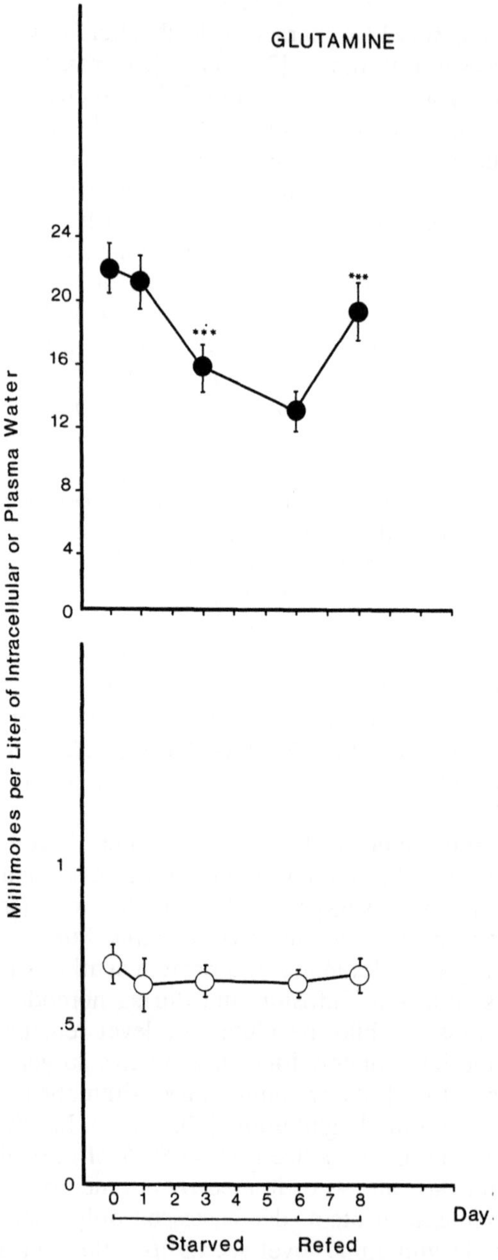

Fig. 2. The concentrations of free glutamine in plasma and in skeletal muscle during 5 days of total starvation followed by 2 days of refeeding. *** denotes significantly different from the paired basal value, ***$p < 0.001$. (From [25] with permission)

and protein metabolism associated with muscle protein catabolism. Muscle glutamine may be a good and reliable indicator of the degree of wasting in muscle tissue.

Amino Acid Fluxes across Peripheral Tissues

If the concentrations of amino acids in plasma or in whole blood are determined in arterial and venous blood, and the plasma or blood flow across a tissue or an organ can be estimated simultaneously, the amino acid influx or efflux across the organ may be calculated. This technique has been widely used to study peripheral tissues by determinations across the leg or the forearm [38]. As peripheral tissues are mainly made up by muscle, this is widely regarded as a measure of muscle amino acid exchange. The limitation of this approach are highlighted by the difference in results obtained by simultaneous measurements across the leg and forearm [39].

Nevertheless, when meticulously performed in the basal state in healthy volunteers, the technique gives valuable information on amino acid metabolism. In particular the efflux of 3-methylhistidine from muscle gives an estimate of the rate of degradation of contractile proteins. As 3-methylhistidine is formed by methylation of histidine residues in polypeptides after translation and it is not reutilized in protein synthesis or otherwise metabolized in the myofibril, 3-methylhistidine efflux from peripheral tissues is thought to reflect protein degradation. The reliability of such estimates is not controversial, but when the urinary excretion of 3-methylhistidine is extrapolated to the rate of muscle protein breakdown some caution must be recommended [40]. Under well specified circumstances, this is a fair estimate, but when nutritional intake is not controlled the contribution from exogenous sources becomes unknown [41, 42]. Furthermore, contractile proteins in cells other than the myofibrils of skeletal muscle also contribute to 3-methylhistidine in urine [40]. This non-muscular 3-methylhistidine in urine (e.g. from the gut) is large in the rat, but in man it is usually negligible [43]. Most of the amino acids are metabolized by muscle, but the net efflux of aromatic amino acids from muscle may be used as a measure of the net protein degradation, since these amino acids are not metabolized in muscle tissue [44].

Such measurements give valuable information concerning tissue protein metabolism if studied during stable steady state [45]. This is easily obtained in healthy subjects in the basal postabsorptive state [46], but when the circulation is unstable as during stress hormone infusion [13] or in critical illness [47], the variability within the same individual as well as inbetween individuals increases, making the results less easy to interpret. In the postabsorptive state the efflux from peripheral tissues may be divided into thirds; one third glutamine, one third alanine, and one third all other amino acids except glutamate which is taken up across the periphery [38]. This pattern persists also in critical illness, although in quantitative terms the efflux has increased 3–4 fold [47]. During feeding, however, this pattern is altered, especially the later third which is changed into an uptake of all amino acids except alanine and glutamine which are constantly exported from the periphery [47]. Although there is an uptake across the leg or the forearm after food intake integrated over 24 h, there is a net loss of amino acids from the peripheral tissues according to this type of measurement [45, 48]. This demonstrates that the somewhat simplified underlying assumptions are not always completely valid. The most likely explanation for this obviously erroneous result is that plasma proteins are to some extent degraded into amino acids in the periphery, giving a transfer of amino acid residues which is not measured by the arteriovenous difference technique [45]. Anyhow, the technique is very useful in many circumstances for investigating amino acid metabolism, preferably when the physiological state of the subject studied may be well defined. When arteriovenous difference measurements are combined with infusion of labelled amino acids, more precise information is obtained concerning whether or not amino acids are taken up by protein synthesis in the periphery to a different degree or if the release by proteolysis occurs [49]. A clear limitation is the pronounced snap-shot character of the measurement and the invasiveness over time if repeated sampling is desirable.

Incorporation of Labelled Amino Acids into Muscle Proteins

The only direct way of obtaining quantitative estimates of muscle protein synthesis rate is measurement of the incorporation of label into muscle proteins. The labels used are usually amino acids containing stable isotopes, such as ^{13}C, ^{14}C, ^{15}N, ^{2}H or ^{3}H. Such measurements also require knowledge about amino acid metabolism and kinetics, since an accurate estimate of the amount of label in the immediate precursor pool for protein synthesis is critical [50, 51]. With labelled branched-chain amino acids, the labelling of the corresponding ketoacid is often regarded as a reliable reflection of the intramuscular precursor pool [49]. However, this requires a complete mixing of all intracellular amino acids, which obviously does not occur in many circumstances unless special precautions are taken to guarantee that. In the basal state for example, most amino acids present in the immediate precursor pool for protein synthesis, the amino acyl-tRNA pool, are recruited from the degradation of proteins within the same cell [52]. This makes it difficult for an infused tracer to achieve the same abundance in the precursor pool as in the ketoacid pool. Conflicting results have been reported when the isotopic enrichment in the tRNA pool has been studied [53, 54]. This is partly explained by the considerable technical difficulties associated with such measurements [55], but also related to the fact that the results seem to be related to the metabolic state of the tissue. In the basal state, the enrichment of the aminoacyl tRNA pool is lower than of the intracellular free pool or of the plasma amino acid or ketoacid pool [52, 53]. In a tissue that is operated on, on the other hand, the enrichment of the aminoacyl tRNA pool lies between those of plasma and intracellular pools [54].

To overcome the uncertainty of not beeing able to know the enrichment of the precursor pool, the flooding dose technique was introduced [56]. The idea is to administer a large dose of the labelled amino acid, that will flood through all amino acid compartments and give a uniform distribution of the label throughout the body. This uniformity of label has also been demonstrated in human subjects [57], like the linearity of the incorporation rate [58]. In addition, the incorporation rate is not influenced by simultaneous flood of other amino acids and the reproducibility is good [59]. An alternative approach for administering the isotope label is to give a primed constant infusion [60, 61]. With this technique, however, it is not always possible to measure protein synthesis rate accurately, as for example during the administration of a large dose of another amino acid [62]. Also in other situations when amino acid concentrations are changing such as after feeding, does the incorporation rate of the constantly infused label become unreliable. The flooding dose technique is applicable under a wide range of circumstances during which the comparatively short-time period for measurements (90 min in man) is a clearcut advantage [58]. In different laboratories, the constant infusion technique requires from 4 to 30 h to obtain high enough enrichment in muscle protein to permit analysis with sufficient precision [63].

The use of stable isotopic labels permits the use of these kinetic techniques in virtually all circumstances. Although the mass-spectrometry equipment needed for the analyses has traditionally been expensive and technically difficult to handle, modern instruments offer new possibilities in this field.

Physiological and Pathophysiological States

The Effects of Feeding and Fasting

Although feeding and fasting are very fundamental states of physiology, their effects upon muscle protein and amino acid metabolism are not thoroughly known [64]. Starvation creates an amino acid pattern similar to that seen after trauma or in depleted states (Fig. 2), but in contrast to what happens after trauma, the changes are normalized within 2 days [25]. The changes in ribosome configuration also run parallel with a decrease appearing after 2–3 days of starvation [1], and a restitution is seen during 2 days of refeeding [3]. The ribosome parameters are not affected within the first 24–36 h of fasting, however [1]. Also the abundance of mRNA for myosin heavy chain decreases after short term starvation [14]. When protein synthesis rate is measured by the incorporation of ^{13}C-leucine into muscle proteins, the decrease after 3 days of starvation is only marginal (15%) by comparison with the postabsorptive state [65].

The immediate effect of feeding is that most amino acids, preferentially the branched-chain ones, are taken up by muscle tissue [48]. This also influences the concentrations of free amino acids in muscle [66]. The impact is limited to the essential amino acids however, and in quantitative terms the influence is very limited. The ribosome pattern is also very little affected by ordinary feeding hence no diurnal changes are seen [29]. It is more difficult to interpret the results of studies using the incorporation rate of labelled amino acids. Subjects given a flooding dose of ^{13}C-leucine show a very marginal increase during 10 h of feeding small meals [67]. However, a similar feeding pattern causes a 100% increase in the incorporation rate of ^{13}C-leucine when given as a primed constant infusion [61]. This difference in the apparent effect of feeding is most likely to result from the difficulty of correctly estimating the enrichment of the true precursor for protein synthesis when the constant infusion technique is used.

The Effects of Trauma

After elective surgical trauma, there is a 2–3 fold increase in the efflux of free amino acids from the periphery [47]. Intracellularly, this is accompanied by a 40% decrease in concentration of free glutamine and of the basic amino acids in conjunction with an approximately doubling of the branched-chain and aromatic amino acids [20]. Also the concentration and size distribution of ribosomes decreases [4], as does the incorporation of ^{13}C-leucine [35] or d5-phenylalanine [36] into muscle proteins (Fig. 3). This obvious decrease in protein synthesis, as indicated by all available techniques, is fully developed on the third postoperative day. The concentrations of glutamine and ribosomes exhibit a slow gradual decrease [4, 30], while the decline in the incorporation rate of labelled amino acids is already very pronounced (20–30%) at the end of the surgical procedure [35] and on the first postoperative day [36]. The restitution of these changes seems to be a very slow process. The drop in glutamine is invariably still present on the 10th day after elective

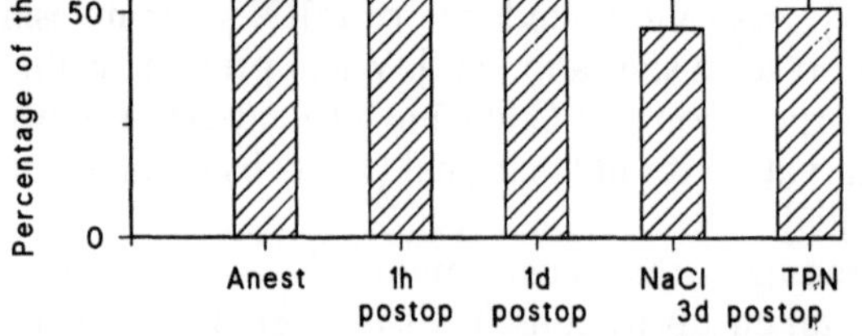

Fig. 3. The postoperative fractional synthesis rate in skeletal muscle as estimated by the incorporation of ^{13}C-leucine or d5-phenylalanine into muscle proteins given as percentage of the paired basal values obtained preoperatively. Synthesis rate is not influenced by anesthesia, but decreases immediately following the operation. Thereafter is continues to decrease on the 1st and 3rd postoperative days regardless of whether conventional intravenous nutrition is given or not. *, **, *** denotes significantly different from the paired basal values, *$p<0.05$, **$p<0.01$, and ***$p<0.001$, respectively. (From [35, 36, 74] with permission)

surgical trauma [2], and thereafter a slow restitution with considerable interindividual variation is seen [31, 68]. Even 30 days postoperatively most patients are not back to their preoperative levels [31]. The ribosome pattern behaves likewise [2]. The drop in the total amount of ribosomes is more pronounced and longstanding, while the relative abundance of polyribosomes is normalized earlier, indicative of an efficient utilization of the existing ribosomes during the restitution phase. Available data concerning the effects on muscle protein degradation, as estimated by the efflux of 3-methylhistidine from peripheral tissues, indicate that elective surgical trauma does not influence protein breakdown [69]. In critical illnes on the other hand, the efflux of 3-methylhistidine increases as a reflection of an elevated degradation rate [70]. In such patients, the drop in muscle glutamine is profound [23], and at least in pancreatitis patients the magnitude of the drop correlates with the mortality rate [22]. Stimultaneously, a drop in the incorporation of d5-phenylalanine into muscle is seen [37]. However, this drop is less pronounced than the drop seen 3 days after surgical trauma. The difference possibly reflects that the depression of protein synthesis is variable inbetween individual muscle proteins.

The effect of feeding upon muscle tissue in the traumatized state is of course not completely understood, as controversies already exist in the basal state. Nevertheless, the changes described above in glutamine, ribosomes or the incorporation of ^{13}C-leucine into muscle protein described above in the postabsorptive state following surgery are present irrespecitve of whether conventional IV nutrition is provided or not [4, 71, 72]. During ongoing conventional IV nutrition, a marginal effect on the incorporation of labelled amino acid may be present [36], but in any case such an effect is not very pronounced in spite of the improvement in whole body nitrogen economy [73]. Also during a hyperinsulinemic clamp, no improvement in muscle protein synthesis rate is seen [74]. However, there may be effects on the protein degradation, but so far the lack of appropriate techniques for investigation has left this question unanswered. Another possibility, which has not yet been investigated, is that provision of nutritional support in the immediate postoperative period shortens the time of the restitution phase.

New Therapies

Glutamine and Alpha-Ketoglutarate

As conventional amino acid solutions for IV use do not contain glutamine, it has been proposed that supplementation with glutamine might improve the effects of IV nutrition in the traumatized state. After all, glutamine is from a quantitative point of view the dominating free amino acid, at least in man. In muscle, glutamine concentration has been shown to be correlated with protein synthesis [33, 34]. Also in rapidly dividing cell populations such as lymphocytes [75] and enterocytes [76], glutamine obviously plays an important role as an energy substrate. Since by definition glutamine is not an essential amino acid for humans, it was initially thought that it could be left out of the amino acid solutions without any detrimental effects. The instability of glutamine in aqueous solution created difficulties when crystalline amino acid mixtures were produced. Before that, when hydrolysates of proteins containing oligopeptides were used [77], the content of glutamine was similar to that in proteins. In several circumstances, conventional parenteral nutrition lacking glutamine has been shown to be very effective. People without a gut could survive for decades, children grew, and malnourished patients could be repleated. However, the effects on some groups of patients were less impressive and this was especially true for muscle tissue. In trauma and critical illness, glutamine shortage and the loss of lean body mass are not influenced by conventional nutrition [23, 72]. The same seems to be the case in malignant disease [78].

To provide glutamine intravenously, it was first given in freshly prepared solutions [8] which was possible since the instability is not immediate. Later on, such preparations have been shown to have a better stability than first anticipated [79]. Glutamate, which is a possible alternative being a precursor, has several drawbacks. It is transported relatively slowly across membranes, giving high plasma concentrations when given in larger amounts. Such high concentrations interfere with glutamate's role as a neurotransmitter and cause adverse effects such as nausea, headache and chest pain, symptoms of the so called chinese restaurant syndrome. If alpha-ketoglutarate, the ketoacid of glutamate is given, on the other hand, no such negative effects occur. α-ketoglutarate is taken up by most tissues [80] and subsequently transferred into the mitochondria, where it can be transformed to glutamate and glutamine, as well as being utilized as an intermediate in the tricarboxylic acid cycle. Another approach for providing glutamine is to use synthetic dipeptides, such as alanyl-glutamine or glycyl-glutamine, which are stable in water solution but hydrolyse quickly after being infused intravenously [81].

Addition of approximately 20 g glutamine per 24 h postoperatively reduces and sometimes even eliminates the decrease in muscle glutamine (Fig. 4) [8, 10, 68, 82]. In addition, the drop in muscle ribosomes is prevented [8, 10, 83] and the whole body nitrogen economy becomes more favorable [8, 10, 82]. This is true when glutamine is added to TPN, but also when glutamine is given together with 200 g of glucose [84]. In a longer perspective, however, it has been demonstrated that these effects only persist as long as extra glutamine is provided [68, 83]. After discontinuation of glutamine supplementation, a delayed drop of muscle glutamine and of ribosomes occurs. When α-ketoglutarate or ornithine-α-ketoglutarate is used similar beneficial effects are seen postoperatively [7, 9, 85, 86]. In critical illness, the effects on muscle glutamine when 20 g glutamine is given daily are less impressive [87]. When a much larger dose of glutamine (60 g) is administered each day, a clear increase of the depleted muscle glutamine is reported [88], but whether or not critically ill subjects can handle such a large dose of glutamine without any hazards is still an open question. α-ketoglutarate on the other hand

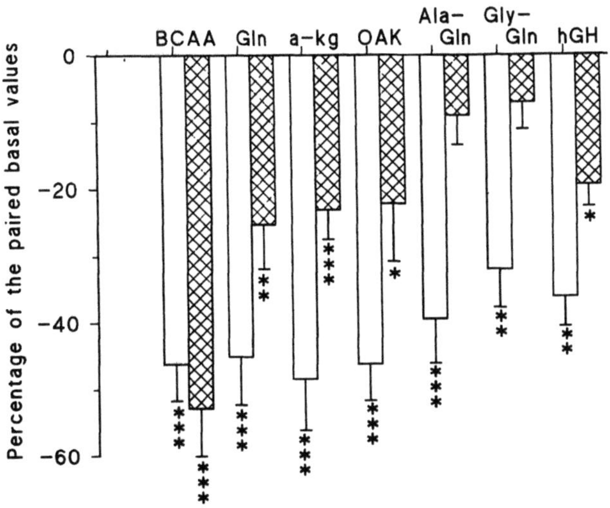

Fig. 4. The concentration of free glutamine in skeletal muscle on the 3rd postoperative day given as percentage of the paired basal preoperative values. All patients were given TPN and some groups were supplemented extra amounts of branched-chain amino acids, glutamine, α-ketoglutarate, ornithine-α-ketoglutarate, alanyl-glutamine, glycyl-glutamine or recombinant human growth hormone. *, **, *** denotes significantly different from the paired basal values, $^*p<0.05$, $^{**}p<0.01$, and $^{***}p<0.001$, respectively. (From [8–11, 25, 68, 85] with permission)

causes a 70% rise in muscle glutamine after 5 days of a 20 g per day treatment [89]. This demonstrates that α-ketoglutarate may be a more physiological substrate than glutamine itself. In clinical investigations, extra glutamine is also shown to have beneficial effects on infectious parameters in bonemarrow transplant patients [90]. All these data refer to glutamine or glutamine analogues administered by the IV route. The possible effects of enterally provided glutamine is quite an open question, since at this time no documentation exists on that point today in human subjects.

Growth Hormone

As growing animals or children exhibit a better healing capacity and a more rapid recovery compared to adult man, the possibility of beneficial effects of growth hormone (GH) treatment was suggested early on [91]. Before extracts from human hypophyses were prepared, the results were not very conclusive, but when human GH could be given, beneficial effects on substrate utilization, nitrogen economy and recovery were reported in patients with burns [92, 93]. Effects on muscle protein metabolism were not studied in man until synthetic human GH became available. During a normocaloric hyponitrogenous diet, healthy volunteers showed a drop in non-essential muscle amino acids together with a decrease in muscle ribosomes [94]. These changes are restored back to normal by the addition of daily injections of GH. After elective surgery, a large number of investigations have shown an improvement of nitrogen balance [11, 95–99]. Although there is a great likelyhood that this will also mean positive effects on muscle protein metabolism, so far experimental data to support this are few. The decreases in free glutamine (Fig. 4) and ribosome concentration in muscle after surgical trauma are attenuated [11] as well as the increase of glutamine efflux from peripheral tissues [98]. In addition, a semiquantitative estimate of muscle strength indicates a favorable effect of GH postoperatively [98]. The effect on whole body nitrogen economy, as shown by the lower urea production rate, is possibly related to an enhanced export of glutamate from the liver [100]. The effects on muscle tissue are not so well characterized at present. It is highly likely that insulin-like growth factor 1 (IGF-1), whose production and release is stimulated by GH, is the active substance. Posttraumatic muscle catabolism is counteracted, and as a result the export of glutamine does not increase. It is still not settled if this is a beneficial effect or not. Muscle tissue obviously benefits, but this may be at the expense of other tissues. Perhaps the export of muscle glutamine is critical, and if an elevation of this export is not possible, important metabolic processes may be impaired. Hence, it may very well prove that clinical use of GH as an adjuvant to nutritional therapy requires the simultaneous supply of glutamine or an analogue to glutamine.

Other Possible Substances

Over the years, several suggestions on how to save muscle protein during critical illness have been put forward. However, very little evidence from human studies to support these proposals has appeared. The response to surgical trauma can be eliminated with an epidural blockade, when muscle glutamine levels are maintained [101]. If, however, the duration of the block is short, no attenuation of the depletion of muscle glutamine is seen [84]. Anabolic steroids have also been suggested and an effect upon the postoperative nitrogen balance is demonstrated [102], but despite the misuse of this type of substance to expand muscle mass or muscle performance, no objective data on this exist in man. Arginine, w3-fatty acids, nucleotides, and medium-chain fatty acids have all been suggested as beneficial nutritional substances. The effects on muscle tissue in man, however, have not been elucidated. Provision of extra amounts of branched-chain amino acids has, at least commercially, been a great success. Unfortunately scientific evidences of beneficial effects in man have not been presented. A stimulatory effect of leucine on muscle protein synthesis in growing animals has been shown [103, 104], but in adult animals no such effect is reported [103]. In man, conflicting results have appeared concerning the possible effect on nitrogen balance. A consensus conference in Miami Beach (1985) was very hesitant regarding any such effects [105]. The only investigation actually looking at muscle free amino acids [85] and ribosomes [106] postoperatively in man showed no effects of branched-chain amino acid supplemented TPN following surgery, except for higher levels of the branched-chain amino acids than usual in muscle (Fig. 4).

Conclusion

Although muscle tissue may not in itself be the functionally limiting factor for critically ill patients, it definitely plays an important role. Muscle depletion does lead to loss of function and consequently results in difficulties in mobilizing the patients, and a prolonged hospital stay. Muscle tissue lost over a short period of critical illness is regained only very slowly during months and years. In elderly subjects, the muscle protein lost may never be restored. In addition, depletion of muscle tissue influences morbidity and mortality more directly. This occurs when amino acid export from skeletal muscle tissue ceases because of inability to produce more. At that time also the myocardium has become depleted and the threatening cardiac failure may lead to death. So far there is no evidence that this process can be prevented by conventional nutritional therapy. However, there are indications that the rate of muscle depletion can be reduced by nutritional support which thereby helps the patient to "buy time" for other, curative treatments to work. If nitrogen economy is a reflection of this process, enteral feeding seems to be superior to conventional parenteral feeding. Addition of new substrates and adjuvant treatments may, though, improve the efficacy of nutritional support. In this perspective, the influence of nutritional treatment on the biochemical changes in muscle is a useful indicator of the mechanism of the effect. However, studies of such biochemical changes will be helpful in designing new therapies. It is doubtful that a single new substrate or any other change to the traditional therapy will have much influence on the overall rates of mortality and/or morbidity. However, their use may even prove life saving for individual patients. Such patients may not be possible to identify in clinical practice, so the biochemical studies of muscle tissue may be the only way to define and optimize the nutrition given to critically ill patients.

References

1. Wernerman J, von der Decken A, Vinnars E (1985) Size distribution of ribosomes in biopsy specimens of human skeletal muscle during starvation. Metabolism 34:665–669
2. Petersson B, Wernerman J, Waller SO, von der Decken A, Vinnars E (1990) Elective abdominal surgery depresses muscle protein synthesis and increases subjective fatigue for more than 30 days. Br J Surg 77:796–800

3. Wernerman J, von der Decken A, Vinnars E (1986) Polyribosome concentration in human skeletal muscle after starvation and parenteral and enteral refeeding. Metabolism 35:447–451
4. Wernerman J, von der Decken A, Vinnars E (1986) Protein synthesis in skeletal muscle after abdominal surgery: The effect of total parenteral nutrition. JPEN 10:578–582
5. Löfberg EHA, Wernerman J, Norée LO, von der Decken A, Vinnars E (1991) Ribosome and free amino acid content in muscle during hemodialysis. Kidney Int 39:984–989
6. Wernerman J, Botta D, Hammarqvist F, Thunell S, von der Decken A, Vinnars E (1989) Stress hormones depress human skeletal muscle protein synthesis as assessed by the concentration and size distribution of ribosomes in percutaneous biopsy specimens. Clin Sci 77:611–616
7. Wernerman J, Hammarqvist F, von der Decken A, Vinnars E (1987) Ornithine-alpha-ketoglutarate improves skeletal muscle protein synthesis as assessed by ribosome analysis and nitrogen balance postoperatively. Ann Surg 206:674–678
8. Hammarqvist F, Wernerman J, Ali MR, von der Decken A, Vinnars E (1989) Addition of glutamine to total parenteral nutrition after elective abdominal surgery spares free glutamine in muscle, counteracts the fall in muscle protein synthesis, and improves nitrogen balance. Ann Surg 209:455–461
9. Hammarqvist F, Wernerman J, von der Decken A, Vinnars E (1991) Alpha-ketoglutarate preserves protein synthesis and free glutamine in skeletal muscle after surgery. Surgery 109:28–36
10. Hammarqvist F, Wernerman J, von der Decken A, Vinnars E (1990) Alanyl-glutamine counteracts the depletion of free glutamine and the postoperative decline in protein synthesis in skeletal muscle. Ann Surg 212:637–644
11. Hammarqvist F, Strömberg C, von der Decken A, Vinnars E, Wernerman J (1992) Biosynthetic growth hormone preserves both muscle protein synthesis, the decrease in muscle free glutamine and improves whole body nitrogen economy postoperatively. Ann Surg 216:184–191
12. Wernerman J, von der Decken A, Vinnars E (1986) The interpretation of ribosome determinations to assess protein synthesis in human skeletal muscle. Infusionstherapie 13:162–165
13. Wernerman J, von der Decken A, Vinnars E (1985) The diurnal pattern of protein synthesis in human skeletal muscle. Clin Nutr 4:203–205
14. Blomqvist B, von der Decken A, Vinnars E, Wernerman J (1991) Starvation changes muscle myosin heavy chain messenger RNA accumulation. J Biochem Nutr 11:223–231
15. Everett AW, Umeda PK, Sinha AM, Rabinowitz M, Zak R (1986) Expression of myosin heavy chains during thyroid hormone-induced cardiac growth. Federation Proc 45:2568–2572
16. Fong Y, Rosenbaum M, Tracey KJ, et al (1989) Recombinant growth hormone enhances muscle myosin heavy-chain mRNA accumulation and amino acid accural in humans. Proc Natl Acad Sci USA 86:3371–3374
17. Fong Y, Moldawer LL, Marano MA, et al (1989) Starvation leads to decreased levels of mRNA for myofibrillar proteins. J Surg Res 46:457–461
18. Bergström J, Fürst P, Norée LO, Vinnars E (1974) Intracellular free amino acid concentration in human muscle tissue. J Appl Physiol 36:693–697
19. Fürst P (1984) Regulation of intracellular metabolism of amino acids. In: F Bozetti, R Dionigi (eds) Nutrition in cancer and trauma sepsis. Karger, Basel, pp 21–53
20. Vinnars E, Bergström J, Fürst P (1975) Influence of the postoperative state on the intracellular free amino acids in human muscle tissue. Ann Surg 182:665–671
21. Askanazi J, Carpentier YA, Elwyn DH, et al (1980) Influence of total parenteral nutrition on fuel utilization in injury and sepsis. Ann Surg 191:40–46
22. Roth E, Funovics J, Mühlbacher F, et al (1982) Metabolic disorders in severe abdominal sepsis: Glutamine deficiency in skeletal muscle. Clin Nutr 1:25–42

23. Gamrin L, Hultman E, Vinnars E, Wernerman J (1991) The effects of stress hormones in combination with an amino acid infusion on protein synthesis and amino acid concentration in skeletal muscle. Clin Nutr 10 (suppl):29
24. Askanazi J, Elwyn DH, Kinney JM, Gump FE, Michelsen CB, Stinchfield FE (1978) Muscle and plasma amino acids after injury: The role of inactivity. Ann Surg 188:797–803
25. Vinnars E, Bergström J, Fürst P (1987) Effects of starvation on plasma and muscle amino acid concentration in normal subjects. Clin Nutr 6 (Suppl):62
26. Sandstedt S, Symreng T, Larsson J (1985) Changes in muscle and plasma amino acid metabolism in severe malnutrition: The influence of total parenteral nutrition. Clin Nutr 4:13–19
27. Sandstedt S, Lennmarken C, Symreng T, Vinnars E (1985) The effect of pre-operative total parenteral nutrition on energy-rich phosphates, electrolytes and free amino acids in skeletal muscle of malnoursihed patients with gastric carcinoma. Br J Surg 72:920-924
28. Bergström J, Fürst P, Norée LO, Vinnars E (1978) Intracellular free amino acids in muscle tissue of patients with chronic uremia: Effect of peritoneal dialysis and infusion of essential amino acids. Clin Sci Mol Med 54:51–60
29. Wernerman J, von der Decken A, Vinnars E (1985) The diurnal pattern of protein synthesis in human skeletal muscle. Clin Nutr 4:203–205
30. Essén P, Wernerman J, Sonnenfeld T, Thunell S, Vinnars E (1992) Free amino acids in plasma and muscle during 24 hours post-operatively: A descriptive study. Clin Physiol 12:165–179
31. Petersson B, Vinnars E, Waller SO, Wernerman J (1992) Long-term changes in muscle free amino acid levels after elective abdominal surgery. Br J Surg 79:212–216
32. Askanazi J, Carpentier YA, Michelsen CB, et al (1980) Muscle and plasma amino acids following injury: Influence of intercurrent infection. Ann Surg 191:78–85
33. Jepson MM, Bates PC, Broadbent P, Pell JM, Millward DJ (1988) Relationship between glutamine concentration and protein synthesis in rat skeletal muscle. Am J Physiol 255:E166–E172
34. Wernerman J, Hammarqvist F, Vinnars E (1990) Alpha-ketoglutarate and postoperative muscle catabolism. Lancet 335:701–703
35. Essén P, McNurlan MA, Wernerman J, Vinnars E, Garlick PJ (1992) Uncomplicated surgery but not general anesthesia decreases muscle protein synthesis. Am J Physiol 262:E253–E260
36. Tjäder I, Essén P, McNurlan MA, Garlick PJ, Wernerman J (1992) Protein synthesis rate in human skeletal muscle decreases 24 hours after abdominal surgery irrespective of intravenous nutrition. Clin Nutr 11 (Suppl):49
37. Essén P, McNurlan MA, Tjäder I, et al (1992) Tissue protein synthesis in the ciritcal ill patient. Clin Nutr 11 (Suppl):1
38. Felig P, Wahren J (1971) Amino acid metabolism in exercising man. J Clin Invest 50:2703–2714
39. Lundholm K, Bennegård K, Zachrisson H, et al (1987) Transport kinetics of amino acids across the resting human leg. J Clin Invest 80:763–771
40. Millward DJ, Bates PC, Grimble GK, Brown JG, Nathan M, Rennie MJ (1988) Quantitative importance of non-skeletal-muscle sources of N-methyl-histidine in urine. Biochem J 190:225–228
41. Young VR, Haverberg LN, Bilmazes C, Munro HN (1973) Potential use of 3-methylhistidine excretion as an index of progressing reduction in muscle protein catabolism during starvation. Metabolism 22:1429–1436
42. Sjölin J, Hjort G, Friman G, Hambreus L (1987) Urinary excretion of 1-methylhistidine: A qualitative indicator of exogenous 3-methylhistidine and intake of meats from various sources. Metabolism 36:1175–1184
43. Sjölin J, Stjernström H, Henneberg S, et al (1989) Splanchnic and peripheral release of 3-methylhistidine in relation to its urinary excretion in human infection. Metabolism 38:23–29

44. Young VR (1970) The role of skeletal and cardiac muscle in the regulation of protein metabolism. In: Munro HN (ed) Mammalian protein metabolism Vol IV. Academic Press, New York, pp 585–674
45. Wernerman J, Vinnars E (1987) The effect of trauma and surgery on interorgan fluxes of amino acids. Clin Sci 73:129–133
46. Wahren J, Felig P, Hagenfeldt J (1976) Effect of protein ingestion on splanchnic and leg metabolism in normal man and in patients with diabetes mellitus. J Clin Invest 57:987–999
47. Clowes GHA, Randell HT, Cha CJ (1980) Amino acid and energy metabolism in septic and traumatized. JPEN 4:195–203
48. Elia M, Livesey G (1983) Effects of ingested steak and infused leucine on forelimb metabolism in man, and the fate of the carbon skeletons and amino groups of branched-chain amino acids. Clin Sci 64:517–526
49. Cheng KN, Dworzak F, Ford CG, Rennie MJ, Halliday D (1985) Direct determination of leucine metabolism and protein breakdown in humans using L-[1-^{13}C, ^{15}N]-leucine and the forearm model. Eur J Clin Invest 15:349–354
50. Garlick PJ, Wernerman J (1993) Responses of protein metabolism to trauma. In: Cooper G, Dudley H, Little R, Meynard R, Heineman R (eds) Scientific Foundations of Trauma. Oxford (in press)
51. Waterlow JC, Garlick PJ, Millward DJ (1978) Protein turnover in the whole body and in whole tissues. In: Waterlow JC, Garlick PJ, Millward DJ (eds) Protein turnover in mammalian tissues and in the whole body. North Holland, Amsterdam, pp 443–479
52. Biolo G, Chinkes D, Zhang XJ, Wolfe RR (1992) In vivo determination of the relationship between amino acid transmembrane transport and protein kinetics in muscle. JPEN 16:23S
53. Baumann PQ, Stirewalt WS, O'Rourke BD, Nair KS (1993) Protein precursor ^{13}C-leucine enrichment in swine thigh muscle, heart and liver. In: Nair KS (ed) Protein metabolism in diabetes mellitus. Smith Gordon, London (in press)
54. Watt PW, Lindsay Y, Scrimgeour CM, et al (1991) Isolation of aminoacyl-tRNA and its labelling with stable-isotope tracers: Use in studies of human tissue protein synthesis. Proc Natl Acad Sci USA 88:5892–5896
55. Airhart J, Vidrich A, Khairrallah EA (1974) Compartmentation of free amino acids for protein synthesis in rat liver. Biochem J 140:539–548
56. Garlick PJ, McNurlan MA, Preedy VR (1980) A rapid and convenient method for measuring the rate of protein synthesis in tissues by injection of [^{3}H]phenylalanine. Biochem J 192:719–723
57. Garlick PJ, Wernerman J, McNurlan MA, et al (1989) Measurement of the rate of protein synthesis in muscle of postabsorptive young men by injection of a flooding dose of [1-^{13}C]leucine. Clin Sci 77:329–336
58. Garlick PJ, Wernerman J, McNurlan MA, Essén P (1993) Measurement of tissue protein synthesis from the incorporation of labelled amino acids. Am J Physiol (in press)
59. McNurlan M, Essén, P, Heys SD, Buchan V, Garlick P, Wernerman J (1991) Measurement of protein synthesis in human skeletal muscle: Further investigation of the "flooding" technique. Clin Sci 81:557–564
60. Rennie MJ, Edwards RHT, Halliday D, Matthews DE, Wolman SL, Millward DJ (1982) Muscle protein synthesis measured by stable isotope techniques in man: The effects of feeding and fasting. Clin Sci 63:519–523
61. Halliday D, Pacy PJ, Cheng KN, et al (1988) Rate of protein synthesis in skeletal muscle of normal man and patients with muscular dystrophy: A reassessment. Clin Sci 74:237–240
62. Jahoor F, Zhang XJ, Baba H, Sakurai Y, Wolfe RR (1992) Comparison of constant infusion and flooding dose techniques to measure muscle protein synthesis rate in dogs. J Nutr 122:878–887
63. Smith K, Rennie M (1990) Protein turnover and amino acid metabolism in human skeletal muscle. Clin Endocr Metab 3:461–498

64. Garlick PJ, Wernerman J, McNurlan MA, Essés P (1990) What is the normal response of protein turnover to nutrient supply? Clin Nutr 9:294–296
65. Essén P, McNurlan MA, Wernerman J, Milne E, Vinnars E, Garlick P (1992) Short term starvation decreases skeletal muscle protein synthesis rate in man. Clin Physiol 12:1–13
66. Bergström J, Fürst P, Vinnars E (1990) Effect of test meal, without and with protein on muscle and plasma free amino acids. Clin Sci 79:331–337
67. McNurlan M, Essén P, Milne E, Vinnars E, Garlick P, Wernerman J (1993) Temporal responses of protein synthesis in human skeletal muscle to feeding. Br J Nutr 69:117–126
68. Petersson B, Waller SO, Vinnars E, Wernerman J (1990) Glycyl-glutamine in postoperative TPN reduces and postpones the decrease in muscle glutamine. Clin Nutr 9 (Suppl):88
69. Rennie MJ, Bennegård K, Edén E, Emery PW, Lundholm K (1984) Urinary excreation and efflux from the leg of 3-methylhistidine before and after major surgical operation. Metabolism 33:250–256
70. Sjölin J, Stjernström H, Friman G, Larsson J, Wahren J (1990) Total and net muscle protein breakdown in infection determined by amino effluxes. Am J Physiol 258:E856–E863
71. Essén P, McNurlan MA, Sonnenfeld T, Milne E, Vinnars E, Wernerman J (1993) Muscle protein synthesis postoperatively: The effect of intravenous nutrition. Eur J Surg (in press)
72. Vinnars E, Holmström B, Schildt B, Odebäck AC, Fürst P (1983) Metabolic effects of four intravenous nutritional regimens in patients undergoing elective surgery. II: Muscle amino acids and energy-rich phosphates. Clin Nutr 2:3–11
73. Ewerth S, Allgén LG, Fürst P, et al (1983) Metabolic effects of four intravenous nutritional regimens after elective surgery I: Clinical data and biochemistry. Clin Nutr 1:313–324
74. Thorell A, Essén P, Ljungqvist O, et al (1992) Postoperative insulin resistance and muscle protein synthesis rate. J Clin Nutr 11 (Suppl):48
75. Newsholme EA, Crabtree B, Ardawi MSM (1985) Glutamine metabolism in lymphocytes: Its biochemical, physiological and clinical importance. Q J Exp Physiol 70:473–489
76. Souba WW, Smith RJ, Wilmore DW (1985) Glutamine metabolism by the intestinal tract. JPEN 9:608–617
77. Elman R (1939) Time factor in retention of nitrogen after intravenous injection of a mixture of amino acids. Proc Soc Exper Biol Med 40:484–487
78. Drott C, Unsgaard B, Scherstén T, Lundholm K (1988) Total parenteral nutrition as an adjuvant to patients undergoing chemotherapy for testicular carcinoma: Protection of body composition – A randomized, prospective study. Surgery 103:499–506
79. Khan K, Hardy G, McElroy B, Elia M (1991) The stability of L-glutamine in total parenteral nutrition solutions. Clin Nutr 10:193–198
80. Roth-Merten A, Karner J, Winkler S, Valentini L, Schaupp K, Roth E (1990) Influence of alpha-ketoglutarate infusion on glutamine and glutamine metabolism. Clin Nutr 9:46–47
81. Stehle P (1991) Das Synthetische Dipeptid L-alanyl-L-glutamine: Ein neues Substrat für die klinische Ernährungstherapie. In: Klinische Ernährung 35, W. Zuckschwerdt Verlag, München pp 1–72
82. Stehle P, Zanders J, Mertes N, et al (1989) Effect of parenteral glutamine peptide supplements on muscle glutamine loss and nitrogen balance after major surgery. Lancet 1:231–233
83. Petersson B, Waller SO, von der Decken A, Vinnars E, Wernerman J (1991) The long-term effect of postoperative TPN supplemented with glycyl-glutamine on protein synthesis in skeletal muscle. Clin Nutr 10 (Suppl):10

84. Blomqvist B, von der Decken A, Hammarqvist F, Wernerman J (1992) Glutamininfusion motverkar minskning av fritt glutamin i muskel efter höftproteskirurgi. Hygiea 101:109
85. Hammarqvist F, Wernerman J, Ali MR, Vinnars E (1990) Effects of an amino acid solution enriched with either branched-chain amino acids or ornithine-alpha-ketoglutarate on the postoperative intracellular amino acid concentration of skeletal muscle. Br J Surg 77:214–218
86. Vesterberg K, Leander U, Fürst P, Vinnars E (1987) Nitrogen sparing effect of Ornicetil in the immediate postoperative state – plasma and muscle amino acids. Clin Nutr 6:213–219
87. Karner J, Roth E (1990) Alanyl-glutamine infusions to patients with acute pancreatitis. Clin Nutr 9:43–44
88. Roth E, Winkler S, Hölzenbein T, Valentini L, Karner J (1992) High load of alanylglutamine in two patients with acute pancreatitis. Clin Nutr 11 (Suppl):82
89. Petersson B, Gamrin L, Hammarqvist F, Vinnars E, Wernerman J (1992) Alphaketoglutarate given together with TPN improves the free glutamine levels in glutamine-depleted intensive care patients. Clin Nutr 11 (Suppl):26
90. Ziegler TR, Young LS, Benefell K, et al (1992) Clinical and metabolic efficacy of glutamine-supplemented parenteral nutrition after bone marrow transplantation. Ann Int Med 116:821–828
91. Cuthbertson DP, Shaw GB, Young FG (1941) The anterior pituitary gland and protein metabolism. II. The influence of anterior pituitary extract on the metabolic response of the rat to injury. J Endocrinol 2:468–474
92. Liljedahl SO, Gemzell CA, Plantin LO (1961) Effect of human growth hormone in patients with severe burns. Acta Chir Scand 122:1–14
93. Soroff HS, Pearson E, Green NL, Artz CP (1960) The effect of growth hormone on nitrogen balance at various levels of intake in burned patients. Surg Gynecol Obstet 111:259–273
94. Lundeberg S, Belfrage M, Wernerman J, von der Decken A, Thunell S, Vinnars E (1991) Growth hormone improves muscle protein metabolism and whole body nitrogen economy in man during a hyponitrogenous diet. Metabolism 40:315–322
95. Ward HC, Halliday D, Sim AJW (1987) Protein and energy metabolism with biosynthetic human growth hormone after gastrointestinal surgery. Ann Surg 206:56–61
96. Mjaaland M, Unneberg K, Horwedt R, Revhaug A (1991) Nitrogen retention caused by growth hormone in patients undergoing gastrointestinal surgery with epidural analgesia and parenteral nutrition. Eur J Surg 157:21–27
97. Ziegler TR, Lorraine SY, Ferrari-Baliviera E, Demling RH, Wilmore D (1990) Use of human growth hormone combined with nutritional support in a critical care unit. JPEN 14:574–581
98. Jiang ZM, He GZ, Zhang SY, Wang XR, Yang NF, Zhu Y (1989) Low-dose growth hormone and hypocaloric nutrition attenuate the protein-catabolic response after major operation. Ann Surg 210:513–525
99. Jauch KW, Hermann A, Hartland W, Schidberg FW (1992) Dose-dependent effects of human-growth-hormone (rHGH) on postoperative substrate metabolism. Clin Nutr 11 (Suppl):9
100. Welbourne T, Joshi S, McVie R (1989) Growth hormone effects on hepatic glutamate handling in vivo. Am J Physiol 257:E959–E962
101. Christensen T, Waaben J, Lindeburg T, Vesterberg K, Vinnars E, Kehlet H (1986) Epidural analgesia attenuates postoperative changes in muscle amino acids. Acta Chir Scand 152:407–411
102. Michelsen CB, Askanazi J, Kinney JM, Gump FE, Elwyn DH (1982) Effect of an anabolic steroid on nitrogen balance and amino acid patterns after total hip replacement. J Trauma 22:410–413
103. Li JB, Jefferson LS (1978) Influence of amino acid availability on protein turnover in performed skeletal muscle. Biochim Biophys Acta 566:351–359

104. Garlick PJ, Grant I (1988) Amino acid infusion increases the sensitivity of muscle protein synthesis in vivo to insulin: Effect of branched-chain amino acids. Biochem J 254:579–584
105. Brennan MF, Cerra F, Daly JM, et al (1986) Branched-chain amino acids in stress and injury. JPEN 10:446–452
106. Hammarqvist F, Wernerman J, von der Decken A, Vinnars E (1988) The effect of branched-chain amino acids upon postoperative muscle protein synthesis and nitrogen balance. Clin Nutr 7:171–175

Enhancing Wound Healing in Severely Burned Patients

D. A. Gilpin, M. J. Muller, and D. N. Herndon

Introduction

Wound healing is often delayed in severely burned patients due to changes in hormone balance, metabolism and immune function. With early wound closure, the hypermetabolic response and risk of infection are reduced. This chapter will discuss some endocrinology and metabolism associated with burn injuries and present some experimental evidence on the benefits of recombinant human growth hormone (GH) in burned children.

The initial response to a burn injury is often focused on maintaining body function by selective preservation of essential organ systems. The initial response to a severe burn injury has been termed the ebb phase and the later response the flow phase. The ebb phase begins immediately after injury and is characterized by a fall in insulin and an increase in catecholamines and glucagon levels. Anti-diuretic hormone (ADH) and aldosterone are released in response to pain. These hormonal changes are associated with a rise in blood sugar, lactate and free fatty acid levels, and a fall in the metabolic rate, core temperature, cardiac output and oxygen consumption. Although the regulators of the ebb phase are not fully understood, the responses elicited within the first 24 h are critical for survival. After these initial responses, there is a prolonged flow phase which may last weeks or months depending upon the severity of injury.

Flow Phase

Endocrinology

The flow phase, or chronic hypermetabolic period of the stress response, was initially described by Cuthbertson in 1942 [1] who identified many changes attributable to catabolism in patients suffering from lower limb fractures. The flow phase is associated with an increase in ACTH, cortisol and insulin increases in catecholamine and glucagon levels (Fig. 1). Catecholamines from peripheral nerve endings and the adrenal medulla act upon α- and β-adrenoreceptors located on the cell membrane. Norepinephrine exerts its effect mainly upon α-receptors while epinephrine acts primarily upon β-receptors. α-adrenoreceptor stimulation inhibits insulin and glucagon production,

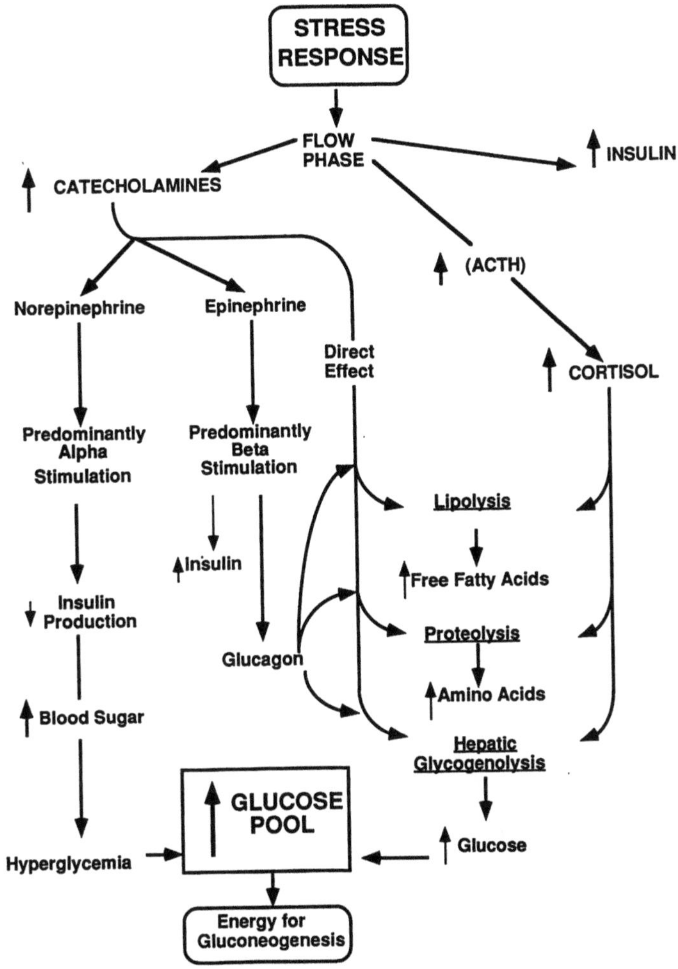

Fig. 1. The flow, or chronic hypermetabolic phase of the stress response occurs within 24 h of injury and is associated with the mobilization of the hormone depicted. The result of this hormonal interaction is an increased glucose level for use as metabolic fuel. Paradoxically, catabolism produces glucose which is used to fuel further catabolism

whereas β-adrenoreceptor stimulation has a stimulating effect on insulin and glucagon production. Catecholamines directly stimulate hepatic glycogenolysis, gluconeogenesis, and lipolysis. β-adrenergic receptor stimulation of the pancreas stimulates glucagon production leading to an increase in gluconeogenesis, proteolysis and lipolysis and, like cortisol, has an anti-insulin effect. The net result is that catecholamines directly and indirectly produce increased glucose, free fatty acids, and amino acids. Cortisol, produced through the hypothalamic-pituitary-adrenal axis, remains elevated for the duration of stress and also stimulates hepatic glycogenolysis, peripheral lipolysis, and skeletal muscle proteolysis resulting in an elevation in blood glucose and the mobilization of fatty and amino acids. The anti-insulin effect of cortisol is additive to the hyperglycemia caused by glycogenolysis.

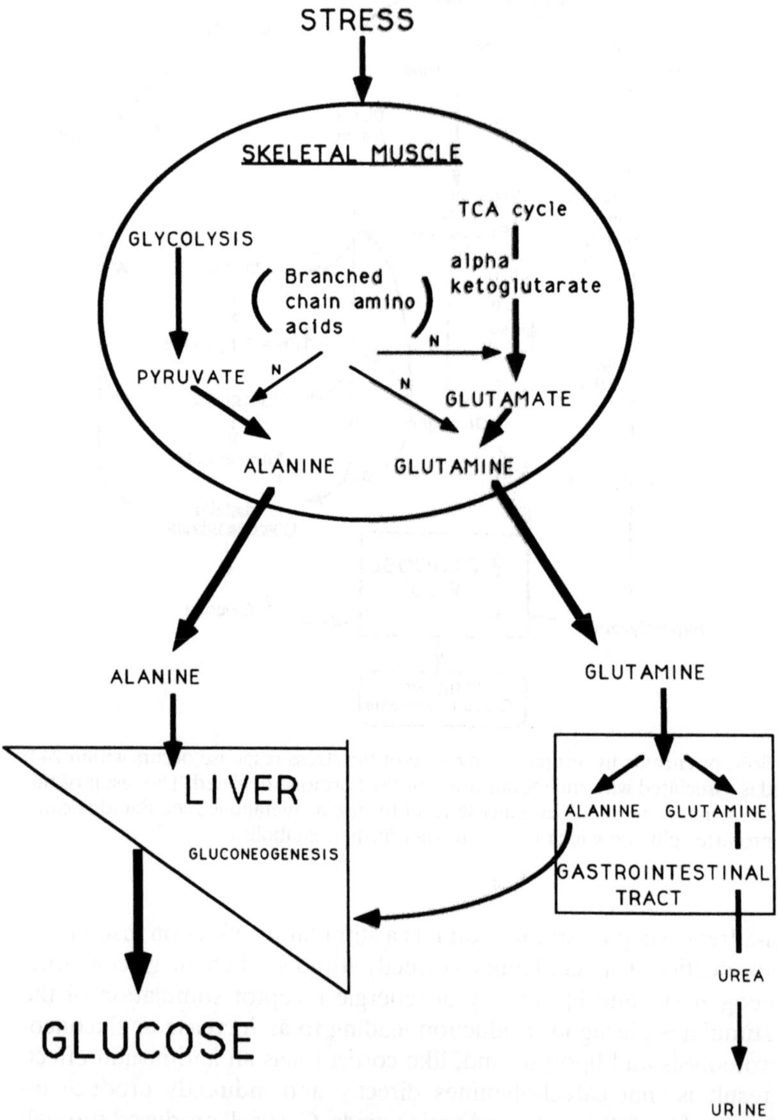

Fig. 2. Proposed mechanism for utilization of branched-chain amino acids, valine, leucine and isoleucine to alanine and glutamine, and their subsequent conversion to glucose

Metabolism

Substrate for hepatic gluconeogenesis is produced by peripheral proteolysis, principally in skeletal muscle. Lactate, pyruvate and alanine are intermediates in this process and require the expenditure of high energy phosphate bonds for both their production and subsequent conversion to glucose. Fat and glucose produced from hepatic gluconeogenesis are burned as fuels for further glucose production. During starvation, hypoglycemia stimulates glucagon and catecholamine production which signals the liver to convert glycogen to glucose. However, the limited supply of glycogen is rapidly depleted and substrate must then be obtained from muscle proteolysis and energy from peripheral fat lipolysis. Protein is degraded to amino acids, and fat to acetyl Co enzyme A which must combine with acetoacetate in order to enter the tricarboxylic acid (TCA) cycle. As plasma glucose and subsequently acetoacetate concentrations fall, the level of acetyl Co enzyme A rises. This substrate is then shunted into another pathway producing β-hydroxybutyrate, acetoacetate and acetone. In most tissues, elevated ketone bodies inhibit proteolysis and decrease glucose utilization leading to a decrease in proteolysis and an increase in lipolysis. In the stress response, elevated levels of catabolic hormones maintain gluconeogenesis, proteolysis and lipolysis preventing the usual conversion of protein metabolism to fat metabolism. The resulting hyperglycemia does not, however, inhibit insulin and glucagon production, while alanine and glutamine are present in skeletal muscle in relatively small quantities compared to other amino acids. Following stress, there is an increase in the release of these two amino acids from muscle which is greater than expected compared to other amino acids. It is thought that the branched-chain amino acids valine, leucine and isoleucine supply nitrogen for transamination of pyruvate to produce alanine which is subsequently utilized for glucose production. Concomitantly, glutamate is converted to glutamine by the action of glutamine synthetase before further conversion to alanine and ammonia in the gastrointestinal tract. Alanine is transported to the liver for gluconeogenesis, and ammonia is converted to urea and subsequently excreted in the urine (Fig. 2). Cortisol has been shown to enhance this pathway [3]. Thus, the various hormonal interactions produce a pool of molecular raw materials which can be used to build proteins for immune function and wound healing [1–8].

Protein Kinetics and Lipolysis

During the flow phase, there is a negative nitrogen balance due to protein loss and changes in the relative rates of synthesis of protein, carbohydrate and lipids. It has been shown that catabolism is associated with a change in the relative rates of synthesis and breakdown, rather than cessation of one or the other [9–11]. Further the administration of protein also influences protein kinetics. Alanine, released from skeletal muscle of injured limbs in proportion to the extent of injury [12], is transported to the liver for subsequent gluconeogenesis or protein synthesis. The hyperglycemia that occurs following injury is usually proportional to the severity of trauma [13]. Its etiology may be due to increased gluconeogenesis rather than any alteration in glucose utilization.

Substrate cycling is a process whereby macromolecules such as lipids, are degraded into their constituent components and transported via the circulation to other sites to be reformed into macromolecules, frequently the same as the parent molecule. Substrate cycling is one way in which energy is utilized but in a "wasteful" manner. Elevated catecholamines have been demonstrated in both the ebb and the flow phases of the trauma response and have been correlated with the severity of lipolysis in burned children. The reduction in the quantity of available fat for fuel, secondary to extensive fascial excision of burned tissue is thought to influence proteolysis. When lipolytic rate is maximal, due to chronic elevation of catecholamines and the source of lipid is limited, substrate availability becomes a problem. Inadequate fuel for gluconeogenesis causes a rise in proteolysis which may be refractory to calorie supplementation. The short-term use of β-blockers can reduce the rate of lipolysis in burned patients [14, 15]. Weight loss in burn patients is dependent upon both the severity of burn and time post-injury [16]. Thus as depicted in Fig. 3, weight is not lost at a fixed rate.

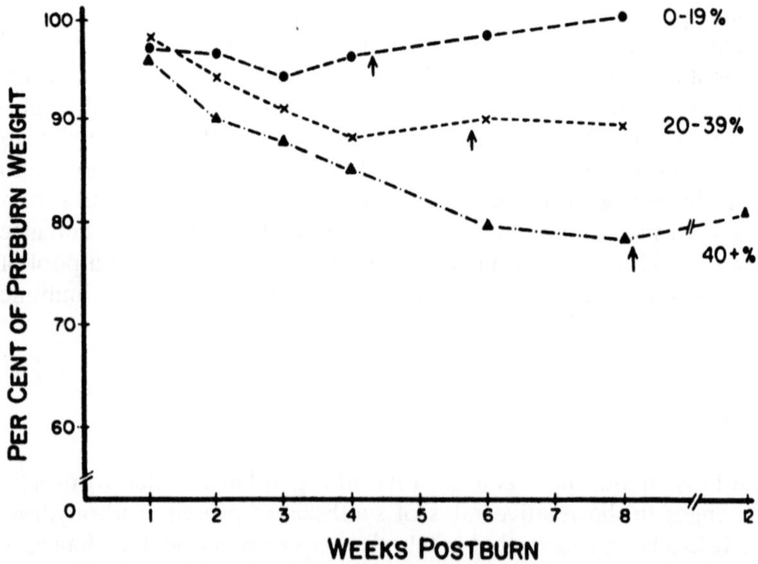

Fig. 3. Graph illustrating percentage weight loss of body weight against time following burn (weeks). Three groups of differing burn sizes are illustrated 0–19%, 20–39%, 40%. Weight loss increases with burn size. (From [16] with permission)

Hypermetabolism

Hypermetabolism is associated with a rise in the basal metabolic rate (BMR) characterized by increased oxygen consumption, elevated core temperature, and an increased urinary excretion of phosphorus, potassium, nitrogen, and sulphur. Initially, it was assumed that hyperthermia was an attempt by the body to enhance healing, since wounds re-epithelialize best at temperatures around 40°C [17]. It is now known that severely burned patients have a particularly high catabolic response. Thyroid stimulating hormone (TSH) and T_3/T_4 levels are often normal or even depressed in burned patients which suggests that the rise in BMR is not mediated through thyroid hormone [5]. Studies using guinea pigs indicate that while thyroid hormones may not be elevated in the stress response, they may influence wound healing. In these studies, thyroidectomized guinea pigs were given intra-peritoneal thyroid hormone in graded doses on a daily basis and then given a 50% scald burn [10]. Results showed thyroid hormones do not account for the increase in oxygen consumption after thermal injury, further at high or low doses, TH can inhibit re-epithelialization in burned thyroidectomized animals, but when given an intermediate dose wound healing was enhanced [18].

Evaporative water and heat losses are proportional to the size of the open burn wound. It has been suggested that the rise in BMR is an attempt to compensate for heat loss due to evaporation. Zawacki et al. [19] demonstrated that when burn wounds were covered with impermeable dressings, to eliminate evaporative water loss, patients still suffered with an elevated BMR [19]. He concluded that while evaporative water loss may be a contributory factor toward increasing BMR, it was not the only influence. These conclusions were independently confirmed by Neely et al. [20]. Wilmore et al. [21] demonstrated that the rise in BMR was proportional to burn size and reached a plateau of twice normal with a 50% total body surface area (TBSA) burn. He further showed that patients preferred an elevated environmental temperature, and that by increasing the temperature metabolic rate decreased for any given burn size. However, even with elevated temperatures, the BMR remained markedly elevated. It was thus concluded that the metabolic rate was temperature sensitive but not temperature dependent. In other studies, involving early burn wound excision as compared to conservative management with open dressing techniques, the BMR increased with burn size and reached a maximum of 50% above normal in patients with a 50% TBSA burn [22]. No further increase in BMR occurred unless the patient became septic. BMR may be increased to maximum during a combination of stresses such as thermal injury and sepsis, however, once the BMR reset is functioning maximally, further stress may lead to death. These findings indicate during the hypermetabolic state there is a rise in the hypothalamic set point by approximately 1–2°C which remains elevated until the burn wound is completely closed [23].

Elaborate studies measuring arteriovenous oxygen differences have shown no difference in the relative oxygen consumption between burned and unburned limbs. While oxygen consumption of the body as a whole was increased, the oxygen utilization in the injured limb and that of the viscera remained the same [21]. Glucose consumption by the injured limb, however, increased relative to the un-injured limb. In the burn wound, glucose is metabolized to lactate and pyruvate by glycolysis and transported to the liver for conversion to glucose. The reason for a large production of lactate, despite adequate oxygen saturation and blood flow probably reflects the anaerobic environment of the wound consisting of macrophages, fibroblasts, and angiogenic tissues [24]. Increased glucose consumption by the wound initially consumes glucose obtained from hepatic glycogen stores and later from lipolysis and proteolysis of skeletal muscle leading to a negative nitrogen balance and total body weight loss. The chance of survival may be reduced when body weight loss is greater than 20% [25].

The role of the central nervous system in the stress response has been demonstrated in patients who have spinal injuries and in those who are brain dead. The latter group fail to produce a flow phase, whereas quadriplegic patients show some features, but no hyperpyrexia. Clinical observations suggest that early wound closure is beneficial in reducing the BMR. Studies in which sheep were burned and their wounds excised and totally grafted, showed a reduction in burn-induced hypermetabolism. Wilmore et al. confirmed these observations, however, Rutan et al. in a comparative study of early wound excision vs conservative serial excision, failed to correlate a reduction in hypermetabolism with early excision [25].

Dietary Influences

In the flow phase, burn patients loose large quantities of body protein and fat. Burned pediatric patients demonstrate a significant redistribution of body fat to the torso secondary to catecholamine-induced lipolysis. This redistribution is associated with fatty infiltration of the liver and an increase in omental fat. The ideal nutritional support would maintain energy reserves by the administration of exogenous nutrients at a rate sufficient to keep up with demand. Often, even with continuous feeding, patients cannot keep up with energy requirements for maintaining an elevated metabolic rate. The use of constant infusion enteral drips has partly solved this problem, although many seriously injured patients are unable to tolerate this route. The need to supply adequate calories and protein from the beginning of treatment is thus paramount and can be achieved by total parenteral nutrition (TPN) given through a central jugular or subclavian line. An estimation of the number of calories required is obviously important, and even more so in a pediatric population. Curreri et al. [26] developed a formula for the calculation of calorie estimates in adult burn patients based upon the percentage of the TBSA burned and body weight. This formula: 25 Kcal × body wt(kg) + 40 Kcal × %TBSA burn, has proven to be a reliable guide to caloric requirements in adults. Unfortunately, it cannot be extrapolated to a pediatric population and its use greatly overestimates requirements. Studies show that excessive administration of TPN has a deleterious effect upon the body including abnormal liver function, fatty infiltration of the liver, and cholestasis resulting in hepatitis and jaundice. Lowry and Brennan [27] attempted to clarify the situation and concluded that excessive carbohydrate calories and nitrogen administration are associated with changes in lung function. Other studies showed that calorie to nitrogen ratios of approximately 100/1 may be adequate in maintaining nitrogen balance. Askanazi et al. [28] observed an increase in oxygen consumption in hypermetabolic patients and suggested that "the greater the resting energy expenditure, the more a carbohydrate load effects oxygen consumption". Various modifications were made to the original Curreri formula before Hildreth and Carvajal [29] devised a formula based upon the burned surface area for pediatric patients treated by serial burn wound excision.

Maintenance calories + calories required for injury is equal to
1800 Kcal/m^2 TBSA/day + 2200 Kcal/m^2 TBSAB@/day.
@TBSAB = Total body surface area burned

A subsequent study, comparing the two formulae for calorie requirements in children treated by early excision [30] showed that an overestimation in calorie requirements was made in both. Studies on over 100 patients treated during a 5 year period, suggested that the Hildreth formula should be modified to account for patient age (Table 1) [31–33]

Hormonal Manipulation of the Stress Response

Following injury, catecholamine levels remain significantly elevated until the burn wound is closed [13]. Cardiovascular manifestations of elevated catecholamines include: increased systemic peripheral resistance secondary to vasoconstriction, skeletal muscle vasodilation, and increased heart rate and contractility [34]. Chronically elevated catecholamines are thought to be detrimental with myocarditis, cardiomyopathy and accelerated atheroma for-

Table 1. Summary of calorie requirements in burned children in different age groups

	Maintenance calories (TBSA m^2)[a]	Calorie allowance for injury (TBSAB)[b]
General	1800 Kcal/m^2·day	+2200 Kcal/m^2·day
Children 13–20 years	1500 Kcal/m^2·day	+1500 Kcal/m^2·day
Children <12 years	1800 Kcal/m^2·day	+1300 Kcal/m^2·day
Children <1 year	2100 Kcal/m^2·day	+1000 Kcal/m^2·day

[a] TBSA = Total body surface area
[b] TBSAB = Total body surface area burned

mation reported as a result [35]. Minifee et al. [36] using propranolol on severely burned patients, showed that both peripheral oxygen delivery and cardiac oxygen utilization were unchanged and that mean arterial blood pressure, pressure work index, and rate pressure products were all decreased. It is known that the IV administration of catecholamines as part of a triple hormone simulation test mediates, at least in part, the increased BMR [37]. Wilmore et al. [13] showed a decreased BMR in those treated with α- and β-blockers. In the complete absence of the catecholamine contribution to the stress response, high doses of propranolol have been shown to be fatal in mice and rats [38, 39]. To ensure safety in humans, Honeycutt et al. [40] assessed the ability of burn patients to respond to cold stress appropriately during propranolol blockade. Their results indicated that despite a reduction in heart rate, patients were still able to respond to cold stress. Further, isoproterenol produced an appropriate increase in heart rate in burned patients treated with propranolol (Fig. 4). Waymack [41] suggested that the presence of severe sepsis accounts for the inability to respond to cold stress and is associated with increased mortality. This may occur due to further stimulation of a system that is already functioning maximally [40].

Propranolol reduces heart rate if given in adequate dose. When propranolol was given to burned children every 8 h for 5 days, cardiac work was reduced without influencing oxygen delivery. Metabolic rate, however, was not reduced in this study and protein catabolism increased [42]. The increase in protein mobilization was felt to be secondary to a reduction in adrenergic blockade of lipolysis and the subsequent need for fuel. Adequate nutritional support is required to offset the decreased lipolytic and increased proteolytic effects of propranolol. It has been suggested that the increase in proteolysis

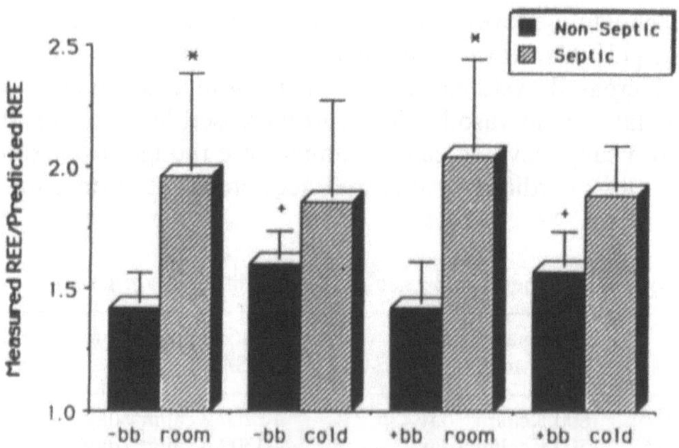

Fig. 4. Measured REE versus predicted REE for nonseptic and septic hypermetabolic patients with (+bb) and without (−bb) β-blockade and before and after cold stress. * = significant difference at $p < 0.05$ for septic patients compared with nonseptic patients. + = significant difference at $p < 0.05$ between nonseptic patients at cold temperature and nonseptic patients at room temperature (mean ± SEM). (From [40] with permission)

with propranolol administration is due to a reduction in the anabolic effects of catecholamines resulting from blockade. Studies of alanine and glutamine metabolism suggest that epinephrine may reduce the liberation of these amino acids from skeletal muscle [43]. Even though catecholamines may have predominantly catabolic effects on fat, they also exert some anabolic effect on protein economy. This finding has been confirmed by recent studies using an IV infusion of propranolol. In two groups, burn patients and volunteers, arteriovenous measurements of limb lactate levels and blood flow characteristics were made. Propranolol was shown to reduce limb lactate levels and peripheral blood flow in both groups. The reduction in blood flow was thought to be due to inhibition of catecholamine-induced vasodilation [44].

The stress response is characterized by the interplay of catabolic and anabolic hormones. At present 4 hormones, GH, insulin, IGF-1 and the catecholamines, are considered to have anabolic functions. The actions of insulin and GH are listed in Fig. 5. The anabolic effects of GH have been known for over 35 years through the work of Liljedahl et al. and Soroff et al. [45–47] who confirmed the nitrogen retaining characteristics of GH in stressed patients. They all recognized the potential usefulness of a naturally occurring anabolic hormone in attenuating the catabolic response [8]. It was not until 1974 when Wilmore et al. [48] studied the anabolic effects of human pituitary GH along with a high caloric intake in thermally injured patients and suggested a therapeutic role for anabolic manipulation. He postulated that "ni-

INSULIN

Actions	Inhibited by	Stimulated by
1. ↑ cellular entry of amino acids, K^+ and glucose in insulin sensitive cells.	α agonists	β agonists
2. ↑ glycogen synthesis	β blockers	glucagon
3. ↓ gluconeogenesis	insulin	ketone bodies
4. ↓ proteolysis; ↑ protein synthesis	K^+ depletion	glucose
5. ↓ lipolysis; low insulin levels favor free fatty acid production & ketone body formation.	lactic acid	amino acids (e.g., leucine)

GROWTH HORMONE

Actions	Inhibited by	Stimulated by
1. contributes to a positive nitrogen balance by increasing P, K & N retention.	Growth hormone	hypoglycemia
2. ↑ blood sugar, ↑ antiinsulin effect & ↓ glucose uptake by some cells	free fatty acids	stress
3. ↑ lipolysis	glucose	exercise
4. ↑ insulin production via hyperglycemia	cortisol	glucagon
5. ↓ proteolysis; ↑ protein synthesis		↑ amino acid levels

Fig. 5. Principle actions and stimulating and inhibiting features of the two major anabolic hormones, insulin and growth hormone

trogen sparing, could be achieved after injury by the administration, or the stimulation, of anabolic hormones to blunt the catabolic response." These findings were later confirmed using GH extracted from human pituitary glands obtained post-mortem [48]. In addition, he found that with GH both insulin and free fatty acids levels were elevated and that insulin resistance increased. It was thus concluded that the administration of GH, along with adequate calorie intake to provide fuel for hypermetabolism, reduced nitrogen loss. The production of recombinant GH through genetic engineering has helped in the investigation of the anabolic effects of this hormone. Further work by Jiang et al. [49], and independently by Ponting et al. [50], confirmed that a positive nitrogen balance could be achieved using recombinant GH. The quantity and duration of administration of central TPN could also be reduced, thereby reducing the risk of complications. Further studies have shown that a positive nitrogen balance can also be achieved using peripheral TPN and GH [51–52].

GH produces hyperglycemia and insulin resistance. Insulin itself is an anabolic hormone and if given in sufficient doses may interact with GH. Gore et al. [53] showed that insulin alone could produce a positive nitrogen balance in stressed patients. Insulin given along with GH was not found to enhance protein kinetics above that observed with GH alone [53]. This is a particularly significant finding since GH treatment exacerbates existing stress-induced hyperglycemia necessitating insulin administration. In contrast, other investigators have found that the combination of insulin and GH produced an effect that was greater than with insulin or GH alone [54]. The use of insulin alone for treating the anabolic effects would not be very practical due to the high dose continuous glucose infusion required to maintain euglycemia. Fleming et al. [55] measured hormone levels in burn patients and showed that exogenously administered rhGH produced elevations in glucagon, catecholamine and free fatty acid levels. Insulin and insulin-like growth factor (IGF-1) were also increased significantly [56]. While the precise role of IGF-1 in the stress response remains to be identified, GH produces a significant increase in IGF-1 production.

Growth Hormone, IGF-1, Wound Healing and the Future

GH has been used to enhance the donor site healing time in burned children after split skin grafting [57]. The effect of rhGH on donor site healing was studied in a double-blind randomized protocol over a 3 year period. Entrance criteria to this study included the following; age between 2–18 years, flame or scald burn greater than 40% TBSA of which 20% had to be third-degree or more, absence of associated head, chest or musculoskeletal trauma, and admission to the unit within 7 days of burn. Children fulfilling the above criteria were given rhGH, Nutropin®, (Genentech, San Francisco, CA), 0.2 mg/kg·day or placebo (0.9% saline) intramuscularly or subcutaneously at approximately the same time each day until donor sites were healed. Nutropin is at present not commercially available.

Children who failed to meet entrance criteria for the double-blind study, was given commercially available Protropin® (Genentech, San Francisco, CA), 0.2 mg/kg·day in an unblinded therapeutic protocol (Table 2). Previous investigations have shown the beneficial effect of rhGH on donor site healing [57]. The purpose of the double-blind study was to confirm the findings of the former investigation and to retrospectively compare Nutropin® to Protropin® in clinical efficacy. Donor site healing was assessed daily by a trained evaluator commencing on the third post-operative day. Using aseptic techniques, the 4 corners of the fine mesh gauze, used for donor site dressing, were gently lifted and minimal tension applied to determine the adherence of the dressing to underlying tissue. The results are presented in Table 3. Initially, there were 45 patients in the double-blind study, 25 placebo and 20 receiving Nutropin. On subsequent analysis, 9 out of 20 required significant insulin (>2 IU insulin per day for >2 weeks), and were excluded so that any

Table 2. Characteristics of patients receiving protropin

Age (yr)	Sex	TBSA % burn	3rd degree % burn	Reason for exclusion from double-blind study
7.1	F	27	26	TBSA burn <40%
0.6	M	46	25	Age <2yr
1.5	F	55	47	Age <2yr
1.3	M	60	60	Age <2yr
1.8	M	62	60	Age <2yr
1.3	F	46	46	Age <2yr
2.0	F	67	67	medico-legal case
4.5	M	56	40	no follow up available
2.0	F	40	35	no follow up available
4.2	F	80	80	no follow up available
12.0	M	40	40	no follow up available
1.2	M	90	90	Age <2yr

Table 3. Patient characteristics, burn size, and length of hospital stay normalized for 3rd degree burn size

	n	Age (yr)	Sex % males	TBSA % burn	3rd degree % burn	LOS (days)	Healing time (days)
Placebo	25	8.4 ± 4.9	72	66 ± 14	55 ± 20	52 ± 27	8.3 ± 2.0
Nutropin@	11	5.4 ± 4.0	73	58 ± 13	49 ± 16	34 ± 11	6.4 ± 1.2[a]
Protropin@	12	3.3 ± 3.2[a]	50	56 ± 17	51 ± 20	41 ± 16	6.0 ± 1.1[a]

LOS: length of stay (mean ± SD). No significant differences could be shown between groups for sex and burn size at $p < 0.05$.

[a] significant difference at $p < 0.05$ compared to placebo.

anabollic influence of insulin would not interfere with the effect of rhGH. No patient in the placebo group required insulin: 13 patients were given Protropin, none of whom needed insulin. The healing time for the initial donor site was significantly less in the Nutropin (6.5 days) compared to placebo group (8.3 days). Similarly, the 2nd donor site healing time was less in the Nutropin group compared to placebo. The Protropin group also showed a reduction in healing time compared to placebo. There was a significant difference between placebo and Protropin groups for age (Table 2).

Both Nutropin and Protropin significantly reduces the healing time of donor sites after split skin grafting. This will benefit the patient by increasing the availability of autograft skin for wound closure. More rapid burn wound closure will not only reduce the susceptibility to wound and systemic sepsis, but may also lead to more rapid rehabilitation and, therefore, a reduction in the length of the hospital stay. Data presented in Table 3 does not show any significant difference between groups for length of stay possibly because it has multiple contributing factors of which donor site healing is only one. An increased availability of autograft skin for wound closure may lead to a reduction in hypermetabolism and therefore aid the healing process in major burns.

Previous studies have shown reductions in whole body and isolated limb protein catabolism with GH administration. Propranolol has been shown to be of value when directed at specific cardiovascular responses, however, its catabolic influences are undesirable. Clenbuterol, a selective β_2 agonist has been shown to reduce the catabolic effects induced by the use of propranolol [58, 59]. Currently, pharmacological modulation with specific β-agonists and specific cardiac β-blockers in addition to rhGH administration may have some benefit in clinical management. IGF-1 and other growth factors could also have value in modulating the stress response.

Conclusion

Advances in fluid resuscitation immediately after burn injury has led to a reduced mortality rate in severely burned children. Over the past 15 years, various pharmacological and hormonal methods have been used to alter the metabolic state following burn. These techniques have helped both in our basic understanding of the stress response and in reducing patient mortality.

References

1. Cuthbertson DP (1979) The metabolic response to injury and its nutritional implications: Retrospective and prospective. JPEN 3:108–130
2. Ganong WF (1991) Review of medical physiology (15th ed), Chapter 13. The autonomic nervous system pp 210–211; Chapter 19: Endocrine functions of the pancreas and the regulation of carbohydrate metabolism pp 312–333, Lange Medical Books, Los Altos, CA

3. Wilmore DW (1986) Chapters 2: Homeostasis: Bodily changes in trauma and surgery; pp 23–37 and Fischer JE Chapter 7: Metabolism in surgical patients: Protein, carbohydrate, and fat utilzation by oral and parenteral routes. pp 116–150. In: Sabiston D (ed) Textbook of surgery; The molecular basis of modern surgical practice, (13th ed) WB Saunders, Philadelphia, PA
4. Dolecek R (1990) The endocrine and metabolic response to burn injuries: Mechanisms and clinical applications. In: Dolecek R, Brizio-Molteni L, Molteni A, Traber D (eds) Endocrinology of thermal injury. Pathophysiologic mechanisms and clinical interpretation. Leo & Febiger, Philadelphia, PA, pp 28–45
5. Arturson MG (1985) The pathophysiology of severe thermal injury. J Burn Care Rehabil 6:129–146
6. Wilmore DW, Aulick LH (1978) Metabolic changes in burned patients. Surg Clinics N Am 58:1173–1187
7. Wilmore DW (1976) Hormonal responses and their effect on metabolism. Surg Clinics N Am 56:999–1018
8. Herndon DN, Curreri PW (1978) Metabolic response to thermal injury and its nutritional support. Cutis 22:501–514
9. Crane CW, Picou D, Smith R, Waterflow JC (1977) Protein turnover in patients before and after elective orthopaedic operations. Br J Surg 64:129–133
10. Herrmann VM, Clarke D, Wilmore DW, Moore FD (1980) Protein metabolism: Effect of disease and altered intake on the stable ^{15}N curve. Surg Forum 31:92–94
11. Birkhahn RH, Long CL, Fitkin D, Jeevanandam M, Blakemore WS (1981) Whole-body protein metabolism due to trauma in man as estimated by L-[^{15}N]-alanine. Am J Physiol 241:E64–E71
12. Aulick H, Wilmore DW (1979) Increased peripheral amino acid release following thermal injury. Surgery 85:560–565
13. Long CL, Spencer JL, Kinney JM, Geiger JW (1971) Carbohydrate metabolism in man: Effect of elective operations and major injury. J Appl Physiol 31:110–116
14. Wolfe RR, Herndon DN, Peters EJ, Jahoor F, Desai MH, Holland OB (1987) Regulation of lipolysis in severely burned children. Ann Surg 206:214–221
15. Wolfe RR, Herndon DN, Jahoor F, Miyoshi H, Wolfe M (1987) Effect of severe burn injury on substrate cycling by glucose and fatty acids. N Engl J Med 317:403–408
16. Newsome TW, Mason AD, Pruitt BA (1973) Weight loss following thermal injury. Ann Surg 178:215–217
17. Gimbel NS, Farris W (1966) Skin grafting. The influence of surface temperature on the epithelization rate of split thickness skin donor sites. Arch Surg 92:554–557
18. Herndon DN, Wilmore DW, Mason AD, Curreri PW (1979) Increased rates of wound healing in burned guinea pigs treated with L-Thyroxine. Surg Forum 30:95–97
19. Zawacki BE, Spitzer KW, Mason AD, Johns LA (1969) Does increased evaporative water loss cause hypermetabolism in burned patients? Ann Surg 171:236–240
20. Neely WA, Petro AG, Holloman GH, Rushton FW, Turner MD, Hardy JD (1973) Researches on the cause of burn hypermetabolism. Ann Surg 179:291–294
21. Wilmore DW, Long JM, Mason AD, Skreen RW, Pruitt BA (1974) Catecholamines: Mediator of the hypermetabolic response to thermal injury. Ann Surg 180:653–669
22. Rutan TC, Herndon DN, Van Osten T, Abston S (1986) Metabolic rate alterations in early excision and grafting versus conservative treatment. J Trauma 26:140–142
23. Wilmore DW, Orcutt TW, Mason AD, Pruitt BA (1975) Alterations in hypothalamic function following thermal injury. J Trauma 15:697–703
24. Falcone PA, Caldwell MD (1990) Wound metabolism. Clinics Plast Surg 17:443–456
25. Kinney JM, Long CL, Gump FE, Duke JH (1968) Tissue composition of weight loss in surgical patients. I. Elective Operations. Ann Surg 168:459–473
26. Curreri PW, Richmond D, Marvin J, Baxter CR (1979) Dietary requirements of patients with major burns. J Am Diet Ass 65:415–417
27. Lowry SF, Brennan MF (1979) Abnormal liver function during parenteral nutrition: Relation to infusion excess. J Surg Res 26:300–307

28. Askanazi J, Rosenbaum SH, Hyman AI, Silverberg PA, Milic-Emili J, Kinney JM (1980) Respiratory changes induced by the large glucose loads of total parenteral nutrition. JAMA 243:1444–1447
29. Hildreth MA, Carvajal HF (1982) Caloric requirements in burned children: A simple formula to estimate daily caloric requirements. J Burn Care Rehabil 3:78–80
30. Hildreth MA, Herndon DN, Parks DH, Desai MH, Rutan T (1987) Evaluation of a caloric requirement formula in burned children treated with early excision. J Trauma 27:188–189
31. Hildreth MA, Herndon DN, Desai MH, Duke MA (1988) Re-assessing caloric requirements in pediatric burn patients. J Burn Care Rehabil 9:616–618
32. Hildreth MA, Herndon DN, Desai MH, Duke MA (1989) Caloric needs of adolescent patients with burns. J Burn Care Rehabil 10:523–526
33. Hildreth MA, Herndon DN, Desai MH, Broemeling LD (1990) Current treatment reduces calories required to maintain weight in pediatric patients with burns. J Burn Care Rehabil 11:405–409
34. Herndon DN, Barrow RE, Rutan TC, Minifee P, Jahoor F, Wolfe RR (1988) Effect of propranolol administration on hemodynamic and metabolic responses of burned pediatric patients. Ann Surg 208:484–492
35. Joshi VV (1970) Effects of burns on the heart. JAMA 211:2130–2134
36. Minifee PK, Barow RE, Abston S, Desai M, Herndon DN (1989) Improved myocardial oxygen utilization following propranolol infusion in adolescents with postburn hypermetabolism. J Paediatric Surg 24:806–811
37. Bessey PQ, Watters JM, Aoki TT, Wilmore DW (1984) Combined hormonal infusion stimulates the metabolic response to injury. Ann Surg 200:264–280
38. Herndon DN, Wilmore DW, Mason AD, Pruitt BA (1977) Humoral mediators of non-temperature dependent hypermetabolism in 50% burned adult rats. Surg Forum 28:37–39
39. Estler CJ, Ammon HPT (1969) The importance of the adrenergic beta-receptors for thermogenesis and survival of acutely cold-exposed mice. Can J Physiol Pharmacol 47:427–433
40. Honeycutt D, Barrow R, Herndon DN (1992) Cold stress response in patients with severe burns after beta-blockade. J Burn Care Rehabil 13:181–186
41. Waymack JP (1989) The effect of ibuprofen on post-burn metabolism and immunologic function. J Surg Res 46:172–176
42. Herndon DN, Barrow RE, Rutan TC, Minifee P, Jahoor F, Wolfe RR (1988) Effect of propranolol administration on hemodynamic and metabolic responses of burned pediatric patients. Ann Surg 208:484–492
43. Garber AJ, Karl IE, Kipnis DM (1976) Alanine and glutamine synthesis and release from skeletal muscle. (IV) Beta-adrenergic inhibition of amino acid release. J Biol Chem 251:851–857
44. Gore DC, Honeycutt D, Jahoor F, Barrow RE, Wolfe RR, Herndon DN (1991) Propranolol diminishes extremity blood flow in burned patients. Ann Surg 213:568–574
45. Liljedahl SO, Gemzell CA, Plantin LO, Birke G (1961) Effect of human growth hormone in patients with severe burns. Acta Chir Scand 122:1–14
46. Soroff HS, Rozin RR, Mooty J, et al (1967) Role of human growth hormone in the response to trauma. I. Metabolic effects following burns. Ann Surg 166:739–752
47. Soroff HS, Pearson E, Green NL, Artz CP (1960) The effect of growth hormone on nitrogen balance at various levels of intake in burned patients. Surg Gynecol Obstet 111:259–273
48. Wilmore DW, Moylan JA, Bristow BF, Mason AD, Pruitt BA (1974) Anabolic effects of human growth hormone and high caloric feeding following thermal injury. Surg Gynecol Obstet 138:875–884
49. Jiang ZM, He GZ, Zhang SY, et al (1989) Low dose growth hormone and hypocaloric nutrition attenuate the protein-catabolic response after major operation. Ann Surg 210:513–525

50. Ponting GA, Halliday D, Teale JD, Sim AJW (1988) Postoperative positive nitrogen balance with intravenous hyponutrition and growth hormone. Lancet 1:438–439
51. McK Manson J, Wilmore DW (1986) Positive nitrogen balance with human growth hormone and hypocaloric intravenous feeding. Surgery 100:188–197
52. Ziegler TR, Young RD, McK Manson J, Wilmore DW (1988) Metabolic effects of recombinant growth hormone in patients receiving parenteral nutrition. Ann Surg 208:6–16
53. Gore DC, Honeycutt D, Jahoor F, Wolfe RR, Herndon DN (1991) Effect of exogenous growth hormone on whole-body and isolated limb protein kinetics in burned patients. Arch Surg 126:38–43
54. Wolfe RF, Pearlstone DB, Newman E, et al (1992) Growth hormone and insulin reverse net whole-body and skeletal muscle protein catabolism in cancer patientes. Ann Surg 216:280–290
55. Fleming RYD, Rutan RL, Jahoor F, Barrow RE, Wolfe RR, Herndon DN (1992) Effect of recombinant human growth hormone on catabolic hormones and free fatty acids following thermal injury. J Trauma 32:698–703
56. Strock LL, Singh H, Abdullah A, Miller JA, Herndon DN (1990) The effect of insulin-like growth factor I on postburn hypermetabolism. Surgery 108:161–164
57. Herndon DN, Barrow RE, Kunkel KR, Broemeling L, Rutan RL (1990) Effects of recombinant human growth hormone on donor site healing in severely burned children. Ann Surg 212:424–431
58. Maclennan PA, Edwards RHT (1989) Effects of clenbuterol and propranolol on muscle mass. J Biochem 264:573–579
59. Carter WJ, Dang ASQ, Faas FH, Lynch ME (1991) Effects of clenbuterol on skeletal mass, body composition, and recovery from surgical stress in senescent rats. Metabolism 40:855–860

Organ Specific Nutrients and Associated Therapy: Growth Factors – Growth Hormone

L. S. Young, T. A. Byrne, and D. W. Wilmore

Introduction

Alterations in body composition commonly occur following critical illness and these changes are associated with expansion of the extracellular fluid compartment, reduction of body adipose tissue and a loss of lean body mass. Fat stores are present to be used as an available energy source and hence fat is mobilized and oxidized during life threatening illness to facilitate homeostasis and tissue repair. Lean tissue is composed of hydrated protein, and this represents the structural and functional components of the body. Protein breakdown is accelerated during critical illness and this response is characterized by the increased ureagenesis and renal excretion of this and other end-products of nitrogen (N) metabolism. This accelerated loss of N contributes to the negative N balance associated with acute illness, and if this net loss of nitrogen from the body persists over an extended period of time, decreased strength and activity occur and prolonged convalescence results.

It has been thought that providing nutritional support, either by the enteral or parenteral route, would greatly reduce or reverse the protein catabolic state. However, serial determinations of body composition coupled with measurements of substrate flux have emphasized how difficult it is to maintain or replete body protein during acute illness. Street et al. [1], for example, vigorously fed 8 septic ICU patients. On average, the subjects received 2716 kcal/day and 22.6 g nitrogen/day. Despite this vigorous support, the patients actually lost 6.2 kg body weight over 10 days: most of this was water, but the subjects also lost 1.5 kg of body protein. In contrast, they gained 2.2 kg of body fat. These findings are not dissimilar to studies in patients with gastrointestinal disease who require vigorous IV nutrition: most of the weight gain was attributable to gain in fat and water, not protein [2].

Why should these critically ill fed patients experience this altered response to nutritional support? Clearly, the hormonal environment plays a role, and this response, coupled with elaboration of cytokine and lipid mediators, favors net protein degradation. However, other factors contribute to this catabolic state. Fever, bed rest, ventilatory support and paralysis, use of drugs which exert catabolic responses (dopamine and glucocorticoids), repeated operation or other invasive procedures and failure to use the GI tract, are all additive factors which promote and support the protein catabolic state.

Clearly, two therapeutic strategies can be adopted: first, the catabolic stimuli can be attenuated, or the anabolic environment can be enhanced.

While this chapter focuses on anabolic support, it should be noted that this approach is most effective only when coupled with a decrease in catabolic stimuli to counteract the catabolic state. We will focus in large part on the work from this laboratory and others using human growth hormone (GH) to enhance the environment. The potential for the use of other growth factors in the catabolic state will also be discussed.

Anabolic Effects of Growth Hormone: Studies in Stable Patients

It has long been known that administration of GH to humans was associated with anabolic effects. Henneman et al. [3, 4] administered pituitary-derived GH to non-deficient adult subjects and children with presumed hypopituitarism. Nitrogen and mineral retention was documented and the proportions of the retained elements were characteristic of lean tissue and bone. Fat mobilization and utilization were observed and glucose intolerance was also noted. Linear growth characteristics occurred in the children.

In the mid-1980's, we examined the relationship between administration of exogenous GH and caloric intake [5]. Normal adults were studied on two occasions while they received a fixed protein, vitamin and mineral infusion. The caloric intake was varied over the course of the study but ranged from 30% of energy requirement to 100% of needs. On one occasion the subjects received daily placebo infusions, and on the other occasion they received GH 10 mg/day. The study periods were separated by two weeks and during the two study periods, each subject received isocaloric and isonitrogenous feedings. During the hypocaloric feedings, the subjects receiving placebo injections were in negative N balance, but maintained N equilibrium when 100% of the energy was provided. However, during the period of GH administration, the subjects were in positive N balance, regardless of the level of energy provided (Table 1). The retention of N, potassium and phosphorus occurred in a ratio similar to that found in skeletal muscle. Stimulation of

Table 1. The effects of varying intravenous calorie intake and GH on nitrogen balance

Intake		Nitrogen balance	
Total calories[a] (kcal/day)	Nitrogen (g/day)	Placebo (g/day)	GH (g/day)
753 (30)	11.3	−3.6	+1.1
1071 (50)	11.3	−2.6	+1.7
2281 (100)	11.3	−0.4	+3.4

[a] Numbers in parentheses represent the percentage of daily energy requirements

protein synthesis and fat oxidation occurred in the presence of increased levels of GH, insulin-like growth factor-1 (IGF-1) and insulin.

Similar studies have been performed in patients with GI fistula [6] and in obese individuals [7]: the lean body mass was protected and in some cases repleted during GH administration, even in the face of hypocaloric feedings.

Two randomized trials have been performed to confirm these and other anabolic effects of GH in well characterized stable patients. In the first group, patients with benign intestinal or pancreatic disease requiring at least

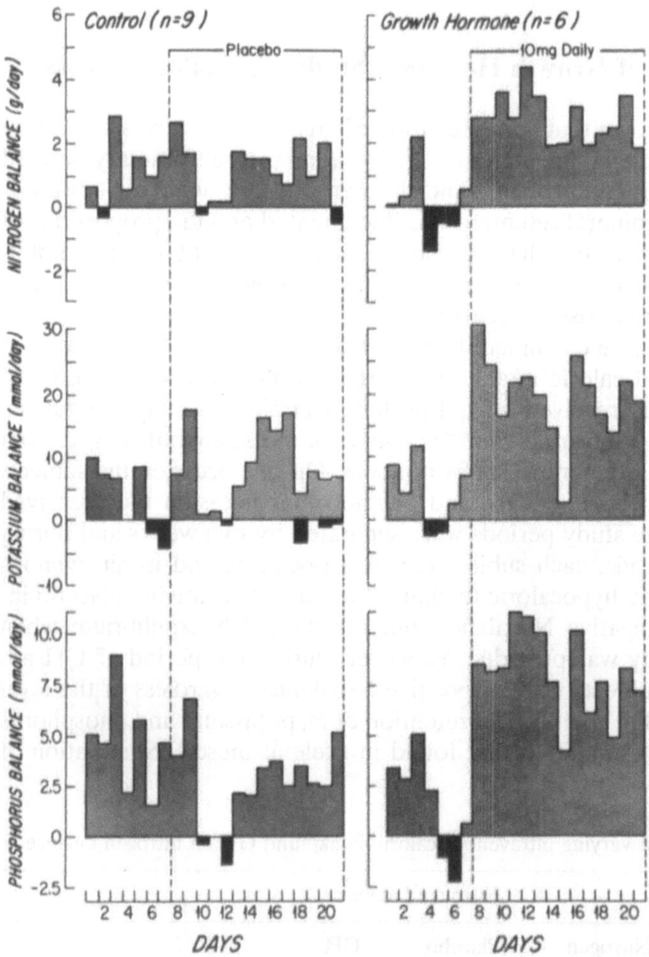

Fig. 1. The effects of placebo or GH on balance of nitrogen, potasium and phosphorus. Intake is comparable throughout the study and positive balance is plotted upward (stipped bars) and negative balance is shown (black bars). During the initial control week, both groups were in nutrient equilibrium. With treatment, the control group remained in equilibrium while the GH group showed a significant increase in net positive balance ($p<0.05$). (From [8] with permission)

3 weeks of TPN were randomized after the first week of a standard feeding to receive either GH or placebo [8]. The subjects received about 30 kcal/kg·day and 1.5 g protein/kg·day through the study. The subjects who received placebo plus IV nutrition maintained relatively stable balance of N, potassium and phosphorus over the 3 week period; improvement over time was not observed and in general the subjects were in neutral (0) balance. In contrast, the group treated with GH increased balance of N by 2.4–2.8 g. The cumulative gain in N was also significantly greater in the GH-treated patients over the last two treatment weeks (Fig. 1); cumulative N balance was 2 ± 7 g in controls vs 36 ± 6 g with GH, $p < 0.005$. As with other studies, plasma levels of IGF-1 rose fivefold.

In a second randomized, blinded trial, Jiang et al. [9] treated a group of patients immediately following GI surgery with hypocaloric (20 kcal/kg·day) isonitrogenous feedings containing adequate protein (1 g/kg·day), vitamins and minerals. The subjects were randomized to receive placebo or GH (0.06 mg/kg·day) for 14 days following operation. Nitrogen and mineral balance was enhanced with GH. Forearm flux of amino acids was positive compared to the negative forearm balance of amino acid N observed in the control group. At the end of 14 days, the controls lost fat and lean tissue (approximately 3.5 kg) while the GH-treated individuals lost only adipose tissue (<1 kg). Finally, muscle strength fell 10% in the control group, but was maintained in the GH-treated subjects (Fig. 2).

Other studies of compositional changes have been performed in a group of patients undergoing nutritional rehabilitation and receiving hypercaloric

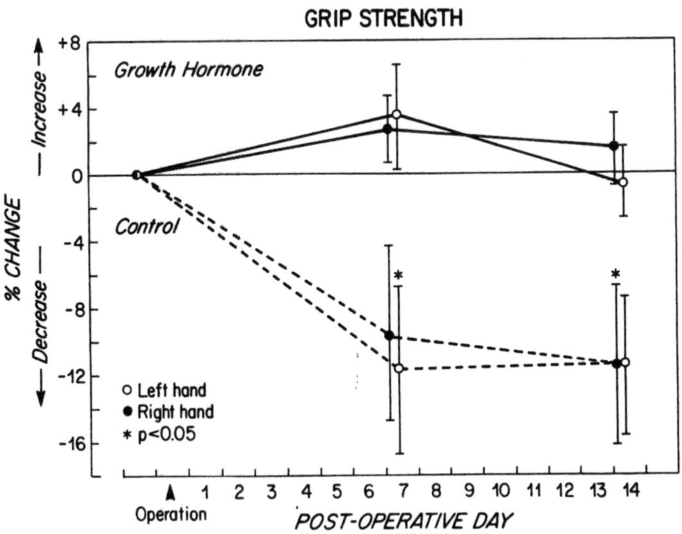

Fig. 2. Changes that occurred in grip strength following operation. The control group decreased grip strength by approximately 10–12% while the GH-treated subjects maintained grip strength. (From [9] with permission)

feedings [10]. All subjects were studied for at least 28 days. Following a one-week equilibration period, the usual parenteral and enteral feedings were adjusted to provide 50 kcal/kg·day and 2 g protein/kg·day. The 14 patients studied were then randomized to continue standard therapy or to receive GH (0.14 mg/kg·day). Lean body mass was assessed by serial dual energy X-ray absorptiometry (DEXA). Body water was determined using dilutional techniques and uptake of minerals, and N was assessed by balance techniques. After 3 weeks of therapy, both groups gained weight (3.9 for standard vs 4.6 kg for GH, NS). However, body compositional studies revealed that a significantly greater percent of the tissue gain in the GH-treated patients was lean when compared to controls (96.8 vs 62.5%). Conversely, there was greater fat gain in the controls than in the GH group (33 vs 1%). Calculation of cumulative N balance confirmed the efficacy of this anabolic therapy when compared with standard. Balance techniques showed that there was a 20.3 g protein gain/kg lean body mass in the GH group when compared to 9.5 g/kg lean body mass in controls (Table 2) ($p<0.04$). Thus, GH therapy may be an effective means to shorter convalescence and accelerate rehabilitation of patients recovering from major illnesses.

Because a major proportion of lean body mass is skeletal muscle, it would seem possible to determine gain in both skeletal muscle structure and function associated with GH therapy. Such has been the case. As previously noted, GH administration was associated with forearm amino acid uptake and maintenance of muscle strength in the postoperative period. In chronic stable patients, arm and leg circumferences have increased with time and this is not accompanied by increased skinfold thickness [10]. Leg resistance, measured by bioelectrical impedance, fell with time. This decrease in resistance indicates an increase in leg water which could be associated with the accretion of lean tissue. Finally, actual leg lean tissue mass, as determined by DEXA, increased while fat mass remains relatively unchanged (Table 3). These changes all indicate an overall gain has occurred in leg skeletal muscle.

Table 2. The effect of hypercaloric feedings and GH on changes in body composition. (Mean ± SEM)

N	Standard therapy 4	GH 10
Weight gain (kg)	2.9 ± 0.1	4.6 ± 0.8
Lean body mass gain (kg)	1.82 ± 0.52	4.13 ± 0.57[a]
% of total gain as lean (%)	62.5 ± 18.5	96.8 ± 5.9[a]
% of total gain as fat (%)	32.9 ± 16.5	1.0 ± 5.5[a]
% lean as water		
before	0.75 ± 0.01	0.77 ± 0.02
after	0.76 ± 0.01	0.76 ± 0.02

[a] $p<0.05$ *vs* standard

Table 3. Leg measurement before and after GH therapy

	Before	After
Leg weight (kg)	8.35	9.26
Thigh circumference (cm)	41.1	45.5
Calf circumference (cm)	24.2	26.5
Electronic resistance (Ω)	229	221
Lean tissue (kg)	6.5	7.2
Fat tissue (kg)	1.5	1.7
Bone (kg)	0.35	0.36

GH Use in Critically Ill Patients

Most of the available data previously discussed are studies performed in relatively stable adults with finite disease processes studied over moderately long periods of time. GH effects were then compared with results obtained from subjects receiving placebo injection. This approach is more difficult when studying ICU patients, and hence fewer investigations are available to assess GH effects in more severely ill catabolic patients. However, it is worthwhile to review the information that is available in order to plan future studies.

Effects of GH on Nitrogen and Mineral Balance

Studies performed between the late 1950's and the 1970's demonstrated the anabolic effects of a short (often one week) course of pituitary-derived GH in adult burn patients. Doses of crude preparations were given daily (range 10–20 mg/day) and improved N balance was observed [11]. These effects were primarily related to the increase in food intake which occurred in association with the therapy. Soroff and associates [12] performed a series of elegant studies in burn patients, performing N and mineral balance studies in both the early and late convalescence periods of injury. The retention of N and other intracellular minerals was much more apparent when GH was given during the convalescent stage of recovery rather than shortly after the injury.

When nutrient therapy was fixed or clamped at hypercaloric levels, GH reduced the high rates of N loss observed in burn patients [13]. Both N and potassium were retained in a ratio similar to that found in skeletal muscle, and hyperinsulinemia was also observed.

More recently, Ziegler et al. [14] administered 10 mg GH daily for up to 6 weeks to patients with severe burn injury. GH was well tolerated by these ICU patients, and minor fluid retention and hyperglycemia was observed. Nitrogen excretion fell by $\approx 30\%$ (Table 4) and IGF-1 levels rose approxi-

Table 4. Nutrient intake and excretion: long-term GH adaptation

Study week	(kcal/day)	Nitrogen (g/day)		Urea (g/day)
	In	In	Exc	Exc
Control	2660±356	16.3±3.1	16.4±2.8	13.4±2.6
GH wk 1	2536±341	15.4±2.4	11.8±1.9[a]	9.1±1.6[a]
GH wk 2	2291±278	14.2±2.5	10.0±1.8[a]	7.6±1.4[a]
GH wk 3	2578±195	16.9±2.2	8.9±1.7[a]	7.1±1.5[a]

[a] $p<0.01$ *vs* control by ANOVA (Scheffe *F*-test); $n=7$, mean±SEM

mately fivefold. It was thought by the physicians and nursing staff that accelerated wound healing occurred along with enhanced physical performance and improved self care.

GH and Wound Healing

Other investigators have commented on the effect GH has on improving wound healing, and we also observed early wound closure in non-randomized trials. These observations were confirmed in a prospective, randomized trial in adults requiring skin grafts [15]. The donor skin was obtained from the anterior thigh of each patient by the same physician using the same dermatome set at the same thickness, and the donor sites were observed daily and assessed to determine rate of epithelization and time of final wound closure. Half the patient group received daily placebo injections and the other half received GH. The patients receiving GH demonstrated a reduction in donor site healing time of 2–4 days when compared to placebo-treated controls. These results are similar to the findings reported by Herndon et al. [16] who gave GH 0.2 mg/kg·day or placebo to burned children (average burn size ≈60% total body surface). In this study, there was a significant increase in healing time which resulted in a net reduction in hospitalization of 14 days.

Effects of GH on Body Fluid Distribution

Retention of sodium and water commonly occurs following critical illness. GH administration also results in mild fluid retention, which is usually observed for only the initial 3–5 days after the initiation of administration. To determine the effect of GH on fluid distribution in critically ill intensive care patients, individuals were selected, matched and studied over a two-week period, during which they continued to receive standard ICU support with or without GH [17]. Body water compartments were measured using traditional dilution methodology: total body water (TBW) was determined by the dilution of heavy water (D_2O) and extracellular fluid was measured by measuring the dilution of sodium bromide.

Nineteen subjects were studied; the two groups were well balanced as to their age, extent of illness, nutritional support and organ system failure. Neither group lost significant amounts of weight or body water over the two-week study period. However, a marked expansion of the extracellular fluid compartment occurred in the control group, and this caused an abnormal ratio of ECF/TBW and a reduction of intracellular fluid, consistent with tissue breakdown and loss of intracellular constituents (Fig. 3). In contrast, the GH-treated patients maintained ECW and ICW, indicating preservation of body cell mass and normalization of the ratio of ECW/TBW. This data is consistent with the known anabolic effects of GH and demonstrates that the GH anabolic effects can be observed in ICU patients with complex disease processes.

GH and the Treatment of Organ Failure

Organ failure, whether single or multiple (MOF), is associated with a series of complex alterations which occur in the patient's normal metabolism. Because of the heterogeneity of the patients that exhibit MOF, little clear-cut data has emerged to demonstrate the efficacy of anabolic factors in this situation. There is, however, some data which may be useful in considering treatment with GH in the patient with single or multiorgan failure. In this section, we will discuss the role of GH in renal, pulmonary and intestinal failure. Finally, we will review the results of a trial which evaluated GH in MOF patients.

Renal failure. There are many reasons why GH should intuitively be beneficial to patients with renal failure. GH decreases ureagenesis, stimulates protein synthesis and maintains the intracellular concentrations of potassium and phosphate. Thus, subjects with normal renal function have lower plasma levels of blood urea N, potassium and phosphate, and their renal excretory

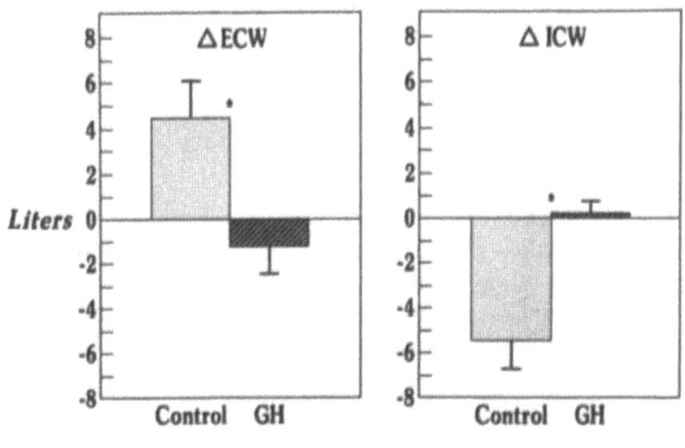

Fig. 3. The change which occurred in critically ill patients over 2 weeks of standard nutritional support, with or without GH. All subjects monitored their weight and TBW throughout the study period. The control subjects gained ECW and lost ICW, while both were stabilized in the GH group. *$p < 0.01$ between groups. (From [17] with permission)

requirements for N and minerals are reduced [6]. In catabolic patients with acute renal failure, the urea N and potassium levels can be controlled, the patient can be more vigorously fed, and the requirement for dialysis or hemofiltration lessened.

These effects were clearly demonstrated in a group of 5 clinically stable adult patients requiring maintenance hemodialysis for end-stage renal failure [18]. The dialysis prescription, pharmacologic therapy and nutrition were kept constant over the three-week period of study. The subjects were followed for an initial control week and then were treated with GH (5 or 10 mg every other day) after each dialysis session. All clinical signs remained stable throughout the two weeks of treatment. The blood urea N fell 20–25%, and urea kinetic modeling demonstrated a significant reduction in urea generation and protein catabolic rate (Table 5). These studies demonstrate that GH may promote the protein synthetic efficiency of dietary protein, while lessening the need for chronic dialysis. Similar effects of GH appear to occur in critically ill patients with acute renal failure.

GH and pulmonary dysfunction. GH has many desirable pharmacologic characteristics which may serve to optimize respiratory function. First, GH shifts oxidative metabolism from carbohydrate to fat utilization; this effect even occurs in the fed state [19]. This, in general, is characterized by a reduced RQ and a diminished rate of carbon dioxide production. This metabolic effect should reduce the respiratory work required to excrete carbon dioxide from the body.

The second beneficial characteristic is the enhancement of protein synthesis and muscle strength which occurs with GH administration. As previously mentioned, these effects have been demonstrated for forearm and leg skeletal muscle. We have studied 4 patients following acute spinal cord injury who have required prolonged ventilatory support. With the administration of GH, tidal volume, vital capacity and inspiratory pressure have all gradually improved over a period of weeks [14]. The patients could gradually be

Table 5. The effect of GH on food intake and urea kinetics in subjects on chronic hemodialysis. (Mean ± SEM)

	Control	GH	
		Week 1	Week 2
Calorie intake (kcal/kg/day)	25±2	24±2	23±2
Protein intake (g/kg/day)	0.92±0.03	0.89±0.04	0.90±0.05
Predialysis blood urea nitrogen (mmol/L)	23±3	19±1 [a]	18±2 [a]
Urea generation (g/day)	6.8±1.0	4.8±0.6 [a]	4.5±0.7 [a]
Protein catabolic rate (g/kg/day)	1.1±0.1	0.9±0.1 [a]	0.8±0.1 [a]

[a] $p<0.01$ *vs* control week

weaned from the ventilator and all were subsequently transferred to a spinal cord rehabilatory unit.

These findings are similar to those studies by Clements and associates in patients with chronic obstructive lung disease [20]. With GH treatment, tidal volume, inspiratory and expiratory pressure increased, and oxygenation improved. Unfortunately, with withdrawal of the drug, pulmonary function gradually returned to baseline.

It is not known if differences in time to wean individuals from a ventilator could be detected in ICU patients treated in a randomized study. The major obstacle to such a study is the heterogeneity of the population and the complications associated with the primary illness.

GH in multiorgan failure (MOF). Several years ago, a multicenter trial was organized as a pilot study to evaluate the effect of GH in ICU patients with 2 or more failed organs [21]. In this blinded study, GH was administered at doses of 0.0–0.3 mg/kg·day to 26 patients; a variety of clinical criteria and IGF-1 responses were assessed at baseline and at weekly intervals thereafter. Thirteen patients died (50% mortality) and the administration of GH did not affect outcome. However, a rise in IGF-1 (2 standard deviations above pretreatment baseline) was associated with survival ($p = 0.04$, Fisher's exact test, one-sided). The IGF-1 response could be predicted by the pretreatment transferrin, alkaline phosphatase and total bilirubin concentrations (Table 6). Age, serum creatinine, prealbumin, enzymes reflecting liver function or serum T_4 concentration were not predictive of a response. Since tests of hepatic function were associated with prediction of an IGF-1 response, it appears that the synthetic capacity of the liver may be the limiting organ to allow an appropriate response when GH is administered to a patient with MOF. This is because the capacity of the liver to synthesize IGF-1 is necessary for GH to manifest its anabolic capacity. This is consistent with data obtained from other critically ill patients which demonstrate that the IGF-1 response following GH administration may be inversely related to the severity of the illness [22]. Administration of IGF-1 may be necessary to mediate an anabolic effect in these and other similar patients.

Table 6. The effect of elevation in IGF-1 following GH administration to patients with MOF (Mean ± SEM)

N	IGF-1 Response 13	No IGF-1 Response 9	p-value
Age (yrs)	45 ± 6	66 ± 5	0.016
Transferrin (mg/dl)	143 ± 14	111 ± 8	0.055
Bilirubin, total (mg/100 ml)	2.62 ± 1.45	4.73 ± 1.00	0.289
Survival (%, survivors/total)	69 (9/13)	22 (2/9)	0.04

Use of Other Growth Factors in Critically Ill Patients

This discussion has primarily focused on the use and potential benefits of GH in critically ill catabolic patients. It has already been noted that many of the anabolic effects of GH are thought to be mediated through the generation of IGF-1. Patients with severe hepatic dysfunction associated with MOF [21] or other critical illness [22] may be unable to synthesize adequate quantities of IGF-1 (primarily in the liver), and current teaching would suggest that GH would be ineffective in these individuals. IGF-1 infusions may be indicated, but reasonably large doses of this factor may be necessary to induce a protein anabolic effect in catabolic humans [23, 24]. IGF-1 may be useful in catabolic patients with elevated blood glucose levels such as those with diabetes mellitus or individuals receiving large doses of glucocorticoids. Particular benefit might be derived in the wound healing effects of this growth factor [25].

Other factors will undoubtedly play a role in the future care of the critically ill. Hematopoietic and leukocyte growth factors are already used extensively in patients undergoing extensive chemotherapy. Likewise, factors which stimulate changes in specific cell populations to enhance immunity (the interleukins and γ-interferon) have also been used in patients with cancer and in immunosuppressed surgical patients. Finally, specific factors may be given to cause growth of specific tissues. Epidermal growth factor may facilitate epithelial coverage of large wounds and also stimulate growth of enterocytes. A variety of factors have been described to stimulate hepatic growth, which may be useful to stimulate rapid growth following segmental transplantation. The administration of specific growth factors to stimulate growth in nerves, bone and other tissue may also be used in the future.

Route of factor administration may be important and topical application, local injection and regional infusion may all be more effective and cost efficient than systemic administration.

Because these factors deal with specific organ growth, the suitable mix of nutrients should be provided to allow optimal expression of the growth factor effects. To date, little is known about nutrient-growth factor interaction.

Finally, a combination of factors may be the most effective method of treatment. For example, GH could be administered to a patient with an extensive burn injury, the resulting hyperglycemia would be treated by an infusion of IGF-1. Simultaneously, epidermal growth factor, which was incorporated in dressings applied to the burns, would be delivered topically to enhance epithelialization. By giving lower doses of substances which augment each other, significant side effects can be diminished. The reduced cost of hospitalization and the enhanced recuperative time would provide more than enough of a cost savings to justify the agents used.

Conclusion

Growth factors have been provided through bioengineering techniques and are now being used in the care of critically ill patients. Growth hormone may serve as the model to stimulate anabolism in the catabolic setting. Other factors may be forthcoming and, when used for specific indications, may greatly enhance recovery and shorten hospitalization.

References

1. Streat SJ, Beddoe AG, Hill GL (1987) Aggressive nutritional support does not prevent protein loss despite fat gain in septic intensive care patients. J Trauma 27:262–266
2. Smith RC, Burkinshaw L, Hill GL (1982) Optimal energy and nitrogen intake for gastroenterological patients requiring intravenous nutrition. Gastroenterology 82:445–452
3. Henneman DH, Henneman PH (1960) Effects of human growth hormone on levels of blood and urinary carbohydrate and fat metabolites in man. J Clin Invest 39:1239–1245
4. Henneman PH, Forbes AP, Moldawer M, Dempsey EF, Carrol EL (1960) Effects of human growth hormone in man. J Clin Invest 39:1223–1238
5. Manson J McK, Wilmore DW (1986) Positive nitrogen balance with human growth hormone and hypocaloric intravenous feeding. Surgery 100:188–197
6. Ziegler TR, Young LS, Manson J McK, Wilmore DW (1988) Metabolic effects of recombinant human growth hormone in patients receiving parenteral nutrition. Ann Surg 208:6–16
7. Clemmons DR, Snyder DK, Williams R, Underwood LE (1987) Growth hormone conserves lean body mass during dietary restriction in obese subjects. J Clin Endocrinol Metab 64:878–883
8. Ziegler TR, Rombeau J, Young LS, et al (1992) Recombinant human growth hormone enhances the metabolic efficacy of parenteral nutrition: A double-blind, randomized, controlled study. J Clin Endocrinol Metab 74:865–873
9. Jiang ZM, He GZ, Zhang SY, et al (1989) Low-dose growth hormone and hypocaloric nutrition attenuate the protein-catabolic response after major operation. Ann Surg 210:513–524
10. Byrne TA, Morrissey TB, Gatzen C, et al (1993) Anabolic therapy with growth hormone accelerates gain in lean tissue in surgical patients requiring nutritional rehabilitation. Ann. Surgery (in press.)
11. Liljedahl S, Gemzell C, Plantin L, Birkin G (1961) Effect of human growth hormone in patients with severe burns. Acta Chir Scand 122:1–14
12. Soroff HS, Rozin RR, Mooty J, Lister J, Raben MS (1967) Role of human growth hormone in the response to trauma. I. Metabolic effects following burns. Ann Surg 166:739–752
13. Wilmore DW, Moylan JA, Bristow BF, Mason AD, Pruitt BA (1974) Anabolic effects of human growth hormone and high caloric feedings following thermal injury. Surg Gynecol Obstet 138:875–884
14. Ziegler TR, Young LS, Ferrari-Baliviera E, Demling RH, Wilmore DW (1990) Use of human growth hormone combined with nutritional support in a critical care unit. JPEN 14:574–581
15. Shernan SK, Demling RH, LaLonde C, Lowe D, Eriksson E, Wilmore DW (1989) Growth hormone enhances re-epithelialization of human split-thickness skin graft donor sites. Surg Forum 40:37–39

16. Herndon DN, Barrow RE, Kunkel KR, Broemeling L, Rutan RL (1990) Effects of recombinant human growth hormone on donor-site healing in severely burned children. Ann Surg 212:424–429
17. Gatzen C, Scheltinga MR, Kimbrough TD, Jacobs DO, Wilmore DW (1992) Growth hormone attenuates the abnormal distribution of body water in critically ill surgical patients. Surgery 112:181–187
18. Ziegler TR, Lazarus JM, Young LS, Hakim R, Wilmore DW (1991) Effects of recombinant human growth hormone in adults receiving maintenance hemodialysis. J Am Soc Nephrol 2:1130–1135
19. Manson J McK, Smith RJ, Wilmore DW (1988) Growth hormone stimulates protein synthesis during hypocaloric parenteral nutrition: Role of hormonal-substrate environment. Ann Surg 208:136–142
20. Pape GS, Friedman M, Underwood LE, Clemmons DR (1991) The effect of growth hormone on weight gain and pulmonary function in patients with chronic obstructive lung disease. Chest 99:1495–1500
21. Lowe D, Cerra F, Shernan S, Lowry S, Wilmore DW (1991) Hepatic synthesis of IGF-1 following growth hormone administration predicts survival following multiorgan failure. Presented at a Conference of Infection/Inflammation Mechanisms and Therapeutic Approaches. March 6–9, Munich, Germany
22. Kimbrough TD, Shernan S, Ziegler TR, Scheltinga M, Wilmore DW (1991) Insulin-like growth factor I (IGF-1) response is comparable following intravenous and subcutaneous administration of growth hormone. J Surg Res 51:472–476
23. Mauras N, Horber FF, Haymond MW (1992) Low dose recombinant human insulin-like growth factor-1 fails to affect protein anabolism but inhibits islet cell secretion in humans. J Clin Endocrinol Metab 75:1192–1197
24. Clemmons DR (1992) Role of insulin-like growth factor-1 in reversing catabolism. J Clin Endocrinol Metab (Editorial) 75:1183–1185
25. Suh DY, Hunt TK, Spencer EM (1992) Insulin-like growth factor-1 reverses the impairment of wound healing induced by corticosteroids in rats. Endocrinology 131:2399–2403

Preventing Complications

Parenteral versus Enteral Nutrition

G. P. Zaloga

Introduction

The supply of adequate cellular nutrients is important for optimal recovery from illness. Nutrients may be supplied via the parenteral or enteral routes. Although techniques are available for delivery of both enteral and parenteral nutrients, the composition and types of nutrients which can be delivered via each route are different. Accumulating data also indicates that nutrients have different physiologic actions when delivered via different routes. In this chapter, we review and summarize studies comparing both the physiologic actions and clinical effects of parenteral and enteral nutrition.

Nutrient Availability

The major classes of nutrients include proteins, carbohydrates, lipids, nucleic acids, minerals, vitamins, and trace elements (Table 1). Parenteral (TPN)

Table 1. Nutrients found in enteral and parenteral formulae

	Parenteral	Enteral nutrition
Protein		
Intact	No	Yes
Peptides	No	Yes
Amino acids	Yes	Yes
Glutamine	No	Yes
Arginine	Yes	Yes
Cysteine	No	Yes
Carbohydrate		
Simple	Yes	Yes
Complex (i.e. fiber)	No	Yes
Lipids		
Long chain omega-6	Yes	Yes
Long chain omega-3	No	Yes
Medium chain	No	Yes
Nucleotides	No	Yes

and enteral nutrition (EN) deliver minerals, vitamins, and trace elements in similar amounts. However, they differ considerably in their ability to deliver proteins, carbohydrates, lipids, and nucleic acids.

Protein is available as intact protein, hydrolyzed protein (i.e. peptides), and amino acids [1]. TPN uses only amino acids as its nitrogen (N) source. Glutamate and aspartate are not administered intravenously (in most formulae) because these "excitatory" amino acids have a variety of toxic effects upon cells (especially the central nervous system) [2, 3]. Glutamine and asparagine are not delivered in TPN because these amino acids break down in solution, liberating ammonia and "excitatory" amino acids. However, recent evidence indicates that glutamine is a major fuel for the GI tract and plays a major role in the maintenance of the immune system [4–6]. Body demands for this amino acid exceed endogenous supply during stress and critical illness. Thus, glutamine is now considered to be "semi-essential". Arginine is present in low concentrations in TPN formulae. Arginine is important for wound healing, N balance, and immune function [7–9]. Similar to glutamine, arginine demands exceed endogenous supply during severe illness and stress. TPN formulae also lack cysteine, an important amino acid in the synthesis of glutathione (γ-glutamylcysteinylglycine).

Recent results suggest that intact protein and peptides are better N sources for the body than are amino acids [1]. Peptides possess biologic activities which are important for normal physiologic activity. Studies have demonstrated a role for peptides in maintenance of the GI tract, support of liver function, stimulation of hormonal responses, N utilization, growth, and wound repair [1]. Intact protein (which is digested to peptides) and peptides are only available for use in EN support.

Complex carbohydrate, in the form of fiber, produces unique effects upon GI tract structure and function [10–12]. Certain fibers are metabolized to short-chain fatty acids, which are preferencial fuels for the colon [11, 12]. In addition, bulk fiber is important for stimulating gut motility (assuring distal nutrient flow) and maintenance. Complex carbohydrate is only available with EN.

Long-chain Ω-6 polyunsaturated fatty acids (i.e. linoleic acid) are precursors to arachidonic acid, which upon subsequent metabolism produce prostaglandins and leukotrienes (of the 2 series). These lipids have profound affects upon cardiovascular and immune function [13, 14]. Reducing the quantity of Ω-6 long-chain fatty acids in the diet may be associated with improved immune function and reduced infections [13–16]. Lipids used during TPN support are high in linoleic acid (50–66%). On the other hand, lipid formulations used for EN are lower in linoleic acid content. Improved immune function and reduced infection rates during EN may partially relate to lipid content.

Nucleotides may play a beneficial role in stimulation of the immune system [17]. Nucleotides are absent from TPN formulae. Although absent from most enteral formulae, nucleotides are present in some enteral diets

In summary, TPN formulae lack many important nutrients. EN provides many of these nutrients.

Studies of Enteral versus Parenteral Nutrition

Animal Studies (Table 2)

Kudsk et al. (18, 19] randomized rats to receive dextrose-amino acid solutions via the parenteral or enteral route. Following 12–14 days of feeding, animals were subjected to *Escherichia coli*-hemoglobin peritonitis. Survival was significantly higher in enterally fed malnourished [18] and well nourished [19] rats. Mortality (2 day) in malnourished animals was 60% for IV feeding and 40% for enteral feeding [18]. Similarly, mortality (2 day) in well nourished animals was 80% with IV nutrition and 40% with enteral feeding [19]. Petersen and coworkers [20] studied normal and protein depleted rats. Survival following *E. coli* hemoglobin peritonitis was 66% in normal animals as opposed to 15% in protein depleted rats. Protein depleted rats refed with regular diets had a 53% survival while rats repleted with IV hyperalimentation had a survival of 0–5%.

Kudsk et al. [21] studied the effect of enteral and parenteral feeding on body composition in malnourished rats. Following protein depletion, animals were fed dextrose-amino acid solutions for 14 days via the enteral or parenteral routes. Parenterally fed animals gained more weight with greater fat formation than the enteral group but had lower intestinal mass and nitrogen.

Zaloga et al. [22] evaluated survival in rats following hemorrhagic hypotension fed via the parenteral and enteral routes. Mortality (24 h) was significantly increased in animals receiving TPN (63%) compared to peptide-based enteral diets (0%). Interestingly, mortality was 0% in animals receiving enteral and IV saline.

Zaloga and coworkers [23] administered high dose methotrexate to rats receiving parenteral and enteral nutrition. Mortality was 100% in parenterally fed animals compared to 50% in animals fed a defined formula enteral diet and 25% in animals receiving chow. All tissues (i.e. mesenteric lymph

Table 2. Animal studies comparing enteral and parenteral nutrition

Ref	Animal	Model	Mortality
[18]	Rat	*E. coli* peritonitis	60% TPN; 40% EN
[19]	Rat	*E. coli* peritonitis	80% TPN; 40% EN
[20]	Rat	*E. coli* peritonitis	95–100% TPN; 47% EN
[22]	Rat	Hemorrhagic shock	63% TPN; 0% EN
[23]	Rat	Methotrexate	100% TPN; 25–50% EN

nodes, liver, spleen, lung) in the parenterally fed animals contained large quantities of bacteria while most tissues in chow animals were free of bacteria. Tissue bacterial counts were intermediate in animals fed the defined formula diet.

These data indicate that IV feeding is associated with higher mortalities in animals following peritonitis, hemorrhage, and high dose methotrexate. TPN is associated with increased bacterial translocation and tissue dissemination following methotrexate. In addition, IV feeding does not improve survival in protein depleted animals with peritonitis. On the other hand, enteral feeding does improve outcome following peritonitis in protein depleted animals.

Human Studies (Table 3)

Trauma. Adams and co-workers [24] compared the efficacy of enteral and parenteral nutrition in 46 trauma patients. Patients were randomized during admission laparotomy to central venous TPN (n=23) or EN via jejunostomy (n=23; intact protein formulae). Nutritional support began on the first postoperative day and the study continued for a maximum of 14 days. There were no significant differences between groups for injury severity, hours to full nutritional support, number of days on nutritional support, average daily caloric intakes, N balance, or complication rates. TPN patients had more hyperglycemia while enterally fed patients had more diarrhea (48 vs 26%). The cost of delivering EN was less than that for TPN. The cost difference for delivering nutritional support between groups (accounting for line and tube placement) was $ 2,383 per patient. The authors concluded that early postoperative jejunostomy feeding was safe and efficacious for multiple trauma patients.

Peterson et al. [25] investigated isocaloric, isonitrogenous total EN (TEN; amino acid based diet) versus TPN in 46 trauma patients. Patients with an abdominal trauma index (ATI) between 15 and 40 were randomized to TEN or TPN. Acute phase proteins increased more in TPN patients. Visceral protein levels (albumin, transferrin, retinol binding protein) increased to a greater extent in TEN patients. Clinical outcomes analyzed by route of nutritional support were comparable for ICU and hospital stay. Septic complications were more common in TPN patients (2/21 vs 8/25; $p=0.08$). The authors concluded that postinjury TEN attenuated reprioritization of hepatic protein synthesis in patients sustaining major trauma. In a follow up study, Moore et al. [26] reported on 59 patients randomized to TEN or TPN. Visceral protein levels improved more in the TEN than TPN group. Overall septic morbidity was 17% in the TEN group and 37% in the TPN group. There were 6/30 (20%) pneumonias in the TPN group and 0/29 (0%) in the TEN group. The authors concluded that TEN was well tolerated in the severely injured patient and that early feeding via the gut reduced septic complications in the stressed patient.

Kudsk et al. [27] randomized 98 patients with an ATI of at least 15 to

Table 3. Human studies comparing EN and TPN

Ref	No.	Result
Trauma		
[24]	46	EN and TPN equally effective; TPN more expensive
[25]	46	Better visceral proteins with EN; More sepsis with TPN
[26]	59	Better visceral proteins with EN; More sepsis with TPN
[27]	98	Sepsis higher with TPN
[28]	META 8 trials	Sepsis higher with TPN
Neuro		
[30]	38	Survival better with early nutrition
[31]	45	No differences between EN and TPN
[32]	41	No differences in outcome between EN and TPN
Perioperative		
[33]	META 18 trials	Routine use of TPN not justified
[45]	34	Pre-op TPN vs No Pre-op TPN; No differences
[46]	24	TPN vs EN; TPN had higher cost
[47]	15	TPN vs EN; No differences noted
[48]	28	TPN vs EN; No differences noted
[29]	20	TPN vs EN; No differnces except TPN higher cost
[49]	395	TPN vs oral; More infections with TPN
[50]	66	TPN vs EN; No differences noted
Cancer		Chemotheraphy and Radiotherapy
[51]	17 trials	TPN vs oral; Sepsis higher with TPN
[52]	28 trials	TPN vs oral; Sepsis higher with TPN
[53]	META 12 trials	TPN vs oral; TPN associated with decreased survival, lower tumor response, higher infection rate
Bone marrow		
[54]	137	TPN vs fluids; Better survival with TPN
[55]	57	TPN vs EN; No differences, TPN cost more

enteral (peptide based formula) or parenteral feeding within 24 h of injury. Groups were matched for severity of injury, age, and mechanism of injury. Length of hospital stay was comparable between groups. One patient died in each group. Septic morbidity was defined as pneumonia, intra-abdominal abscess, empyema, line sepsis, or fasciitis occurring during the first 15 days of hospitalization. Septic morbidity was significantly lower in the enteral group (24 vs 76%). The enteral group had fewer pneumonias (11.8 vs 31%), intra-abdominal abscesses (1.9 vs 13.3%), and line sepsis (1.9 vs 13.3%).

Moore and co-workers [28] reported results form 8 prospective randomized trials comparing the efficacy of early enteral (amino acid based diet) versus early TPN in high risk surgery patients. Two of these trials were published previously [26, 29]. The data were analyzed by meta-analysis. TEN and TPN groups were comparable. Septic complications were lower in TEN patients (18 vs 35%; $p=0.01$). TEN patients had a lower incidence of pneumonia, intra-abdominal abscesses, and catheter sepsis.

Neuro-Injury. Rapp and colleagues [30] compared the effects of early TPN to delayed EN on outcome in patients following head injury. Thirty eight head injured patients were randomily assigned to receive TPN or standard EN. Eight of 18 (44%) delayed EN patients died within 18 days of injury, whereas none of the TPN patients dies within this period. TPN patients had improved N balances and higher serum albumin levels. The authors concluded that early nutrition could improve survival following head injury. This study primarily compares early to delayed feeding. It is difficult to draw conclusions regarding route of nutrient delivery since the parenteral and enteral groups were not comparable for nutritional support.

Hadley et al. [31] randomized 45 acute head injury patients to TPN or EN (intact protein formula). TPN patients had significantly higher mean daily N intakes. However, there were no differences between groups for maintenance of serum albumin levels, weight loss, incidence of infection, N balance, and outcome.

Young et al. [32] studied 41 brain-injured patients randomized to TPN or EN (intact protein formulae). The TPN group received significantly more protein (1.35 vs 0.91 g/kg·day) and calories (76 vs 59% of requirements) than the enteral group. Nitrogen balance was significantly better in the TPN patients. The incidence of infections and sepsis was not significantly different between groups. Early (<18 days of injury) and late (>18 days of injury) deaths were not statistically different between groups. Ten of 23 (43%) of the TPN patients and 10 of 28 (36%) of the enteral patients died. The authors concluded that more patients in the TPN group had favorable outcomes (43.5 vs 32.1% at 6 months). However, the definition of favorable neurologic outcome was arbitrary and based upon a Glasgow Coma Scale (GCS). Five patients (22%) in the TPN group had peak admission GCS of 5 or less, while 10 patients in the enteral group (36%) had admission GCS of 5 or less. One would not have expected the enteral group to have done as well neurologically. Thus, despite lower calories and protein intake, there was no difference in outcome between patients receiving enteral or parentereal nutrition.

Perioperative nutritional support. Detsky et al. [33] used meta-analysis to evaluate the results of 18 controlled trials (1966–1986) that measured the effectiveness of perioperative TPN. Many of the trials suffered from poor methodologies. In 4 studies, TPN was administered only during the postoperative period; in 5, only during the preoperative period; and in 10, during both preoperative and postoperative periods. In 15 studies, patients with GI malignancies were involved; in 1, head and neck cancers; and in 1 bladder cancer. Most studies compared TPN to oral diet (not tube feeding). The evidence suggested that "routine use of perioperative TPN in unselected patients having major surgery was not justified". There was no significant reduction in complication rates or mortality. The health and public policy committee of the American College of Physicians [34] published a position paper on perioperative TPN in 1987. The committee agreed that "routine use of perioperative TPN for unselected patients having major surgery was not justified". The committee called for further trials in subgroups of high risk patients (i.e. severely malnourished patients having major surgery, postoperative patients with complications which result in prolonged periods of inadequate nutritional intake). The committee also suggested that some of these patients may be able to receive their nutrients through enteral feeding tubes.

We will review selected studies from the meta-analysis.

- Moghissi et al. [35] studied patients with carcinoma of the esophagus (with dysphagia) randomized to preoperative TPN (n=10; 34–36 kcal/kg·day and 0.18–0.20 g nitrogen/kg·day) or no TPN (6 kcal/kg·day and no nitrogen). The TPN group had better N balance and weight gain. No significant differences in complications or mortality were reported.
- Holter et al. [36] randomized patients with GI malignancies to perioperative TPN or no preoperative TPN. There were no differences in complications or mortality.
- Heatley et al. [37] randomized patients with cancer of the esophagus and stomach to hospital diet or hospital diet plus parenteral nutrition (amino acids, ethanol, sorbitol). There was no difference in mortality. However, complication rate (primarily wound infections) was lower in the patients receiving supplemental parenteral nutrition.
- Thompson et al. [38] randomized 21 patients with GI cancers and weight loss (>10%) to TPN (n=12; starting an average of 8 days before surgery) or no TPN (n=9). There were no differences between groups for postoperative complications or mortality.
- Muller and associates [39] randomized 125 patients with GI cancer to preoperative TPN (n=66) or hospital diet (n=59). The diet group had more malnourished patients (62 vs 41%). The overall major complication rate was 30% in the control group and 20% in the TPN group. The mortality rates were 18.6% in the control group and 4.5% in the TPN group.
- Lim et al. [40] randomized 24 patients with esophageal carcinoma to TPN (n=12) or gastrostomy feedings (n=12; blenderized diet). The TPN group attained earlier balance. The percent increase in serum albumin was similar between groups. Two patients (17%) in the TPN group developed catheter sepsis and one patient developed thrombosis of the subclavian vein. One gastrostomy patient had a mild wound infection. One patient died in

the TPN group and two died in the gastrostomy group. There were no significant differences in complications between groups. TPN was significantly more expensive than enteral feeding.

- Abel et al. [41] randomized malnourished patients undergoing cardiac surgery to postoperative TPN (n=24) or diet (n=20) (this study is part of the meta-analysis). A separate group of well nourished patients undergoing cardiac surgery were also studied. TPN was continued for 5–6 days postoperatively (average daily intake 1000 kcal, 5 g nitrogen). Oral intake was allowed as soon as the patients were extubated. The malnourished patients had more complications than the well nourished patients. In addition, the TPN malnourished patients had more complications than the non-TPN malnourished patients.
- Collins et al. [42] studied 30 patients undergoing abdominal perineal resections. Patients were divided into 3 matched groups: IV fluids, postoperative IV amino acids, and postoperative TPN. There were no significant differences between groups for septic morbidity or mortality. The TPN group had better wound healing and decreased hospital stay.
- The retrospective study by Mullen et al. [43] was also included in the meta-analysis [33]. Mullen studied patients referred to the nutritional support service who underwent major intra-abdominal or intrathoracic surgery. The study was not randomized. The decision to use TPN was made by the primary surgeon. Patients not receiving preoperative TPN served as the control group. Patients were retrospectively stratified by PNI. Data were reported on 145 patients (50 TPN, 95 controls). Nine patients developed complications (18%) and 2 died (4%) in the TPN group. Thirty-seven patients developed complications (38.9%) and 27 died (29.4%) in the control group. Significant differences between groups was demonstrated only for those patients identified as high risk by a PNI≥50%. Preoperative nutritional support was associated with a reduction in complications, sepsis, and mortality.
- Daly et al. [44] also retrospectively assessed the effect of preoperative TPN in malnourished patients with esophageal cancer. Patients receiving preoperative TPN had lower wound infection rates compared to patients not receiving preoperative TPN.
- Smith et al. [45] randomized 34 surgery patients with a PNI >30% to preoperative TPN (10 days) or surgery without preoperative nutritional support (controls). This study was not part of the meta-analysis [33]. Patients underwent major GI surgery. Preoperative nutritional support in these malnourished patients was associated with weight gain, increased triceps skinfold, improved delayed skin hypersensitivity responses, and improved PNI (5.5%). There were 3 major complications and 1 death in the preoperative nutrition group, and 6 major complications and 3 deaths in the control group (not significant). Average hospital stay was 38 days in the control group and 44 days in the treatment group. This study did not compare TPN to EN but rather preoperative IV nutritional support to no preoperative IV nutritional support.

It is important to note that these studies did not evaluate parenteral versus enteral nutrition. They evaluated perioperative parenteral nutrition versus no perioperative parenteral nutrition. The control groups had access to food but it is unclear how much they received.

- McArdle et al. [46] studied 24 surgical patients (i.e. burns, trauma, cancer, head injury, respiratory failure) with >15% weight loss in a prospective randomized study. Patients were randomized to receive TPN solution (amino acids and dextrose) via the intravenous or enteral routes. Both groups achieved N balance by the 3rd day of nutritional support. Serum insulin levels were higher and free fatty acid levels lower (decreased fat mobilization) in the parenterally fed patients. The cost of delivering the enteral solution was 50% less than the cost of the parenteral solution. Complications and outcome were not reported.
- Muggia-Sullam et al. [47] studied 15 patients undergoing abdominal surgery. Patients received an elemental diet via needle catheter jejunostomy or TPN (non-randomized). Both nutritional groups were similar for N balance, body weight preservation, and visceral protein levels. No data is presented for complications.
- Fletcher et al. [48] randomized 28 patients undergoing aortic grafting for aneurysm or occlusive disease to standard IV fluids, TPN, or early postoperative enteral feeding. Nitrogen balance was similar in the parenteral and enteral groups. As expected, both nutritional groups had better N balances than the IV fluid group. There were no deaths. There were no significant differences between groups for complications or length of stay.
- Bower et al. [29] randomized 20 patients underdoing major upper-GI or pancreaticobiliary surgery to postoperative nutritional support by TPN or EN (amino acid based formula; needle catheter jejunostomy). Both routes of nutritional support provided adequate nutrition, although N balance was better in the TPN group. Serum albumin and transferrin levels decreased more in the TPN group. Prealbumin decreased more in the enteral group. SGOT and SGPT increased to a greater extent in the TPN group. There were no difference in complications between groups. The enteral nutrition was cheaper.
- The Veterans Affairs Total Parenteral Nutrition Cooperative Study Group evaluated perioperative TPN in 395 malnourished surgery patients [49]. Patients who required laparotomy or noncardiac thoracotomy were randomily assigned to receive either TPN for 7–15 days before surgery and 3 days afterwards, or no perioperative TPN (diet alone). Patients were monitored for complications for 90 days after surgery. The rates of complications during the first 30 days after surgery were similar between groups (25.5% TPN, 24.6% control group). Mortality rates (90 day) were similar between groups (13.4% TPN, 10.5% control group). However, there were more infectious complications in the TPN group than controls (14.1 vs 6.4%, $p=0.01$). Severely malnourished patients who received TPN had fewer complications than controls (5 vs 43%). The TPN group averaged

2944 kcal/day in the preoperative period while the control group received 1280 kcal/day. Some have argued that the increased infectious complications in the TPN group may have resulted from overfeeding. However, it must also be pointed out that this study did not compare isocaloric isonitrogenous enteral to parenteral nutrition. Many would also argue that EN (via feeding tube) could be used for nutritional support in all the malnourished patients, and there was little if any need for TPN in these patients.

- Cerra et al. [50] randomized 66 surgery patients with sepsis and persistent hypermetabolism to TPN or EN. They reported no reduction in the incidence of MOF or mortality between groups. The authors concluded that the route of nutrient delivery had little effect on outcome after organ failure developed.

In summary, the routine use of preoperative TPN appears unjustified in unselected patients. In addition, routine perioperative use of TPN does not decrease surgical complications, infections, or outcome. However, it is more costly than perioperative EN.

Cancer. Retrospective and uncontrolled trials have reported benefit from TPN in patients with cancer. However, therapeutic efficacy can only be established by careful prospective, randomized, controlled trials. In 1984, Koretz [51] evaluated survival data, tumor response, and therapeutic toxicity from 17 randomized controlled trials using TPN as an adjunct to chemotherapy and radiation therapy. Most of the control groups received oral nutrition (diet). TPN did not improve survival, tumor response, or toxicity. Sepsis was more common in patients receiving TPN. Klein et al. [52] evaluated 28 prospective randomized controlled clinical trials of TPN in cancer patients in 1986. Control patients were treated with diet in most trials. The authors concluded that TPN may be useful (reduces surgical complications and mortality) when used preoperatively in patients with GI tract cancer. No significant benefit from TPN could be demonstrated for survival, treatment tolerance, treatment toxicity, or tumor response in patients receiving chemotherapy or radiotherapy. There was a significant increase in infections ($P<0.0001$) in TPN patients receiving chemotherapy.

A position paper from the American College of Physicians evaluated TPN in patients receiving cancer chemotherapy in 1989 [53]. Meta-analysis was used to pool the results from 12 randomized controlled trials. Patients receiving TPN support were 81% as likely to survive as control patients ($p=0.05$), 68% as likely to achieve complete or partial tumor response ($p=0.12$), and 40% more likely to develop a significant infection ($p<0.0001$). The report concluded, "parenteral nutritional support was associated with net harm, and no conditions could be defined in which such treatment appeared to be of benefit".

Bone marrow transplantation. Weisdorf et al. [54] studied the impact of TPN (n=71) versus IV fluids (n=66) on the clinical outcome of well nourished patients receiving bone marrow transplants for malignant disease. The study period began 1 week prior to marrow transplant and continued for 4 weeks posttransplant. All patients were encouraged to maintain enteral intake during the study. Calorie and protein intake was significantly higher in the TPN treated patients. In addition, 61% of the control patients were eventually treated with IV nutrition (average start 21 days posttransplant). Survival was significantly longer in the patients receiving TPN than in control patients (2 year survival for TPN=50% and controls=35%). Time to relapse and disease free survival were significantly longer in the TPN patients. There was no difference between groups for engraftment, graft-versus-host-disease, or hospital days. Time-to-bacteremia was not significantly different for the two groups when all patients were included. However, in patients receiving allogenic transplants, the incidence of bacteremia was higher in TPN patients [72 vs 48%, p=0.001). This study evaluated the role of TPN supplementation to an enteral diet. It was not a comparison of isocaloric isonitrogenous parenteral versus enteral diets. The study suggested that improved nutrient intake could improve survival after bone marrow transplantation.

Szeluga et al. [55] compared TPN (n=27) to EN (n=30) in a prospective randomized trial of patients receiving bone marrow transplants. EN was provided by oral supplements and/or tube feeding. TPN was associated with more days of diuretic use, more frequent hyperglycemia, and more frequent catheter removal (prompted by catheter related complications), but less frequent hypomagnesemia. There were no significant differences in the rate of hematopoietic recovery, length of hospitalization, or survival, but nutrition related costs were 2.3 times greater in the TPN group. The authors concluded that TPN was not superior to enteral feeding and recommended that TPN be reserved for bone marrow transplant patients who demonstrate intolerance to enteral feeding.

Inflammatory bowel disease. TPN is frequently employed as primary therapy for patients with severe inflammatory bowel disease (IBD). Recent attention has also focused on the use of EN as primary therapy for patients with IBD (primarily Crohn's disease). Few studies of nutritional support of IBD compare isocaloric isonitrogenous parenteral and enteral nutrition. Most studies are retrospective and uncontrolled. They are difficult to interpret because of small size and many patients received different medications (i. e. corticosteroids). In most of the controlled studies, the control group received corticosteroids while the nutrition therapy group did not. Some studies attempted to evaluate nutritional therapy as an adjunct to medical or surgical therapy. Others evaluated the nutritional therapy as primary therapy for the disease.

To compare the benefits of TPN vs EN for induction of remission in Crohn's disease, we tabulated know studies of TPN and EN (with element diets) in patients with Crohn's disease (Tables 4 and 5). TPN (Table 4) was associated with a 65% early (in hospital) remission rate and a 41% long-term (3–64 month) remission rate. Elemental enteral diets were associated with a 68% early remission rate and 47% long-term remission rate (Table 5). These results were not statistically different from each other. To further evaluate route of nutritional support in the treatment of Crohn's disease, we evaluated only prospective controlled studies (Table 6). Seven studies compared TPN to control diets [56–62]. Both short (74 and 76%) and long-term (40 and 41%) remission rates were similar with both nutritional regimens (Table 6). In addition, elemental diets were not better than control diets for inducing remission in Crohn's disease (Tables 5 and 6). Abad-Lacruz et al. [63] evaluated liver function in 29 patients with IBD randomized to total TEN or TPN. Patients receiving EN had better liver function (measured by serum bilirubin and albumin levels) and less hepatic damage (measured by alkaline phosphatase, GGT, AST and ALT).

Patients with active ulcerative colitis respond poorly to TPN. The majority of patients continue to have active disease. Only 4 of 22 (18%) patients treated with TPN by Sitzmann et al. [64] had acceptable response to therapy.

Table 4. TPN in the treatment of Crohn's disease

Series	No.	Short-term remission	Long-term remission	Type
Anderson (1973)	8	7 (88%)	1 (13%)	R
Fischer (1973)	7	3 (43%)	–	R
Vogel (1974)	8	8 (100%)	4 (50%)	R
Reilly (1976)	23	14 (61%)	–	R
Dean (1976)	11	4 (36%)	–	R
Hartford (1978)	30	23 (77%)	4/21 (19%)	R
Mullen (1978)	50	19 (38%)	–	R
Milewski (1980)	7	2 (29%)	–	R
Bos (1980)	86	24 (28%)	7 (8%)	R
Houcke (1980)	36	27 (75%)	22 (61%)	R
Holm (1981)	8	7 (88%)	7 (88%)	R
Shiloni (1983)	9	9 (100%)	6 (67%)	R
Ostro (1985)	100	77 (77%)	50/93 (54%)	R
Elson (1980)	20	13 (65%)	8 (40%)	P
Greenberg (1981)	43	33 (77%)	29 (67%)	P
Muller (1983)	30	25 (83%)	17 (57%)	P
Lerebours (1986)	20	19 (95%)	3 (15%)	P
Dickinson (1980)	6	4 (67%)	1 (17%)	PC
Lochs (1983)	10	6 (60%)	5 (50%)	PC
Greenberg (1985)	17	12 (71%)	8 (47%)	PC
McIntyre (1986)	9	9 (100%)	3 (33%)	PC
Greenberg (1988)	17	12 (71%)	5 (29%)	PR
Jones (1987)	16	14 (88%)	–	PR
Cravo (1991)	24	18 (75%)	12/23 (52%)	PR
Totals		389/595 (65%)	192/464 (41%)	

R = retrospective, P = prospective, PC = prospective controlled, PR = prospective randomized

Table 5. Elemental diets in the treatment of Crohn's disease

Series	No.	Short-term remission	Long-term remission	Type
Voitk (1973)	7	3 (43%)	–	R
Rocchio (1974)	25	10 (40%)	–	R
Axelsson (1977)	11	8 (73%)	4 (36%)	R
O'Morain (1980)	27	24 (89%)	18 (67%)	P
Lochs (1978)	15	15 (60%)	12 (48%)	P
O'Morain (1984)	11	9 (82%)	8 (73%)	PC
Saverymutti (1985)	21	15 (71%)	–	PC
Greenberg (1985)	19	11 (58%)	2 (11%)	PC
Jones (1987)	16	14 (88%)	–	PR
Giaffer (1990)	16	12 (75%)	–	PC
Totals		121/178 (68%)	44/93 (47%)	

R=retrospective, P=prospective, PC=prospective controlled, PR=prospective randomized

In a prospective controlled trial, Dickinson et al. [56] reported no difference in clinical response between conventional medical therapy (with diet) and TPN. In hospital, remission rates were 57% for controls versus 46% for TPN. One year follow up revealed 36% of controls and 31% of TPN patients to be in remission. McIntyre et al. [59] reported a 58% in hospital remission rate in control diet patients and 40% in TPN patients. Long-term remission rates were 25 and 13%, respectively.

Malnutrition is a risk factor for patients undergoing operative procedures. Although there are a lack of controlled trials evaluating perioperative nutritional support in patients with IBD, preoperative nutritional support may benefit many of these patients. Patients with significant underlying malnutrition are those most likely to benefit from preoperative nutritional support. The best route to deliver nutrients remains undefined.

These studies support the conclusion that nutritional therapy can reverse the nutritional deficits caused by IBD and aid in the healing process. However, these studies do not support a role for nutritional therapy as primary therapy for IBM. In addition, TPN may result in bowel starvation rather than bowel rest [65].

On the basis of these clinical studies, it appears that TPN offers little advantage over EN plus medical therapy (i. e. corticosteroids, sulfasalazine) for the treatment of IBD in most patients. Enteral nutrition is preferable to TPN as initial therapy for IBD. TPN should be reserved for patients who do not tolerate EN, patients with short guts, patients with bowel obstruction, and patients with high-output fistulas.

Intestinal Fistulae. GI fistulae may develop as a result of abdominal surgery, inflammatory bowel disease, cancer, pancreatitis, radiation, trauma, and oth-

Table 6. TPN vs EN in the treatment of Crohn's disease (prospective, controlled studies)

Series	Group	Short-term remission	Long-term remission
Parenteral			
Dickson (1980)	Control	3/3	0/3
	TPN	4/6	1/6
Lochs (1983)	Control	6/10	6/10
	TPN	6/10	5/10
Greenberg (1985)	Control	9/15	6/15
	TPN	12/17	8/17
McIntyre (1986)	Control	5/7	2/7
	TPN	9/9	3/9
Jones (1987)	Enteral	14/16	–
	TPN	14/16	–
Greenberg (1988)	DFD	11/19	6/19
	TPN	12/17	5/17
	TPN + Food	9/15	5/15
Cravo (1991)	Control	35/42	18/38
	DFD	11/15	4/13
	TPN	18/24	12/23
Totals	Controls	83/112 (74%)	38/96 (40%)
	TPN	75/99 (76%)	34/83 (41%)
Enteral			
O'Morain (1984)	Control	8/10	7/10
	elemental	9/11	8/11
Saverymutti (1985)	Control	16/16	–
	elemental	15/21	–
Greenberg (1985)	Control	9/15	6/15
	elemental	11/19	2/19
Malchow (1990)	Control	32/44	–
	PEP-DIET	21/51	–
Giaffer (1990)	Control	5/14	–
	elemental	12/16	–
Totals	Control	70/99 (71%)	13/25 (52%)
	enteral	68/118 (58%)	10/30 (33%)

TPN = parenteral nutrition, DFD = defined formula diet, PEP-DIET = peptide based diet

er etiologies. The reported mortality rate of patients with GI fistulae is 6–67% [66]. Most patients with fistulae are malnourished or become malnourished secondary to anorexia, infection and sepsis, protein losses, or inability to tolerate enteral diets. Adequate nutritional support is an integral part of the management of these patients. Mortality is higher in malnourished patients compared to well nourished patients with enterocutaneous fistuale [66].

Many clinicians routinely treat patients with GI fistulae with TPN. TPN is believed to improve nutritional status, close the fistulae, and improve outcome. TPN decreases fluid losses from fistula. Hamilton et al. [67] reported that TPN decreased fistula output by 80–85% within 2–3 days. Wolfe et al. [68] studied enterocutaneous fistulae in the dog. Fistula output decreased by 81% with an elemental diet and 93% with TPN. On the other hand, Fischer [69] noted only a 31.5% decrease in fistula output with TPN.

Fistula closure rates average around 50–59% using enteral feeding [70–72]. Fistula closure rates have been reported to be as high as 73–89% with TPN [73, 74]. However, prospective controlled randomized studies evaluating TPN vs EN on closure rate and mortality in patients with GI fistulae have not been performed. Reber et al. [75] compared 82 fistula patients treated between 1968–1971 (35% receiving IV nutrition) with 104 patients treated between 1972–1977 (71% receiving IV nutrition). Spontaneous fistula closure rates were 26 (1968–1971) and 35% (1972–1977). Mortality rates were 22 and 29%, respectively. These differences were not significant. Soeters et al. [76] reviewed 404 patients with GI fistulae. Mortality was 15.1% from 1960–1970 (before TPN) and 25.6% from 1970–1975 (after the introduction of TPN). The major cause of death was uncontrolled sepsis. Spontaneous closure rates increased from 10 to 23.3%. Similarly, Deitel et al. [77] compared outcome in patients with fistulae, before and after TPN. Mortality decreased from 40 to 9.3%, and closure rate increased from 34.4 to 81%. Most studies indicate that increased spontaneous closure rates of fistulae can be achieved with TPN. Although some reports have shown decreased mortality with TPN, mortality figures in several large series range from 6.5–22% with TPN, and 15–28% without TPN [66].

The anatomical location of a fistula and the volume of drainage should determine the optimal means of nutritional support. Patients with high output fistula and high small bowel fistula (i.e. upper jejenum) are difficult to replete with EN. These patients may better be repleted with TPN. EN (perhaps with elemental diets) should be tried in most of the remaining patients. Distal or colonic fistulae can usually be supported with enteral feedings. High upper GI fistula (i.e. stomach, duodenum) patients can be fed by placing a feeding tube 30–40 cm beyond the fistula. Radiation induced fistulae and fistulae in patients with Crohn's disease are less likely to close and are associated with high mortalities. These patients frequently require surgery.

Pancreatitis. The pancreas possesses both exocrine and endocrine functions. It secretes bicarbonate, electrolytes, digestive enzymes (i.e. amylase, lipase, phospholipase, trypsin, chymotrypsin) and hormones (i.e. insulin, glucagon, somatostatin). Because it is the major source of digestive enzymes and insulin, malfunction of the pancreas has important nutritional implications. Pancreatic secretion is stimulated by vagal efferents from the brain in response to sight, smell, or taste of food (cephalic phase), stimulation of the pancreas due to food in the stomach (gastric phase), and the presence of acid or food in the intestine (intestinal phase). Undigested proteins have little or no stimulatory effect upon pancreatic secretion. On the other hand, peptides and amino acids have a strong stimulatory effect. Pancreatic secretion is inhibited by the consumption of hypertonic glucose solutions and GI hormones (i.e. glucagon, somatostatin, pancreatic polypeptide). Infusion of trypsin and chymotrypsin into the duodenum inhibits pancreatic secretion [78, 79].

Elemental (amino acid, low fat) diets cause less stimulation of pancreatic exocrine secretion than complex diets. Oral consumption of nutrients stimulates more pancreatic secretion than intragastric administration. Administration of nutrients into the stomach stimulates more pancreatic secretion than infusion into the duodenum; duodenal infusion stimulates more secretion than jejunal administration. Jujunal administration results in pancreatic juice that is "enzyme poor". In addition, acidic diets stimulate more pancreatic secretion than basic diets. It is clear that use of the GI tract for nutritional support induces some pancreatic secretion. Stimulation can be minimized by infusion of elemental neutral pH diets into the proximal jejunum. Elemental enteral diets also have a smaller trophic effect upon the pancreas and GI tract than complex diets.

Intravenous glucose (i.e. 25–40%) inhibits secretin and cholecystokinin-induced pancreatic secretory output (i.e. fluid, protein, amylase, lipase). Intravenous infusion of glucose, amino acids, and fat stimulates little if any pancreatic secretion [80–82]. The secretory response to IV nutrition is less than that to intraduodenal administration of elemental diets [70–82]. Thus, enteral diets induce more pancreatic stimulation than IV diets.

Chronic pancreatitis results in a loss of exocrine function. These patients are usually managed with EN. Limitation of dietary fat intake can help prevent steatorrhea. Vitamin and mineral deficiencies can usually be treated with oral supplements. Malabsorption frequentlly results from insufficient pancreatic enzyme secretion. Enzyme supplementation aids in nutrient digestion and absorption. It can also help reduce pain [83, 84]

Acute pancreatitis presents as a systemic illness characterized by pain, fluid and electrolyte imbalance, shock, organ failure, and even death. This systemic response is felt to result from the release of pancreatic enzymes, bioactive digestion products, and cytokines. During recovery from an attack of acute pancreatitis, the patient is at risk for nutritional depletion, immune compromise, and infection/sepsis. Many of these patients have been traditionally fed using TPN. TPN provides nutritional support and can "rest" the pancreas.

If continued production of pancreatic enzymes during acute pancreatitis is responsible for systemic manifestations and complications, then suppression of these enzymes may ameliorate the severity of the attack. Some evidence suggests that pancreatic enzyme production is already low as a result of pancreatitis. Few studies have compared TPN to enteral feeding in patients with acute pancreatitis. Goodgame et al. [85] reported data from a retrospective study of 46 cases of acute pancreatitis treated with TPN (mortality 20%). Results were compared to complications and mortality (23%) found in the medical literature. They concluded that TPN had little effect on disease pathophysiology as judged by mortality and morbidity. TPN was associated with a higher incidence of catheter-related sepsis. Similar conclusions were drawn from a retrospective analysis by Grant et al. [86]. In a more recent uncontrolled retrospective analysis of 67 patients with acute pancreatitis, Kalfarentzos et al. [87] reported an overall complication rate of 55.2% and mortality of 24% in paitents treated with TPN. An increased incidence of catheter-related sepsis was also reported. Sax and associates [88] performed a randomized, prospective trial of early TPN in acute pancreatitis. Patients were randomized to conventional therapy (i.e. IV fluids, analgesics, antacids, NG suction) or conventional therapy plus TPN (dextrose plus amino acids initially, 10% lipid added when triglycerides normal). Patients not eating in 7 days were crossed over to TPN. TPN patients maintained better N balance. However, early institution of TPN had no advantage over conventional therapy. Catheter-related sepsis was higher in the TPN group (10.5 vs 1.5%). Days to full oral intake ($p<0.06$) and length of hospitalization ($p<0.04$) were longer in the TPN group. Total hospital charges were greater in the TPN patients.

Overall, at the present time, there is no data to indicate that TPN alters the course of acute pancreatitis. EN is the preferred method for initial nutritional support of patients with pancreatitis. Acute pancreatitis has been successfully managed with EN [89, 90].

Metabolic Effects of Parenteral and Enteral Nutrition

Gastrointestinal Tract and Liver

Luminal nutrients are important for maintenance of normal GI tract structure and function. Luminal nutrients directly stimulate the gut. They also produce indirect effects via stimulation of gut trophic hormones. Intravenous feeding is associated with loss of gut weight, mucosal protein and DNA content, villous height, glucose absorption, and mucosal enzyme activities [91–99]. TPN is also associated with atrophy of the pancreas [92, 100]. Thompson et al. [94] measured diamine oxidase (DAO) activity, an intestinal mucosal enzyme which serves as a marker of gut cellular maturity and integrity, in animals given TPN or enteral diets. DAO activity decreased with TPN and correlated with a decrease in gut mass.

Intestinal growth and development may be delayed in premature neonates given IV nutrition. Immature sucking rats given TPN during weaning demonstrate delayed intestinal growth, decreased mucosal mass, and reduced enzyme activity [101–103]. These effects are reversed by EN [102].

Guedon et al. [93] performed duodenal endoscopic biopsies in 7 adults with inflammatory bowel disease placed on TPN and corticosteroids. The patients had moderate weight loss at the time of study. Following 21 days of TPN, there were significant decreases in disaccharidase (72–83%) and peptidase (23–78%) enzyme activities. These activities increased after oral refeeding. There were also significant decreases in microvillus height (13%) in comparison with pre-TPN values. No data were presented from normal controls for comparison. Biasco et al. [104] followed an adult patient with serial jejunal biopsies after intestinal resection for superior mesenteric artery thrombosis. Intestinal hypoplasia was found after 30 days of TPN; cell proliferation and intestinal hyperplasia occurred within 14 days of oral refeeding.

Greene et al. [105] studied 16 infants with protracted diarrhea and malnutrition who were allocated to TPN or parenteral nutrition plus enteral feedings. The enterally fed group had earlier recovery of intestinal sucrase and maltase activities and shorter hospital stay (34 vs 46 days). Orenstein [106] prospectively randomized infants with intractable diarrhea to parenteral or enteral nutrition. Parenteral and enteral nutrition produced similar weight gain. However, enteral feeding was associated with faster resolution of malabsorption and diarrhea, fewer complications, and less expensive hospitalization.

Gut trophic hormones are also important for maintaining the integrity of the GI tract. Adams et al. [107] constructed isolated bowel loops in rats. Structural hypoplasia occurred in intact and isolated intestines in animals fed with TPN. However, intestinal integrity was maintained in both intact and isolated gut of enterally fed animals. These findings indicated that some systemic (i.e. hormonal) factor(s) affected gut mass. Intravenous feeding results in lower level of gut trophic hormones compared with enteral feeding. These hormones include gastrin [92, 108, 109], cholecystokinin and secretin [110], insulin [111], enteroglucagon [109, 111, 112], motilin [109], neutrotensin [109], and epidermal growth factor [113, 114]. Administration of gastrin [108], cholecystokinin and secretin [110], and epidermal growth factor [113, 114] have been shown to improve gut mass and/or function during TPN. Saito et al. [115] have also shown that EN, compared to TPN, diminishes the secretion of catabolic hormones (i.e. VMA, cortisol, glucagon) following burn injury in animals.

Elevations in serum aminotransferases, bilirubin, and bile salts are frequently seen in patients receiving TPN. These findings suggest that TPN may have deleterious effects on hepatic function. Knodell et al. [116, 117] evaluated the effect of enteral and parenteral nutrition on liver function in rats. Hepatic microsomal cytochrome P-450 oxidase activity and capacity for demethylation of meperidine and hydroxylation of pentobarbital were significantly reduced in TPN animals. Katayama et al. [118] randomized rats to parenteral or enteral nutrition (using the same formula) and measured hepatic energy charge (EC) and mitochondrial phosphorylation rates (PR). The TPN group showed a deterioration of hepatic PR and EC. Charland et al. [119] also randomized rats to parenteral or enteral feeding and found that TPN was associated with a decrease in hepatic cytochrome P-450 activity. These data suggest that the route of delivery of nutrients may have significant impact upon liver function.

Bacterial Translocation

The intestinal mucosa and immune system function as major defense barriers, preventing bacteria and endotoxin contained within the gut from invading distant organs. Bacterial translocation is reported to occur in animals following endotoxin [120], hemorrhage [121], trauma [122], burn injury [123], and methotrexate [23].

Alverdy et al. [124] randomized animals to food, oral TPN fluid, or IV TPN. Animals were fed for two weeks. Two thirds of the TPN animals had culture-positive mesenteric lymph nodes compared with one third of oral TPN animals, and none of the food group. Spaeth et al. [125] divided rats into three groups: food, oral-TPN, and IV-TPN. Bacterial translocation occurred in 60% of IV and oral TPN fed animals. Translocation did not occur in animals receiving food. The addition of oral cellulose powder to the oral and IV TPN groups reduced bacterial translocation to 8 and 0%. Thus, oral administration of fiber appeared to maintain the intestinal barrier and reduced bacterial translocation. We [23] randomized methotrexate treated animals to TPN or enteral diets. Bacterial translocation and mortality were significantly greater in TPN animals. These data suggest that TPN promotes bacterial translocation in animals.

Many have questioned the role of bacterial translocation in human disease. However, recent studies suggest that bacterial/toxin translocation occurs in humans following injury [125–128]. Reed et al. [126] harvested mesenteric lymph nodes from 25 patients undergoing exploratory celiotomy for abdominal injury. Six patients (25%) had bacteria in their lymph nodes by culture. However, all patients received preoperative antibiotics. Brathwaite et al. [127] sampled portal venous blood (PVB) and mesenteric lymph nodes (MLN) from 10 patients with trauma. PVB was culture positive in 2 patients (20%), and MLN were culture positive in 1 patient (10%). However, when MLN were reacted with monoclonal antibody to *E. coli* beta-galactosidases, all the MLN were positive. Reed et al. [128] confirmed these findings. They harvested MLN from 16 patients with abdominal trauma. All received preoperative antibiotics. One patient had bacteria in the MLN by culture, 9 by electron microscopy, and 3 by both techniques. Overall, bacteria were identified in the MLN in 13/16 (81%) patients. These studies indicate that bacteria/toxins may be present in MLN (indicating translocation) even though cultures are negative. Clearly, preoperative antibiotics may interfere with culture results. Together, these data indicate that bacterial translocation is common in humans after abdominal trauma.

Immunity

Immune responsiveness was assessed in animals fed orally or intravenously for 7 days [129]. Lymphocyte reactivity to concanavalin A remained unchanged over 7 days in oral fed rats. On the other hand, lymphocyte reactivity was depressed by 60% in TPN fed animals. Renk et al. [130] measured lymphocyte response to concanavalin A and phytohemagglutinin in traumatized rats (bilateral femoral fracture) randomized to TPN or EN. Lymphocyte responses were depressed in both groups one day after injury. Lymphocyte responses returned to normal by 7 days postinjury in the enteral group but not the TPN group. Alverdy and coworkers [131] measured secretory IgA in animals fed intravenously or enterally. Secretory IgA levels were significantly higher in enterally fed animals.

Immune response of patients receiving TPN vs EN has not been evaluated in prospective randomized trials. However, there is worry that the lipid composition (i.e. high in long-chain Ω-6 fatty acids) and protein composition (i.e. amino acids, no glutamine, low arginine) of TPN may result in suppression of immune responses.

Miscellaneous

A number of studies (human and animal) have evaluated the effect of TPN and EN on N balance during stress. Overall, studies indicate that protein and calories administered via the enteral route result in the same or better N balance than when administered via the parenteral route [132, 133].

Delany et al. [134] evaluated wound healing in rats fed for 6 days via the parenteral and enteral routes. There were no significant differences between groups for weight change, N balance, colonic bursting strenght, or skin incision bursting strength. Similar results were obtained by Zaloga et al. [135].

Differences in the response to infection may exist between enterally and parenterally fed individuals. Mortality from infection is higher in animals [18–23] and humans [53] fed with TPN versus EN. The acute phase protein response to infection [25] and catabolic hormone secretion [115] are higher in animals fed with TPN compared to EN. Endotoxin triggers many of the hemodynamic, metabolic, and immune responses associated with injury and infection. To determine whether TPN altered the host response to infection, Fong et al. [136] administered endotoxin to human volunteers (prospective, randomized) maintained on 1 week of EN or TPN. In response to endotoxin, parenterally fed patients developed higher body temperature, higher heart rates, and lower blood pressures. Individuals receiving TPN had higher stress hormone responses (i.e. epinephrine, glucagon, CRP), hepatic venous TNF levels, lactate levels, and greater peripheral amino acid mobilization. These data indicate that TPN produces alterations in the host response to "infection" independent of nutritional status.

Conclusions

We have reviewed a large quantity of data comparing EN and TPN. Results have been grouped into three major categories: nutrient availability, studies of enteral vs parenteral nutrition (animal and human), and metabolic effects of enteral vs parenteral nutrition.

The following conclusions are based upon the data presented

1. TPN and EN differ in their ability to deliver proteins, carbohydrates and fats. TPN formulae lack many important nutrients (i.e. glutamine, peptides, complex carbohydrates such as fiber, medium-and short-chain fatty acids, Ω-3 long chain fatty acids, and nucleotides).
2. Prospective randomized studies of infection in animals demonstrate higher mortality in animals fed with TPN compared to EN.
3. TPN (compared to EN) is associated with a higher rate of sepsis in humans following trauma.
4. EN and TPN are associated with similar outcomes following head injury.
5. Routine use of perioperative TPN in unselected patients having major surgery is not justified.
6. EN is as good or better than TPN in patients following surgery. EN is safe, cheaper than TPN, and may be associated with a lower infection rate.
7. TPN is associated with lower survival, poorer tumor response, and more infections in unselected patients receiving chemotherapy or radiotherapy for cancer.
8. TPN has no beneficial effects on the course of inflammatory bowel disease or pancreatitis. EN should be the primary mode of nutritional support in these patients.
9. TPN and EN are of equal efficacy in most patients with GI fistula. However, some patients with fistula (i.e. high output, high jejunal, pancreatric) may benefit from TPN.
10. When compared to EN, TPN induces gut atrophy, liver dysfunction, gut bacterial translocation (animals), and immune dysfunction.

In summary, EN is superior to TPN as a means of nutritional support in most patients. The primary indication for use of TPN is failure of EN.

References

1. Zaloga GP (1993) Studies comparing intact protein, peptide, and amino acid formulas. In: Bounous G (ed) Uses of elemental diets in clinical situations, CRC Press, Boca Raton, pp 201–217
2. Buchan AM (1990) Do NMDA antagonists protect against cerebral ischemia: Are clinical trials warranted? Cerebrovasc Brain Metab Rev 2:1–26
3. Weiss JH, Hartley DM, Koh J, Choi DW (1990) The calcium channel blocker nifedipine attenuates slow excitatory amino acid neurotoxicity. Science 247:1474–1477
4. Proceedings of an international glutamine symposium (1990) Glutamine metabolism in health and disease – Basic science and clinical aspects. JPEN 14 (Suppl):39–46

5. Hwang TL, O'Dwyer ST, Smith RJ, et al (1986) Preservation of small bowel mucosa using gutamine enriched parenteral nutrition. Surg Forum 37:56–58
6. Souba WW, Smith RJ, Wilmore DW (1985) Glutamine metabolism by the intestinal tract. JPEN 9:608–617
7. Barbul A (1986) Arginine – Biochemistry, physiology, and therapeutic implications. JPEN 10:227–238
8. Barbul A (1990) Arginine and immune function. Nutrition 6 (Suppl):53–58
9. Barbul A, Fishel RS, Shimazu S, et al (1985) Intravenous hyperalimentation with high arginine levels improves wound healing and immune function. J Surg Res 31:328–334
10. Palacio JC, Rombeau JL (1990) Dietary fiver – A brief review and potential application to enteral nutrition. Nutr Clin Pract 5:99–106
11. Settle RG (1988) Short-chain fatty acids and their potential role in nutritional support. JPEN 12:104S-107S
12. Rombeau JL (1988) Colonic infusions of short-chain fatty acids. JPEN 12:102S–103S
13. Zaloga GP (1991) Nutrition and prevention of systemic infection. Critical Care – State of the Art 12:31–79
14. Kinsella JE, Lokish B (1990) Dietary lipids, eicosanoids, and the immune system. Crit Care Med 18 (Suppl):94–113
15. Meydani SN, Nicolosi RJ, Hayes KC (1985) Effect of long term feeding of corn oil or coconut oil on immune response and prostaglandin E2 synthesis on squirrel and cebus monkeys. Nutr Res 5:993–1002
16. Wan JMF, Teo TC, Babayan VK, et al (1988) Lipids and the development of immune dysfunction and infection. JPEN 12:43S
17. Van Buren CT, Rudolph FB, Kulkarni A, Pizzini R, Fanslow WC, Kumar S (1990) Reversal of immunosuppression induced by a protein-fee diet. Comparison of nucleotides, fish oil, and arginine. Crit Care Med 18:S114–S117
18. Kudsk KA, Carpenter G, Petersen S, Sheldon GF (1981) Effect of enteral and parenteral feeding in malnourished rats with E. coli-hemoglobin peritonitis. J Surg Res 31:105–110
19. Kudsk KA, Stone JM, Carpenter G, Sheldon GF (1983) Enteral and parenteral feeding influences mortality after hemoglobin E. coli peritonitis in normal rats. J Trauma 23:605–609
20. Petersen SR, Kudsk KA, Carpenter G, Sheldon GF (1981) Malnutrition and immunocompetence: Increased mortality following an infectious challenge during hyperalimentation. J Trauma 21:528–533
21. Kudsk KA, Stone JM, Carpenter G, Sheldon GF (1982) Effects of enteral and parenteral feeding of malnourished rats on body composition. J Trauma 22:904–906
22. Zaloga GP, Knowles R, Black KW, Prielipp R (1991) Total parenteral nutrition increases mortality after hermorrhage. Crit Care Med 19:54–59
23. Zaloga GP, Roberts P, Black KW, Prielipp R (1993) Gut bacterial translocation/ dissemination explains the increased mortality produced by parenteral nutrition following methotrexate. Circ Shock (in press)
24. Adams S, Dellinger EP, Wertz MJ, Oreskovich MR, Simonowitz D, Johansen K (1986) Enteral versus parenteral nutritional support following laparotomy for trauma: A randomized prospective trial. J Trauma 26:882–891
25. Peterson VM, Moore EE, Jones TN, et al (1988) Total enteral nutrition versus total parenteral nutrition after major torso injury: Attenuation of hepatic protein reprioritization. Surgery 104:199–207
26. Moore FA, Moore EE, Jones TN, McCroskey BL, Peterson VM (1989) TEN versus TPN following major abdominal trauma – Reduced septic morbidity. J Trauma 29:916–923
27. Kudsk KA, Croce MA, Fabian TC, et al (1992) Enteral versus parenteral feeding: Effects on septic morbidity after blunt and penetrating abdominal trauma. Ann Surg 215:503–513

28. Moore FA, Feliciano DV, Andrassy RJ, et al. (1992) Early enteral feeding, compared with parenteral, reduces postoperative septic complications. The results of a meta-analysis. Ann Surg 216:172–183
29. Bower RH, Talamini MA, Sax H, Hamilton F, Fischer JE (1986) Postoperative enteral vs parenteral nutrition. Arch Surg 121:1040–1045
30. Rapp RP, Young B, Twyman D, et al (1983) The favorable effect of early parenteral feeding on survival in head-injured patients. J Neurosurg 58:906–912
31. Hadley MN, Grahm TW, Harrington T, Schiller WR, McDermott MK, Posillico DB (1986) Nutritional support and neurotrauma: A critical review of early nutrition in forty-five acute head injury patients. Neurosurgery 19: 367–372
32. Young B, Ott L, Twyman D, et al (1987) The effect of nutritional support on outcome from severe head injury. J Neurosurg 67:668–676
33. Detsky AS, Baker JP, O'Rourke K, Goel V (1987) Perioperative parenteral nutrition: A meta-analysis. Ann Intern Med 107:195–203
34. Health and public policy committee (1987) Perioperative parenteral nutrition. Ann Intern Med 107:252–253
35. Moghissi K, Hornshaw J, Teasdale PR, Dawes EA (1977) Parenteral nutrition in carcinoma of the esophagus treated with surgery: Nitrogen balance and clinical studies. Br J Surg 64:125–128
36. Holter AR, Fischer JE (1977) The effects of hyperalimentation on complications in patients with carcinoma and weight loss. J Surg Res 23:31–34
37. Heatley RV, Lewis MH, Williams RHP (1979) Pre-operative intravenous feeding: A controlled trial. Postgrad Med J 55:541–545
38. Thompson BR, Julian TB, Stremple JT (1981) Peri-operative total parenteral nutrition in patients with gastrointestinal cancer. J Surg Res 30:497–500
39. Muller JM, Dienst C, Brenner U, Pichlmaier H (1982) Preoperative parenteral feeding in patients with gastrointestinal carcinoma. Lancet 1:68–71
40. Lim STK, Choa RG, Lam KH, Wong J, Ong GB (1981) Total parenteral nutrition versus gastrostomy in the preoperative preparation of patients with carcinoma of the oesophagus. Br J Surg 68:69–72
41. Abel RM, Fischer JE, Buckley MJ, et al (1976) Malnutrition in cardiac surgical patients. Results of a prospective randomized evaluation of early postoperative parenteral nutrition. Arch Surg 111:45–50
42. Collins JP, Oxby CB, Hill GL (1978) Intravenous amino acids and intravenous hyperalimentation as protein sparing therapy after major surgery. A controlled clinical study. Lancet 1:788–791
43. Mullen JL, Buzby GP, Matthews DC, Smale BF, Rosato EF (1980) Reduction of operative morbidity and mortality by combined preoperative and postoperative nutritional support. Ann Surg 192:604–613
44. Daly JM, Massar E, Giacco G, et al (1982) Parenteral nutrition in esophageal cancer patients. Ann Surg 196:203–208
45. Smith RC, Hartemink R (1988) Improvement of nutritional measures during preoperative parenteral nutrition in patients selected by the prognostic nutritional index: A randomized controlled trial. JPEN 12:587–591
46. McArdle AH, Palmason C, Morency I, Brown RA (1981) A rationale for enteral feeding as the preferable route for hyperalimentation. Surgery 90:616–623
47. Muggia-Sullam M, Bower RH, Murphy RF, Joffe SN, Fischer JE (1985) Postoperative enteral versus parenteral nutritional support in gastrointestinal surgery. Am J Surg 149:106–111
48. Fletcher JP, Little JM (1986) A comparison of parenteral nutrition and early postoperative enteral feeding on the nitrogen balance after major surgery. Surgery 100:21–24
49. The veterans affairs total parenteral nutrition cooperative study group (1991) Perioperative total parenteral nutrition in surgical patients. N Engl J Med 325:525–532
50. Cerra FB, McPherson JP, Konstantinides FN, et al (1988) Enteral nutrition does not prevent multiple organ failure syndrome (MOFS) after sepsis. Surgery 104:727–733

51. Koretz RL (1984) Parenteral nutrition: Is it oncologically logical? J Clin Oncology 2:534–538
52. Klein S, Simes J, Blackburn GL (1986) Total parenteral nutrition and cancer clinical trials. Cancer 58:1378–1386
53. Position paper (1989) Parenteral nutrition in patients receiving cancer chemotherapy. Ann Intern Med 110:734–736
54. Weisdorf SA, Lysne J, Wind D, et al (1987) Positive effect of prophylactic total parenteral nutrition on long-term outcome of bone marrow transplantation. Transplantation 43:833–838
55. Szeluga DJ, Stuart RK, Brookmeyer R, Utermohlen V, Santos GW (1987) Nutritional support of bone marrow transplant recipients: A prospective randomized clinical trial comparing total parenteral nutrition to an enteral feeding program. Cancer Res 47:3309–3316
56. Dickinson RJ, Ashton MG, Axon ATR, Smith RC, Yeung CK, Hill GL (1980) Controlled trial of intravenous hyperalimentation and total bowel rest as an adjunct to the routine therapy of acute colitis. Gastroenterology 79:1199–1204
57. Lochs H, Meryn S, Marosi L, et al (1983) Has total bowel rest a beneficial effect in the treatment of Crohn's disease? Clin Nutr 21:61–64
58. Greenberg GR, Fleming CR, Jeejeebhoy KN, et al (1985) Controlled trial of bowel rest and nutritional support in the management of Crohn's disease. Gastroenterology 88:140
59. McIntyre PB, Powell-Tuck J, Wood SR, et al (1986) Controlled trial of bowel rest in the treatment of severe acute colitis. Gut 27:481–485
60. Jones VA (1987) Comparison of total parenteral nutrition and elemental diet in induction of remission of Crohn's disease. Dig Dis Sci 32 (Suppl):100–107
61. Greenberg GR, Fleming CR, Jeejeebhoy KN, Rosenberg IH, Sales D, Tremaine WJ (1988) Controlled trial of bowel rest and nutritional support in the management of Crohn's disease. Gut 29:1309–1315
62. Cravo M, Camilo ME, Correia JP (1991) Nutritional support in Crohn's disease: Which route? Am J Gastroenterol 86:317–321
63. Abad-Lacruz A, Gonzalez-Huis F, Esteve M, et al (1990) Liver function tests abnormalities in patients with inflammatory bowel disease receiving artificial nutrition: A prospective randomized study of total enteral nutriton vs total parenteral nutrition. JPEN 14:618–621
64. Sitzmann JV, Converse RL, Bayless TM (1990) Favorable response to parenteral nutrition and medical therapy in Crohn's colitis. Gastroenterology 99:1647–1652
65. Culpepper-Morgan JA, Floch MH (1991) Bowel rest or bowel starvation: Defining the role of nutritional support in the treatment of inflammatory bowel diseases. Am J Gastroenterol 86:269–271
66. Tarazi R, Steiger E (1988) Enterocutaneous fistulas. In: Kinney JM, Jeejeebhoy KN, Hill GL, Owen OE (eds) Nutrition and metabolism in patient care. WB Saunders, Philadelphia pp 243–257
67. Hamilton RF, Davis WC, Stephenson DV, et al (1971) Effects of hyperalimentation on upper gastrointestinal tract secretions. Arch Surg 102:340–352
68. Wolfe BM, Keltner RM, Willman VL (1972) Intestinal fistula output in regular, elemental, and intravenous alimentation. Am J Surg 124:803–806
69. Fischer JF (1975) The management of high-output intestinal fistulas. Adv Surg 9:139–176
70. Voitk AJ, Echave V, Brown RA, McArdle AH, Gurd FN (1973) Elemental diet in the treatment of fistulas of the alimentary tract. Surg Gynecol Obstet 137:68–72
71. Rocchio MA, Cha C, Haas KF, Randall HT (1974) Use of chemically defined diets in the management of patients with high output gastrointestinal cutaneous fistulas. Am J Surg 127:148–156
72. Bury KD, Stephens RV, Randall HT (1971) Use of a chemically defined liquid elemental diet. Am J Surg 121:174–183
73. Graham JA (1977) Conservative treatment of gastrointestinal fistulas. Surg Gynecol Obstet 144:512–514

74. Silberman H, Granson M, Fong G, et al (1980) Management of external gastrointestinal fistulas with glucose and lipids. Surg Gynecol Obstet 150:856–858
75. Reber HA, Roberts C, Way LW, Dunphy JE (1978) Management of external gastrointestinal fistulas. Ann Surg 188:460–467
76. Soeters PB, Ebeid AM, Fischer JE (1979) Review of 404 patients with gastrointestinal fistulas: Impact of parenteral nutrition. Ann Surg 190:189–202
77. Deitel M (1976) Nutritional management of external gastrointestinal fistulas. Can J Surg 19:505–511
78. Slaff J, Jacobson D, Tillman CR, et al (1984) Protease-specific suppression of pancreatic exocrine secretion. Gastroenterology 87:44–52
79. Green GM, Lyman RL (1972) Feedback regulation of pancreatic enzyme secretion as a mechanism for trypsin inhibitor-induced hypersecretion in rats. Proc Exp Biol Med 140:6–12
80. Kelly GA, Nahrwold DL (1976) Pancreatic secretion in response to an elemental diet and intravenous hyperalimentation. Surg Gynecol Obstet 143:87–91
81. Stabile BE, Debas HT (1981) Intravenous versus intraduodenal amino acids, fats, and glucose as stimulants of pancreatic secretion. Surg Forum 32:224–226
82. Stabile BE, Borzatta M, Stubbs RS (1984) Pancreatic secretory responses to intravenous hyperalimentation and intraduodenal elemental and full liquid diets. JPEN 8:377–380
83. Sarles H, Sahel J, Staub JL, et al (1979) Chronic pancreatitis. In: Howat HT, Sarles H (eds) The exocrine pancreas. WB Saunders, London, pp 402–439
84. Isaksson G, Ihse I (1983) Pain reduction by oral pancreatic enzyme preparation in chronic pancreatitis. Dig Dis Sci 28:97–102
85. Goodgame JT, Fischer JE (1977) Parenteral nutrition in the treatment of acute pancreatitis: Effect on complications and mortality. Ann Surg 186:651–658
86. Grant JP, James S, Grabowski V, et al (1984) Total parenteral nutrition in pancreatic disease. Ann Surg 200:627–631
87. Kalfarentzos FE, Karavias DD, Karatzas TM, Alevizatos BA, Androulakis JA (1991) Total parenteral nutrition in severe acute pancreatitis. J Am Coll Nutr 10:156–162
88. Sax HC, Warner BW, Talamini MA, et al (1987) Early total parenteral nutrition in acute pancreatitis: Lack of beneficial effects. Am J Surg 153:117–124
89. McArdle AH, Echave W, Brown RA, et al (1974) Effect of elemental diet on pancreatic secretion. Am J Surg 128:690–692
90. Voitk A, Brown RA, Echave V, et al (1973) Use of an elemental diet in the treatment of uncomplicated pancreatitis. Am J Surg 125:223–227
91. Levine GM, Deren JJ, Steiger E, Zinno R (1974) Role of oral intake in maintenance of gut mass and disaccharide activity. Gastroenterology 67:975–982
92. Johnson LR, Copeland EM, Dudrick SJ, Lichtenberger LM, Castro GA (1975) Gastroenterology 68:1177–1183
93. Guedon C, Schmitz J, Lerebours E, et al (1986) Decreased brush border hydrolase activities without gross morphologic changes in human intestinal mucosa after prolonged total parenteral nutrition of adults. Gastroenterology 90:373–378
94. Thompson JS, Vaughan WP, Forst CF, Jacobs DL, Weekly JS, Rikkers LF (1987) The effect of the route of nutrient delivery on gut structure and diamine oxidase levels. JPEN 11:28–32
95. Hughes CA, Dowling RH (1980) Speed of onset of adaptive mucosal hypoplasia and hypofunction in the intestine of parenterally fed rats. Clin Sci 59:317–327
96. Kotler DP, Levine GM, Shiau YF (1981) Effects of luminal nutrition and metabolic status on in-vivo glucose absorption. Am J Physiol 240:G432–G436
97. Hosoda N, Nishi M, Nakagawa M, Hiramatsu Y, Hioki K, Yamamoto M (1989) Structural and functional alterations in the gut of parenterally or enterally fed rats. J Surg Res 47:129–133
98. Czernichow B, Galluser M, Hasselmann M. Doffoel M, Raul F (1992) Effects of amino acids in mixtures given by enteral or parenteral route on intestinal morphology and hydrolases in rats. JPEN 16:259–263

99. Morin CL, Ling V, Bourassa D (1980) Small intestinal and colonic changes induced by a chemically defined diet. Dig Dis Sci 25:123–128
100. Hughes CA, Prince A, Dowling RH (1980) Speed of change in pancreatic mass and in intestinal bacteriology of parenterally fed rats. Clin Sci 59:329–336
101. Castillo RO, Pittler A, Costa F (1988) Intestinal maturation in the rat: The role of enteral nutrients. JPEN 12:490–495
102. Ford WD, Boelhouwer RU, King WW, deVries JE, Ross JS, Malt RA (1984) Total parenteral nutrition inhibits intestinal adaptive hyperplasia in young rats: Reversal by feeding. Surgery 96:527–534
103. Morgan W, Yardley J, Luk G, Niemiec P, Dudgeon D (1987) Total parenteral nutrition and intestinal development: A neonatal model. J Ped Surg 22:541–545
104. Biasco G, Callegari C, Lami F, Minarini A, Miglioli M, Barbara L (1984) Intestinal morphologic changes during oral refeeding in a patient previously treated with total parenteral nutrition for short bowel resection. Am J Gastroenterol 79:585–588
105. Greene HL, McCabe DR, Merenstein GB (1975) Protracted diarrhea and malnutrition in infancy: Changes in intestinal morphology and disaccharidase activities during treatment with total intravenous nutrition or oral elemental diets. J Peds 87:695–704
106. Orenstein SR (1986) Enteral versus parenteral therapy for intractable diarrhea of infancy: A prospective randomized trial. J Peds 109:277–286
107. Adams PR, Copeland EM, Dudrick SJ, Johnson LR, Castro GA (1978) Maintenance of gut mass in bypassed bowel of orally vs parenterally nourished rats. J Surg Res 24:421–427
108. Johnson LW, Lichtenberger LM, Copeland EM, Dudrick SJ, Castro GA (1975) Action of gastrin on gastrointestinal structure and function. Gastroenterology 68:1184–1192
109. Aynsley-Green A, Lucas A, Lawson GR, Bloom SR (1990) Gut hormones and regulatory peptides in relation to enteral feeding, gastroenteritis, and necrotizing enterocolitis in infancy. J Peds 117:24–32
110. Hughes CA, Bates T, Dowling RH (1978) Cholecystokinin and secretin prevent the intestinal mucosal hypoplasia of total parenteral nutrition in the dog. Gastroenterology 75:34–41
111. Lickley HLA, Track NS, Vranic M, Bury KD (1978) Metabolic response to enteral and parenteral nutrition. Am J Surg 135:172–175
112. Sagor GR, Ghatei MA, Al-Mukhtar MYT, Wright NA, Bloom SR (1983) Evidence for a humoral mechanism after small intestinal resection. Gastroenterology 84:902–906
113. Jacobs DO, Evans DA, Mealy K, O'Dwyer ST, Smith RJ, Wilmore DW (1988) Combined effects of glutamine and epidermal growth factor on the rat intestine. Surgery 104:358–364
114. Bragg LE, Hollingsed TC, Thompson JS (1990) Urogastrone reduces gut atrophy during parenteral alimentation. JPEN 14:283–286
115. Saito H, Trocki O, Alexander JW, Kopcha R, Heyd T, Joffe SN (1987) The effect of route of nutrient administration on the nutritional state, catabolic hormone secretion, and gut mucosal integrity after burn injury. JPEN 11:1–7
116. Knodell RG, Steele NM, Cerra FB, Gross JB, Solomon TE (1984) Effects of parenteral and enteral hyperalimentation on hepatic drug metabolism in the rat. J Pharmacol Exp Ther 229:589–597
117. Knodell RG, Spector MH, Brooks DA, Keller FX, Kyner WT (1980) Alterations in penobarbital pharmacokinetics in response to parenteral and enteral alimentation in the rat. Gastroenterology 79:1211–1216
118. Katayama T, Tanaka M, Tanaka K, et al (1990) Alterations in hepatic mitochondrial function during total parenteral nutrition in immature rats. JPEN 14:640–645
119. Charland SL, Dickerson RN, Rajter JJ, Settle RG (1991) The effect of sepsis on hepatic cytochrome P-450 activity in parenterally fed rats. Clin Res 39:682A
120. Deitch EA, Specian RD, Berg RD (1991) Endotoxin-induced bacterial translocation and mucosal permeability: Role of xanthine oxidase, complement activation, and macrophage products. Crit Care Med 19:785–791

121. Baker JW, Deitch EA, Li M, Berg RD, Specian RD (1988) Hemorrhagic shock induces bacterial translocation from the gut. J Trauma 28:896–906
122. Deitch EA, Bridges RM (1987) Effect of stress and trauma on bacterial translocation from the gut. J Surg Res 42:536–542
123. Maejima K, Deitch E, Berg R (1984) Promotion by burn stress of the translocation of bacteria from the gastrointestinal tracts of mice. Arch Surg 119:166–172
124. Alverdy JC, Aoys E, Moss GS (1988) Total parenteral nutrition promotes bacterial translocation from the gut. Surgery 104:185–190
125. Spaeth G, Berg RD, Specian RD, Deitch EA (1990) Food without fiber promotes bacterial translocation from the gut. Surgery 108:240–247
126. Reed L, Martin M, Kocka F, Barrett R, Barrett J (1992) Bacterial translocation following abdominal injury. Circ Shock 37:57
127. Brathwaite CEM, Ross S, Nagele R, Mure A, Field C, O'Malley KO (1992) Significance of bacterial translocation after multiple trauma with hemorrhagic shock. Circ Shock 37:50
128. Reed L, Martin M, Manglano R, Newson B, Barrett J (1991) Bacterial translocation following abdominal trauma in humans. Crit Care Med 19:S95
129. Birkhahn RH, Renk CM (1984) Immune response and leucine oxidation in oral and intravenous fed rats. Am J Clin Nutr 39:45–53
130. Renk CM, Owens DR, Birkhahn RH, Long CL. Blakemore WS (1980) Effect of intravenous or oral feeding on immunocompetence in traumatized rats. JPEN 4:587
131. Alverdy J, Chi HS, Sheldon GF (1985) The effect of parenteral nutrition on gastrointestinal immunity: The importance of enteral stimulation. Ann Surg 202:681–684
132. Rowlands BJ, Giddings AEB, Johnston AOB, Hindmarsh JT, Clark RG (1977) Nitrogen-sparing effect of different feeding regimens in patients after operation. Br J Anaesth 49:781–787
133. Hulten L, Andersson H, Bosaeus I, et al (1980) Enteral alimentation in the early postoperative course. JPEN 4:455–459
134. Delany HM, Teh E, Dwarka B, Levenson SM (1991) Infusion of enteral vs parenteral nutrients using high-concentration branch-chain amino acids: Effect on wound healing in the postoperative rat. JPEN 15:464–468
135. Zaloga GP, Bortenschlager L, Black K (1992) Early postoperative administration of enteral or parenteral nutrients improves wound healing. JPEN 16 (Suppl):28S
136. Fong Y, Marano MA, Barber A, et al (1989) Total parenteral nutrition and bowel rest modify the metabolic response to endotoxin in humans. Ann Surg 210:449–457

The Importance of the Gut as a Central Organ in the Pathogenesis of MOF

M. P. Fink

Introduction

In 1988, Wilmore et al. [1] proposed that the intestinal tract plays a central role in the pathophysiologic responses to severe injury or infection. Others, including Deitch and colleagues [2], Border et al. [3], and Meakins and Marshall [4], also have championed this concept. The barest outlines for the gut hypothesis for multiple organ dysfunction (MOF) can be summarized as follows: "derangements in the barrier function of the gut permit the dissemination of intraluminal microbes and/or microbial products to mesenteric lymph nodes (MLN) or other organs (particularly the liver), which are downstream from the intestinal tract". The pathological dissemination of microbes or microbial products beyond the confines of the intestinal lumen leads to pathological modulation of immune cells. This results in excessive release of a wide variety of pro-inflammatory mediators, including cytokines, such as IL-1 and TNFα, and lipids, like PAF, which can promote organ injury via numerous mechanisms.

The "gut hypothesis" is attractive, in part, because it might explain why hypermetabolism and fetal organ system dysfunction occur in a sizeable number of critically ill patients, even in the absence of a discrete focus of infection [5, 6]. Moreover, this hypothesis is supported by a large body of data from studies using animal models of critical illness. There is a remarkable paucity of clinical data, however, that support the gut hypothesis of MOF. Indeed, some results obtained by studying patients conflict with findings obtained in animal models. Thus, the true importance of the gut as a central organ in the pathogenesis of MOF remains very much an open question. This chapter will review some of the recent data pertinent to this field.

Microbial Translocation

Definition and Mechanisms

Microbial translocation has been defined as the passage of viable and nonviable microbes, microbial products, or even inert particles, from the lumen of the intestine to extra-luminal locations [7, 8]. In most studies, the extent of translocation has been quantitated by enumerating viable colony-forming units in MLN or other organs. Recent studies by Alexander et al. [9] however, suggest that this methodology grossly underestimates the true number of translocating organisms, since the majority of microbes migrating to tissues such as MLN or the spleen are killed. Because nonviable microbes or microbial products may be as important as viable organisms as stimuli for the release of pro-inflammatory mediators or as modulators of immune responsiveness, it may be preferable, at least in animal studies, to assess the degree of translocation by loading the intestinal tract with radionuclide-labelled bacteria or endotoxin, and measuring the subsequent appearance of radioactivity in tissue samples or blood [9–11]. This methodology also permits the investigator to disassociate pathological alterations in the extent of microbial passage across the intestinal epithelium from changes in the ability of the host to kill microbes in extraluminal sites.

The mechanism(s) responsible for translocation have not been elucidated with certainty. Based upon data obtained from models of thermal injury, hemorrhage, or endotoxemia in rodents, Deitch and colleagues [12–14] have proposed that translocation occurs via microscopic disruptions in the integrity of the epithelium (i.e. via a paracellular route). These workers have presented evidence supporting that the disruptions in the intestinal epithelium are mediated by oxidants generated by the xanthine-xanthine oxidase system [12, 13].

Other data suggest that intact organisms and macromolecules can traverse the epithelium via a transcellular route. It is well-established that the uptake of macromolecules by enterocytes is a physiologic phenomenon. Uptake of antigens by the gut is a critical event in the development of mucosal immunity [15]. The transepithelial passage of certain macromolecules, e. g. maternally-derived immunoglobulins during the neonatal period, is a receptor-mediated process [16]. The binding of other macromolecules to the mucosal surface is a nonspecific and nonsaturable phenomenon that appears to be closely linked to the subsequent uptake of the substance by enterocytes [17]. The normal uptake of macromolecules by enterocytes is an energy-dependent process [18]. Absorption of macromolecules, such as horseradish peroxidase, occurs via endocytosis [20, 21]. Macromolecules that are taken up by enterocytes are rapidly transported across the epithelium into mesenteric lymph and portal venous blood [19]. Although uptake of macromolecules by gut epithelium occurs normally, enhanced transcellular passage of a marker protein (horseradish peroxidase) has been documented under pathologic conditions, such as thermal injury [20].

In addition to macromolecules, recent evidence suggests that intact microorganisms also can traverse the epithelium via a transcellular route. Wells et al. [21] showed that intestinal overgrowth of *Enterococcus faecalis* in rats promotes translocation of this organism across histologically intact mucosa. Transmission electron and fluorescent microscopic techniques localized cocci and diplococci within, but not between, epithelial cells [21]. The intracellular cocci were shown to be localized within membrane-bound vacuoles. Similar data have been obtained by Alexander et al. [22].

Enhanced microbial translocation has been demonstrated in experimental animals after a variety of insults, including total parenteral nutrition (TPN) [23], burn trauma [9, 11], endotoxemia [13], hemorrhage [10, 12], and sterile inflammation induced by intraperitoneal administration of zymosan [24]. When measured by enumerating viable colony-forming units in MLN or other organs, increased translocation in these models of critical illness can reflect changes in intraluminal microbial ecology, enhanced transepithelial passage of micro-organisms, and/or diminished killing of microbes by the host's immune system. The relative importance of these various factors, and the mechanisms which underly them, remain the subjects of intense investigation.

Some studies suggest that mesenteric ischemia is an important factor leading to enhanced translocation due to thermal injury or endotoxemia [25–29]. Other authors have questioned this notion [30]. Certainly, in some models of enhanced translocation, such as antibiotic decontamination of the gut followed by oral administration of *E. coli* or *E. faecalis*, gut ischemia is not mechanistically important [21]. Conceivably, mesenteric ischemia might promote the transepithelial passage of microbes, impair immune responsiveness, or both. If the migration of organisms or macromolecules across the mucosa is transcellular and energy-dependent, however, then it is difficult to understand why this phenomenon should be increased by ischemia. Alternatively, if transmucosal passage occurs because of microscopic breaks in the integrity of the epithelial sheet, then ischemic necrosis of enterocytes and/or oxidant-mediated damage to the epithelium during reperfusion are probably critical events. It also is quite possible that mesenteric hypoperfusion is immunosuppressive, but the effects of ischemia or ischemia/reperfusion on the microbicidal efficiency of the gut-associated immune network has received relatively little attention.

The adherence of microbes (or macromolecules) to enterocytes is probably a necessary early step in the process of transcellular translocation [17, 21]. Results obtained recently by Alverdy and colleagues [31, 32] suggest that a common factor in many models of increased bacterial translocation may be enhanced adherence of bacteria to mucosa due to deficient intraluminal levels of IgA. The major source of intraluminal IgA is secretory IgA in bile [33], and the amount of IgA secreted into bile is markedly diminished in a variety of conditions associated with enhanced translocation, including TPN (with glutamine-deficient formulae) [34], thermal injury [33], glucocorticoid administration [32], and endotoxemia [31]. Bile duct ligation also increases bacterial translocation [35], possibly by interrupting the delivery of secretory IgA into the foregut.

Role of Translocation in the Development of MOF; Studies using animals

At present, really good animal models of MOF are unavailable. Nevertheless, data are accumulating that suggest that microbial translocation and/or gut-derived endotoxemia contribute to mortality in certain laboratory models of critical illness. For example, using a model of hemorrhagic shock, Rush and colleagues [36, 37] have shown that survival is modestly, but significantly, better in germ-free as compared to conventional rats. These results, however, are discordant with findings made by Zweifach et al. [38] and McNulty and Linares [39] more than 30 years ago. Rush's group believes that in the older studies, inadequate resuscitation was responsible for the failure to demonstrate improved survival after hemorrhage in germ-free animals.

Gaffin and colleagues have documented elevated circulating endotoxin levels in experimental animals subjected to superior mesenteric arterial ischemia and reperfusion [40], heat stroke [41], and arterial hypoxemia [42]. In these studies, no endotoxin has been detectable in plasma samples from appropriate controls. By using nonabsorbable antibiotics to "decontaminate" the gut, this group has provided evidence that the gut is the source of endotoxemia after mesenteric ischemia [40]. In addition, these authors have shown that administration of a polyvalent preparation of (anti-O) anti-endotoxin antibodies improves survival in rabbits subjected to mesenteric ischemia and reperfusion [43], cats subjected to hemorrhagic shock [44], and monkeys subjected to heat stroke [45]. Thus, at least in these models, systemic absorption of gut-derived endotoxins appears to play a critical role in the development of systemic complications that lead to mortality.

The role of bacterial translocation in MOF also has been addressed in several recent studies, which have employed a model of sterile inflammation induced by intraperitoneal zymosan in rats. In this model, which was developed by Goris et al. [46], about a third of the animals die within 72–96 h. Among animals surviving through day 12, organ weights are increased and blood lactate and alkaline phosphatase concentrations are elevated [46]. In germ-free rats, early deaths are not observed [46], suggesting that translocation of microbes or microbial products may be an etiologic factor contributing to mortality. This notion is further supported by findings recently reported by Deitch et al. [47], who showed that systemic administration of cefoxitin, an antibiotic active against gram-negative enteric bacilli, prevents early deaths in a murine model of zymosan-induced sterile peritonitis. In this study, the effect of cefoxitin on bacterial translocation during the early period after zymosan challenge was not assessed, but both Deitch's group [24, 47] and Goris' group [48] have documented that translocation occurs in this model in the absence of antibiotics. Findings similar those obtained by Shreveport group were reported recently by Goris et al. [48] who found that bowel decontamination with streptomycin abrogated early mortality in rats injected intraperitoneally with sterile zymosan. Interestingly, in this study, decontamination with another antibiotic with excellent activity against facultative enteric organisms, trimethoprim, was not found to provide protection against zymosan-induced early mortality. No explanation has been provided for the discrepancy in the results obtained with streptomycin or cefoxitin, on the one hand, and trimethoprim, on the other.

In another recent study, Fukushima et al. [40] hypothesized that oral administration of analogues of PGE might diminish translocation after thermal injury in mice. This hypothesis is plausible in view of the known GI cytoprotective effects of these compounds [50]. In their study, Fukushima et al. made several observations: 1) PGE analogues improve survival in this burn injury model; 2) PGE analogues diminish the extent of bacterial translocation, as assessed by measuring radioactivity in blood after oral administration of C^{14}-labelled *E. coli*; and 3) there is a significant inverse correlation ($r=0.415$, $p<0.05$) between the degree of translocation to blood and the length of survival. Thus, in this model, the degree of translocation seems to be a determinant of outcome. Alternatively, PGE analogues may improve survival and limit translocation, in the absence of a causal relationship between the two phenomena.

Evidence that Pathological Translocation occurs in Humans

Although MLN obtained from patients with inflammatory bowel disease or intestinal obstruction frequently harbor viable bacteria [51, 52], data supporting the idea that pathological translocation is important in critically ill humans are quite limited. Marshall et al. [6] provided some circumstantial evidence in support of the gut hypothesis, when they showed that the microbial species most commonly responsible for nosocomial infections in critically ill surgical patients (i.e. *Candida albicans*, Pseudomonas sp., and entercocci) were the same as those commonly isolated from the proximal intestine of these patients. Additionally, in a study of 50 trauma patients, Rush et al. [53] reported that blood cultures drawn within 3 h of admission were positive in 56% of those patients with profound arterial hypotension, whereas only 4% were positive in the subgroup not in shock. In this study, however, most of the isolates were gram-positive, rather than the gram-negative enteric bacilli most commonly isolated in animal studies of bacterial translocation after hemorrhage. Furthermore, most of the patients with profound hemorrhagic shock died in less than 24 h, rendering it impossible to determine whether positive blood cultures on admission are a predictor of the later development of MOF.

In contrast to the data from Rush's group, Moore et al. [54] were unable to detect elevated endotoxin levels in portal venous or systemic blood samples obtained over the first 5 days of hospitalization from 20 victims of major abdominal trauma. Although 9 (2%) of 424 systemic and portal venous blood cultures were positive over the 5-day period of observation, many of the isolates were probably contaminants. Cultures of ileocolic MLN obtained from 4 of 12 patients were positive, although in one case, the isolated organism (coagulase-negative *Staphylococcus*) was probably a contaminant.

Another study that casts doubt on the importance of translocation in the development of MOF in trauma victims was performed by Reitzman et al. [55]. These investigators obtained biopsies of MLN at the time of laparotomy from 25 trauma patients and 4 patients with primary GI diseases. None of the trauma patients had positive MLN cultures, whereas 3 of the 4 patients with primary GI problems had enteric organisms isolated. Despite having negative MLN cultures, 40% of the trauma patients had major complications, including pulmonary infections and ARDS. Two of the trauma patients subsequently developed gram-negative bacteremias.

Mucosal Permeability

Definition: Physiological and Pharmacological Regulation

Increased intestinal epithelial permeability is another phenomenon that may have a bearing on the role of the gut in MOF. Permeability refers to the passage of hydrophilic compounds across the epithelial barrier. The lipid membrane of the enterocyte is quite impermeable to hydrophilic molecules. Nevertheless, highly water-soluble componds can permeate the intestinal epithelium quite readily by traversing the paracellular pathway formed by the tight junctions between cells [56]. Formerly, it was thought that only small hydrophilic molecules (Stokes radius <11.5 A) are capable of paracellular permeation under normal conditions [56]. Recently, however, convincing evidence has been presented that convective and diffusional movement of inulin, a hydrophilic macromolecule (molecular weight = 5000 D, Stokes radius 14–20 A), also occurs in the normal rat intestine [57].

Paracellular intestinal permeability to hydrophilic molecules is dynamically regulated by functional changes in the tight junctions, or zonula occludens (ZO), between adjacent epithelial cells [56]. The barrier function of the ZO, in turn, apparently is regulated by perturbations in the actomyosin cytoskeleton [56]. Under physiological conditions, intestinal epithelial permeability is increased by activation of the Na^+-coupled cotransporters on the apical membrane of the cell by intraluminal substrates, such as glucose or amino acids [58]. Certain drugs, such as pharmacological doses of L-tryptophan [59] and cyclo-oxygenase inhibitors [57, 60] increase gut epithelial permeability, whereas other drugs, such as prostaglandin E analogues [57], decrease paracellular conductance of water-soluble probes. In general, direct exposure of intestinal epithelium to lipopolysaccharide (LPS) or cytokines does not appear to affect permeability, although prolonged incubation of a model epithelium (cultured monolayers of T_{84} cells) to interferon-γ significantly impairs barrier function [61].

Recently, Kubes [62] showed that pharmacological inhibition of nitric oxide synthase (NOS) markedly, but reversibly, increases small intestinal permeability in the cat. This study is of considerable interest, because NOS inhibitors have been used experimentally to treat septic shock [63–65]. Kubes data raise the possibility that such therapy might precipitate or exacerbate derangements in the barrier function of the gut.

Alterations in Mucosal Permeability in Animal Models of Critical Illness

Increases in intestinal permeability have been demonstrated in numerous animal models of critical illness, including: intestinal ischemia and reperfusion in rats, pigs, and dogs [66–70]; thermal injury in rats [71]; TPN in rats [72]; and endotoxemia in rats and pigs [70, 73–75]. The mechanisms responsible for mucosal hyperpermeability in these models have not been established with certainty. In the most stringent models, such as prolonged intestinal ischemia followed by reperfusion, the main mechanism is probably frank disruption of the epithelial covering of the mucosa [69]. In other, milder models of critical illnesses, derangements in permeability probably result from functional changes in the ZO, rather than epithelial necrosis. Results obtained by Deitch et al. [73] suggest that endotoxin-induced changes in permeability are due to oxidants generated by the xanthine-xanthine oxidase system. Our group has presented data suggesting that mucosal hyperpermeability due to endotoxicosis is mediated, in part, by mesenteric hypoperfusion, although modest degrees of mesenteric ischemia, in the absence of LPS administration, do not cause derangements in gut barrier function [88]. Recent results from our laboratory suggest that mucosal acidosis, irrespective of cause, is a major factor contributing to hyperpermeability in shock states (unpublished observations).

Based upon the preceding discussion, it is reasonable to ask: what is the relationship between microbial translocation and mucosal hyperpermeability? Only a few published studies have addressed this issue. Deitch et al. [73] found that changes in translocation and permeability tended to correlate in a rat model of endotoxicosis. In contrast, Illig et al. [72] showed that 10 days of TPN in rats causes mucosal atrophy and hyperpermeability, but does not increase bacterial translocation.

Clinical Implications of Mucosal Hyperpermeability in Critically Ill Patients

It has been hypothesized that increased paracellular permeability of the intestinal mucosa might permit systemic absorption of microbial byproducts or other luminal toxins. Such products might include LPS, bacterial N-formyl-methionyl oligopeptides [76], or bacterial cell wall polymers (peptidoglycan-polysaccharides) [77]. The last named compounds are of particular interest, since they have been shown to have pro-inflammatory properties [78] and cause hepatic injury in rats [77].

Although mucosal hyperpermeability to hydrophilic solutes has been demonstrated in numerous animal models of critical illness, clinical data are far more limited. Wilmore's group has documented increased permeability to the hydrophilic probe, lactulose, in volunteers injected with a tiny dose of LPS [79] and burn patients with septic complications [80]. Deitch [81] reported that gut permeability is increased in burn patients shortly after injury, an observation which has been confirmed recently by Ryan et al. [82]. Harris et al. [83] showed that permeability is increased in many patients with a variety of critical illnesses. It is noteworthy that these workers found that the degree of gut hyperpermeability bore no relationship to severity of illness (APACHE II score), sepsis score, or survival.

Conclusion

Despite intensive investigation by numerous groups all over the world, the true role of gut barrier failure in critical illness remains to be established. Recent studies suggest that increased microbial translocation is a major determinant of survival in animal models of acute illness and inflammation, but unambiguous clinical confirmation for this notion has yet to be obtained. Increased mucosal permeability to hydrophilic probes clearly has been demonstrated in both animal models and humans with critical illnesses, but, again, the true clinical significance of this phenomenon is unknown.

References

1. Wilmore DW, Smith RJ, O'Dwyer ST, Jacobs DO, Ziegler TR, Wang XD (1988) The gut: A central organ after surgical stress. Surgery 104:917–923
2. Mainous MR, Deitch EA (1992) Bacterial translocation and its potential role in the pathogenesis of multiple organ failure. J Intensive Care Med 7:101–108
3. Border JR, Hasset JM, LaDuca J, et al. (1987) Gut origin septic states in blunt multiple trauma (ISS=40) in the ICU. Ann Surg 206:427–448
4. Carrico CJ, Meakins JL, Marshall JC, Fry D, Maier RV (1985) Multiple-organ-failure syndrome. Arch Surg 121:196–208
5. Goris RJ, Beokhorst PA, Nuytinck KS (1985) Multiple organ failure: Generalized autodestructive inflammation. Arch Surg 120:1109–1115
6. Marshall JC, Christou NV, Horn R, Meakins JL (1988) The microbiology of multiple organ failure: The proximal gastrointestinal tract as an occult reservoir of pathogens. Arch Surg 123:309–315
7. Alexander JW, Boyce ST, Babcock GF, et al (1990) The process of microbial translocation. Ann Surg 212:496–512
8. Mora EM, Cardona MA, Simmons RL (1991) Enteric bacteria and ingested inert particles translocate to intraperitoneal prosthetic materials. Arch Surg 126:157–163
9. Alexander JW, Gianotti L, Pyles T, Carey MA, Babcock GF (1991) Distribution and survival of Escherichia coli translocating from the intestine after thermal injury. Ann Surg 213:558–567

10. Redan JA, Rush BF, McCullough JN, et al (1990) Organ distribution of radiolabelled enteric Escherichia coli during and after hemorrhagic shock. Ann Surg 211:663–668
11. O'Brien R, Murdoch J, Kuehn R, Marshall JC (1992) The effect of albumin or crystalloid resuscitation on bacterial translocation and endotoxin absorption following experimental burn injury. J Surg Res 52:161–166
12. Deitch EA, Bridges W, Baker J, et al (1988) Hemorrhagic shock-induced bacterial translocation is reduced by xanthine oxidase inhibition or inactivation. Surgery 104:191–198
13. Deitch EA, Ma L, Ma JW, et al (1989) Inhibition of endotoxin-induced bacterial translocation in mice. J Clin Invest 184:36–42
14. Deitch EA, Morrison J, Berg R, Specian RD (1990) Effect of hemorrhagic shock on bacterial translocation, intestinal morphology, and intestinal permeability in conventional and antibiotic-decontaminated rats. Crit Care Med 18:529–536
15. Bienenstock J, Befus AD (1980) Mucosal immunology. Immunology 41:249–270
16. Casanova JE (1992) Transepithelial transport of macromolecules. Chest 101:55S–58S
17. Sterns M, Walker WA (1984) Food proteins and gut mucosal barrier. I. Bunding and uptake of cow's milk proteins by adult rat jejunum in vitro. Am J Physiol 246:556–562
18. Walker WA, Cornell R, Davenport LM, Isselbacher KJ (1972) Macromolecular absorption: Mechanism of horseradish peroxidase uptake and transport in adult and neonatal rat intestine. J Cell Biol 54:195–205
19. Warshaw AL, Walker WA, Cornell R, Isselbacher KJ (1971) Small intestinal permeability to macromolecules. Transmission of horseradish peroxidase into mesenteric lymph and portal blood. Lab Invest 25:675–684
20. Carter EA, Gonnell A, Tompkins RG (1992) Increased transcellular permeability of rat small intestine after thermal injury. Burns 18:117–120
21. Wells CL, Jechorek RP, Erlandsen SL (1990) Evidence for the translocation of Enterococcus faecalis across the mouse intestinal tract. J Infect Dis 162:82–90
22. Alexander JW, Boyce ST, Babcock GF, et al (1990) The process of microbial translocation. Ann Surg 212:496–512
23. Alverdy J, Aoys E, Moss GS (1988) Total parenteral nutrition promotes bacterial translocation from the gut. Surgery 104:185–190
24. Mainous MR, Tso P, Berg RD, Deitch EA (1991) Studies of the route, magnitude, and time course of bacterial translocation in a model of systemic inflammation. Arch Surg 126:33–37
25. Navaratnam NRL, Morris SE, Traber DL, et al (1990) Endotoxin increases mesenteric vascular resistance and bacterial translocation. J Trauma 30:1104–1115
26. Tokyay R, Loick HM, Traber DL, et al (1992) Effects of thromboxane synthetase on postburn mesenteric vascular resistance and the role of bacterial translocation in a chronic porcine model. Surg Gynecol Obstet 174:125–132
27. Morris SE, Navaratnam N, Townsend CM, Herndon DN (1988) Bacterial translocation and mesenteric blood flow in a large animal model after cutaneous thermal and smoke inhalation injury. Surg Forum 39:189–190
28. Saydjari R, Beerthuizen GIJM, Townsend CM, et al (1991) Bacterial translocation and its relationship to visceral blood flow, gut mucosal ornithine decarboxylase activity, and DNA in pigs. J Trauma 31:639–644
29. Sheng ZY, Dong YL, Wang XH (1992) Bacterial translocation and multiple system organ failure in bowel ischemia and reperfusion. J Trauma 32:148–153
30. Jones WG II, Barber AE, Minei JP, Fahey TJ III, Shires GT III, Shires GT (1991) Differential pathophysiologic of bacterial translocation after thermal injury and sepsis. Ann Surg 214:24–30
31. Alverdy JC, Aoys E (1992) The effect of dexamethasone and endotoxin administration on biliary IgA and bacterial adherence. J Surg Res 53:450–454
32. Alverdy J, Aoys E (1991) The effect of glucocorticoid administration on bacterial translocation: Evidence for an acquired mucosal immunodeficient state. Ann Surg 214:719–723
33. Cappeller WA, Bloch KJ, Hatz RA, et al (1992) Reduction in biliary IgA after burn injury: Role of diminished delivery via the thoracic duct and of enhanced loss from the systemic circulation. Ann Surg 215:338–343

34. Alverdy JA, Aoys E, Weiss-Carrington P, Burke DA (1992) The effect of glutamine-enriched TPN on gut immune cellularity. J Surg Res 52:34–38
35. Deitch EA, Sittig K, Li M, Berg R, Specian RD (1990) Obstructive jaundice promotes bacterial translocation. Am J Surg 159:79–84
36. Rush BF Jr, Redan JA, Flanagan JJ, et al (1989) Does the bacteremia observed in hemorrhagic shock have clinical significance? A study in germ-free animals. Ann Surg 210:342–347
37. Bruce CJ, Rush BF Jr, Ferraro FJ, Murphy TF, Hsieh JT, Machiedo GW (1992) The effect of the germ-free state on survival following hemorrhagic shock. A study in germ-free and germ-bearing rats. Surg Form 53:47–49
38. Zweifach BW, Gordon HA, Wagner M, Reyniers JA (1958) Irreversible hemorrhagic shock in germ-free rats. J Exp Med 107:437–450
39. McNulty WP Jr, Linares R (1960) Hemorrhagic shock of germ-free rats. Am J Physiol 198:141–144
40. Gathiram P, Wells MT, Brock-Utne JG, Gaffin SL (1988) Oral administered non-absorbable antibiotics prevent endotoxemia in primates following intestinal ischemia. J Surg Res 45:187–193
41. Gathiram P, Gaffin SL, Brock-Utne JG, Wells MT (1987) Time course of endotoxemia and cardiovascular changes in heat-stressed primates. Aviation Space Environ Med 58:1071–1075
42. Gaffin SL, Brock-Utne JG, Zanotti A, Wells MT (1986) Hypoxia-induced endotoxemia in primates: Role of reticuloendothelial system function and anti-lipopolysaccharide plasma. Aviation Space Environ Med 57:1044–1049
43. Zanotti AM, Gaffin SL (1985) Prophylaxis of superior mesenteric artery occlusion shock in rabbits by antilipopolysaccharide (anti-LPS) antibodies. J Surg Res 38:113–115
44. Gaffin SL, Grinberg Z, Abraham C, Birkhan J, Shechter Y (1981) Protection against hemorrhagic shock in the cat by human plasma containing endotoxin-specific antibodies. J Surg Res 31:18–21
45. Gathiram P, Wells MT, Brock-Utne JG, Gaffin SL (1987) Antilipopolysaccharide improves survival in primates subjected to heat stroke. Circ Shock 23:157–164
46. Goris RJA, Boekholtz WKF, van Bebber IPT, Nuytinck JKS, Schillings PHM (1986) Multiple-organ failure and sepsis without bacteria. Arch Surg 121:897–901
47. Deitch EA, Kemper AC, Specian RD, Berg RD (1992) A study of the relationships among survival, gut-origin sepsis, and bacterial translocation in a model of systemic inflammation. J Trauma 32:141–147
48. Goris RJA, van Bebber IPT, Mollen RHM, Koopman JP (1991) Does selective decontamination of the gastrointestinal tract prevent multiple organ failure? An experimental study. Arch Surg 126:561–565
49. Fukushima R, Gianotti L, Alexander JW, Pyles T (1992) The degree of bacterial translocation is a determinant factor for mortality after burn injury and is improved by prostaglandin analogs. Ann Surg 216:438–445
50. Miller TA (1983) Protective effects of prostaglandins against gastric mucosal damage: Current knowledge and proposed mechanisms. Am J Physiol 243:601–623
51. Deitch EA (1989) Simple intestinal obstruction causes bacterial translocation in man. Arch Surg 124:699–701
52. Ambrose NS, Johnson M, Burdon DW, Keighley MRB (1984) Incidence of pathogenic bacteria from mesenteric lymph nodes and ileal serosa during Crohn's disease surgery. Br J Surg 71:623–625
53. Rush BF, Sori AJ, Murphy TF, et al (1988) Endotoxemia and bacteremia during hemorrhagic shock. Ann Surg 207:549–554
54. Moore FA, Moore EE, Poggetti R, et al (1991) Gut bacterial translocation via the portal vein: A clinical perspective with major torso trauma. J Trauma 31:629–638
55. Peitzman AB, Udekwu AO, Ochoa J, Smith S (1991) Bacterial translocation in trauma patients. J Trauma 31:1083–1087

56. Madara JL (1989) Loosening of tight junctions: Lessons from the intestine. J Clin Invest 83:1089–1094
57. Ma TY, Hollander D, Erickson RA, Truong H, Krugliak P (1991) Is the small intestinal epithelium truly "tight" to inulin permeation? Am J Physiol 260:G669–G676
58. Pappenheimer JR, Volpp K (1992) Transmucosal impedance of small intestine: Correlation with transport of sugars and amino acids. Am J Physiol 263:C480–C493
59. Madara JL, Carlson S (1991) Supraphysiologic L-tryptophan elicits cytoskeletal and macromolecular permeability alterations in hamster small intestinal epithelium in vitro. J Clin Invest 87:454–462
60. Bjaranson I, Williams P, Smethurst P, Peters TJ, Levi AJ (1986) Effect of nonsteroidal anti-inflammatory drugs and prostaglandins on the permeability of the human small intestine. Gut 27:1292–1297
61. Madara JL, Stafford J (1989) Interferon-γ directly affects barrier function of cultured intestinal epithelial monolayers. J Clin Invest 83:724–727
62. Kubes P (1992) Nitric oxide modulates epithelial permeability in the feline small intestine. Am J Physiol 262:G1138–G1142
63. Petros A, Bennett D, Vallance P (1991) Effect of nitric oxide synthase inhibitors on hypotension in patients with septic shock. Lancet 338:1557–1558
64. Lubbe AS, Garrison RN, Cryer HM, Alsip NL, Harris PD (1992) EDRF as a possible mediator of sepsis-induced arteriolar dilation of skeletal muscle. Am J Physiol 262:H880–H887
65. Meyer J, Traber LD, Nelson S, et al (1992) Reversal of hyperdynamic response to continuous endotoxin administration by inhibition of NO synthesis. J Appl Physiol 73:324–328
66. Bulkley GB, Kvietys PR, Parks DA, Perry MA, Granger DN (1985) Relationship of blood flow and oxygen consumption to ischemic injury in the canine small intestine. Gastroenterol 89:852–857
67. Langer JC, Sohal SS (1992) Increased mucosal permeability after intestinal ischemia-reperfusion injury is mediated by local tissue factors. J Ped Surg 27:329–332
68. Horton JW (1992) Alterations in intestinal permeability and blood flow in a new model of mesenteric ischemia. Circ Shock 36:134–139
69. Salzman A, Wollert PS, Wang H, et al (1993) Intraluminal oxygenation ameliorates ischemia/reperfusion-induced hyperpermeability in pigs. Circ Shock (in press)
70. Fink MP, Antonsson JB, Wang H, Rothschild HR (1991) Increased intestinal permeability in endotoxic pigs. Limited role for mesenteric hypoperfusion. Arch Surg 126:211–218
71. Epstein MD, Tchervenkow JI, Alexander JW, Johnson JR, Vester JW (1991) Increased gut permeability following burn trauma. Arch Surg 126:198–200
72. Illig KA, Ryan CK, Hardy DJ, Rhodes J, Locke W, Sax HC (1992) Total parenteral nutrition-induced changes in gut mucosal function: Atrophy alone is not the issue. Surgery 112:631–637
73. Deitch EA, Specian RD, Berg RD (1991) Endotoxin-induced bacterial translocation and mucosal permeability: Role of xanthine oxidase, complement activation, and macrophage products. Crit Care Med 19:785–791
74. Fink MP, Kaups KL, Wang H, Rothschild HR (1991) Maintenance of superior mesenteric arterial perfusion prevents increased intestinal mucosal permeability in endotoxic pigs. Surgery 110:154–161
75. Fink MP, Kaups KL, Wang H, Rothschild HR (1992) Ibuprofen improves survival but does not ameliorate increased gut mucosal permeability in endotoxic pigs. Arch Surg 127:49–54
76. Ferry DM, Butt TJ, Broom MF, Hunter J, Chadwick VS (1989) Bacterial chemotactic oligopeptides and the intestinal mucosal barrier. Gastroenterology 97:61–67
77. Lichtman SN, Okoruwa EE, Keku J, Schwab JH, Sartor RB (1992) Degradation of endogenous bacterial cell wall polymers by the muralytic enzyme mutanolysin prevents hepatobiliary injury in genetically susceptible rats with experimental intestinal bacterial overgrowth. J Clin Invest 90:1313–1322

78. Stimpson SA, Schwab JH, Janusz MJ, Anderle SK, Brown RR, Cromartie WJ (1986) Acute and chronic inflammation induced by peptidoglycan structures and polysaccharide complexes. In: Seidle PH, Schleifer KH (eds) Biological properties of peptidoglycan. Walter de Gruyter, Berlin, pp 273–290
79. O'Dwyer S, Michie HR, Zeigler TR, Revhaug A, Smith RJ, Wilmore DW (1988) A single dose of endotoxin increases intestinal permeability in healthy humans. Arch Surg 123:1459–1464
80. Ziegler TR, Smith RJ, O'Dwyer ST, Demling RH, Wilmore DW (1988) Increased intestinal permeability associated with infection in burn patients. Arch Surg 123:1313–1319
81. Deitch EA (1990) Intestinal permeability in burn patients shortly after injury. Surgery 107:411–416
82. Ryan CM, Yarmush ML, Burke JF, Tompkins RG (1992) Increase permeability early after burns correlates with the extent of burn injury. Crit Care Med 20:1508–1512
83. Harris CE, Griffiths RD, Freestone N, Billington D, Atherton ST, Macmillan RR (1992) Intestinal permeability in the critically ill. Intensive Care Med 18:38–41

Altering Bowel Contents with Lactulose and other Substances prevents Endotoxemia

P. A. M. van Leeuwen, M. A. Boermeester, and A. P. J. Houdijk

Introduction

Obstructive jaundice and liver disease are often complicated by severe infection or sepsis, especially after surgical procedures, reflected in a considerable percentage of mortality. This increased susceptibility to infection is considered to be caused by an impairment of the reticuloendothelial system (RES), together with an increased resorption of endotoxin from the gut [1].

Endotoxins are present in large quantities in the human gut without any harmful effects. The intestinal wall and associated immune system maintain an effective barrier between the gut lumen and the systemic circulation. Translocation of small amounts of endotoxins is regarded as physiological and can easily be cleared by a normal functioning RES [2, 3]. The RES of the liver is comprised mainly of the Kupffer cells, and provides a major fraction of the systemic phagocytic clearance. Impaired liver function, as seen in obstructive jaundice, cirrhosis and other liver diseases, is characterized by a diminished RES phagocytic function and depletion of opsonins (e.g. fibronectin).

A combination of an insufficient gut barrier and a depression of the RES can result in a systemic endotoxemia. Endotoxemia in turn results in organ dysfunction, further impairment of the gut mucosal barrier, and depression of the humoral and cellulair immune system [4–9]. Moreover, since the RES is also predominantly responsible for clearing the blood of procoagulant factors, and systemic endotoxins induce a microvascular procoagulant state, RES dysfunction can contribute to the development of excessive coagulation [10].

A transient depression of the RES is found following burn, trauma, surgery, and even anesthesia. However, a longer lasting depression is seen after liver resection and in obstructive jaundice [1, 11]. This chapter provides evidence that the systemic complications, seen after liver surgery and after surgery in obstructive jaundice, are related to gut-derived endotoxin, and can be prevented by preoperative treatment with an endotoxin-binding agent.

Gut Barrier Function

The gastrointestinal (GI) tract is traditionally viewed as a nutrient resorbing system. On the contrary, the gut barrier function against translocation of intraluminal bacteria and endotoxin to the systemic circulation was given less attention, but appears to be of similar importance. Integrity of the intestinal structures that preserve this barrier function determines whether translocation of endogenous bacteria or endotoxin can be prevented. Translocation of bacteria from the intestinal lumen does not normally occur in a healthy gut. However, very small amounts of gut-derived endotoxin can be detected in the portal vein of healthy humans. The integrity of the gut is maintained by a variety of barrier mechanisms, including the mechanical barrier of mucosa and mucus, an ecologic balance of normal intestinal microflora, immunological defense mechanisms, intestinal peristalsis, and intraluminal secretion of saliva, gastric and bile acids.

The maintenance of a normal cellular structure of the gut wall prevents transepithelial migration of particles from the intestinal lumen, and preservation of the tight junctions between the epithelial cells prevents movements through the paracellular channels. A thick mucus layer sustains this epithelial barrier function. The mucosal epithelium is a dynamic, rapidly dividing tissue, therefore highly dependent on adequate nutritional supply. Changes in composition, amount and even administration route of nutrition can easily affect the integrity of the mucosa. When the nutritional supply is insufficient, mucosal atrophy will follow, with a decrease in villus-crypt height and activity of brush border enzymes.

The normal equilibrium between the resident intestinal microorganisms prevents overgrowth of individual bacterial species. This internal protective mechanism of the normal gut flora against colonization of certain bacteria is termed "colonization resistance". The intestinal anaerobic population is mainly gut wall associated and attached to the mucosal cells by receptor binding. Disruption of the anaerobic layer exposed the binding sites to aerobic bacteria. Attachment of potential pathogenic aerobic bacteria to the mucosal surface is regarded as the initial event and a prerequisite in the pathogenesis of systemic infection [12].

Immunological defense mechanisms involve intraepithelial and lamina propria lymphocytes, lymphoid follicles, Peyer's patches, macrophages of the lamina propria and mesenteric lymph nodes (MLN). This intestinal immune system is referred to as gut associated lymphoid tissue (GALT). Peyer's patches are particularly important because of their antigen-sampling function through specialized M-cells. These sampled antigens are presented to lymphocytes within the Peyer's patch. Antigen-stimulated lymphocytes leave the intestinal tract, migrate through the MLN, the thoracic duct and reach the systemic circulation. After transforming into plasma cells, capable of IgA production, these cells "home back" to the intestinal tract, where IgA is secreted directly intraluminally and in bile. IgA can bind to bacteria or endotoxin and this complex is excreted in the faeces. This complicated process leads to development of an immune tolerance, suppressing unnecessary immune responses which could otherwise trigger an inflammatory response and lead to mucosal damage. The physiological translocation of minute amounts of endotoxin may well be part of this normal antigen-sampling process of

GALT. Besides a high concentration of IgA, bile is also important because of the capability of bile acids to bind endotoxin. Absence of bile acids during obstructive jaundice increases the risk for endotoxin translocation.

Critically ill patients are exposed to gut barrier compromising events, which attack one or more of the basic defense mechanisms. Impaired peristalsis, inhibition of gastric acids by H_2 receptor antagonists, antibiotics or parenteral nutrition (TPN) all can disturb the microbial balance. Moreover, sepsis, endotoxemia, shock, use of TPN or surgery, which commonly occur in these patients, all increase mucosal permeability, thus facilitating translocation of endotoxin [1, 13]. This increased permeability is most likely based on a decrease in mucosal blood flow. The intestinal mucosa is very sensitive to changes in blood flow. The entire mucosa accounts for 80% and the mucosal villus and crypt cells for 50–60% of the total intestinal flow, needed for their high metabolic activity [14], which explains their particular sensivity to hemodynamic changes. The gut mucosa is one of the first tissues to be affected by a decrease in arterial blood pressure [15]. The hairpin vascular loop in the villus, with close contact between arterioles en venules, allows stealing of oxygen to the venules before reaching the villus tip. As a response to stress, the oxygen delivery to vital organs, such as the brain and the heart, is preserved at the expense of other organs and tissues. The splanchnic blood flow is the major target for this compensatory response [16]. A recent study from our group examined organ blood flow in a jaundiced rat model. With the microsphere method, an analysis was made of organ blood flow 24 h after surgical stress. We [17] found a significant decreased blood flow through the small bowel, colon, pancreas and spleen in jaundiced rats compared to the control group. In contrast, blood flow through brain and heart was not affected. Clearly, these critically ill rats exhibit an impaired perfusion of the splanchnic bed to preserve flow through vital organs, when exposed to stress.

Hemodynamic instability and concomitant periods of hypotension are commonly observed in severely ill patients. During critical illness, hypotension and/or shock leads to the release of vasopressin and angiotensin, which causes splanchnic vasoconstriction, despite a markedly increased need for oxygen delivery [18]. Even a 10% loss of circulating plasma volume can result in a 40% reduction of splanchnic flow [19]. The gut mucosa is rapidly exposed to the effects of an inadequate blood and oxygen supply. Impaired mucosal oxygenation then will cause disruption of the mucosa. Additionally, ischemic mucosa is highly susceptible to the action of proteolytic enzymes present in the intestinal lumen. Translocation of endotoxin is promoted by an increased mucosal permeability associated with ischemic mucosal damage. When oxygen supply is restored during reperfusion, accumulating damage of the mucosa occurs due to formation of cytotoxic oxygen radicals. Oxygen radicals activate local neutrophils, which then release cytotoxic oxygen intermediates and proteolytic enzymes, again damaging the gut mucosa.

Therapeutic use of vasoactive agents like norepinephrine during systemic hypotension may contribute to vasoconstriction of intestinal blood vessels, causing a decreased splanchnic perfusion. Enteral nutritional intake is of major importance in the preservation of adequate intestinal blood flow. This effect is established by mechanical stimulation, secretion of pancreatic enzymes and bile acids, and by induction of an increased mucosal metabolism. Critically ill and postoperative patients are frequently regarded as intolerant for enteral intake and therefore receive TPN. TPN or rather absent luminal intake decreases intestinal blood flow. An additional compromising effect of TPN is caused by a concomittant decrease in bile secretion, which further decreases blood flow [14]. Absence of bile IgA and bile acids further impairs the patient's gut barrier function. Malnourishment of surgical or injured patients, in combination with hemodynamic instability and use of vasopressors, predispose these patients to exaggerated translocation of endotoxin.

An even more complicating event is observed by Deitch et al. [20] who found that translocation of bacterial particles leads to immune suppression of GALT cells. These results were confirmed by Mc Gee et al. [21] who demonstrated an increased proliferation of suppressor T lymphocytes in GALT caused by gut-derived endotoxin. The initially impaired gut barrier function in critically ill patients, who display mucosal damage, is thus compromised even more by the immunodepressive effects of translocating endotoxins on GALT. Moreover, this underlines the major importance of the hepatic RES, being the last defense line before entrance to the systemic circulation.

Endotoxin Translocation and the Reticuloendothelial System

Reticuloendothelial cells are found in the liver, spleen and bone marrow. The major part of these cells is compromised by the phagocytic cells lining the liver sinusoids. Endothelial cells and resident macrophages or Kupffer cells of the sinusoidal lining play a crucial role in the removal of particles from the portal blood. Sinusoidal endothelial cells have shown to inactive particles, especially immune complexes, as effectively as Kupffer cells by endocytosis. However, Kupffer cells are the major site of endotoxin detoxification. Phagocytosis of endotoxin by Kupffer cells involves binding to complement (C3) receptors. Kupffer cells reside in the liver for a few weeks and their population is restored from circulating monocytes. In response to injury or partial hepatectomy, Kupffer cells can divide and proliferate locally to restore the hepatic phagocytic function.

Translocation of physiological amounts of endogenous endotoxin may be important in stimulating the RES and maintaining normal phagocytic capacity [22]. Maintaining the integrity of the RES is essential to protect the host against gut-derived endotoxin. Chronic endotoxin administration has proven to stimulate the RES and to induce the development of tolerance to certain levels of endotoxin [23, 24]. However, high levels of portal endotoxin immediately result in a transient decrease in RES phagocytic capacity [24]. This depression lasts 12 to 18h, followed by a rapid recovery. Transient RES depression is most likely mediated by a decreased activity of C3 receptors on Kupffer cells, possibly due to endotoxin overload. Depression of the RES, as seen shortly after high portal levels of endotoxin, results in spillover of endotoxin to the systemic circulation. In addition, Marshall et al. [25] found evidence for an immunosuppressive influence of activated Kupffer cells on systemic immunity. This effect coincided with extraction of large numbers of pathogenic particles by the RES. Thus, depression of systemic immunity after an endotoxin challenge to the liver may result from spilled endotoxins and/or immunoregulatory effects of endotoxin-activated Kupffer cells. In conclusion, the early period after an endotoxin load appears to be critical towards the RES phagocytic function, as well as the systemic immunocompetent cells.

A transient depression of RES function is found in patients recovering from trauma, burn injury, major surgery or shock. These critically ill patients often display a decrease in hepatic blood flow up to 50%, which can be caused by systemic hypotension or shunting of blood from the splanchnic bed during normo-, hypo- or hyperdynamic responses [26]. An overload of endotoxin from the gut and a low hepatic flow both contribute to an impaired RES capacity and can easily result in systemic endotoxemia in these patients. Also liver failure, as seen in jaundiced or cirrhotic patients, leads to RES failure and enhances the ability of endotoxin to reach the systemic circulation. The effects of systemic spillover can be limited, though not completely abolished, by circulating serum proteins as BPI (bactericidal/permeability-increasing protein), LBP (LPS-binding protein) and HDL (high density lipoprotein), which can bind and inactivate endotoxin.

Within 24 h after the initial event, RES function is restored to normal or even elevated levels. Endotoxins are thought to prime the Kupffer cells of the RES during this second phase, resulting in a hyperreactive state of these cells. These primed Kupffer cells can rapidly produce large amounts of inflammatory mediators. Experimental work of Keller et al. [27] generated the idea that endotoxin-stimulated release of mediators by Kupffer cells impairs hepatocyte function. Normal acute phase protein synthesis, which is an important defensive reaction during inflammation, is subsequently decreased. Recent studies have revealed that binding of endotoxin to monocytes and macrophages involves specialized (CD14) receptors [28]. These receptors recognize complexes of LPS and LBP; in contrast to C3 receptors on macrophages which bind to complement-opsonized endotoxin. LBP-LPS complexes have an increased capacity, compared to LPS alone, to stimulate monocytes and macrophages. Binding of this complex to the CD14 receptors on the cell surface induces production of inflammatory mediators, like TNF and IL-1. Altered monocyte behavior in production of mediators is observed after massive tissue injury and during severe sepsis. A suppressed IL-1 and IL-8 production was found and correlated to the severity of the injury. The production of TNF and IL-6 was upregulated in these patients [29]. This characterizes the complexity of changes in mediator release after monocyte overactivation by excessive amounts of circulating endotoxin. Generally, initial

RES depression is followed by a hyperreactive state of the RES with release of inflammatory mediators, leading to a generalized inflammatory response. It is possible that depressed RES phagocytosis and increased induction of mediator production by Kupffer cells exist at the same time, but involve different receptor mechanisms. More research needs to be done in this area to unravel this complex process.

Hepatic Failure and Mortality after Liver Resection

We have summarized the results of experimental work that clearly indicate a relationship between hepatic RES function and endotoxin of gut origin. Major surgery in general results in an increased translocation of endotoxin across the gut wall to the portal vein and the MLN and in a depression of the RES [30–33]. Partial hepatectomy, which results in fewer hepatocytes and, even more important, fewer Kupffer cells, compromises the ability of the liver to clear endotoxin even further. Impaired functioning of the remnant liver after partial resection may be caused by systemic inflammatory responses.

We postulated that hepatic failure after liver resection is related to gut-derived endotoxemia. To test this concept we performed a series of experiments in which we manipulated the bowel endotoxin contents. Male Wistar rats (220–230 grams) were randomized to receive oral gavage twice daily with endotoxin-binding or-reducing drugs: 1) neomycin/cefazolin; 2) lactulose; and 3) cholestyramine; control rats received saline. After 7 days of gavage, the animals were subjected to either a 70% partial hepatectomy or a SHAM operation. At time 0 (preresection), 10, 20 and 30 h (after resection) aortic blood was obtained for determination of ammonia, glutamine and en-

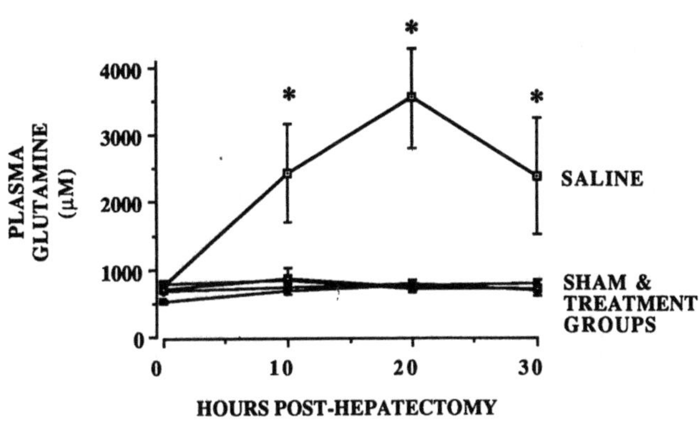

Fig. 1. Plasma glutamine concentrations in conventional rats after hepatectomy or SHAM operation. (mean ± SEM)
*$p < 0.05$ saline-treated hepatectomized vs SHAM and treatment groups (two factor ANOVA, linear contrast)

dotoxin levels. In selected animals, portal vein or inferior caval blood was obtained to evaluate the glutamine and ammonia exchange across the intestine and hind limb. Germ-free rats also underwent a partial hepatectomy or SHAM operation, and blood was obtained for glutamine and ammonia exchange at 0 and 20h. Results show that liver resection in the saline pretreated rats elicited a six fold increase in plasma glutamine (Fig. 1), a significant increase in glutamine uptake and ammonia release by the gut, concomittant with an increased release of glutamine from the hind limb (Table 1). The mortality rate in this group was 40%. Pretreatment with the various drugs reduced systemic endotoxemia and maintained normal glutamine and ammonia levels. Additionally, no deaths occurred in the three treated groups. Germ-free rats showed similar values as seen in treated groups.

These results suggest that intestinal bacteria and endotoxin play an important role in the pathophysiology of postresection hepatic failure and catabolic responses. These observations can be explained by the following mechanisms. After liver resection, a functional local inflammatory response provides for an adequate stimulus for liver regeneration. Endotoxin plays a leading role in this regenerative process. A study by Cornell [34] demonstrated that binding of intestinal endotoxin with cholestyramine decreased the hepatic regenerative activity. Thus, endotoxin from the gut seems to amplify liver regeneration. Kupffer cells of the remnant liver are in a primed state shortly after liver resection, reflected in the release of large amounts of TNF, which is a potent stimulus for the hepatocyte DNA synthesis [35, 36]. The local endotoxin-induced inflammatory response with concomittant increased TNF production by Kupffer cells may be essential for a rapid recovery of the liver capacity. However, an overshoot of endotoxin exaggerates the inflammatory response, leads to hepatic failure, and elicits systemic effects like catabolism. This results in muscle proteolysis with accelerated release of glutamine from muscle stores.

During sepsis, plasma glutamine levels are only slightly higher due to the enormous compensating capacity of the liver [37]. This capacity for glutamine uptake is diminished after liver resection, resulting in high plasma concentrations. Gut utilization of glutamine increases as plasma levels become

Table 1. Arterial-venous differences post-hepatectomy

	N	Saline	Cholestyramine
Arterial-Portal Glutamine (microM)	7	540±96[a]	213±12
Arterial-Portal Ammonia (microg/ml)	6	−5.9±1.2[a]	−2.4±0.4
Arterial-hind limb Glutamine (microM)	6	−379±150[a]	−66±16

[a] $p<0.05$ saline vs cholestyramine by unpaired t-test
− (minus) = release

elevated, leading to a high production of ammonia by the gut mucosa. Under normal circumstances, ammonia is efficiently cleared from the blood and converted to urea by the liver. However, the ability of the resected liver to convert ammonia to urea is also impaired, resulting in high systemic ammonia concentrations and progressive ammonia intoxication. Pretreatment with endotoxin-binding or -reducing agents blunts the catabolic response and enhances survival.

The Effect of Liver Resection on Immune Function

Secondary infection is a leading cause of mortality in patients who are recovering from major surgery. A compromised functioning of the immune system shortly after traumatic injury, including burn injury and major surgery, renders these patients susceptible to infection [38–40]. An intact cellular immune response is apparently required for adequate resistance to infection, since clinical anergy, a reflection of deficient T lymphocyte responsiveness, is associated with an increased risk of sepsis in surgically traumatized patients [41].

Over the last decade, experimental work indicated that endotoxin is the primary mediator of this posttraumatic immunosuppression. This concept is fortified by the results of a recent study, in which administration of a small dosis of endotoxin to healthy volunteers could elaborate a cellular immunosuppression [42]. Moreover, Polymyxin B, a known endotoxin-binding drug, was able to preserve immune function in burn patients [43]. In the liver-resected patient, alterations in the intestinal mucosal barrier may allow large amounts of endotoxin to enter the circulation. It is unclear whether alterations of cell-mediated immunity after major surgery promote systemic endotoxemia and further amplify translocation of endotoxin, or, alternatively, whether excessive endotoxin translocation in turn elicits immunosuppression.

In the present study, we monitored *ex vivo* immune function after major liver resection, since the loss of part of the hepatic RES adds to the already compromised cell-mediated immunity of the patient. Male Wistar rats were randomized in treated and non-treated groups. After a 7-day period of oral gavage with cholestyramine or saline, rats of each group were subjected to either a 70% partial hepatectomy or a SHAM operation, Twenty-four hours later the spleen was removed in order to harvest spleen cells. A mixed population of spleen cells was subsequently stimulated by the T-cell mitogens PHA (phytohemagglutinin) and Con-A (concanavalin A), and by LPS, predominantly a B-cell mitogen. Proliferative responses were determined by measurement of ^{3}H thymidine incorporation. Liver surgery clearly resulted in a significant depression of response to PHA, Con A and LPS of, respectively, 72.6±7.6, 22.9±7.5, and 53.2±9.6% compared to SHAM values, indicating a depression of both T- and B-cell immune function (Fig. 2, 3 and 4). Responses of cholestyramine-treated SHAM rats were not significantly differ-

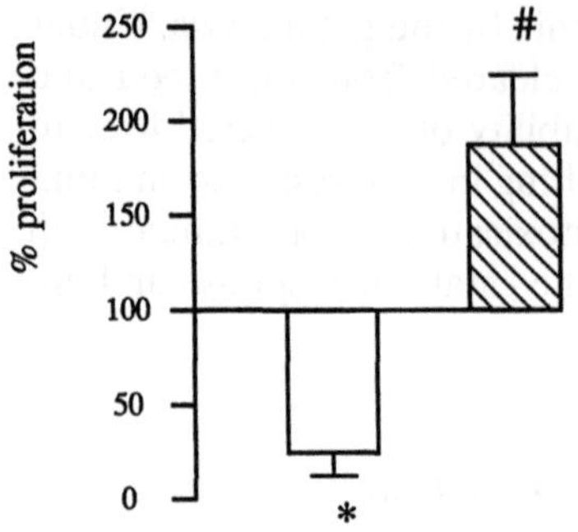

Fig. 2. Proliferative response of total spleen cells to PHA mitogen, expressed as percentage proliferation (mean ± SEM) of saline-treated (HEP-SAL, open bars) and cholestyramine-treated (HEP-CHOL, hatched bars) rats after partial hepatectomy. Mean proliferation measured in saline-SHAM rats was set at a 100% level. Percentage proliferation for each hepatectomized rat: [response to mitogen (cpm) less background/mean response to mitogen (cpm) less background for all saline-SHAM rats] × 100.
*$p < 0.0001$ HEP-SAL vs SHAM. #$p < 0.001$ HEP-CHOL vs HEP-SAL; p = ns HEP-CHOL vs SHAM (ANOVA)

ent from saline-SHAM rats, and are therefore not shown. The proliferative responses of the cholestyramine-treated hepatectomized rats were highly significantly enhanced compared to the saline-treated hepatectomized rats, and were comparable to SHAM values (Fig. 2, 3 and 4).

These data show that liver surgery can result in an impairment of cellular and humoral immunity, and may well explain the postoperative infections seen in these patients. Pretreatment with cholestyramine prevented immunosuppression after liver resection, accomplishing an adequate (slightly, though not significantly enhanced) proliferative response of lymphocytes to the various mitogens. Moreover, preservation of immune functions through binding

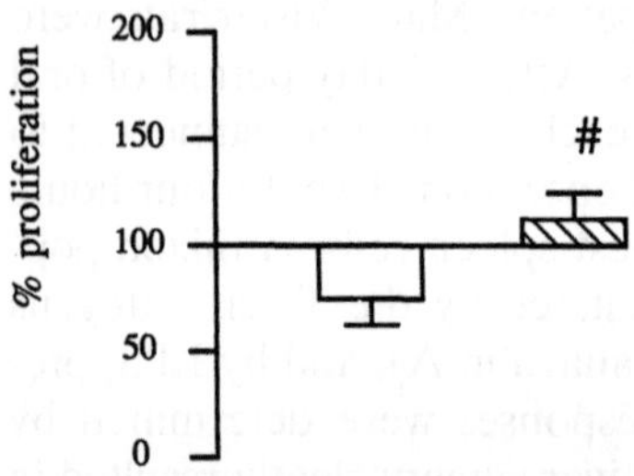

Fig. 3. Proliferative response of total spleen cells to ConA mitogen, expressed as percentage proliferation (mean ± SEM) of saline-treated (HEP-SAL, open bars) and cholestyramine-treated (HEP-CHOL, hatched bars) rats after partial hepatectomy vs SHAM 100% level.
#$p < 0.01$ HEP-CHOL vs HEP-SAL; p = ns HEP-CHOL vs SHAM (ANOVA)

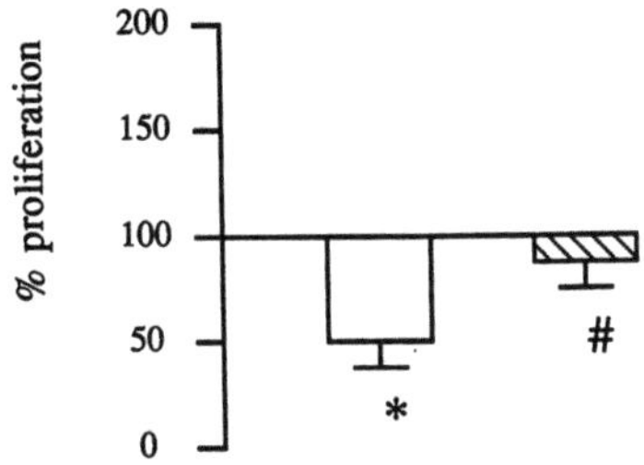

Fig. 4. Proliferative response of total spleen cells to LPS, expressed as percentage proliferation (mean ± SEM) of saline-treated (HEP-SAL, open bars) and cholestyramine-treated (HEP-CHOL, hatched bars) rats after partial hepatectomy vs SHAM 100% level. *$p<0.0005$ HEP-SAL vs SHAM. #$p<0.05$ HEP-CHOL vs HEP-SAL; p = ns HEP-CHOL vs SHAM (ANOVA)

of intestinal endotoxin with cholestyramine indicates that translocation of gut-derived endotoxin is of major importance in the pathogenesis of postsurgical immunosuppression.

Hemodynamic Disturbances following Surgery in Obstructive Jaundice

Surgery in patients with obstructive jaundice is associated with an overall mortality of 16%. In 9% of such patients, acute renal failure develops which increases mortality rates to 75% [44]. Renal failure in postoperative patients with obstructive jaundice is correlated with hemodynamic disturbances, finally resulting in hypotension, shock, and reduced renal blood flow [45, 46]. In addition, several authors have shown the occurrence of systemic endotoxemia in the presence of renal failure in obstructive jaundice and suggested a causative relation [47, 48].

In a recent study, performed at our institute, the relationship between gut-derived endotoxemia, hemodynamic disturbances and renal failure in obstructive jaundice was investigated. In order to prevent endotoxemia, male Wistar rats received cholestyramine (CHOL) twice daily by oral gavage; control rats received saline (SAL). This treatment was continued until the end of the experiment. On day 7, the groups were randomized to receive a bile duct ligation (BDL) or a SHAM operation. This resulted in 4 groups i.e. SHAM-SAL, SHAM-CHOL, BDL-SAL, and BDL-CHOL. On day 20, all rats were subjected to a surgical trauma by means of a xyphoidectomy. The following day, systemic hemodynamics and organ blood flows were measured using the radiolabelled microsphere technique.

Compared to SHAM animals (SHAM-SAL and SHAM-CHOL combined because of comparable results) profound alterations were observed in systemic hemodynamics in the BDL-SAL group (Table 2). Despite a compensatory increase in cardiac output (CO), mean arterial pressure (MAP) was

Table 2. Systemic hemodynamics

	SHAM (n=20)	BDL-SAL (n=10)	BDL-CHOL (n=10)
CO, ml/min	85.5±4.8[a]	98.9±2.8[d]	115.7±4.6[g]
MAP, mmHg	121±5[b]	106±3[e]	119±4
HR, bpm	358±9[c]	304±9[f]	332±8[h]

SHAM vs BDL-SAL [a] $p<0.05$, [b] $p<0.05$, [c] $p<0.001$. BDL-SAL vs BDL-CHOL [d] $p<0.01$, [e] $p<0.05$, [f] $p<0.05$. BDL-CHOL vs SHAM [g] $p<0.0005$, [h] $p<0.05$.
(mean±SEM) (Student's T-test using the Bonferroni correction for multiple comparisons).

Table 3. Renal blood flow

	SHAM	BDL-SAL	BDL-CHOL
RBF, ml/min/g	6.56±0.50	4.41±0.40[a]	5.65±0.42[c]
Total RBF, ml/min	14.78±0.63	11.24±0.95[b]	14.58±0.73[d]

BDL-SAL vs SHAM [a] $p<0.01$, [b] $p<0.01$. BDL-CHOL vs BDL-SAL [c] $p<0.05$, [d] $p<0.01$.
(Student's T-test using the Bonferroni correction for multiple comparisons). (mean±SEM).

significantly reduced due to a significant decrease in heart rate (HR). In contrast, BDL-CHOL rats had a normal MAP resulting from an increase in HR and CO. Renal blood flow tissue was significantly reduced in BDL-SAL rats compared to the SHAM group, while cholestyramine prevented this decrease, thus preserving normal renal blood flow (Table 3). Also, total renal blood flow showed a significant reduction; cholestyramine, although, preserved total flow at SHAM levels.

These data demonstrate that factors closely related to renal organ failure following surgery in obstructive jaundice, namely hypotension and reduced renal blood flow, can be prevented by pretreatment with the gut-endotoxin binder cholestyramine. Endotoxin of gut origin should be considered the major factor in the etiology of postoperative hemodynamic alterations in obstructive jaundice.

Conclusion

These data demonstrate clearly that breakdown of both the mucosal barrier and the RES capacity can result in systemic disturbances, likely to be induced by gut-derived endotoxemia. Surgery itself can impair intestinal defense mechanisms against intraluminal bacteria and their endotoxins. However, a normal functioning RES, in collaboration with systemic defense mechanisms like the serum proteins LPB and HDL, is capable of clearing this overshoot of endotoxin.

Depression of the RES, as seen in obstructive jaundice, compromises the host defense mechanisms against systemic spillover of endotoxin. Complications like renal failure are clearly related to gut-derived systemic endotoxins, and are prevented by pretreatment with endotoxin binders. The same mechanism applies for the postoperative complications seen after liver surgery. Secondary infections still account for a high percentage of morbidity and mortality in the postoperative period following liver surgery, and are likely to be related to endotoxins originating from the gut. The effect of liver resection on the intestinal barrier has not been thoroughly studied, though it is conceivable that the local inflammatory response, which triggers liver regeneration and is induced by activated macrophages, results in a significant production of TNF. This TNF release may well cause a major disruption of the intestinal mucosa, increase intestinal oxygen extraction rate and decrease mucosal flow. These effects enhance translocation of endotoxin, which in turn amplifies TNF production by Kupffer cells and depresses the immune system, resulting in an exaggerated inflammatory response with increased catabolism and coagulation-fibrinolysis disturbances.

Future therapeutic strategies should concentrate on prevention of postoperative complications by treatment with endotoxin binding agents before the triggering event. This implicates that preoperative treatment should be preferred, preventing the majority of expensive postoperative therapeutic interventions and intensive care. In addition, early postoperative feeding through the enteral route should be given more attention. Starvation combined with endotoxin-triggering moments due to surgical stress aggravates translocation of endotoxin to MLN, liver and spleen. Especially protein malnutrition, but also TPN, leads to an impaired gut mucosal barrier and decreased primary immune responses. Pretreatment with endotoxin binders for at least a week prior to major surgery, combined with early enteral feeding after the operation, could prevent the majority of postoperative complications and reduce the number of hospitalization days.

References

1. Van Leeuwen PAM, Boermeester MA, Houdijk APJ, et al (1993) Clinical significance of translocation. Gut (in press)
2. Jacob AI, Goldberg PH, Bloom D, Degenshein GA, Korin PJ (1977) Endotoxin and bacteria in portal blood. Gastroenterology 72:1268–1270
3. Nolan JP (1981) Endotoxin, RES function and liver injury. Hepatology 1:458–465
4. Bradfield JWB (1973) Control of spillover. The importance of Kupffer cell function in clinical medicine. Lancet 2:883–886
5. Sullivan BJ, Swallow CJ, Girotti MJ, Rotstein OD (1991) Bacterial translocation induces procoagulant activity in tissue macrophages. A potential mechanism for end-organ dysfunction. Arch Surg 126:586–590

6. O'Dwyer ST, Michie HR, Ziegler TR, Revhaug A, Smith RJ, Wilmore DW (1988) A single dose of endotoxin increases intestinal permeability in healthy humans. Arch Surg 123:1459–1464
7. Deitch EA, Berg RD, Specian R (1987) Endotoxin promotes the translocation of bacteria from the gut. Arch Surg 122:185–190
8. Van Deventer SJH, Ten Cate JW, Tytgat GNJ (1988) Intestinal endotoxemia. Gastroenterology 94:825–831
9. Rodrick ML, Grbic JT, Moss N, et al (1987) Endotoxin in vivo may cause a functional blockade of in vitro cellular immune responses. Surg Forum 38:98–100
10. Kaplan JE (1980) The role of the reticuloendothelial system in control of hemostatic and thrombotic mechanisms. In: Altura BM, Saba TM (eds) Pathophysiology of the reticuloendothelial system. Raven Press, New York, pp 111–131
11. Greve JW, Gouma DJ, Soeters PB, Buurman WA (1990) Suppression of cellular immunity on obstructive jaundice is caused by endotoxins. Gastroenterology 98:478–485
12. Beachey EH (1981) Bacterial adherence adhesin-receptor interactions mediating the attachment of bacteria to mucosal surfaces. J Infect Dis 143:325–345
13. Deitch EA (1990) The role of intestinal barrier failure and bacterial translocation in the development of systemic infection and multiple organ failure. Arch Surg 125:403–404
14. Granger DN, Richardson PDI, Kvietys PR, Mortillaro NA (1980) Intestinal blood flow. Gastroenterology 78:837–863
15. Nelson DP, King CE, Dodd SL, Schumacker PT, Cain SM (1987) Systemic and intestinal limits of O_2 extraction in the dog. J Appl Physiol 63:387–394
16. Antonsson JB, Fiddian-Green RG (1991) The role of the gut and multiple system organ failure. Eur J Surg 157:3–12
17. Houdijk APJ, Van Leeuwen PAM, Van Lambalgen AA, Bading JR, Boermeester MA, Wesdorp RIC (1993) Preoperative enteral cholestyramine prevents hemodynamic disturbances following surgery in obstructive jaundice (in press)
18. McNeill JR, Stark RD, Greeway CV (1970) Intestinal vasoconstriction after hemorrhage: Roles of vasopressin and angiotensin. Am J Physiol 219:1342–1347
19. Gilmour DG, Aitkenhead AR, Hothersall AP, et al (1980) The effect of hypovolemia on colon blood flow in the dog. Br J Surg 67:82–87
20. Deitch EA, Xu D, Qi X, Berg RD (1991) Bacterial translocation from the gut impairs systemic immunity. Surgery 109:269–276
21. Mc Ghee JR, Kiyono H, Alley CD (1984) Gut bacterial endotoxin: Influence on gut-associated lymphoreticular tissue and host immune function. Surv Immunol Res 3:241–252
22. Steffan AM, Hirn A (1986) C3 mediated phagocytosis induced in murine Kupffer cells by in vitro activation with endotoxin. Gastro Clin Biol 10:117–121
23. Richards PS, Saba TM (1985) Effect of endotoxin on fibronectin and Kupffer cell activity. Hepatology 5:32–37
24. Loegering DJ, Schneidkraut MJ (1979) Effect of endotoxin on alpha-2-SB-opsonic protein activity and reticuloendothelial system phagocytic function. J Reticuloendothel Soc 26:197–204
25. Marshall JC, Lee C, Meakins JL, Michel RP, Christou NV (1987) Kupffer cell modulation of the systemic immune response. Arch Surg 122:191–196
26. Walvatne G, Cerra FB (1990) Hepatic dysfunction in multiple organ failure. In: Deitch EA (ed) Multiple organ failure. Pathophysiology and basic concepts of therapy. Thieme, New York, pp 241–260
27. Keller GA, West MA, Cerra FB, Simmons RL (1985) Multiple systems organ failure. Modulation of hepatocyte protein synthesis by endotoxin activated Kupffer cells. Ann Surg 201:87–95
28. Ulevitch RJ, Mathison JC, Schumann RR, Tobias PS (1990) A new model of macrophage stimulation by bacterial lipopolysaccharide. J Trauma 30:189–192
29. Faist E, Storck M, Hultner L, et al (1992) Functional analysis of monocyte activity through synthesis patterns of proinflammatory cytokines and neopterin in patients in surgical intensive care. Surgery 112:562–572

30. Van Leeuwen PAM, Hong RW, Rounds JD, Rodrick ML, Wilmore DW (1991) Hepatic failure and coma after liver resection is reversed by manipulation of gut contents: The role of endotoxin. Surgery 110:169–175
31. Nakagawa K, Matsubara S, Ouchi K, Owada Y, Yajima Y (1986) Endotoxemia after abdominal surgery. Tohoku J Exp Med 150:273–280
32. Schildt BW (1970) Function of RES after thermal and mechanical trauma in mice. Acta Chir Scand 136:359–364
33. Saba TM (1975) RES systemic host defense after surgery and traumatic shock. Circ Shock 2:91–108
34. Cornell RP (1985) Restriction of gut-derived endotoxin impairs DNA synthesis for liver regeneration. Am J Physiol 249:R563–R569
35. Satoh A, Adachi K, Yamazaki M, Mizuno D (1991) TNF-driven inflammation during mouse liver regeneration after partial hepatectomy and its role in growth regulation of liver. Mol Biother 3:136–147
36. Feingold KR, Barker ME, Jones AL, Grunfeld C (1991) Localization of tumor necrosis factor-stimulated DNA synthesis in the liver. Hepatology 13:773–779
37. Souba WW, Herskowitz K, Salloum RM (1990) Gut glutamine metabolism. JPEN 14:45–50
38. Slade MS, Simmons RL, Yunis E, et al (1975) Immunodepression after major surgery in normal patients. Surgery 78:363–372
39. Christou NV, Mannick JA, West MA, Kasper DL (1987) Cellular immune dysfunction in response to injury. Arch Surg 122:240–241
40. Wolfe JHN, Wu AVO, O'Connor NE, Saporoschetz I, Mannick JA (1982) Anergy, immunosuppressive serum, and impaired lymphocyte blastogenesis in burn patients. Arch Surg 117:1266–1271
41. Moss N, Gough DB, Jordan A, Grbic JT, Rodrick ML, Mannick JA (1988) Correlation of susceptibility to sepsis with suppression of cell mediated immunity. Surgery 104:882–887
42. Rodrick ML, Michie HR, Moss NM, et al (1989) In vivo infusion of a single dose of endotoxin in healthy humans causes in vitro alterations of both T-cell and adherent cell functions. In: Faist E (ed) Host defense dysfunction in trauma shock and sepsis. Springer-Verlag, Berlin Heidelberg, pp 475–483
43. Munster AM, Winchurch RA, Thupari JM, Ernst CB (1986) Reversal of postburn immunosuppression with low-dose Polymyxin B. Br J Trauma 26:995–998
44. Wait RB, Kahng KU (1989) Renal failure complicating obstructive jaundice. Am J Surg 157:256–263
45. Green J, Beyar R, Bomzon L, Finberg JPM, Better OS (1984) Jaundice, the circulation and the kidney. Nephrol 37:145–152
46. Wardle EN, Wright NA (1970) Endotoxin and acute renal failure associated with obstructive jaundice. Br Med J 4:472–474
47. Bailey ME (1976) Endotoxin, bile salts and renal function in obstructive jaundice. Br J Surg 63:774–778
48. Wilkinson SP, Moodie H, Stamatakis JD, Kakkar VV, Williams R (1976) Endotoxemia and renal failure in cirrhosis and obstructive jaundice. Br Med J 2:1415–1418

Metabolic Support: Modulation of Purine Metabolism

J. M. Boeynaems

Introduction

As the major substrate of energy-consuming reactions, ATP plays a key role in cell metabolism. Hypoxia and ischemia impair the mitochondrial process of oxidative phosphorylation, resulting in a net catabolism of ATP. A primary goal of metabolic support should thus be the preservation of cellular ATP levels. One possible strategy is the enhancement of natural homeostatic mechanisms designed to decrease energy demand and to increase energy supply. At least 3 of these mechanisms involve purines themselves. The drop in cell ATP and the accompanying rise in ADP result in the allosteric activation of phosphofructokinase, a key enzyme in the glycolytic pathway, which under hypoxia, provides an alternative to oxidative phosphorylation as a source of ATP. This reciprocal change also induces the opening of a particular set of K^+ channels, resulting in hyperpolarization and decreased activity of excitable cells. AMP, which accumulates inside hypoxic cells, activates a specific AMP-dependent protein kinase which inhibits key enzymes in the biosynthesis of fatty acids and cholesterol. Finally, ATP catabolism leads to the accumulation of adenosine in the interstitial fluid. Activation of A_1 adenosine receptors reduces the O_2 demand of neurons and cardiomyocytes, whereas O_2 supply is increased via the activation of vascular A_2 adenosine receptors. Several pharmacological tools are becoming available to enhance these physiological mechanisms of protection: K^+ channels openers, adenosine analogues, blockers of adenosine uptake, inhibitors of adenosine deaminase and allosteric enhancers of adenosine receptors. A number of animal studies indicate that these agents may indeed exert a cardio- and neuroprotective action.

Adenine Nucleotides and the Energetic Status of the Cell

Under normal basal conditions, the generàtion of ATP, by oxidative phosphorylation and glycolysis, equals its consumption by various reactions catalyzed by ATPases and kinases. The cellular levels of the various adenine nucleotides have roughly the following values:

- [ATP]: 5 mM
- [ADP]: 1 mM
- [AMP]: 0.15 mM.

The terminal phosphate groups of both ATP and ADP have a large standard energy of hydrolysis (7.3 kcal/mol), whereas the single phosphate group in AMP contains much less energy (3.4 kcal/mol). From an energetic point of view, it is thus useful to quantitate the distribution of the various nucleotides in the adenylate system with the so-called "energy charge" index, which has the following value:

$$0.5\,\frac{[\mathrm{ADP}]+2[\mathrm{ATP}]}{[\mathrm{AMP}]+[\mathrm{ADP}]+[\mathrm{ATP}]}$$

If all the adenine nucleotides in the cell would be ATP, the energy charge would have a theoretical value of 1. In general cells have an energy charge of about 0.85. If the cell capacity to generate ATP does no longer meet its consumption, there will be a net catabolism ATP (Fig. 1). The energy charge will fall, as ADP and AMP accumulate. Furthermore, AMP will be degraded into adenosine by a cytosolic 5'-nucleotidase which is activated allosterically by ADP [1]. This allosteric regulation results in a more-than-linear increase in adenosine formation rate when ATP falls.

ATP-dependent Potassium Channels

The opposite allosteric regulatory effects of ATP and ADP on several enzymes are well known. In particular, phosphofructokinase, a key enzyme in the glycolytic pathway, is activated by ADP and inhibited by ATP. This regulatory mechanism is responsible for the reciprocal relationship between oxidative phosphorylation and glycolysis. The inhibition of glucose consump-

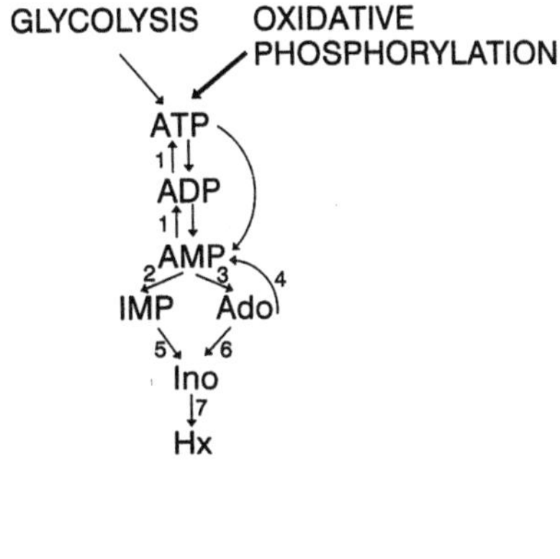

Fig. 1. Cellular metabolism of ATP. ATP is produced mainly by oxidative phosphorylation and to a lesser extent by glycolysis. It can also be resynthesized from ADP by adenylate kinase (1). Other enzymes on the diagram include: (2) AMP deaminase, (3) 5: 5′-nucleotidases, (4) adenosine kinase, (6) adenosine deaminase, and (7) purine nucleoside phosphorylase. Ado = adenosine; Ino = inosine; Hx = hypoxanthine

tion by oxygen consumption is known as the Pasteur effect. Conversely under anaerobiosis and during hypoxia, there is a compensatory increase in the rate of glycolysis. More recently, another homeostatic mechanism was identified: a subset of membrane K^+ channels are regulated reciprocally by ATP and ADP [2]. They open when ATP falls and/or when ADP rises. These channels will thus open under conditions of hypoxia and ischemia. The resulting hyperpolarization will reduce the electrical activity of excitable cells. In the heart, the mechanical activity and hence the energy demand will be decreased [3]. In addition of being regulated by the ATP/ADP ratio, these channels are the target of pharmacological agents: they are closed by sulfonylureas and opened by the potassium channels openers, such as pinacidil and chromakalim. The potential cardioprotective action of these last agents will be discussed later.

AMP-activated Protein Kinase

Like ADP, AMP produces an allosteric activation of some key enzymes in cell metabolism, such as phosphofructokinase. In addition, at least one regulatory mechanism specific for AMP has been identified [4]. AMP activates a protein kinase which phosphorylates and thereby inactivates two key enzymes in lipid biosynthesis: acetyl CoA carboxylase and 3-hydroxy-3-methylglutaryl-CoA reductase involved in the synthesis of fatty acids and cholesterol, respectively. By reducing the synthesis of lipids, the AMP-activated protein kinase will decrease the energy demand under hypoxia or ischemia.

Control of Adenosine Concentration in the Interstitial Fluid

Various factors interplay to control the concentration of adenosine in the interstitial fluid:

- adenosine is formed from AMP by the action of a *5'-nucleotidase*, either in the cytosol or extracellularly on the surface of the plasma membrane;
- adenosine is transported across the plasma membrane by a process of facilitated diffusion mediated by a *nucleoside transporter* which can operate in both directions; this transporter is inhibited by various pharmacological agents (dipyridamole, dilazep, mioflazine ,..);
- inside the cells, adenosine is transformed either into AMP by *adenosine kinase* or into inosine by *adenosine deaminase*; adenosine kinase can be inhibited by 5'-amino-5'-deoxyadenosine, and adenosine deaminase by 2'-deoxycoformycin; and
- interstitial adenosine is also degraded into inosine by an extracellular form of adenosine deaminase and it is washed away by the blood flow via uptake into endothelial cells.

Several mechanisms can lead to the appearance of adenosine in the interstitial fluid. One mechanism involves the release of ATP /and or ADP from cells followed by their sequential degradation by ectonucleotidases (ecto-ATPase, ecto-ADPase, 5'-nucleotidase) localized on the cell surface. This mechanism operates in various circumstances:

- during synaptic transmission, the ATP co-stored in vesicles with amines and other neurotransmitters is released by exocytosis [5–7] (Fig. 2);
- aggregating platelets release by exocytosis the content of their dense granules, which includes huge amounts of both ATP and ADP [8] (Fig. 3); and
- vascular endothelial cells may release part of their cytosolic ATP by a process of selective permeabilization, for instance when the shear stress exerted by the blood flow is increased [9].

Other mechanisms might operate in case of ischemia and hypoxia. Two possibilities have been proposed: either adenosine is formed intracellularly from AMP by the cytosolic 5'-nucleotidase [1] and released via the nucleoside transporter [10], or it is formed extracellularly from released AMP by the action of 5'-nucleotidase on the cell surface [11]. Initial studies in the perfused isolated guinea pig heart showed that the hypoxia-induced release of adenosine into the perfusate was decreased during perfusion of an inhibitor of nucleoside transport. These results were taken as evidence that adenosine is formed inside the cardiomyocytes and released in the interstitium via the nucleoside transporter [10]. Another interpretation of these data is

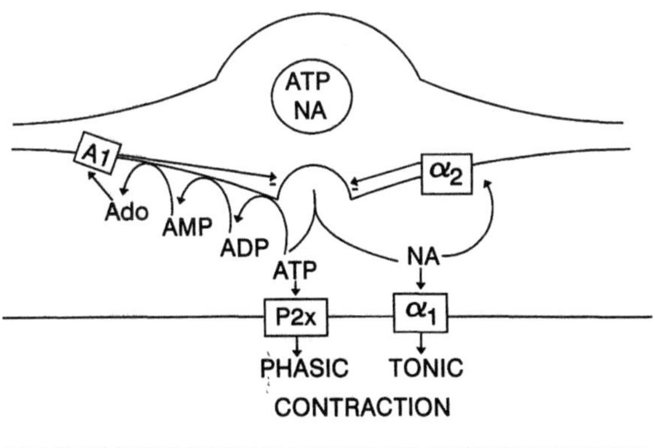

Fig. 2. Role of ATP and adenosine in neurotransmission. ATP is colocalized with amines (for instance in orthosympathetic varicosities) or acetylcholine. At the junction with smooth muscle, both ATP and noradrenaline are cotransmitters involved respectively in phasic and tonic contraction. The sequential degradation of ATP by ectonucleotidases generates adenosine which acts on presynaptic A_1 receptors to inhibit transmitter release. (From [5] with permission)

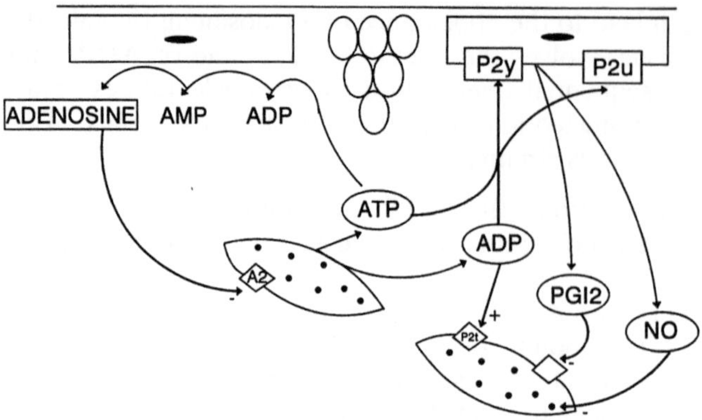

Fig. 3. Role of ATP in the platelet-endothelium interaction. Huge amounts of ATP and ADP are contained in the dense granules of platelets from which they are released during aggregation. ADP recruits additional platelets. ATP and ADP are sequentially degraded by endothelial ectonucleotidases, which ultimately generate adenosine which inhibits platelet aggregation via A_2 receptors. Finally, ATP and ADP activate endothelial receptors to induce the release of both prostacyclin and nitric oxide (NO) which synergize to inhibit platelet aggregation. That feedback mechanism will limit the extent of intravascular platelet aggregation and help localize thrombus formation to areas of endothelial damage

that adenosine is formed in the heart interstitial fluid and that nucleoside transport inhibitors do inhibit the release of adenosine into the perfusate by blocking the uptake into endothelial cells, and not by preventing the release from cardiomyocytes [11] (Fig. 4).

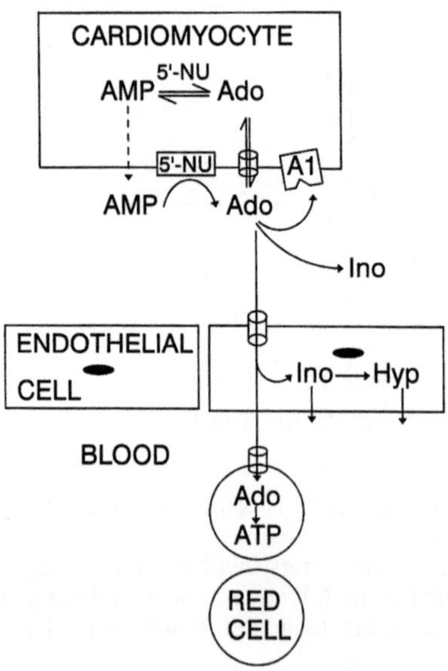

Fig. 4. Accumulation of adenosine in the myocardial interstitial fluid. Adenosine is formed from AMP either intracellularly or extracellularly. It is degraded by adenosine deaminase into inosine. Its uptake into endothelial cells precedes its washout in circulating blood, where it accumulates inside red cells

Whatever the mechanism of its appearance, microdialysis experiments have demonstrated the accumulation of adenosine in the interstitial fluid of the ventricular myocardium, during coronary ischemia in dogs [12]. A more than 10-fold increase, up to 10 μM was observed following coronary occlusion. Similar results have been obtained in cerebral ischemia and hypoxia. Under normal conditions, the concentration of adenosine in rat cortex perfusates and in cerebrospinal fluid was about 50nM [13]. It increased up to 30-fold following hypoxia. The measurement of plasma adenosine is subject to artifacts, involving rapid uptake into endothelial cells and erythrocytes, degradation by adenosine deaminase and *ex vivo* formation from ATP and ADP released by aggregating platelets. When heparinized blood from healthy volunteers is incubated at 37°C, the half-life of adenosine is about 1 sec [14]. By the way, this ultra-short half-life excludes an hormonal role for adenosine, which can only act as a local mediator. Feldman et al. [15] recently reported measurements of adenosine in coronary sinus blood, collected with a double-lumen metabolic catheter allowing blood to be mixed with a stop solution at the catheter tip. The stop solution contained dipyridamole (in order to block exchanges of adenosine across cell membranes), erythro-9(2-hydroxy-3-nonyl)-adenine (EHNA, an inhibitor of adenosine deaminase) and α,β-methylene-adenosine 5'-diphosphate (an inhibitor of 5'-nucleotidase) in addition to heparin and EDTA. With this method, the baseline value was 0.13 μM. During atrial pacing, this value did not change significantly in normal subjects, but was doubled in patients with coronary artery disease.

Adenosine Receptors and Metabolic Control

At least 5 subtypes of adenosine receptors have been cloned and sequenced in the last 3 years: A_1 receptors [16], A_{2a} receptors [17], 2 isoforms of A_{2b} receptors expressed in fibroblasts and brain, respectively [18], and A_3 receptors [19]. All these receptors are structurally related and belong to the superfamily of receptors which are coupled to G proteins and contain 7 transmembrane domains. A_3 receptors, expressed mostly in testis, have pharmacological properties quite different from all the other subtypes and their function remains a mystery [19]. A_{2a} receptors, which are responsive to nM concentrations of adenosine, are expressed selectively in the striatum, where they play a role in the control of dopaminergic transmission. Only A_1 and A_{2b} receptors are relevant in terms of metabolic control. A_1 receptors are coupled via G_i protein to at least 3 distinct effector mechanisms: inhibition of adenylate cyclase, opening of K^+ channels, and closure of Ca^{2+} channels [20]. Opening of K^+ channels explains why adenosine decreases heart rate and conduction, whereas the inhibition of neurotransmitter release by adenosine results from the closure of Ca^{2+} channels. A_2 receptors are coupled via the regulatory protein G_S to the stimulation of adenylate cyclase [20]. Adenosine is an agonist and methylxanthines are competitive antagonists of both types of receptors. Recently however, some pharmacological agents able to discriminate between A_1 and A_2 receptors have become available: examples include N-cyclopentyladenosine, a selective agonist of A_1 receptors, and 1,3-dipropyl-8-cyclopentyl-xanthine, a preferential antagonist of A_1 receptors [21].

It has been known for a long time that organs regulate their own blood flow: a typical example is the dilation of coronary arteries in response to hypoxia. In 1963, Berne [22] proposed his famous hypothesis that the hypoxic dilation of coronary arteries is mediated by adenosine. A broader concept of the role of adenosine in metabolic control has emerged recently (Fig. 5) [23]. According to this theory, the accumulation of adenosine in the interstitial fluid is inversely related to the energy charge of surrounding cells. Both A_1 and A_2 receptors are designed to restore the energy charge to its normal value, A_1 receptors mainly via a decrease in energy demand, and A_2 receptors via an increase in energy supply. The activation of A_1 receptors on cardiomyocytes reduces both the rate and the force of contraction thereby decreasing the work of the heart. In the central nervous system, A_1 receptor activation decreases the release of neurotransmitters, the neuronal firing rate, the locomotor activity, and the body temperature. On the other hand, the vasodilatory action of adenosine in various vascular beds is mediated by A_2 receptors. From an evolutionary point of view, it is interesting to notice that adenosine plays in mammals a role similar to that of "alarmones", such as diadenosine tetraphosphate or cyclic AMP, in bacteria. As defined by Stephen et al. [24], an alarmone is a low molecular weight compound that accumulates in response to metabolic stress and acts homeostatically to increase probability of cell survival.

Some of the homeostatic mechanisms described earlier are interrelated. Recent studies have indeed established a link between the receptors of adenosine and the ATP-dependent K^+ channels. Challenging the Berne hypothesis, they concluded accumulation of adenosine is not a prerequisite for hypoxic vasodilation, which can be induced directly by the drop of ATP level

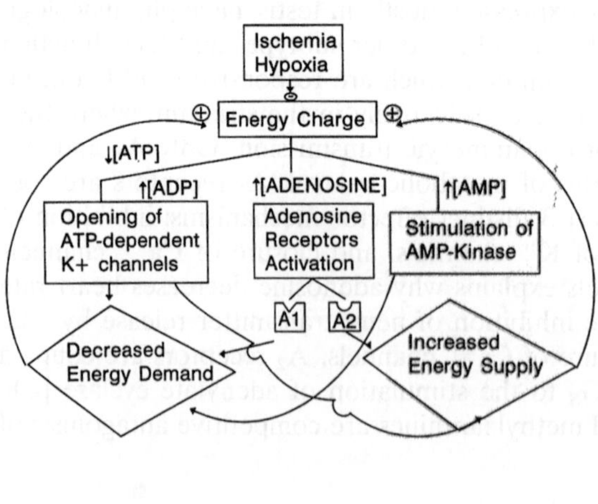

Fig. 5. Global picture of various homeostatic mechanisms involved in the restoration of the energy charge during ischemia and hypoxia

in coronary smooth muscle cells. However the two mechanisms are not really exclusive of each other, since they found that the vasodilatory action of adenosine was also inhibited by glibenclamide. Independently, Kirsch et al. [26] demonstrated that in rat ventricular myocytes, the A_1 receptors are coupled *inter alia* to ATP-dependent K^+ channels. These channels are thus subject to multiple regulations. Both a drop of the intracellular ATP level and the activation of adenosine receptors by extracellular adenosine can induce their opening. Both mechanisms are likely to cooperate in case of hypoxia and ischemia.

ATP-dependent Potassium Channels and Cardioprotection

Low concentrations of K^+ channel openers such as pinacidil or cromakalim synergize with a drop in intracellular ATP to open the ATP-dependent potassium channels. Pretreatment of rat hearts with cromakalim reduced the consequences of an experimental ischemia: the release of LDH was decreased and the contractile function during reperfusion was improved [27]. At a 10 μM concentration which does not depress cardiac function, cromakalim partially preserved the ATP level in the ischemic heart. After a 20 min period of ischemia, the energy charge had fallen from the 0.9 baseline value to 0.2 in the control group, and only to 0.45 in the treated group. In another study, anesthetized dogs were submitted to an occlusion of the left circumflex coronary artery for 90 min, followed by a 5 h reperfusion period: at that time the infarct size was determined by an histochemical technique [28]. Pretreatment of the dogs with a non-hypotensive dose of aprikalim, another K^+ channel opener, reduced the size of the infarct by 38%. On the contrary, glibenclamide, a blocker of ATP-dependent K^+ channels increased the infarct size by 38% and abolished the protective effect of aprikalim. In conclusion, these two studies demonstrate that the protective action medited by ATP-dependent K^+ channels, when ATP level drops during ischemia or hypoxia, can be enhanced by K^+ channels openers, at low doses which do not exert an hypotensive or negative inotropic effect.

Adenosine and Adenosine Analogues for Metabolic Support

The group of Mentzer [29–32] has investigated the metabolic and functional effects of exogenous adenosine during ischemia and reperfusion of the isolated perfused rat heart model. Global ischemia led to myocardial contracture which was detectable after a 9 min delay. Perfusion of these hearts with adenosine (100 μM) prior to the onset of ischemia delayed the contracture, which appeared after 18 min. After a 30 min ischemia, the hearts were reperfused for 45 min. At that time, the control hearts had only recovered 54% of the preischemic left ventricular developed pressure, whereas recovery was 75% in the heart perfused with adenosine before ischemia [30]. This functional improvement was associated with an increase in the cellular level of ATP. In control hearts, the preischemic ATP level was 24 μmol/g (dry weight); that value dropped to 9 after 10 min ischemia and to 5 at the end of the reperfusion period. In adenosine perfused hearts, these levels were respectively 26, 12, and 9. Adenosine might have acted as an ATP precursor: it is indeed well known that the exposure of cultured cells to adenosine gives rise to an expansion of the cellular ATP pool [33]. However, the preservation by adenosine of ATP level in ischemic myocardium involved a completely different mechanism: the stimulation of the glycolytic production of ATP as a consequence of A_1 receptor activation [31, 32].

Adenosine and various analogues have been shown to exert a neuroprotective action in various experimental models. An incomplete brain ischemia in rats induces a delayed and extensive loss of neurons. 2-Chloroadenosine was injected stereotaxically in the hippocampus at the time of ischemia and after 4 and 10 h. As a result, only 55% of the neurons were lost, as compared to 90% on the contralateral untreated side [34]. The cerebroventricular injection of the A_1 agonist cyclohexyladenosine to gerbils, shortly after bilateral carotid occlusion, increased survival [35]. After 10 days, 53% of the animals in the treated group were alive against only 10% in the control group. It is now well established that neuronal damage following ischemia or trauma occurs in two phases: a first one directly related to the causal event, and a second one involving the release of excitatory neurotransmitters which behave as excitotoxins, killing neurons by exciting them too much for too long. One major mechanism involved in the neuroprotective action of adenosine is the inhibition of the release of the excitatory neurotransmitter glutamate [36–38].

So far, the therapeutic application of adenosine has been restricted to the treatment of supraventricular tachycardia. This action of adenosine is mediated by A_1 receptors and involves a blockade at the atrioventricular node, which is very short since the half-life of adenosine in the circulation is a few seconds. Several metabolically stable analogues of adenosine have been synthesized, but none has reached the clinical trials and for many the preclinical development ended in failure. One reason is the ubiquity of adenosine receptors and the related risk of unacceptable side-effects: hypotension as a result of A_2 receptor activation, and atrioventricular block due to A_1 receptor activation [39]. Therefore, the concept has emerged that it would be much better to use agents devoid of action *per se* but able to enhance the effects of endogenous adenosine, when and where its production is increased.

Adenosine Enhancers

There are several possibilities to enhance the action of adenosine. At least three classes of drugs should be considered:

1. *inhibitors of nucleoside uptake:* they block the transporter involved in the facilitated diffusion of adenosine across cell membranes and therefore enhance the interstial accumulation of adenosine;
2. *inhibitors of adenosine deaminase:* they block the degradation of adenosine into inosine which is inactive at adenosine receptors; and
3. *allosteric enhancers:* these compounds enhance the binding of adenosine to its receptors and their resulting activation.

Several inhibitors of adenosine uptake have been identified: nitrobenzylthioinosine, dipyridamole, dilazep, mioflazine ... The usefulness of these compounds is limited by a poor oral bioavailability, especially for dipyridamole and dilazep, and their lack of specificity: dipyridamole also inhibits phosphodiesterases, and dilazep has calcium-antagonist properties [40]. There is some evidence that these drugs can indeed enhance the action of endogenous adenosine. Intravenous dilazep has a powerful dilating action on coronary arteries and decreases peripheral resistance in man [41]. In dogs, oral mioflazine exerts a significant hypnotic action [42]. There are preliminary indications that an analog of mioflazine (R 75231), which does not cross the blood brain barrier, might exert a cardioprotective action [39].

Inhibitors of adenosine deaminase include 2'-deoxycoformycin and erythro-9-(2-hydroxy-3-nonyl)adenine (EHNA). NMR measurements of renal ATP after bilateral occlusion of rat renal arteries indicate that an intramuscular injection of 2'-deoxycoformycin (2 mg/kg, 24 h prior to the occlusion) increased by 20% the residual ATP at the end of ischemia, and accelerated the postischemic restoration of ATP, so that after 2 h, it was 83% of the preischemic value in treated rats and only 63% in control animals [43]. In a similar way, intraarterial EHNA accelerated the restoration of myocardial ATP following a coronary occlusion in dogs [44].

Allosteric enhancers represent a more remote possibility. During the screening of potential adenosine receptors ligands, some compounds exhibiting unexpected properties were identified [45]. At high concentrations, they behaved as competitive antagonists of A_1 receptors. However at lower concentrations, they enhanced the binding of adenosine and the resulting activation of A_1 receptors. It is believed that these compounds interact with a regulatory site on the receptor, distinct from the adenosine binding site, and exert their action through an allosteric mechanism. So far this concept has not left the field of *in vitro* studies and no candidate for clinical development is yet available.

Conclusion

During this overview of purine-related homeostatic mechanisms involved in physiological metabolic support, several pharmacological targets have been identified. Among the various pharmacological agents which have been presented, potassium channel openers represent probably the most practical possibility today. The promises of nucleoside uptake inhibitors have not been fulfilled yet, mostly because of bioavailability problems. Adenosine deaminase inhibitors and allosteric enhancers of adenosine receptors represent interesting possibilities for the future.

References

1. Skladanowski AC, Newby AC (1990) Partial purification and properties of an AMP-specific soluble 5'-nucleotidase from pigeon heart. Biochem J 268:117–122
2. Noma A (1983) ATP-regulated K^+ channels in cardiac muscle. Nature 305:147–148
3. Escandre D, Cavero I (1992) K^+ channels openers and "natural" cardioprotection. TIPS 13:269–271
4. Hardie DG, Carling D, Sim ATR (1989) The AMP-activated protein kinase: A multi-substrate regulator of lipid metabolism. TIBS 14:20–23
5. Sneddon P, Westfall DP (1984) Pharmacological evidence that adenosine triphosphate and noradrenaline are cotransmitters in the guinea-pig vas deferens. J Physiol 347:561–580
6. Edwards FA, Gibb AJ, Colquhoun D (1992) ATP receptor-mediated synaptic currents in the central nervous system. Nature 359:144–147
7. Evans RJ, Derkach V, Surprenant A (1992) ATP mediates fast synaptic transmission in mammalian neurons. Nature 357:503–505
8. Boeynaems JM, Pearson JD (1990) P2 purinoceptors on vascular endothelial cells: Physiological significance and transduction mechanisms. TIPS 11:34–37
9. Pearson JD, Gordon JL (1979) Vascular endothelial and smooth muscle cells in culture selectively release adenine nucleotides. Nature 281:384–386
10. Schütz W, Schrader J, Gerlach E (1991) Different sites of adenosine formation in the heart. Am J Physiol 240:H963–H970
11. Van Belle H, Goossens F, Wynants J (1987) Formation and release of purine catabolites during hypoperfusion, anoxia, and ischemia. Am J Physiol 252:H886–H893
12. Van Wylen DGL, Willis J, Sodhi J, Weiss RJ, Lasley RD, Mentzer RM (1990) Cardiac microdialysis to estimate interstitial adenosine and coronary blood flow. Am J Physiol 258:H1642–H1649
13. Phillis JW, Walter GA, Simpson RE (1991) Purine release from the hypoxic/ischemic rat cerebral cortex: Manipulation of adenosine levels. In: Imai S, Nakazawa M (eds) Role of adenosine and adenine nucleotides in the biological system. Elsevier Science Publishers, pp. 661–671
14. Möser GH, Schrader J, Deussen A (1989) Turnover of adenosine in plasma of human and dog blood. Am J Physiol 256:C799–C806
15. Feldman MD, Ayers CR, Lehman MR, et al (1992) Improved detection of ischemia-induced increases in coronary sinus adenosine in patients with coronary artery disease. Clin Chem 38:256–262
16. Libert F, Schiffman S, Lefort A, et al (1991) The orphan receptor cDNA RCD7 encodes an A_1 adenosine receptor. EMBO J 10:1677–1682
17. Maenhaut C, Van Sande J, Libert F, et al (1990) RCD8 codes for an adenosine A_2 receptor with physiological constitutive activity. Biochem Biophys Res Commun 173:1169–1178

18. Piece KD, Furlong TJ, Selbie LA, Shine J (1992) Molecular cloning and expression of an adenosine A_{2b} receptor from human brain. Biochem Biophys Res Commun 187:86–93
19. Zhou QY, Li C, Olah ME, Johnson RA, Stiles GL, Civelli O (1992) Molecular cloning and characterization of an adenosine receptor: The A_3 adenosine receptor. Proc Natl Acad Sci USA 89:7432–7436
20. Stiles GL (1992) Adenosine receptors. J Biol Chem 267:6451–6454
21. Martinson EA, Johnson RA, Wells JN (1987) Potent adenosine receptor antagonists that are selective for the A_1 receptor subtype. Mol Pharmacol 131:247–252
22. Berne RM (1964) Regulation of coronary blood flow. Physiol Rev 44:1–29
23. Bruns RF (1991) Role of adenosine in energy supply/demand balance. Nuclesides and Nucleotides 10:931–943
24. Stephens JC, Artz SW, Ames BN (1975) ppGpp: Positive effector for histidine operon transcription and general signal for amino acid deficiency. Proc Natl Acad Sci USA 72:4389–4393
25. Daut J, Maier-Rudolph W, von Beckerath N, Mehrke G, Günther K, Goedel-Meinen L (1990) Hypoxic dilation of coronary arteries is mediated by ATP-sensitive potassium channels. Science 247:1341–1344
26. Kirsch GE, Codina J, Birnbaumer L, Brown AM (1990) Coupling of ATP-sensitive K^+ channels to Al receptors by G proteins in rat ventricular myocytes. Am J Physiol 259:H820–H826
27. Grover GJ, Newburger J, Sleph PG, et al (1991) Cardioprotective effects of the potassium channel opener cromakalin: Stereoselectivity and effects of myocardial adenine nucleotides. J Pharmacol Exp Therapeutics 257:156–162
28. Auchampach JA, Maruyama M, Cavero I, Gross GJ (1991) The new K^+ channel opener aprikalim (RP 52891) reduces experimental infarcts size in dogs in the absence of hemodynamic changes. J Pharmacol Exp Therapeutics 259:961–967
29. Mentzer RM, Lasley RD, Van Wylen DGL (1991) A new role for adenosine: Modulation of myocardial tolerance to ischemia. In: Imai S, Nakazawa M (eds) Adenosine and adenine nucleotides in the biological system. Elsevier Science Publishers, pp. 547–556
30. Lasley R, Mentzer RM (1992) Adenosine improves recovery postischemic myocardial function via an adenosine A_1 receptor mechanism. Am J Physiol 263:H1460–H1465
31. Mainwaring R, Lasley R, Rubio R, Wyatt DA, Mentzer RM (1988) Adenosine stimulates glucose uptake in the isolated rat heart. Surgery 103:445–449
32. Wyatt DA, Edmunds MC, Rubio R, Berne RM, Lasley RD, Mentzer RM (1989) Adenosine stimulates glycolytic flux in isolated perfused rat hearts by A_1-adenosine receptors. Am J Physiol 257:H1952–H1957
33. Klenow H, Ostergaard E (1988) Adenosine induction of rapid catabolism of adenine ribonucleotides and independent elevation of the ATP content in quiescent mouse fibroblasts. J Cell Physiol 137:565–570
34. Evans MC, Swan JH, Meldrum BS (1987) An adenosine analogue, 2-chloroadenosine, protects against long-term development of ischaemic cell loss in the rat hippocampus. Neuroscience (Lett) 83:287–292
35. von Lubitz DKEJ, Dambrosia JM, Redmond DJ (1989) Protective effect of cytohexyl adenosine in treatment of cerebral ischemia in gerbils. Neuroscience 30:451–462
36. Dolphin AC, Archer ER (1983) An adenosine agonist inhibit and a cyclic AMP analogue enhances the release of glutamate but not GABA from slices of rat dentate gyrus. Neuroscience (Lett) 43:49–54
37. Corradetti R, Lo Conte G, Moroni F, Passani MB, Pepeu G (1984) Adenosine decreases asparate and glutamate release from rat hippocampal slices. Eur J Pharmacol 104:19–26
38. Arvin B, Neville LF, Pan J, Roberts PJ (1989) 2-chloroadenosine attenuates kainic acid-induced toxicity within the rat striatum: Relationship to release of glutamate and $Ca2^+$ influx. Br J Pharmacol 98:225–235
39. Jacobson KA, Trivedi BK, Churchill PC, Williams M (1991) Novel therapeutics acting via purine receptors. Biochem Pharmacol 41:1399–1410

40. Van Belle H (1988) In vivo effects of inhibitors of adenosine uptake. In: Paton D (ed) Adenosine and adenine nucleotides: Physiology and pharmacology. Taylor and Francis, pp. 251–258
41. Marzilli M, Simonetti I, Levantesi D, et al (1984) Effects of dilazep on coronary and systemic hemodynamics in humans. Am Heart J 108:276–285
42. Waugier A, Van Belle H, Van der Broeck WAE, Janssen PAJ (1987) Sleep improvement in dogs after oral administration of mioflazine, a nucleoside transport inhibitor. Psychopharmacology 91:434–440
43. Stromski ME, van Waarde A, Avison MJ, et al (1988) Metabolic and functional consequences of inhibiting adenosine deaminase during renal ischemia in rats. J Clin Invest 82:1694–1699
44. Henrichs KJ, Matsuoka H, Schaper W (1988) Enhanced postischemic ATP repletion by pharmacological inhibition of nucleoside washout and catabolism. J Cardiovascular Pharmacol 11:694–700
45. Bruns RF, Fergus JH (1990) Allosteric enhancement of adenosine A_1 receptor binding and function by 2-amino-3-benzoylthiophenes. Mol Pharmacol 38:939–949

Metabolic Responses to Anti-Cytokine Therapies

S. F. Lowry

Introduction

Severe injury or invasive infection induce complex alterations of host metabolic and immunologic function. Although it is evident that these are dynamic processes serving as necessary adjuncts to the normal evolution of repair, their propagation may become severely dysfunctional in the setting of complicated injury or organ failure. Despite the clinical application of advanced technology for anti-microbial therapy, organ support, and nutrition, the mechanisms underlying the evolution of such adverse events have generally proven elusive. This discussion will selectively review current understanding of the *potential* role for inflammatory mediators as proximal determinants of the acute and chronic host metabolic responses to injury or infection. Where possible, observations derived from human systems will be utilized and, additionally, data suggesting the *potential* influence of anti-cytokine therapies upon these events will be provided.

The Dynamics of Injured Host Response

The initial (ebb) phase following injury is accompanied by responses generally reflective of immune cell activation. (Fig. 1). Successful early resuscitation and clinical management serves to usher in a period of increased energy expenditure and substrate turnover which, more often than not, co-exists with a state of immune system under-responsiveness. In those subjects destined for early recovery, these host response parameters return toward normal conditions in concert with traditional clinical hallmarks of improvement. A severe initial insult, or the evolution of complications may obviate early resolution of these host metabolic and immune responses [1, 2]. The evolution of solid organ failure and clinical evidence of immune incompetence portends a disatrous clinical cycle of complications, such as repeated or sustained infection [2]. Recent data would argue for the eventual attenuation of such heightened activity, as examplified by the suppression of monocyte soluble cytokine production during the early flow phase. However, this suppression, if prolonged, portends poorly for outcome of critical illness.

The metabolic consequences of prolonged injury also trends toward continued erosion of energy stores and lean tissue mass, a process not readily

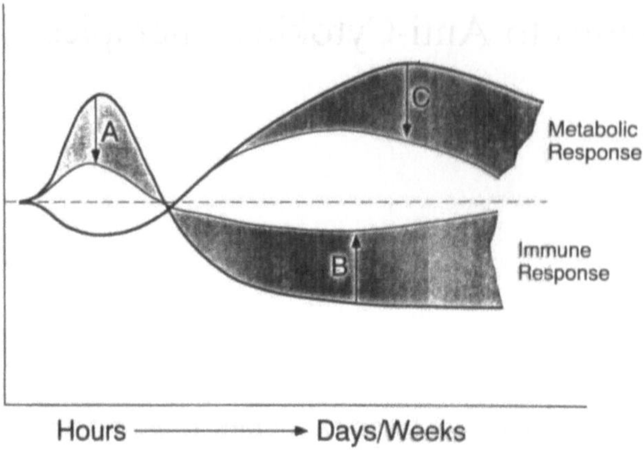

Fig. 1. Relationship between initial acute immune activation (A), and subsequent flow phase immune hyporesponsiveness (B) or hypermetabolic conditions (C)

reversible by conventional means of nutritional support. It is this divergence of host homeostatic processes which most clearly correlates with progressive organ dysfunction and mortality in severely injured or infected patients. While a causal relationship between determination of nutritional status and immune function remains an attractive theory, clear demonstration of a cause and effect relationship has proven elusive [1].

Recent insights have arisen from both the basic and clinical science levels as to the biochemical mechanisms for such changes [3, 4]. In several cases, the rapidity of this technology transfer has prompted the clinical application of therapies directed toward inflammatory mediators believed responsible for the acute sequelae of injury as well as for those adverse host responses eventuating in organ failure and demise [5, 6]. If current theory is correct, the early, as well as, late immune and metabolic consequences of severe injury and infection might both be influenced by such therapies.

The extent of metabolic [1, 7] and immune [8] dysfunction achieved during the flow phase response to injury or infection is well documented. However, given the dynamic nature of the injury/repair/complication cycle which frequently supervenes, antecedent or concurrent diseases, as well as clinical interventions such as nutrient provision [9], may also influence the magnitude of eventual substrate turnover and immune function responses. Additional mechanisms for endogenous regulation of inflammatory mediator activity also exist [6]. It is likely that such clinical therapies also influence the host capacity for effective counter-regulation. Whether nutritional variables are of importance in mediator antagonism, as they appear to be for agonist activity, remains to be determined.

The early immunologic and metabolic events attending severe injury or infection appear to be driven by the individual and synergistic activities of both classical macroendocrine hormones and microendocrine mediators. Both endocrine stress hormone components [8] and pro-inflammatory cytokine influences are exerted upon immune function [10]. Unfortunately, much

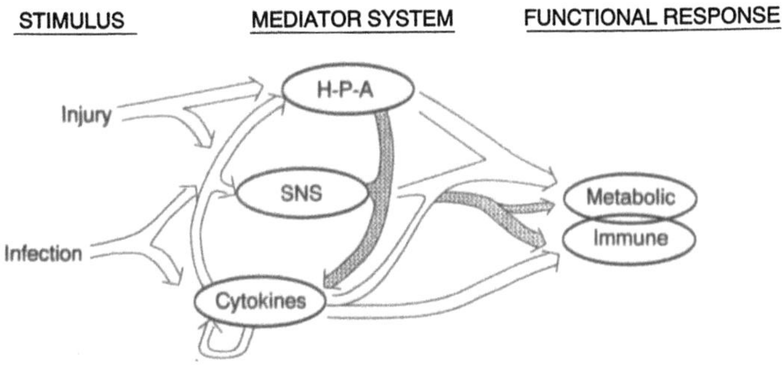

Fig. 2. The potential relationship between injury stimulae, hypothalamic/pituitary/adrenal (H-P-A), sympathetic nervous system (SNS) and cytokines as impacting upon metabolic and imune function. Open bars = amplification – dark bars = attenuation

of the relevant *in vivo* biology of their specific influences during post-injury or severe inflammatory conditions remains to be dissected. The dynamic nature of metabolic host mediator responses to dysfunction resulting from severe injury or infection suggests a significant degree of interdependence of the neuro-endocrine hormone axis and components of the pro-inflammatory mediator system (Fig. 2).

The current discussion, in keeping with the theme of this volume, will focus upon the potential influence of these mediators in directing some of the flow phase metabolic events attending injury and severe infection. Although it is recognized that such efforts are founded upon limited data, the current discussion can only anticipate that interventions which successfully counteract cytokine influences may also definitively influence host metabolic responses.

Classical Endocrine Stress Hormone Influences (Table 1)

Critically ill and injured patients readily exhibit a diverse neuro-endocrine stress response. The extent of this response is most evident during the ebb and early flow phase following insult. Frequently, components of this response are also documented over the same temporal scale as the hypermetabolic phase. Whether such hormones, either individually or in combination, initiate or sustain the hypermetabolic/catabolic responses to injury remains a topic of some controversy [1]. Numerous clinical studies attest to the efforts directed toward dissecting the contribution of classical neuro-humoral stress hormone components to post-injury hypermetabolism and substrate turnover [1–14].

The kinetics of body protein metabolism have been most carefully evaluated during the acute post-injury phase [15–21]. The regulation of the syn-

Table 1. Impact of counter-regulatory hormone excess upon circulating substrates and nitrogen balance. (From [11, 12, 22, 23, 26] with permission)

	Glucose/Lactate		Amino acids	Nitrogen balance	Protein (leucine) Turnover
Cortisol	↑	↑[a]	↑[a]	±↓	↑
Epinephrine	↑(↑↑)[a]	↑↑[a]	↓[a]	0	±↓[a]
Epinephrine + Cortisol	↑↑[a]	↑[a]	↑[a]	N.D.	0[a]
Epinephrine + Cortisol + Glucagon	↑↑		↓↓	↓	0,(↑)[b]

Arrows indicate change relative to baseline period – [a] defined only for short (<24 h) time periods – [b] as determined by ^{15}N-glycine method – N.D. not determined

thetic and catabolic components of protein metabolism appear to be sensitive to the phase of injury and, by implication, to the hormonal milieu. Although some have reported that increased adrenergic stimulation may acutely alter the oxidative and synthetic components of protein metabolism, we [22] and others [23] have been unable to confirm any sustained influence of catecholamines upon body protein kinetics without concurrent injury. Indeed, an excess catecholamine stimulus appears to promote a degree of net nitrogen conservation within some regional tissues, such as skeletal muscle [22]. When assessed in injured humans, selective α-adrenergic blockade demonstrates only a modest decrease in net protein catabolism without an attendant influence upon rates of glucose production [24]. Nevertheless, efforts to duplicate this hormonal milieu by exogenous infusions [22], or alternatively at blockade of components of the neuro-humoral response in normal subjects [25], suggest that excessive adrenergic stimulation is insufficient *per se* to fully explain the metabolic consequences of severe injury or infection.

By contrast to any sustained influence of adrenergic influence upon protein kinetics, an extended period of hypercortisolemia does alter the kinetic of protein metabolism in a manner consistent with, but not of the same magnitude to observed clinical scenarios [22, 26]. Indeed, studies of excess cortisol background in normal subjects have, like those investigating isolated catecholamine excess, failed to reproduce the magnitude of nitrogen wasting commonly observed after major injury [11, 12].

Pro-Inflammatory Cytokine Influences (Table 2)

Pro-Inflammatory cytokine activity is most readily associated with systemic hemodynamic and tissue inflammatory reactions. Some evidence does suggest that they may also influence some component of cellular substrate processing reminiscent of that noted after injury or infection [27–30]. Several of the *in vivo* properties of pro-inflammatory cytokines suggesting their direct

Table 2. Acute impact of cytokine administration upon hormonal and metabolic responses: comparison to endotoxinemia and bacteremia

Stimulus (dose) [species]	Glucose	Lactate	Amino acids	T_3/T_4	ACTH	Catechol-amines	Cortisol	Insulin	Glucagon
LPS (500 μg/Kg) [baboons]	0	↑(2–4h)	↓(2–4h)	↓(8h)	0			↓(>4h)	
E. coli (10 μg/Kg) [baboons]	↑(1h) ↓↓(2–8h)	↑(>1h)	↑(8h)			↑(>2h)			↑(8h)
IL-1∝ (10000 μg/Kg)[a] [baboons]	↑(1h) ↓(3h)	↑(>1h)	↓(2h)	↓(>4h)[b]	↑(>4h)[b]			↑(1h) ↓(>2h)[b]	
TNF∝ (0.57×10^5 μ/Kg or 10–100 μg/Kg) [canine]	↑(≤1h) ↓↓(>1h)	↑(>1h)	↑(>2h)		↑(>1h)	↑(1–6h)	↑(>1h)	±↓	↑(>1h)

0=no change – ↑=increased from basal – ↓=decreased from basal – (h)=hrs after stimulus for observed change – [a] no effected observed @ 0.1 μg/Kg dose, except – [b] includes effects observed @ 0.1 μg/Kg dose – ( ) indicates post-Rx time frame for observed responses participation in post-injury flow phase metabolism have been reviewed [3, 31–33].

A summary of hormonal and substrate alterations arising from the exogenous administration of endotoxin or live bacteria is depicted in Table 2. These changes, which occur in concert with endogenous production of pro-inflammatory cytokines, are contrasted with several pre-clinical reports which have utilized exogenous cytokine infusion. It is of interest to note the fidelity of isolated cytokine administration, either TNF or IL-1, to both the direction and temporal sequences of infection-induced hormone and substrate changes. As noted, there is some evidence to suggest a cytokine dose-response relationship with respect to several metabolic response parameters. While similar associations to components of the acute phase response have also been noted in humans, the degree of macroendocrine activation appears largely dose-independent.

In humans, it is also known that administration of tumor necrosis factor (TNF) elicits an increase in energy expenditure as well as enhanced turnover of glucose and free fatty acid pathways [29, 34]. This increased metabolic activity is preceded by increases in counter-regulatory hormone activity [34, 35], although this brief macroendocrine stress response, as discussed previously, does not fully elicit the spectrum of injury-induced substrate turnover [22]. Some elements of both a systemic as well as regional tissue dose response relationship to exogenous TNF appear to exist [28, 29, 36, 37]. Furthermore, the temporal relationship between this early neuro-endocrine activation and later metabolic disruptions, such as increased energy expenditure, suggests the participation of other mediator systems. Clearly, some components of post-injury metabolism, such as generation of an acute phase protein response, are virtually dependent upon pro-inflammatory cytokine activity. Indeed, counter-regulatory hormone influence that attenuates cytokine activity, significantly influences the characteristic injury response [38, 39]. It remains to be determined whether synergistic influences of limited duration between endocrine elements and pro-inflammatory cytokine activity are necessary or sufficient adjuncts for full expression of the injury phenotype.

Unlike TNF, there is limited information referable to the clinical sequelae of exogenous IL-1 administration. Although Phase I and II trials utilizing this agent for therapeutic anti-tumor therapy are currently underway, no reports focusing specifically upon hormonal or metabolic response modification have yet appeared. It might be anticipated, based upon pre-clinical data, that IL-1 may well exhibit the capacity to alter endocrine stress hormone and metabolic responses in a manner similar to TNF.

Compelling evidence attesting to the influence of cytokines upon the metabolic alterations of injured subjects also emanates from observations attained during the *in vivo* blockade of cytokine activity utilizing monoclonal antibodies or receptor antagonists. For example, animals pretreated with a specific anti-TNF antibody prior to challenge with bacteria or endotoxin exhibit not only improved hemodynamic performance, but also a significant attenuation of the systemic substrate alterations and some regional tissue metabolic responses [30, 31]. Such blockade is also associated with diminished catecholamine levels [40], but is without apparent attenuation of the adrenal steroid response. Similarly, concurrent treatment of bacteremic primates with IL-1 receptor antagonist also attenuates several aspects of the host metabolic response [41]. As the extent to which the individual contributions of TNF and IL-1 or other pro-inflammatory cytokines may overlap, it is clear that simultaneous utilization of specific antagonists directed against such cytokines as well as endocrine hormone components are necessary to more fully dissect this complex mediator biology.

The nature of the initial stimulus, as well as other as yet undefined elements, dictate the extent to which endogenous mediator systems are activated. Non-infectious injury and shock is not, at least initially, identified with a systemic pro-inflammatory cytokine (TNF, IL-1) response. While diverse stimulae very likely do result in more global activation of this, or other, mediator classes, more precise details of the temporal relationship between non-infectious challenge and tissue or systemic cytokine activity are necessary.

By contrast, evidence attesting to the parallel activation of these mediator system *in vivo* is readily observed in response to an infectious challenge. Whether resulting from administration of the primary antigen (endotoxin) or the proximal pro-inflammatory cytokine (TNF), full expression of the subsequent classical counter-regulatory stress hormone and cytokine systems is readily observed. Indeed, this mediator background appears sufficient to invoke, albeit briefly, much of the systemic metabolic responses characteristic of the flow phase [35] while also acutely inducing the dynamic activation/suppresion cycle of immune function [42, 43].

The biology of the interdependent macroendocrine and pro-inflammatory mediator systems is also influenced by hormonally and cytokine directed feedback mechanisms as well as endogenously by the capacity for production of cytokine antagonists. We have recently demonstrated the acute *in vivo* attenuation of endotoxin-induced TNF production by antecedent administration of glucocorticoids in humans [38]. While such an influence might well have been predicted by known *in vitro* influence of steroids, the complex nature of amplified TNF production under hypercortisolemic conditions could not have been foreseen. Although such interactions are only partially defined, it is intuitively evident that prolonged activity of all such systems may be inconsistent with maintenance or restoration of reparative processes or organ system function.

The interdependent nature and, to some extent countervailing influences, of the neuro-endocrine and cytokine signalling systems promotes, at least initially, a degree of host metabolic and immunologic modulation appropriate to the magnitude of the injury. If this challenge is of a modest, reparable magnitude and of limited duration, these intial counter-regulatory hormone and cytokine responses promote the mobilization of energy stores and the maintenance of substrate availability for critical organ function. Presumably, the level of natural cytokine antagonists generated, as demonstrated by example during endotoxinemia in Fig. 3, are sufficient only to prevent any unwarranted systemic influences of cytokines while simultaneously providing sufficient activity for wound repair. By contrast, the persistent or excessive stress hormonal and cytokine signals responding to severe or prolonged injury conditions readily overwhelm these natural antagonist systems [44, 45], serving to further erode metabolic and immunologic reserves. Recent data also suggest that responsiveness of the microendocrine (cytokine) system may be differentially affected by unstressed malnutrition [46] as opposed to conditions of undernutrition in association with stress [47]. Although the

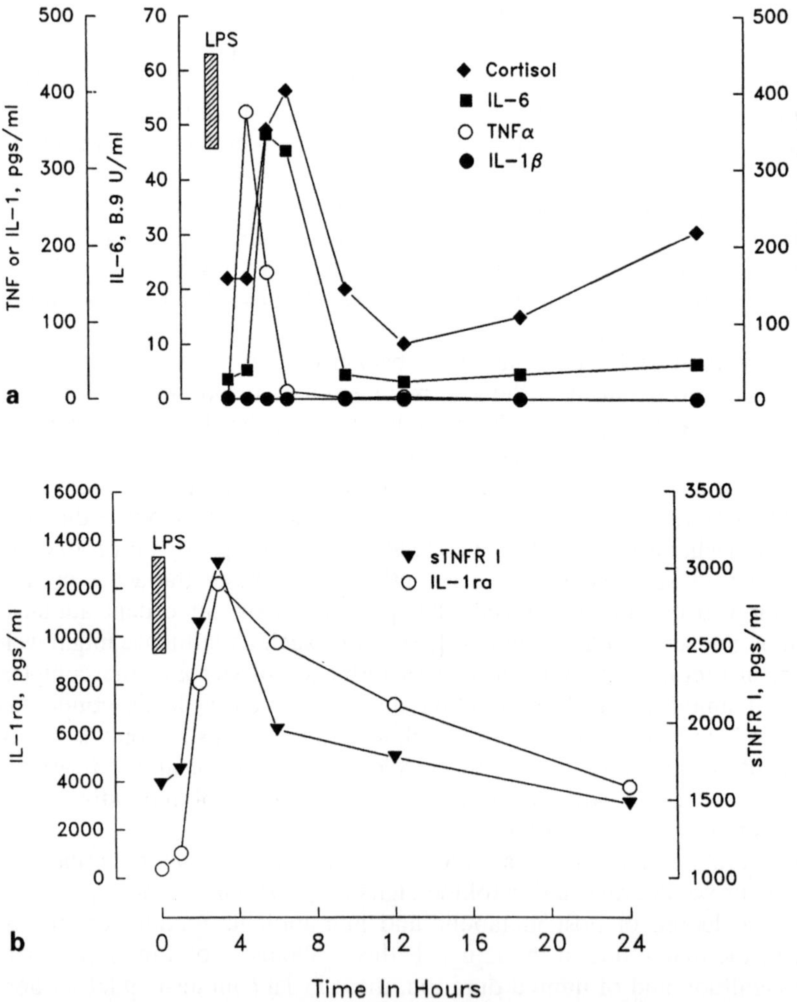

Fig. 3. a Circulating TNF-∝, IL-1β, IL-6 and cortisol levels after LPS administration in normal human subjects. **b** Circulating sTNFR-I and IL-1ra after LPS administration in normal subjects

mechanisms and functional significance for this differential alteration in cytokine responsiveness remain unclear, it has been suggested that this diminished cytokine responsiveness portends poorly for injured patients. Alternatively, in the absence of repeated or ongoing antigenic challenges, the initial attenuation of inflammatory mediator production during stress may be teleologically appropriate for the preservation of metabolic reserves and for limitation of tissue injury.

Therapeutic Considerations

The capacity to influence the adverse systemic und tissue manifestations of ongoing mediator activation via traditional clinical technologies, including nutritional support, have exhibited only marginal benefits. As discussed elsewhere in this volume, a number of strategies directed toward specific nutrient or anabolic growth factor supplementation suggest that additional benefits will accrue from these techniques. Within this context, it could be hypothesized that mediator specific interventions might, if pursued at the appropriate time, be of additional benefit in modulating the otherwise uncontrolled expression of the flow phase biology.

The concept of mediator blockade as a beneficial intervention rests, thus far, largely upon pre-clinical information pertaining to hemodynamic shock and the immediate consequences thereof. While the preliminary results of clinical trials evaluating therapies directed against either TNF or IL-1 have been suggestive of early clinical benefit in septic populations, it has yet to be established that these improvements extend to any significant influence upon

Table 3. Influence of antecedent TNF or IL-1 blockade on responses to E. coli bacteremia

	Pre-E. coli		8 h after E. coli	
	Control	anti-αTNF	Control	anti-TNF
TNF Blockade[a]				
Epinephrine (pg/ml)	165±27	191±25	3.012±861	160±16
Glucose (mg/dl)	82±10	80±7	50±10[c]	76±7
Triglycerides (mg/dl)	55±13	51±9	87±10[c]	47±15[d]
WBC (10^3 cells/μL)	13.2±0.8	12.1±1.1	1.2±0.1[c]	8.2±4.0[d]
IL-1 Blockade[b]				
Glucose (mg/dl)	70±3	75±5	57±7[c]	74±6
Lactate (mg/L)	10±1	9±1	35±12[c]	22±3[c]
WBC (10^3 cells/μL)	14.2±1.3	11.0±1.2	2.5±0.3[c]	2.6±0.2[c]

[a] Adapted from [49 and 53] utilizing a 10 mg/Kg dose of anti-TNF mAb 2 h prior to E. coli

[b] Adapted from [41] utilizing a bolus (10 mg/Kg) and continuous infusion (25 μg/Kg·min) of IL-1ra from 0 to 8 h during E. coli, with permission

[c] $p<0.05$ vs respective pre-E. coli

[d] $p<0.05$ vs respective 8 h after E. coli

metabolic or immune function. The problems inherent in defining such influences rest upon our tenuous understanding of not only the inter-relationship between mediator systems noted above, but also to convincing evidence that excessive, or inappropriate, cytokine activity remains a significant mechanism for these late events. It has yet to be established, with the possible exception of maintenance of adipose tissue stores, that interventions against pro-inflammatory cytokines might benefit host substrate mass [32, 48]. Indeed, some data suggest that interventions designed to restore, rather than attenuate late cytokine production might prove more beneficial to survival. The ultimate influence, if any, deriving from anti-cytokine therapies in clinical sepsis can presently only be speculated. The metabolic and other influences deriving from anti-cytokine treatment of bacteremia in primates is summarized in Table 3. While such results suggest that these therapies may impact upon similar parameters in humans, it must be borne in mind that the studies outlined are presumptive in nature. Hence, results of anti-cytokine therapies in clinical treatment schemes might not exhibit this magnitude of acute host benefit, if any.

Human Studies

Pre-clinical studies would suggest that interventions directed against the cytokine mediators will benefit some patients during the early phase of severe infectious challenge [49]. Prospective clinical trials to address these issues are currently underway. In a manner similar to that achieved with therapy directed against endotoxin [50], anti-cytokine therapies may also prove effective against infection-related mortality and organ system dysfunction. Therapies directed against the more proximal elements of the cytokine cascade, such as TNF or IL-1, are appealing in that these therapies may counteract the early mediators arising from a diverse array of inciting factors, including bacteria, viruses, and severe tissue injury. At present, the clinical scenario most appropriate for application of these antagonists is limited to acute bacterial or endotoxin induced injury. It will be of significant interest to determine whether these interventions effectively abrogate the more extended metabolic consequences attributable to excessive cytokine activity or, as is more likely, demonstrate only a modest impact on the metabolic alterations associated with infection.

Later Interventions

Given the current inability to effectively attenuate the early metabolic disruptions associated with severe injury and the unknown longer term clinical efficacy of anti-cytokine therapies, it is likely that a proportion of critically ill subjects will continue to manifest both systemic and organ specific resistance to such therapies. Consequently, efforts directed at combined therapies against multiple components of the mediator cascade may be advocated as a means of globally interdicting the injury response. As discussed above, our understanding of such therapies respective to their influences upon immunologic and metabolic function remains limited. Given the likelihood that beneficial influences of cytokines and other mediator systems may be adjuncts to the recovery process [51], such interventions may, conceivably, invoke untoward adverse consequences. It also remains to be established whether these patients will benefit from repeated administration of response modifying agents directed against cytokines or other mediator systems. While the failure to influence the late sequelae of injury and sepsis by conventional means lends promise to such strategies, it will be necessary to reassess the balance between the stress hormone and micromediator environment evoked by other prior therapies before such interventions can be logically undertaken.

Superimposed upon the inability to pharmacologically influence post-injury metabolic responses is the frustration derived from the apparent failure of nutrient intake to influence the post-injury response [24]. Although severely injured patients exhibit a degree of insulin resistance as well as increased lipolysis, such subjects appear to adequately oxidize these substrates, and a lack of energy supply does not appear responsible for the continued losses of nitrogen and progressive lean tissue wasting [21]. Given the degree to which neuro-humoral components are known to influence injury-induced metabolic processes, the complete attenuation of such responses might not be expected [19, 24]. Unfortunately, other parameters which are presumptively sensitive to nutrient intake, such as immune and solid organ system functions, are likewise not beneficially influenced in this setting [52, 53]. As the nutrient environment increasingly appears to interface with the endocrine and immunologic systems in complex fashion, doubtless alterations in the composition and manner by which critically ill patients are nourished will prove an additional means of response modification.

Conclusion

Both classic counter-regulatory and neuroendocrine hormones as well as proinflammatory mediators participate in the hypermetabolic response to injury and sepsis. The complete metabolic profile of severe injury or infection cannot be reproduced by the administration of one or more neuro-endocrine hormones, nor in response to specific cytokine or endotoxin administration. Hence, our understanding of the appropriate targets for intervention against the hypermetabolism and associated immune dysfunction of severe sepsis remains limited. Although anti-mediator therapies may prove of some benefit with respect to outcome parameters, our current understanding of the metabolic and immunologic consequences of such blockade remains to be fully elucidated. It will be of interest to determine whether such therapies meaningfully impact upon the hypermetabolic response to sepsis or injury or, alternatively, whether this complex response is independent of the influence exerted by any single inflammatory mediator.

References

1. Lowry SF (1986) The host metabolic response to injury. In: Shires GT, Davis JM (eds) Host defenses Vol. 6, Academic Press, pp. 169–180
2. Cerra FB (1987) Hypermetabolism, organ failure, and metabolic support. Surgery 101:1–14
3. Fong Y, Moldawer LL, Shires GT, Lowry SF (1990) The biological characteristics of cytokines and their implication in surgical injury. Surg Gynecol Obstet 170:363–378
4. Bone RC (1991) The pathogenesis of sepsis. Ann Intern Med 115:457–469
5. Bone RC (1991) A critical evaluation of new agents for the treatment of sepsis. JAMA 266:1686–1691
6. Lowry SF, VanZee KJ, Moldawer LL (1992) Strategies for modulation of systemic and tissue cytokine responses to sepsis. In: Lamy M, Thijs LG (eds) Update in Intensive Care and Emergency Medicine, Vol. 16. Mediators of Sepsis. Springer-Verlag, Berlin, Heidelberg, pp. 345–361
7. Lowry SF (1993) Hormone and cytokine regulation of injury metabolism. In: Vincent JL (ed) Yearbook of Intensive Care and Emergency Medicine 1993, pp. 3–11
8. Calvano SE (1986) Hormonal mediation of immune dysfunction following thermal and traumatic injury. In: Davis JM, Shires GT (eds) Advances in host defense mechanisms. Raven Press, New York pp. 111–142
9. Lowry SF (1990) The route of feeding influences injury responses. J Trauma 30:510–515
10. Vassalli P (1992) The pathophysiology of tumor necrosis factors. In: Paul WE, Fathman CG, Metzger H (eds) Annual Review of Immunology, vol. 10. Annual Reviews Inc., Palo Alto pp. 411–452
11. Bessey PQ, Watters JM, Aoki TT, Wilmore DW (1984) Combined hormonal infusion stimulates the metabolic response to injury. Ann Surg 200:264–281
12. Gelfand RA, Matthews DE, Bier DM, Sherwin RS (1984) Role of counterregulatory hormones in the catabolic response to stress. J Clin Invest 74:2238–2248
13. Stoner HB, Frayn KN, Barton RN, Threlfall CJ, Little RA (1979) The relationships between plasma substrates and hormones and the severity of injury in 277 recently injured patients. Clin Sci 56:563–573
14. Wilmore DW, Long JM, Mason AD, Skreen RW, Pruitt BA (1974) Catecholamines: Mediator of the hypermetabolic response to thermal injury. Ann Surg 180:653–668
15. Lowry SF (1992) Modulating the metabolic response to injury and infection. Proc Nutr Soc 51:267–277
16. Shaw JHF, Wolfe RR (1985) Alanine, urea, and glucose interrelationship in normal subjects and patients with sepsis with stable isotope tracers. Surgery 97:557–567
17. Shaw JHF, Wildbore M, Wolfe RR (1987) Whole body protein kinetics in severely septic patients. Ann Surg 205:288–294
18. Shaw JHF, Wolfe RR (1987) Fatty acid and glycerol kinetics in septic patients and in patients with gastrointestinal cancer. Ann Surg 205:368–376
19. Wolfe RR, Herndon DN, Jahoor F, Miyoshi H, Wolfe M (1987) Effect of severe burn injury on substrate cycling by glucose and fatty acids. N Engl J Med 317:403–408
20. Shaw JHF, Wolfe RR (1989) An integrated analysis of glucose, fat, and protein metabolism in severely traumatized patients. Ann Surg 209:63–72
21. Jahoor F, Shangraw RE, Miyoshi H, Wallfish H, Herndon DN, Wolfe RR (1989) Role of insulin and glucose oxidation in mediating the protein catabolism of burns and sepsis. Am J Physiol 257:E323–E331
22. Fong Y, Albert JD, Tracey KJ, et al (1991) The influence of substrate background on the acute metabolic response to epinephrine and cortisol. J Trauma 31:1467–1476
23. Matthews DE, Pesola G, Campbell RG (1990) Effect of epinephrine on amino acid and energy metabolism in humans. Am J Physiol 258:E948–E956
24. Shaw JHF, Holdaway CM, Humberstone DA (1988) Metabolic intervention in surgical patients: The effect of α or β-blockade on glucose and protein metabolism in surgical patients receiving total parenteral nutrition. Surgery 103:520–525

25. Kraenzlin ME, Keller U, Keller A, Thélin A, Arnaud MJ, Stauffacher W (1989) Elevation of plasma epinephrine concentrations inhibits proteolysis and leucine oxidation in man via β-adrenergic mechanisms. J Clin Invest 84:388–393
26. Beaufrere B, Horber FF, Schwenk WF, et al (1989) Glucocorticosteroids increase leucine oxidation and impair leucine balance in humans. Am J Physiol 257:E712–E721
27. Lee MD, Zentella A, Pekala PH, Cerami A (1987) Effect of endotoxin-induced monokines on glucose metabolism in the muscle cell line L6. Proc Natl Acad Sci USA 84:2590–2594
28. Warren RS, Starnes HF Jr, Gabrilove JL, Oettgen HF, Brennan MF (1987) The acute metabolic effects of tumor necrosis factor administration in humans. Arch Surg 122:1396–1400
29. Starnes HF, Warren RA, Jeevanandam M, et al (1988) Tumor necrosis factor and the acute metabolic response to tissue injury in man. J Clin Invest 82:1321–1325
30. Tracey KJ, Fong Y, Hess D, et al (1988) Cachectin (tumor necrosis factorα, TNF-α) participates in the metabolic derangements induced by gram-negative bacteremia. Surg Forum 39:8–10
31. Tracey KJ, Lowry SF (1989) The role of cytokines in septic shock. In: Tompkins RK (ed) Advances in surgery. Yearbook Medical Publishers, Chicago pp. 21–56
32. Moldawer LL, Lowry SF, Cerami A (1988) Chachectin: Its impact on metabolism and nutritional status. Ann Rev Nutr 8:585–609
33. Klasing KC (1988) Nutritional aspects of leukocytic cytokines. J Nutr 118:1436–1446
34. van der Poll T, Romijn JA, Endert E, Born JJJ, Büller HR, Sauerwein HP (1991) Tumor necrosis factor mimics the metabolic response to acute infection in healthy humans. Am J Physiol 261:E457–E465
35. Fong Y, Marano MA, Moldawer LL, et al (1990) The acute splanchnic and peripheral tissue metabolic response to endotoxin in man. J Clin Invest 85:1896–1904
36. Tracey KJ, Lowry SF, Fahey TJ, et al (1987) Cachectin/tumor necrosis factor induces lethal septic shock and stress hormone responses in the dog. Surg Gynecol Obstet 164:415–422
37. Evans DA, Jacobs DO, Revhaug A, Wilmore DW (1989) The effects of tumor necrosis factor and their selective inhibition by ibuprofen. Ann Surg 209:312–321
38. Rock CS, Coyle SM, Keogh CV, et al (1992) Influence of hypercortisolemia on the acute phase protein response to endotoxin in man. Surgery 112:467–474
39. Barber AE, Coyle SM, Marano MA, et al (1993) Glucocorticoid therapy alters hormonal and cytokine responses to endotoxin in man. J Immunol 150:1999–2006
40. Fischer E, Marano MA, Barber A, et al (1991) Interleukin-1α administration can replicate the hemodynamic and metabolic responses to sublethal endotoxemia. Am J Physiol 261:R442–R452
41. Fischer E, Marano MA, Van Zee KJ, et al (1992) Interleukin-1 receptor blockade improves survival and hemodynamic performance in *E. coli* septic shock, but fails to alter host responses to sublethal endotoxemia. J Clin Invest 89:1551–1557
42. Rhyne CD, Calvano SE, Richardson RP, et al (1987) Functional immune consequences following *in vivo* lipopolysaccharide (LPS) administration to normal human subjects are secondary to an alteration of antigen presenting cells. Surg Forum 38:96–98
43. Richardson RP, Rhyne CD, Fong Y, et al (1989) Peripheral blood leukocyte kinetics following *in vivo* lipopolysaccharide (LPS) administration to normal human subjects: Influence of elicited hormones and cytokines. Ann Surg 210:239–245
44. Fischer E, Van Zee KJ, Marano MA, et al (1992) Interleukin-1 receptor antagonist circulates in experimental inflammation and in human disease. Blood 79:2196–2200
45. VanZee KJ, Kohno T, Fischer E, Rock CS, Moldawer LL, Lowry SF (1992) Tumor necrosis factor (TNF) soluble receptors circulate during experimental and clinical inflammation and can protect against excessive TNFα *in vitro* and *in vivo*. Proc Natl Acad Sci 89:4845–4849
46. Schattner A, Steinbock M, Tepper R, Schonfeld A, Vaisman N, Hahn T (1990) Tumour necrosis factor production and cell-mediated immunity in anorexia nervosa. Clin Exp Immunol 79:62–66

47. Luger A, Graf H, Schwarz H-P, Stummvoll H-K, Luger TA (1986) Decreased serum interleukin 1 activity and monocyte interleukin 1 production in patients with fatal sepsis. Crit Care Med 14:458–461
48. Oliff A, Defeo-Jones D, Boyer M, et al (1987) Tumors secreting human TNF/cachectin induce cachexia in mice. Cell 50:555–563
49. Tracey KJ, Fong Y, Hesse DG, et al (1987) Anti-cachectin/TNF monoclonal antibodies prevent septic shock during lethal bacteremia. Nature 330:662–664
50. Ziegler EJ, Fisher CJ Jr, Sprung CL, et al (1991) Treatment of gram-negative bacteremia and septic shock with HA-IA monoclonal antibody endotoxin: A randomized, double-blind, placebo-controlled trial. N Engl J Med 324:429–436
51. Munoz C, Carlet J, Fitting C, Misset B, Blériot J-P, Cavaillon J-M (1991) Dysregulation of *in vitro* cytokine production by monocytes during sepsis. J Clin Invest 88:1747–1754
52. Herndon DN, Stein MD, Rutan TC, Abston S, Linares H (1987) Failure of TPN supplementation to improve liver function, immunity, and mortality in thermally injured patients. J Trauma 27:195–204
53. Fong Y, Tracy KJ, Moldawer LL, et al (1989) Antibodies to cachectin/TNF reduce interleukin-1β and interleukin-6 appearance during lethal bacteremia. J Exp Med 170:1627–1633

The Maintenance of Antioxidant Defenses during Inflammation

R. F. Grimble

Introduction

Invasion of the body by pathogens, or trauma and chronic neoplastic and inflammatory disease, brings about activation of the immune system. A range of molecules with high biological potency are produced by the system, with the objective of defeating the invasion, destroying damaged and aberrant cells, and restoring tissue function to normal. Cytokines, free radicals and other oxidant products are among these potent molecules. The cytokines comprise the interleukins 1–12 (IL1–12), tumour necrosis factors (TNF) and interferons [1]. Free radicals comprise the superoxide, hydroxyl and nitric oxide radicals. Other oxidant products which are related to free radical biology are hypochlorous acid and hydrogen peroxide [2, 3].

The very nature of these substances potentially exposes the host to damage. However, natural systems exist to afford a high degree of protection of the host against the deleterious effects of cytokines, and free radicals and other oxidant molecules. An increasing body of evidence suggests that enhanced production of all three types of molecule occurs under physiological as well as pathological circumstances. The utilization of oxygen results in production of various reactive oxygen species which have the potential to cause tissue damage. Thus, organisms which utilize oxygen have developed sophisticated anti-oxidant defenses. Strenuous exercise increases free radical and cytokine production [4, 5]. Ovulation is accompanied by increased synthesis of TFN [6]. Mild psychological stress may also enhance IL-1 production [7].

Cytokines, free radicals and other oxidant molecules which are produced as a consequence of activation of the immune system, arise largely from phagocytic cells. These molecules have the ability to enhance each others production. TNF and IL-1 elicit reactive oxygen and nitrogen oxide species from macrophages [8, 9]. Conversely, enhanced TNF production has been observed in experimental situations in which free radical generation is enhanced [10]. Antioxidant defenses are increased by the action of a number of cytokines including IL-1, TNF and IL-6. Thus within mammals, there are attempts to balance oxidant and antioxidant systems even under pathological circumstances. The achievement of a balance may not however occur with total success, as will be seen later in this chanter.

The Nature of Free Radical and other Oxidant Production by Immune Cells

Before considering the oxidant products which are synthesized by the immune system, it is first necessary to consider the consequences of the synthesis of the superoxide radical, which is a major product of the oxidant burst, that occurs when phagocytic cells are activated [2]. Figure 1 gives an overview of possible products from the superoxide radical.

The superoxide radical is the least active of the free radicals, with the exception of the α-tocopherol radical. Superoxide is removed by the action of superoxide dismutases (SOD). Hydrogen peroxide is the product of the reaction and acts as substrate for a number of competing reaction, some of which result in biologically inactive products, and others in substances of greater potency than the original superoxide. Glutathione peroxidase and catalase convert hydrogen peroxide to water. Myeloperoxidase catalyses the reaction of the peroxide, with chloride, to produce a hypochlorite radical. Hydrogen peroxide may also react nonenzymically with superoxide to produce hydroxyl radicals in the presence of trace amounts of iron and other transition metals. In the presence of the same metals, the hydroxyl radical will react with lipids to produce lipid peroxides which rapidly decompose, producing lipid free radicals. The appearance of these substances leads to a chain reaction of lipid peroxidation. The end-products from this sequence of events are cytotoxic aldehydes, such as malonaldehyde, and hydrocarbons such as ethane and pentane. The chain of lipid peroxidation is arrested or broken if α-tocopherol reacts with a peroxyl radical to produce its own radical, which has virtually no reactivity with lipids. Superoxide production is not limited to immune cells. Fibroblasts and endothelial cells are also capable of production [11, 12]. The physiological role of such production in unclear, however fibroblast proliferation is stimulated, suggesting a role in healing and tissue repair [11]. Nitric oxide (NO) is also among the oxidant substances produced by activated immune cells. It is produced as the result of the action of argin-

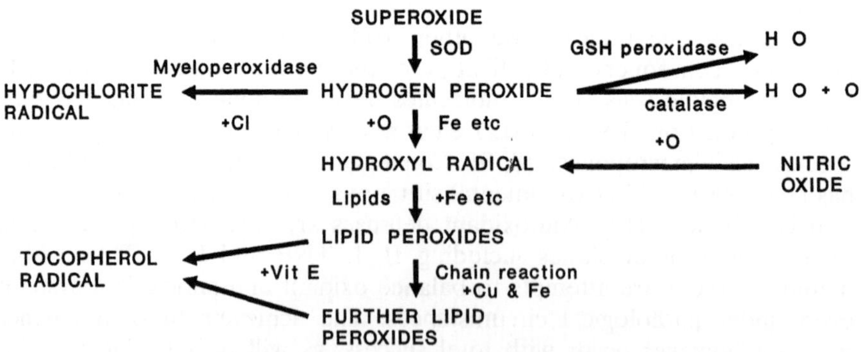

Fig. 1. Metabolism and consequences of superoxide radical formation

ine deimidase on intracellular arginine. NO, like superoxide, can also be produced from other cells such as endothelial cells. The physiological functions of NO in each context is however different. For endothelial cells, NO influences vascular tone by causing vasodilation. For macrophages, NO acts as a killing agent for invading cells. The manner and amount of NO production from each cell source are different. Stimulation of endothelial cells results in rapid, transient production of relatively small amounts of NO, the production does not involve a protein synthetic step. Stimulation of macrophages results in massive, prolonged production after a lag period of several hours. The enhanced production involves a protein synthetic step [3]. Due to the ability of NO to cause vasodilation, production in response to pathogens carries with it the risk of hypotension [13]. Thus, it can be seen from this simplified view of superoxide and NO metabolism that the process carries benefits of killing of pathogens, wound healing, and tissue repair, but also a twofold risk of producing potentially toxic substances and of initiating processes which can lead to cell damage, should antioxidant defenses fail to meet the challenge. The importance of the superoxide and NO radical in the morbidity of severe trauma and sepsis is illustrated by the improved condition which occurs on administering recombinant SOD or a metabolic inhibitor of NO production, n-methyl L-arginine (NMDA) [14, 15].

The cells of the immune system which are mainly responsible for the production of free radicals and other oxidant molecules, are eosinophils and neutrophils. The most potent inducers of free radical and other oxidant molecule production (oxidant or respiratory burst) from neutrophils are phagocytozable microorganisms. A number of physiological secretagogues such as immune complexes, arachidonic acid, leukotrienes and platelet activating factor (PAF) elicit transient release. The amount produced is well below that caused by contact with bacteria. Furthermore, some of the secretagogues are active at concentrations which are unlikely to be present during inflammation.

A wide range of cytokines, including IL-1, IFNγ, and TNFα and β stimulate transient production of reactive oxygen radicals. Cytokines exert their effects at concentrations that are three to five orders of magnitude lower than those required for agents such as leukotrienes or PAF. The ability of polymorphonuclear cells (PMN) to produce oxidant bursts is considerably enhanced when the cells have adhered to surfaces, or have been sensitized by agents such as endotoxin. Adherence of cells to endothelial cells resulted in prolonged production of oxygen radicals in the presence of TNFα that is similar in amounts to that produced by stimulation with bacteria [16]. Production of oxygen radicals by eosinophils in response to TNF is dependent upon adhesion to surfaces [17]. Thus while such sensitization might increase resistance to infection, it might also predispose the patient to oxidant damage. Indeed increased evidence of oxidant damage is present in patients undergoing major inflammatory reactions such as in ARDS [18].

The Actions of Free Radicals and other Oxidant Molecules

There are many ways in which free radicals can exert damaging effects upon bacterial, and malignant and normal cells of the host. Superoxide radicals will, by conversion to hydrogen peroxide, damage cell membrane proteins. The peroxide can rapidly diffuse into cells, inhibit ATP synthesis and produce breaks in the DNA molecule. The latter is more likely to occur in the presence of transition metals which encourage the formation of hydroxyl radicals. Hydrogen peroxide, in the presence of chloride ions and myeloperoxidase, is transformed to hypochlorous acid which will damage the cell membrane by attacking the sulphydryl groups of constituent proteins [19, 20].

A number of studies carried out *in vivo* and *in vitro* suggest that TNF may exert its lethal effects by induction of free radicals. Hydroxyl radical scavengers, anaerobic conditions, and inhibitors of arachidonic acid metabolism, prevent TNF from exerting lethal effects on tumor cell lines *in vitro*. *In vivo*, the lethality of TNF will be increased in animals which have antioxidant defenses impaired by reduction of tissue glutathione concentrations by diethylmaleate. The converse is true, since a reduction in lethality was observed in animals whose defenses were enhanced by feeding N-acetyl cysteine (NAC) [21].

The Nature of Antioxidant Defenses

Defenses are comprised of lipid and water soluble substances and enzymes, while the components of the defenses are derived ultimately from the diet, many are derived directly from the diet. Vitamins E and C, carotenes, and the copper and zinc moities of ceruloplasmin (CP) and metallothionien (MT), fall into this category. Glutathione (GSH) arises to a large extent from dietary supplies of its three constituent amino acids: glycine, cysteine, and glutamate, although *de novo* synthesis of the three amino acids may make a significant contribution. The importance of the dietary contribution is underlined by the major fall in tissue GSH content that occurs when food intake decreases (Fig. 3). The enzyme systems include SOD, glutathione peroxidase and catalase (Fig. 1). The acute phase protein CP also has SOD-like activity [22].

The defenses are strategically placed throughout the body to afford maximum protection from free radicals. Ceruloplasmin, MT, GSH and nutrient antioxidants are present in the circulation. The latter three are also present within the cell. GSH, MT and vitamin C reside within the aqueous parts of the cell. Vitamin E (α-tocopherol) resides within the cell membrane where it acts as the main antioxidant at that location. The vitamin is also present in tissue fluids and within the cell, attached to low density lipoproteins and lipids. The enzyme systems are situated throughout the organelles of the cell.

A number of constituents of antioxidant defenses, which depend upon nutrient intake for their adequacy, interrelate. Tocopherol may be regenerated from its radical by the action of GSH [23] and ascorbic acid [24]. Despite the ubiquitous nature of antioxidant defenses, it is possible for free radical generation to deplete defenses at a local level. This phenomenon is illustrated in rheumatoid arthritis where α-tocopherol concentrations in serum are normal while the antioxidant concentration in synovial fluid is severely depleted [25].

As well as direct defenses which destroy free radicals, indirect systems exist which prevent free radicals from propogating. Hydrogen peroxide which is produced during the metabolism of superoxide is transformed into hydroxyl radicals if trace amounts of transition metals, such as iron and copper, are present to catalyse the action. Thus safe storage of these ions is crucial at all time. Two thirds of the 4 g of iron present in the human body is stored as hemoglobin, one tenth as myoglobin, a smaller portion is bound to transferrin (the iron transport protein), and the remainder is stored bound to intracellular proteins such as ferritin and hemosiderin. The substantial ability of ferritin to bind iron and the fact that transferrin is only 30% saturated with iron, result in virtually no free iron within the cell [26]. Ceruloplasmin also inhibits transition metal ion catalyzed production of radicals by sequestration of metal ions. The biological importance of adequate sequestration of transition metal ions, in conditions in which the immune system is activated, is illustrated in patients who have suffered iron overload as a consequence of their treatment. Such patients exhibited liver damage and joint inflammation [27, 28]. Studies in mice suggest that iron overload increases hepatic synthesis of glutathione, thereby increasing the demand for its constituent amino acids [29].

The importance of adequate transition metal ion binding is also underlined by the potential of iron to convert ascorbic acid from an antioxidant to a prooxidant role. The transformation occurs due to the ability of ascorbic acid to convert unsequestered iron from ferric to ferrous ions. Since oxidation of ascorbic acid can result in hydrogen peroxide, all the necessary components for production of hydroxyl radicals will be in place [25, 26].

Influence of Cytokines on Antioxidant Defenses

As outlined earlier, it is necessary for antioxidant defenses to be enhanced in situations in which the immune system is activated, to protect host tissues from the damaging effects of free radicals and other oxidant substances produced by the system. Cytokines, in particular IL-1, TNF, and IL-6, marshall a number of components of these defenses. Cytokines bring about large increases in glutathione synthesis, thereby enhancing and maintaining the tissue content. The stimulatory effect on synthesis is necessary since glutathione synthesis is greatly dependent upon dietary protein intake. In particular, on the intake if sulphur amino acids. IL-1 and TNF released during inflammation may bring about a substantial fall in food intake, thus the effects of the reduction in substrate intake are circumvented by the stimulatory effects of the cytokines on GSH synthesis. The enzymes involved in the metabolism of the superoxide radical and hydrogen peroxide are increased by the actions of a number of cytokines. For example, IL-1 and TNF induce production of manganese SOD (MnSOD) in pulmonary endothelial cells in rats [30, 31].

In addition to increasing the active antioxidant defenses, cytokines also induce changes which minimize free radical proliferation by inducing the synthesis of the substances which limit the exposure of tissues to iron and copper ions. Cytokines bring about substantial changes in the synthesis of hemoglobin, transferrin, ferritin, CP and MT.

That of the first three, hemoglobin, transferrin and ferritin is increased, thereby exerting close control on iron sequestration. The sequestration may however not be completely assured. At a pH of 6, iron dissociates from ferritin. The pH within close proximity to an activated phagocyte may fall below this value permitting iron to enhance free radical production [25]. The acute phase protein haptoglobin also acts to reduce the possibility of iron to becoming available, in catalytic amounts, by binding to haem, released from the destruction of red blood cells which is a consequence of tissue injury and infection. Circulating CP concentrations are enhanced by a number of inflammatory agents such as endotoxin, IL-1 and TNF [32, 33].

An increasing body of evidence is emerging that cytokines and free radicals enhance each others production. Chaudhri and Clark [10] demonstrated that the ability of endotoxin to stimulate TNF production was enhanced by alloxan, a prooxidant drug, and that the effect could be prevented by administration of butylated hydroxyanisole, an antioxidant, or desferrioxymine an iron chelating agent. Other antioxidant substances may be able to suppress cytokine production in situations in which a prooxidant environment has been created. Ku et al. [34] showed that probucol, a hypocholesterolemic drug with antioxidant properties, was able to suppress IL-1 production from murine peritoneal macrophages, that were incubated with endotoxin. The production of TNF was however unaffected. N-acetyl-cysteine which is a substrate for glutathione synthesis, and an antioxidant in its own right, was however able to inhibit production of TNF by splenocytes from mice injected with endotoxin. IL-6 production by the same tissue was unaffected [35].

Subsequently it was shown that TNF, IL-1 and IL-2 production could be stimulated by hydrogen peroxide *in vitro* [10, 36]. The mechanism underlying the enhansive effects of free radicals upon cytokine production may be the ability of oxidants to stimulate production of the transcription factor NFkB. The factor is involved in production of cytokines from stimulated immune cells [37]. Thus, antioxidant substances may prevent the stimulatory effect of oxidants and oxidant situations on cytokine production at the level of the transcription factor.

Interactions between Nutrition, Cytokines and Antioxidant Defenses

The Increased Demand for Nutrients

The metabolic events which occur during inflammation carry with them a nutritional cost. The nutritional implications of inflammation are set out in Table 1. These nutritional implications include increased demands for protein, specific amino acids, and trace elements. A number of these nutrients are involved in the elaboration and maintainance of antioxidant defenses. In addition, the ability of certain nutrients such as fatty acids to alter the intensity of the inflammatory process may alter both the magnitude of synthesis of antioxidants and oxidant production [38].

A number of studies have shown that a low protein diet reduces the GSH content of liver and lungs [33, 34, 36]. The question arises as to whether the reduction is due to protein deficiency *per se*, or to a deficiency in one of the constituent amino acids of the antioxidant i.e. cysteine, glycine or glutamate. Studies carried out by our group on rats suggest that the adequacy of dietary sulphur amino acid intake can influence tissue GSH content. Furthermore, Hong et al. [39] have shown that glutamine supplementation helps to restore

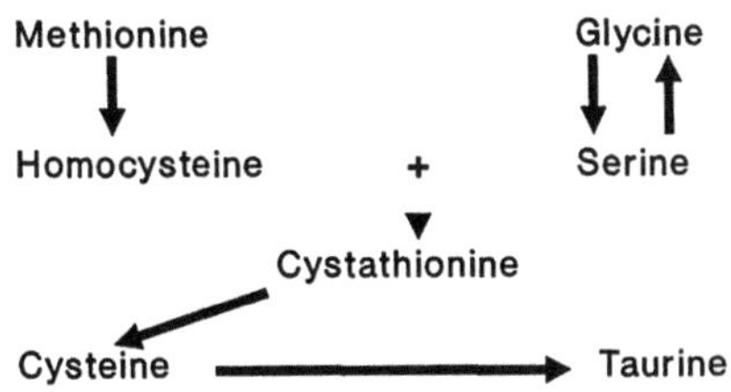

Fig. 2. Metabolic relationship of glycine, serine, cysteine and taurine

Table 1. Nutritional implications of inflammation

Process	Nutrient implication
Fever	Energy requirements
Antioxidant defenses	
– Glutathione	Cysteine, glycine, glutamine
– Antioxidant enzymes	Cu, Mn, Zn, Se
– Nutrient derived	Vitamins A, C, E
Acute phase proteins	Protein, specific amino acids, Cu, Zn, Fe
Connective tissue remodelling	Protein, Glycine, Vitamin C
Hematopoesis	Protein, Vitamin B12, folate, Fe
Inflammatory intensity	n6 to n3 polyunsaturated fatty acid ratio
Immune cell increase and activation	Protein, glutamine, glucose, vitamins, trace elements

liver GSH and plasma content, following acetoaminophen poisoning, in rats consuming a diet with an adequate sulphur amino acid content. Thus, there may be a nutritional hierarchy in the relative importance of nutrient provision, to maintain GSH synthesis. There are several pieces of circumstantial evidence which suggest that the requirement for sulphur amino acids, methionine and cysteine, and amino acids that are metabolically related to them (glycine and serine) are increased during inflammation. Askanazi et al. [40] observed decreases in plasma concentrations of serine, glycine and taurine of 11, 35 and 45%, respectively, in patients with severe trauma and sepsis. As shown in Fig. 2 glycine is a precursor of serine and serine forms the carbon skeleton of cysteine. Several tissue components such as glutathione and metallothionein, which show enhanced syntheses during inflammation are particularly rich in the amino acids related to cysteine (Table 2). Following fractures and burns, urinary sulphur excretion is enhanced to a lesser extent than that of nitrogen [41, 42]. This may indicate preferential retention of sulphur amino acids. The decrease in plasma taurine concentration during sepsis and trauma may likewise indicate diversion of cysteine, from the synthesis of this major end-product, into molecules with a high cysteine content. Indeed in rats given TNF, decreases in urinary sulphate excretion occur in concert with increases in liver and lung glutathione content [43]. We examined the influence of glycine, methionine, cysteine, serine and taurine supplementation on the response of protein depleted rats to TNF injections. Protein depletion was achieved by feeding a diet containing 8% casein instead of 20%. A number of responses to TNF were blunted in animals receiving the 8% diet (Table 3). In animals fed the low protein diet with contained alanine, as an isonitrogenous control for the amino acids interrelated to cysteine, liver glutathione, protein and zinc content did not increase in response to TNF, as it did in animals receiving the 20% casein diet. Furthermore, lung GSH content fell by 42% in the former group in response to the cytokine. No significant change in lung glutathione occurred in animals consuming the high protein diet. Addition of cysteine, and methionine to the low protein diet permitted an increase in GSH content of both liver and lung in response to TNF. While

Table 2. Amino acid composition of proteins and peptides which show increased rates of synthesis during inflammation

(% of residues)	Glycine	Serine	Methionine + Cysteine	Total
C3 complement	6	6	4	16
Haptoglobin	7	5	4	16
Ceruloplasmin	7	6	3	16
C-reactive protein	8	10	3	21
Serum amyloid A	12	9	4	25
Phospholipase A2	5	9	11	25
Collagen	34	3	1	38
Metalothionein	11	13	32	56
Glutathione	33	0	33	66

Table 3. Influence of supplementary glycine, serine, methionine, cysteine and taurine on the response of protein depleted rats to TNFα[a]

Injection diet	Liver [Zn]		Liver [Protein]		Liver [GSH]		Lung [GSH]		Plasma [CP]	
	S	T	S	T	S	T	S	T	S	T
20% Casein	100	124	100	137	100	121	100	95	100	230
8% Cas+ala	91	85	99	102	21	28	71	42	180	353
8% Cas+gly	38	56	106	110	13	28	78	78	133	303
8% Cas+ser	71	85	116	110	33	29	115	74	183	285
8% Cas+met	88	86	72	99	39	105	38	106	192	252
8% Cas+cys	65	92	94	134	79	104	75	110	100	220
8% Cas+tau	85	85	110	106	29	25	96	72	187	365

[a] Values shown are for rats 24 h after an injection of 100 μg/kg TNFα (T) and are expressed as a percentage of the value observed for saline (S) injected rats receiving the 20% casein diet. Amino acid additions to the diets are isonitrogenous and equivalent to 6 g alanine/kg diet

addition of the provider of the carbon skeleton of cysteine (serine), or a major end-product of cysteine (taurine) did not assist an increase in liver GSH content, both reduced the extent of the fall in lung GSH in response to TNF. The data suggest that the sulphur moiety of cysteine is of prime importance in maintaining and enhancing tissue glutathione, in situations in which cytokines such as TNF may be operating.

TNF may play a role in the extensive weight loss observed in cancer and AIDS [44]. It is thus interesting to note that, in asymptomatic HIV-infected individuals, substantial reductions occur in GSH concentrations in plasma, immune cells, and lung endothelial lining fluid [49]. The decreases in tissue GSH in AIDS may therefore indicate the requirement for sulphur amino acids is not being satisfied. There may indeed be an enhanced requirement for cysteine for GSH synthesis in AIDS since alveolar macrophages from such patients are activated and exhibit exaggerated production of oxidants, and urinary malonaldehyde production is enhanced [46, 47]. Furthermore, administration of GSH to the lungs of patients by aerosol resulted in greatly enhanced concentrations of oxidized glutathione in the endothelial lining fluid, suggesting enhanced utilization of this antioxidant [48].

Compensatory Adaptations in Defenses

Our studies suggest that when the nature of the diet limits supplies of substrate for maintaining antioxidant defenses, adaptations occur to maintain defense from the resources available. The data for ceruloplasmin concentrations shown in Table 3 indicates that a compensatory increase occurs in this component of antioxidant defenses, when the ability to synthesize glutathione is impaired by the low protein diet. Compared with the response of well fed animals, an enhanced effect occurred in animals consuming the low protein diet supplemented with alanine. Addition of serine, cysteine and methionine to these diets resulted in a lesser degree of enhancement. Thus when sulphur amino acid intake limits the ability to synthesize GSH, which contains 33% cysteine; ceruloplasmin, which contains 3% of sulphur amino acids, is synthesized in an attempt to maintain antioxidant defenses.

Compensatory increases in components of the antioxidant defenses may also take place in other experimental contexts where defenses are modulated by nutritional means. We studied effects of vitamin E sufficiency on liver and lung GSH concentrations when food intake was decreased. Rats were fed diets deficient in vitamin E, or containing an adequate (50 mg/kg diet) or supplemental (250 mg/kg) level α-tocopherol. The diets were fed in an *ad libitum* amount for 3 weeks prior to 24 h in which feeding continued at 100 or 50 or 25% of the *ad libitum* rate. The data in Fig. 3 show that an enhanced concentrations of hepatic GSH occurs in the vitamin E deficient animals at all levels of food intake, the drive to synthesize GSH overrides the inhibitory effect of reduced sulphur amino acid intake which would occur at the reduced levels of food intake. Lung GSH does not exhibit the same characteristics.

The Effectiveness of Defenses in Nutritional Deficiency

The extent to which such adaptations in antioxidant defenses protect the animals from antioxidant damage is not clear. However, studies carried out by Swords et al. [49] suggest that, at best, the compensatory increase in liver

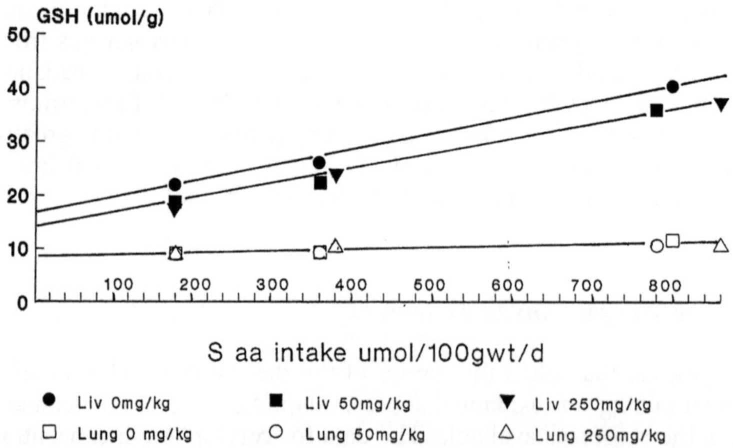

Fig. 3. Influence of sulphur amino acid and vitamin E intake on gluthatione content of liver and lung in rats

GSH would limit, rather than prevent, the increase in oxidant damage which occurs in vitamin E deficiency. As selenium is an important component of glutathione peroxidase, Swords et al. examined the effects of selenium and vitamin E deficiency on lipid peroxidation following endotoxin injections in rats. The investigators also examined the relative effectiveness of vitamin E and selenium supplementation in suppressing the induced lipid peroxidation. Ethane production rose from 0.5 nmol/kgBW/h, in animals receiving adequate vitamin E and selenium, to 5 nmol/kg/h in deficient animals. Treatment with endotoxin increased production to 1 and 15 nmol/kg/h in the well fed and deficient animals. Supplementation of the latter group with selenium and vitamin E reduced production to 4.2 and 1.8 nmol/kg, respectively. Thus vitamin E was more protective than selenium against lipid peroxidation induced by inflammation.

Deficiencies in dietary copper and zinc may also limit antioxidant defenses in a number of ways. Both metals are cofactors in copper-zinc SOD which acts as the first line of defense against the superoxidase free radical (Fig. 1), as well as being components of ceruloplasmin and metalothionein, respectively. In rats, copper deficiency reduced the activity of the enzyme to 11 and 74% of normal activity in liver and lung, respectively. Manganese SOD activity was unchanged in both tissues, while catalase was reduced by 15% in liver by this dietary treatment [50]. Ceruloplasmin activity fell to 18% of normal values. Zinc deficiency had no effect upon the antioxidant enzymes, but reduced liver and lung MT content to 6 and 73% of normal values. Deficiencies in copper and zinc effect CP and MT synthesis, in a different manner, in response to an inflammatory stimulus. In copper deficient rats, synthesis of CP protein in response to IL-1 is unimpaired, while the oxidase activity of the molecule is severely reduced [32]. In zinc deficient rats, the synthesis of MT protein is inhibited [50]. Thus copper deficiency acts posttranscriptionally, while that of zinc acts at the level of transcription. In the study, reduction of CP and MT had little influence on the concentrations of plasma α-tocopherol and ascorbate, however zinc deficiency led to a reduction of 40% and 10% in GSH in liver and lung, respectively. It would appear from this finding that zinc deficiency had the greatest impact on antioxidant defense despite having no effect on SOD activity [50]. Clearly the situation is complex.

It is not clear from the study how the deficiencies in Cu and Zn would influence the effectiveness of the defenses during an inflammatory stress. Exposure to high oxygen concentrations as occurs in care of the premature infant, can cause inflammation of lungs that may be mediated by free radicals and cytokines. Animal models have been used to study this problem. A greater degree of lung damage occurred in the zinc deficient rats when exposed to high oxygen tensions for 7 days, than in rats that were zinc repleted. While increases in lung SOD, glutathione peroxidase and catalase occurred in the latter animals, deficient animals showed none of these changes. In the same animal model, copper deficiency did not prevent the increase in lung CuZn SOD which occurred in response to oxygen exposure, despite major decreases in lung copper content [52]. The data reported in the studies illus-

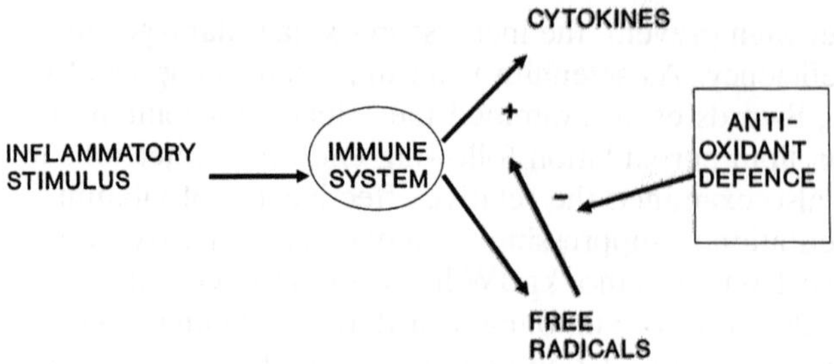

Fig. 4. Influence of antioxidant defenses on the interaction of cytokines and free radicals during inflammation

trate the relative sensitivities of the antioxidant defenses in liver and lung to the dietary intake of precursors. Since free radicals produced as a consequence of cytokine action are able to enhance cytokine production, the question arises as to whether nutrients can indirectly modulate cytokine production by enhancing antioxidant defenses as shown in Fig. 4.

We examined the effects of altering the effectiveness of antioxidant defenses, on the responsiveness to inflammatory agents, by studying the effects of vitamin E sufficiency on the response to endotoxin in rats (Table 4) [53]. Rats were fed diets which contained 0,5 or 250 mg/kg of α-tocopherol for 3 weeks prior to injection. A greater degree of anorexia and increase in α-1-acid glycoprotein occurred in the deficient animals suggesting an enhanced production of cytokines. However infiltration of PMN into lung was similar in all groups after injection with endotoxin. In vitamin E deficient control animals, which had experienced only the minor day-to-day exposure to inflammatory agents in the environment of the animal colony, significantly greater amounts of PMN appeared in lung tissue, than in animals receiving 50 mg/kg α-tocopherol. Animals receiving the supernormal amount of α-

Table 4. Influence of vitamin E status on the response to endotoxin in rats

Diet Vit E (mg/kg)	0		50		250	
Injection	S	E	S	E	S	E
Food intake (g/24 h post injury)	23	3	27	13	24	17
Liver wt (% body wt)	4.0	5.1	3.7	5.1	4.1	5.3
Plasma a-1-acid glycoprotein (units/ml)	22	256	14	157	18	163
Plasma albumin (mg/ml)	34.5	30.9	34.4	28.5	33.4	31.5
Lung PMN (% cells)	9.2	10.6	7.9	10.9	7.0	9.2
Plasma Vit E (mg/ml)	0.32		0.76		0.97	
Red cell Vit E (mg/ml)	0.41		0.73		1.12	

S and E are saline and endotoxin injections, respectively, 800 μg/kg of endotoxin given i.p. Saline injected animals pair fed to intakes of E animals. Effects measured 24 h post-injection. (From [53] with permission)

tocopherol had significantly lower concentrations of PMN in lung than animals given a normal amount of α-tocopherol. Evidence of enhanced responsiveness to endotoxin is also apparent in the study of Omer and Millward [54] in which rats had antioxidant defenses depleted by feeding diets deficient in vitamin E and protein. A greater increase in hepatic protein synthesis and fall in plasma zinc occurred in these, than in animals receiving a diet adequate in these two nutrients.

Conclusion and Clinical Implications

In patients responding to infections, trauma and chronic inflammatory challenges, cytokines orchestrate events to bring about repair and restoration of health. In so doing, cytokines lead to the generation of oxidant molecules which are potentially toxic to the patient. However cytokines also induce defenses against these substances. It is apparent from the studies described above that nutrition may exert substantial effects on antioxidant defenses and cytokine biology (Fig. 5).

The potential for preventing free radicals from leading to overproduction of cytokines by means of the strategy of maintaining and enhancing antioxidant defenses exists. A numer of clinical and laboratory studies, in which the intake of sulphydryl compounds such as cysteine, glutathione and N-acetylcysteine have been enhanced, illustrates this potential. N-acetyl-cysteine (NAC), GSH and cysteine all inhibit NFkB expression in stimulated T-cell lines [55, 56]. N-acetyl-cysteine produced beneficial effects in ARDS patients and in a sheep model of ARDS [57, 58]. It also improved inflammation in healthy smokers, as assessed by examination of bronchoalveolar lavage fluid for eosinophil basic protein, lactoferrin, α-chymotrypsin, and chemotaxis of neutrophils [59]. As NAC has antioxidant properties, it is unclear whether NAC is acting directly, or indirectly, by undergoing deacetylation and delivering cysteine directly to tissues. Certainly the importance of cysteine in optimum immune function is highlighted by the fact that macrophages act as a

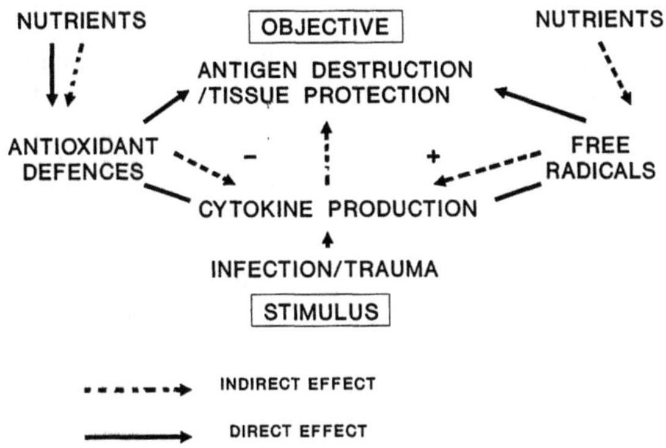

Fig. 5. Effects of nutrients on cytokine and free radical interactions during infection and trauma

cysteine pump to deliver the sulphur amino acid to lymphocytes at variable but controlled rates. Macrophages take up cysteine and cystine from tissue fluid and release cysteine under the action of inflammatory stimuli such as endotoxin and TNF. Close proximity of activated macrophages and lymphocytes facilitates the transfer. In addition to supressing NFkB expression, cysteine enhances a number of lymphocyte functions such as cytotoxic T-cell activity. Uptake of cystine into macrophages is competitively inhibited by glutamate. It is therefore interesting to note that raised plasma glutamates have been observed in AIDS and advanced malignancy, since immunosuppression is apparent in both conditions [60].

The drug diethylthiocarbamate, which has antioxidant capabilities due to glutathione peroxidase like activity, reduces the rate of progression of new opportunistic infections in AIDS. A study in which Zidovudine produced a slowing in the development of AIDS led to a rise in plasma GSH [48]. Vitamin E sufficiency may also play a key part in the antioxidant defenses in AIDS since many of the abnormalities seen in components of the immune system, as a result of HIV infection, are stimulated, or restored, by a high intake of the vitamin e.g. 400 iu/day in man. Feeding studies of normal subjects have shown that α-tocopherol increased delayed type hypersensitivity, and lymphocyte proliferation and IL-2 production in response to mitogens [61].

The inhibitory actions of the sulphydryl compounds on NFkB expression, mentioned earlier on, takes on an additional importance in AIDS since the transcription factor enhances HIV mRNA expression. Thus free radicals cytokines produced during the progression of AIDS will enhance replication of the virus via this route. Since *in vitro* studies have shown that the stimulatory effect of TNF in HIV replication in monocytes can be inhibited by GSH and NAC, the sufficiency of antioxidant defenses take on an additional importance, apart from protecting the patient from the potentially damaging outcome of activation of the immune system by encounters with bacteria, viruses and other inflammatory agents and situations.

References

1. Male D, Roitt I, Rook G (1989) Cell mediated immune responses. In: Roitt, Brostoff, Male (eds) Immunology. Churchill Livingstone. Edinburgh London Melbourne. pp 9.1–9.13
2. Halliwell B (1991) Reactive oxygen species in living systems: Source, biochemistry, and role in human disease. Am J Med 91 (Suppl 3C):14S–22S
3. Marletta MA (1989) Nitric oxide: Biosynthesis and biological significance. TIBS 14:488–492
4. Lindsay MW, Alexander D, Jacobs P (1991) Strenuous exercise: Analogous to the acute-phase response? Clin Sci 81:677–683
5. Mena P, Mayner M, Gutierrez JM, Mayner J, Timon J, Campillo JE (1991) Plasma interleukin concentrations in professional cyclists. Int J Sports Med 12:563–566
6. Adashi EY (1989) Cytokine-mediated regulation of ovarian function: Encounters of a third kind. Endocrinology (Editorial) 124:2043–2045

7. Kluger MJ (1991) Fever: Role of pyrogens and cryogens. Physiological Reviews 71:93–127
8. Lamas S, Michel T, Brenner BM, et al (1991) Nitric oxide synthesis in endothelial cells: Evidence for a pathway inducible by TNFa. Am J Physiol 261:C634–641
9. Farante A, Nandoskar M, Walz A, et al (1988) Effects of tumor necrosis factor alpha and interleukin 1 alpha and beta on human neutrophil migration, respiratory burst and degranulation. Int Arch Allerg Appl Immunol 86:82–91
10. Chaudhri G, Clark IA (1989) Reactive oxygen species facilitate the in vitro and in vivo lipopolysaccharide-induced release of tumor necrosis factor. J Immunol 143:1290–1294
11. Murrell GAC, Francis MJO, Bromley L (1990) Modulation of fibroblast proliferation by oxygen free radicals. Biochem J 265:659–665
12. Matsubara T, Ziff M (1986) Superoxide anion release by human endothelial cells: Synergism between a phorbol ester and a talcum ionophore. J Cell Physiol 127:207–210
13. Ochoa JB, Udekwu AO, Billiar TR, et al (1991) Nitrogen oxide levels in patients after trauma and during sepsis. Ann Surg 214:621–616
14. Kilbourne RG, Gross SS, Jubran A (1990) N-methyl L-arginine inhibits TNF induced hypotension: Implications for involvement of nitric oxide. Proc Natl Acad Sci 87:3622–3632
15. Tikka R, Marzi I, Dike J, Trentz O, Buhren V (1991) Circulating phospholipase A_2 and C reactive protein after polytrauma: Effect of superoxide dismutase. Acta Chir Aust 1:2–4
16. Nathan CF (1987) Neutrophil activation on biological surfaces. Massive secretion of hydrogen peroxide in response to products of macrophages and lymphocytes. J Clin Invest 80:1550–1560
17. Slingaard A, Vercelotti GM, Walker G, Nelson RD, Jacobs HS (1990) Tumor necrosis factor/cachectin stimulates iosinophil oxidant production and toxicity towards human endothelium. J Exp Med 171:2025–2041
18. Baldwin SR, Simon RH, Grim CM, Ketai LH, Box LA, Dievall LJ (1986) Oxidant activity in expired breath of patients with adult respiratory distress syndrome. Lancet 1:11–14
19. Cochrane CG (1991) Cellular injury by oxidants. Am J Med 91 (Suppl 3C):23S–30S
20. Ward PA (1991) Mechanisms of endothelial cell killing by H_2O_2 or products of activated neutrophils. Am J Med 91 (Suppl 3C):89S–94S
21. Zimmerman RJ, Marafino BJ, Chan A, Landre P, Winkelhake L (1989) The role of oxidant injury in tumor cell sensitivity to recombinant human tumor necrosis factor in vivo. J Immunol 142:1405–1409
22. Broadley C, Hoover RL (1989) Ceruloplasmin reduces the adhesion and scavenges superoxide during the interaction of activated polymorphonuclear leukocytes with endothelial cells. Am J Path 135:647–655
23. Taylor CG, Bray TM (1991) Effect of hyperoxia on free radical defense enzymes in the lungs of zinc-deficient rats. J Nutr 121:460–466
24. Wefers, Sies H (1988) The protection by ascorbate and glutathione against microsomal lipid peroxidation is dependent on vitamin. Eur J Biochem 174:353–357
25. Fairburn K, Grootveld M, Ward RS, et al (1992) α-tocopherol, lipids and lipoproteins in knee joint synovial fluid and serum from patients with inflammatory joint disease. Clin Sci 83:657–664
26. Bast A, Haenen GRMM, Doelman CJA (1991) Oxidants and antioxidants: State of the art. Am J Med 91 (Suppl 3C):2S–13S
27. Grootveld M, Bell JD, Halliwell B, Aruoma OL, Bomford A, Sadler PJ (1989) Non-transferrin bound iron in plasma or serum from patients with idiopathic hemochromatosis. Characterisation by high performance liquid chromatography and nuclear magnetic resonance spectroscopy. J Biol Chem 264:4417–4422
28. Winyard PG, Blake DR, Chirico S, Gutteridge JMC, Lunec J (1987) Mechanisms of exacerbation of rheumatoid synovitis by total-dose iron-dextran infusion: In vivo demonstration of iron-promoted oxidant stress. Lancet 1:69–72

29. Ogino T, Kawabala T, Awai M (1989) Stimulation of glutathione synthesis in iron-loaded mice. Biochim Biophys Acta 1006:131–135
30. Visner GA, Dougall WC, Wilson JM, Burr IA, Nick HS (1990) Regulation of manganese superoxide dismutase by lipopolysaccharide, interleukin 1, and tumor necrosis factor. Role in the acute inflammatory response. J Biol Chem 265:2856–2864
31. Wong GHL, Goeddel DV (1988) Induction of manganous superoxide dismutase by tumor necrosis factor: Possible protective mechanisms. Science 242:941–944
32. Barber EF, Cousins RJ (1988) Interleukin-1-stimulated induction of ceruloplasmin synthesis in normal and copper deficient rats. J Nutr 118:375–381
33. Pathirana C, Grimble RF (1992) Taurine and serine supplementation modulates the metabolic response to tumor necrosis factor-a in rats fed a low protein diet. J Nutr 122:1369–1375
34. Ku G, Doherty NS, Schmidt LF, Jackson RL, Dinerstein RJ (1990) Ex vivo lipopolysaccharide-induced interleukin-1 secretion from murine peritoneal macrophages by probucol, a hypocholesterolemic agent with antioxidant properties. FASEB J 4:1645–1653
35. Peristeris P, Clark BD, Gatti S, et al (1992) N-acetyl cysteine and glutathione as inhibitors of tumor necrosis factor production. Cell Immunol 140:390–399
36. Deneke SM, Fanburg BL (1989) Regulation of cellular glutathione. Am J Physiol 257:L163–173
37. Pfizenmaier K, Himmler A, Schütze S, Scheurich P, Kronke M (1992) TNF receptors and TNF signal transduction. The molecules and their emerging role in medicine. In: Beutler B (ed) Tumour Necrosis Factors. Rover Press Ltd, New York, ISBN 0-88167-852-X. pp 439–472
38. Grimble RF (1992) Dietary manipulation of the inflammatory response. Proc Nutr Soc 51:285–294
39. Hong RW, Rounds JD, Helton WS (1992) Glutamine preserves liver glutathione after lethal hepatic injury. Ann Surg 215:114–119
40. Askanazi J, Carpentier YA, Michelsen CB, et al (1980) Muscle and plasma amino acids following injury: Influence of intercurrent infection. Ann Surg 192:78–95
41. Cutherbertson DP (1931) The distribution of N & S in urine during conditions of increased catabolism. Biochem J 25:236–239
42. Larsson J, Liljedahl SO, Martensson J, Nordstrom H, Schildt B, Sorbo B (1982) Urinary excretion of sulfur amino acids and sulfur metabolites in burned patients receiving parenteral nutrition. J Trauma 22:656–663
43. Hunter EAL, Meakins T, Grimble RF (1993) Effects of glycine and arginine supplementation on the metabolic response to tumour necrosis factor in rats fed low protein diets. Proc Nutr Soc 52:90A (Abst)
44. Balkwill F, Burke F, Talbot D (1987) Evidence for TNF/Cachectin production in cancer. Lancet 2:1229–1232
45. Staal FJT, Ela SW, Roederer M, Anderson MT, Herzenberg LA (1992) Glutathione deficiency in human immunodeficiency virus infection. Lancet 1:909–912
46. Crystal RG (1991) Oxidants and respiratory tract epithelial injury: Pathogenesis and strategies for therapeutic intervention. Am J Med 91 (Suppl 3C):39S–44S
47. Sonnerborg A, Carlin G, Akerlund B, Jarstrand C (1988) Increased malondialdehyde in patients with HIV infection. Scand J Inf Dis 20:287–290
48. Baruchel S, Wainberg MA (1992) The role of oxidative stress in disease progression in individuals infected by the human immunodeficiency virus. J Leuk Biol 52:111–114
49. Swords JT, Pope AL, Hoekstra WG (1991) Endotoxin and lipid peroxidation in selenium and vitamin E deficient and adequate rats. J Nutr 121:251–257
50. Taylor CG, Bettger WJ, Bray TM (1988) Effect of dietary zinc or copper deficiency on the primary free radical defense system in rats. J Nutr 118:613–621
51. Cousins RJ, Leinart AS (1988) Tissue specific regulation of zinc metabolism and metalothionein genes by interleukin 1. FASEB J 2:2884–2890
52. Taylor CG, Bray TM (1991) Increased lung copper-zinc superoxide dismutase activity and absence of magnetic resonance imaging detectable lung damage in copper deficient rats exposed to hyperoxia. J Nutr 121:476–479

53. Troughton K, Grimble RF (1993) Vitamin E status modulates the inflammatory response to endotoxin in rats. Proc Nutr Soc 52:84A (Abst)
54. Omer AB, Bates PC, Millward DJ (1988) Effect of combined vitamin E and protein deficiency on the hepatic response of the rat to the Escherichia Coli endotoxin. Proc Nutr Soc 47:10A (Abst)
55. Mihm S, Droge W (1990) Intracellular glutathione level controls DNA binding activity of NFkB like proteins. Immunobiol 181:245–251
56. Mihm S, Ennen J, Pessara U, Kurth R, Droge W (1991) Inhibition of HIV-1 replication and NFkB activity by cysteine and cysteine derivatives. AIDS 5:497–503
57. Bernard GR (1991) N-acetyl cysteine in experimental and clinical lung injury. Am J Med 91 (Suppl 3C):54S–59S
58. Bernard GR, Lucht WD, Niedermeyer ME, Snapper JR, Ogletree ML, Brigham KL (1984) Effect of N-acetyl cysteine on the pulmonary response to endotoxin in the awake sheep and upon in vitro granulocyte function. J Clin Invest 73:1772–1784
59. Eklund A, Eriksson O, Hakansson L, et al (1988) Oral N-acetyl cysteine reduces selected humoral markers of inflammatory cell activity in BAL fluid from healthy smokers: Correlation with cellular variables. Eur Respir 1:832–838
60. Droge W, Eik HP, Gminder H, Mahon S (1991) Modulation of lymphocyte functions and immune response by cysteine and cysteine derivates. Am J Med (Suppl 3C) 91:1405–1445
61. Odelye O, Watson RR (1991) The potential role of vitamin E in the treatment of immunologic abnormalities during acquired immune deficiency syndrome. Prog Food Nut Sci 15:1–19

Disease/Nutrients Interactions

Acute Renal Failure in the ICU: Approaches to Nutritional Support

D. Bihari, I. Mitchell, and R. Chang

Introduction – The Kidney as "Victim"

For many years it has been apparent that the provision of nutritional support is fundamental in the treatment of patients with acute renal failure (ARF). There is now an extensive literature concerning the metabolic abnormalities associated with acute uremia and the possible beneficial effects of various parenteral solutions of amino acids, essential or non-essential, standard or enriched with branch-chain amino acids, in combination with hypertonic glucose [1, 2]. In the last 15 years, however, clinicians who work regularly in the ICU have come to appreciate that most patients with ARF in the ICU do not suffer from a discrete "single organ" failure, i. e. ARF by itself, but rather that any renal dysfunction that occurs – e. g. failure to concentrate the urine or oliguria together with a rising blood urea and serum creatinine, etc ... – is yet another facet of the "multiple organ dysfunction syndrome" (MOF) most commonly related to sepsis, trauma or an inadequate cardiac output [3]. Occasionally, patients with an arteritis and multisystem dysfunction present to the ICU, and it is important to make this diagnosis since specific treatment, e. g. immunosuppression with steroids, cyclophosphamide and/or plasma exchange may be indicated. Whilst undoubtedly these cases are rare, microscopy of the urine (so often forgotten in the ICU and replaced by "stick"" testing) remains critical in the assessment of all patients with oliguria. Nowadays, it seems to us appropriate to distinguish between those conditions in which the kidney is the "prime mover" in a patient's illness i. e. simple uncomplicated renal, single organ, failure, in contrast with those other systemic processes in which the kidney, along with many other organ systems, is the "victim" (Table 1). This distinction between the kidney as "prime mover" and the kidney as "victim" is fundamental in the analysis of the large number of outcome studies that are available [4, 5] and leads immediately to the rejection of the commonly held belief (a belief mainly held by nephrologists) that survival from ARF has not improved in the last 30 years [6, 7]. This is plainly not the case; survival has improved but the casemix of patients treated has changed considerably. In 1985, the European Dialysis and Transplant Association in collaboration with the European Renal Association performed a survey of 114 renal units throughout Europe documenting the etiology and outcome of 474 patients with ARF [8]. This survey demonstrated that only 61 (13%) patients had simple uncomplicated ARF – the kidney as

Table 1. Acute renal failure in the ICU: the kidney as "prime mover" or "victim"

The kideny as "prime mover"	– glomerulonephritis – interstitial nephritis – pigment – obstetric causes – nephrotoxins – vascular problems – vasculitis
The kidney as "victim"	– sepsis – burns – major surgery – multiple trauma – pancreatitis – cardiogenic shock – vasculitis

"prime mover" – but the survival rate in this group was 92%. In contrast, the remaining 413 (87%) patients had a course complicated by one or more of the following: respiratory failure, circulatory failure, jaundice, uncontrolled sepsis and thrombocytopenia. The survival rate in this group was only 40%. Similarly, a careful retrospective study of patients with ARF treated in the Leeds Renal Unit between 1955–1988 clearly demonstrated that the median age of treated patients has increased progressively over the last 30 years and that survival is inversely proportional to age [9]. Moreover, the Leeds group have compared and contrasted the cohort of patients with ARF treated in the decade 1960–1969 with that treated between 1980–1989 [10]. Whilst numbers of patients treated and survival rates in particular are unchanged, 48.7%

Table 2. Acute renal failure after surgery at Guy's Hospital 1964–1992

	Treatment[a]	n	Deaths	Ventilated cases	
				n	Deaths
Cameron (1964–67)	PD/HD	62	40 (65%)		
Stott (1968–73)	HD/PD	109	67 (62%)		
Brown (1969–73)	HD/PD	73	45 (62%)	22	20 (91%)
Neild (1977–78)	HD	28	14 (50%)	21	15 (71%)
Taube[b] (1981–84)	HD/HF	143	91 (64%)	29	22 (76%)[c]
Smithies (1985–86)	HD/HF/CAVHD	20	15 (75%)	31	24 (77%)
Bihari[b] (1990–91)	CVVH/CVVHD			42	32 (76%)
Bihari[b] (1991–92)	CVVH/CVVHD			79	34 (43%)

[a] PD: peritoneal dialysis, HD: hemodialysis, HF: hemofiltration, CAVHD: continuous arteriovenous hemodiafiltration, CVVH: continuous venous-venous hemofiltration.
[b] All cases treated including post-surgery.
[c] Data for 1984 only.

and 36.6% survival for the two cohorts respectively, the mean age of the more recent cohort (1980/1989) was significantly greater: 63.1 compared with 50.9 years. Of vital importance was the observation that, in the early 1960/69 cohort, only 1.7% of patients required mechanical ventilation whereas in the more recent 1980/1989 cohort, 41.1% of patients treated were supported in this way. Clearly, the situation has changed and our own figures from Guy's Hospital support this view (Table 2). Indeed, in our latest series of patients from the 2 year period 1990–1992 in which we have only considered those cases who required both prolonged mechanical ventilation and renal replacement therapy (Table 3), all patients had at least two organ systems in failure. From these observations we conclude that it is artificial and anachronistic, if not even frankly misleading, to consider ARF in the ICU as a discrete metabolic entity. It is no more than a manifestation of MOF, and the metabolic considerations that pertain to this latter condition are exactly the same as those described in the past relating to acute uremia.

Special Metabolic considerations relating to Acute Renal Failure

Hypercatabolism in ARF, best defined by an initially disproportionate increasing level of blood urea in relation to the reduction in renal clearance [11], has been held responsible for a considerable portion of the morbidity – impaired wound healing, immune system dysfunction – and mortality related to the condition [12, 13]. There are a number of factors that underlie the accelerated protein breakdown and negative nitrogen balance of these patients (Table 4) but most of these are familiar from their role in the pathogenesis of the "autocannabolism" of MOF (and have been reviewed else-

Table 3. Survival from severe combined acute respiratory and renal failure at Guy's Hospital 1990/1992. Clinical features of the 121 patients

	June 1st 1990– May 31st 1991	June 1st 1991– May 31st 1992
No of cases requiring ventilation and CVVH(D)	**42**/971[a]	**79**/1123[a]
1. *non-operative cases*	**35** (83%)	**62** (78%)
ward transfers	13 (31%)	18 (23%)
hospital transfers	21 (60%)	41 (52%)
2. *post-operative cases*	**7** (17%)	**17** (22%)
elective surgery	5 (12%)	9 (12%)
emergency surgery	2 (5%)	8 (10%)
ICU survival	**17** (40%)	**46** (58%)
Hospital survival	**10** (**24**%)	**45** (**57**%)

[a] Total number of patients treated in the 12 months.

Table 4. Factors promoting muscle wasting in acute renal failure

1. Azotaemia, metabolic acidosis
2. Circulating inhibitors of protein synthesis
3. Endocrine abnormalites
4. Protease/antiprotease imbalance
5. Blood losses
6. Hemodialysis – nutritional losses, cytokine/protease release from blood membrane interactions
7. Immobilization
8. Underlying diseases or associated illness – sepsis, shock, trauma, rhabdomyolysis

where). Suffice it to say that glucose intolerance is common and the clearance of non-esterified fatty acids (NEFA) and fat emulsions is reduced. There is some suggestion that these metabolic abnormalities are reversed by the treatment of uremia with hemodialysis [2]. It appears that patients with ARF who also require mechanical ventilation show a median level of energy expenditure of 124% (range 90–148%) of basal energy expenditure predicted from the Harris Benedict equation. This is in comparison with 116% (range 95–129%) found in a control group of critically ill ventilated patients who were not in renal failure [2]. Moreover, in this study, the contribution of protein metabolism (calculated from urinary nitrogen and urea production rates) to total energy expenditure (22.3±1.8%) was found to be significantly higher than in those control patients (16.4±1.8%) whose kidneys continued to function. These findings have been confirmed by Bouffard et al. [14] who also found that energy expenditure in mechanically ventilated patients with ARF was 1.19±0.03 times predicted but with large interindividual variations (0.7–1.7 of the predicted resting energy expenditure). The presence or absence of sepsis seems to be the most important factor determining metabolic rate in these cases.

The Effects of the Various Forms of Renal Replacement Therapy on the Metabolic Abnormality associated with Acute Renal Failure

An important consideration in the management of these patients is the effect of the form of renal support together with the administration of any anticoagulation regimen on the metabolic abnormalities that are present. Peritoneal dialysis (PD), for example, very often leads to peritoneal inflammation and additional protein loss directly into the dialysate. Attempts have been made to reduce this unwanted effect by adding amino acids and albumin to the peritoneal dialysate. There have also been reports of "overfeeding" associated with the absorption of glucose from the peritoneal dialysate across the peritoneal membrane [15]. Since PD, however, should be and is rarely used in the support of the critically ill patient (other than in neonates and infants), this is probably of little relevance. On the other hand, intermittent hemodialysis, which until the middle 1980s remained the mainstay of treatment in most ICU, has been extensively studied and is known to have a variety of effects depending upon the membrane (cuprophane vs a more biocompatible material e. g. polyacrylonitrile (PAN) [16] or polysulphone) or buffer (acetate vs bicarbonate) used. Again, we have reviewed this subject in depth elsewhere [17] but in our opinion, the attending intensive care specialist must be aware of these effects in order to prescribe rationally the appropriate renal replacement therapy.

Acetate dialysis in the ICU should no longer be used; there is good evidence that high plasma levels of acetate lead directly to hypotension whereas the use of this buffer leaves the acidosis of uremia relatively undertreated. (The depression of the respiratory drive due to a loss of carbon dioxide (CO_2) into the dialysate is another effect of acetate dialysis but is not a real issue. Indeed, this effect can be quite helpful in some patients with severe acute respiratory failure requiring renal support, since very often these cases are hypoventilated to reduce intrathoracic pressure and minute volume, leading to so-called "permissive hypercapnea".) Hemodialysis with a cuprophane membrane should no longer be used; this form of dialysis results in the activation of both the contact systems (complement, kininogen-kinins, coagulation) and the cellular constituents (white cells and platelets) of blood. In contrast, PAN membranes are considerably more biocompatible and are not associated with the release of cytokines, proteolytic enzymes nor the activation of complement when blood is passed over their surface. Whilst biocompatibility is often thought to be a rather academic (and expensive) consideration, Alvestrand's group [18] were able to demonstrate enhanced release of amino acids from skeletal muscle during sham dialysis in human volunteers with cuprophane membrane, an effect which was not found when PAN membranes were used. This is exactly the effect that the intensive care physician is trying to avoid, and for this reason, we insist in our unit that all renal replacement therapy – technique, the nature of the membrane, duration, fluid balance, and anticoagulation regimen – is carefully prescribed by the attending physician on a daily basis.

Duration of the extracorporeal circulation is important because loss of many nutrients, including free amino acids, water soluble vitamins and glucose, can occur during the period of renal support [19]. From 6 to 10 g of amino acids are removed during the usual hemodialysis treatment of 4–6 h, but there is little information available concerning the effects of the continuous 24 h technique of renal support (continuous arteriovenous/venous-venous hemofiltration ± dialysis [CAVH/CAVHD; CVVH/CVVHD]) using highly permeable, high flux membranes. One study of CAVHD examined nitrogen, lipid and carbohydrate balance in 9 parenterally fed, critically ill patients and documented total daily nitrogen losses at 24.1 g (95% confidence intervals 20.9–27.3 g/24 h). Carbohydrate delivery of course depended upon the dialysate flow rate since these investigators used peritoneal dialysis fluid as their dialysate in their CAVHD system [20]. There remains the possibility that continuous techniques of renal support will remove nutrients at rates unsuspected by the attending clinicians, and further study of this particular problem is required. Against this theoretical objection is the obvious advantage offered by CAVH/D or CVVH/D in terms of fluid balance. Undoubtedly in the past, patients did not receive their allocated nutritional therapy because the PD or the intermittent HD did not generate sufficient "space" to accommodate further fluid infusion. Bartlett [21] was one of the first investigators to emphasize the fact that CAVH has distinct advantages in the nutritional management of surgical patients. He studied 56 patients with acute oliguric ARF complicating MOF who were treated using two management protocols; the first was standard hemodialysis combined with a calorie intake to balance expenditure but with a low protein intake (phase 1), whilst the second was CAVH, similar calorie intake but a high protein diet (phase 2). Survival rates overall were very low: 12 and 28% for phase 1 and phase 2 treatment regimens respectively, p=NS. Nevertheless, CAVH was found to facilitate parenteral nutrition, and patients with positive energy balance did have an improved survival rate compared with those who had a significant energy deficit (37.5 and 9.4%, respectively). A study like this demonstrates the problems of attempting to dissect out the important factors related to improving outcome: parenteral nutrition *per se*, protein content, fluid balance, or the detrimental effects of intermittent hemodialysis!

Finally, some consideration must be given to the anticoagulation regimen and its effects upon metabolism. Heparin is known to increase the activity of lipoprotein lipase, and when used for a prolonged period of time, can cause osteoporosis. On the other hand, prostacyclin (epoprosternol Flolan; Wellcome Foundation, Crewe, UK) is not only an inhibitor of platelet and white cell activation but is also a potent microcirculatory vasodilator. We have found it particularly helpful in the management of these cases since, when used with heparin to anticoagulate an extracorporeal CVVH/CVVHD system (PGI_2 at 2.5–10.0 ng/kg/min), it has a considerable "heparin sparing" effect (only 200–400 units/h heparin being required to maintain circuit patency for upto 72h); this reduces the likelihood of systemic anticoagulation, bleeding, and metabolic abnormalities [22, 23]. Moreover, the associated microcirulatory vasodilatation helps to correct any remaining perfusion deficit that may contribute to the development of MOF [24].

The Nutritional Treatment of Hypercatabolic Acute Renal Failure in the ICU

It is important to emphasize that in the management of a catabolic patient, there is no role for the restriction of protein intake in order to avoid or reduce the frequency of renal support. Whilst a protein restricted died (15–20 g/day) supplemented with essential amino acids (8–12 g/day) may reduce the need for dialysis, this approach should only be used in chronic renal failure, or in the occasional acute patient who is not hypercatabolic. The key issue surrounds treatment with essential amino acids and hypertonic glucose and whether or not it improves survival. On the one hand, Abel [25] has argued that supplemental parenteral nutrition with essential amino acids and hypertonic glucose should be administered to all patients with ARF, whilst on the other, there have been a number of reviews [26] and meta-analyses [27] emphasizing that the efficacy of these solutions remains in question. Toxicity of amino acids has been explored and demonstrated in a number of animal models. It is our view that parenteral nutrition is expensive and has a number of side effects [28], and so is best avoided unless there is a specific contra-indication to enteral nutrition.

Our approach has been to examine the impact of a gut protection protocol on the outcome of patients with acute respiratory and renal failure in our ICU at Guy's Hospital. Our audit was carried out over a 2 year period from June 1990 to May 1992, and included assessment of all admissions (more than 2000 patients) to the ICU (Riyadh Intensive Care Programme v 4.0, Medical Associated Software House Ltd, London, UK) [29]. Data were collected prospectively and included daily APACHE II scores, daily TISS scores and organ failure variables. ICU costs were calculated at £ 27 per daily TISS point. During the first year of the audit period, patients received either total parenteral nutrition (TPN) formulated on a daily basis by the hospital pharmacy (0.2–0.4 gm N/kg/day as Synthamin, Baxter; 25–30 nonprotein kcals/kg/day as glucose 20%/50% with Intralipid 10/20%, KabiVitrium in a 2/1 ratio) or enteral nutrition (EN) (Fortison, Cow and Gate, Trowbridge, UK) to meet calorific requirements as assessed by the ICU dietician. EN was started when the traditional criteria of returning bowel sounds, absence of diarrhea and small volume gastric aspirates were met. H_2 receptor blockers were not used routinely and enteral feeding was discontinued for 6 h overnight to allow stomach re-acidification. During the second year, the gut protection protocol was introduced. This included the routine use of gastric tonometers in all patients who required pulmonary artery catheterisation, normalisation of gastric intramucosal pH (pHi) as an end-point of resuscitation, the administration of a specific splanchnic vasodilator dopexamine to those patients with a persistently low pHi, and a much greater emphasis on the use of EN. Patients only received TPN if an absolute contra-indication existed, or if enteral feeding was considered to have failed.

In the first year (June 1990 to May 1991) there were 42 patients who required both ventilation and renal support. In the year June 1991 to May 1992, there were 79 patients in this category (Table 3). There were no statistically significant differences in age, diagnostic category, mean admission APACHE II score or mean admission Risk of Death (calculated from the APACHE II score and the diagnostic category) between the two groups) (Table 5). In the first year, 17% of patients received EN alone, 33% received TPN alone, 38% received both types of feeding, and 12% received no feed. In the second year, 73% of patients received enteral feed alone, 3% received TPN alone, 8% received both types of feeding, and 16% received no feed. The change in the number of patients receiving EN alone was highly statisti-

Table 5. Survival from severe combined acute respiratory and renal failure at Guy's Hospital 1990/1992. Severity of illness and mortality rates

	June 1st 1990–May 31st 1991	June 1st 1991–May 31st 1992
Numbers of patients	**42** (971)[a]	**79** (1123)[a]
APACHE II scores (means ± SD)	**25.2** ± 6.6 (14.7 ± 6.6)[a]	**21.9** ± 7.3 (14.2 ± 6.2)[a]
Risk of death (%) (means ± SD)	**42.4** ± 23.5 (15.1 ± 17.1)[a]	**35.1** ± 23.4 (13.5 ± 16.2)[a]
Hospital mortality (%)	**76%** (17%)[a]	**43%** (13%)[a]
Standardized mortality ratios (SMR)	**1.79** (1.13)[a]	**1.23** (0.99)[a]

[a] Figures in parentheses refer to the entire cohort of patients treated in the 12 months.

cally significant ($p<0.001$). The mortality for all the patients was significantly reduced from 76% in the first year to 43% in the second year ($p<0.001$). The standardized mortality ratio (SMR), calculated as the ratio of the actual mortality and the expected risk of death, was 1.79 in the first year and 1.23 in the second year. The effective cost per survivor (calculated by dividing the total amount spent on all the patients by the number of survivors) also fell from £ 61,180 in the first year to £ 20,545 in the second year (Table 6). The feeding cost per patient fell from £ 676 in the first year to £ 145 in the second year. The effective feeding cost per survivor fell from £ 2839 to £ 254.

We believe that the change in the numbers receiving EN alone from 17% in the year 1990/91 to 73% in 1991/92 together with the apparent improvement in the standarized mortality ratio underlines the importance of using EN in this group of patients.

Table 6. Survival from severe combined acute respiratory and renal failure at Guy's Hospital 1990/1992. Intensive care costs

	June 1st 1990–May 31st 1991	June 1st 1991–May 31st 1992
Numbers of patients	**42** (971)[a]	**79** (1123)[a]
Total ICU costs	**£ 611,806** (£ 2.17 million)	**£ 924,527** (£ 2.69 million)
Costs per survivor	£ 21,179	£ 10,871
Costs per death	£ 12,500	£ 12,803
Effective cost per survivor	**£ 61,180** (£ 2,696)	**£ 20,545** (£ 2,767)

[a] Figures in parentheses refer to the entire cohort of patients treated in the 12 months and total overall costs.

Conclusion

Acute renal failure in the ICU is not a disease nor a metabolic state, it is part of a syndrome occurring in a heterogenous population of patients and usually reflects the development of multiple organ failure. There are a number of principles to be considered concerning the nutritional management of these cases – not least the importance of preserving blood flow to the gut! There is no evidence that parenteral nutrition of any composition improves outcome and many unwanted side-effects have been associated with standard TPN. We have demonstrated that the vast majority of cases can be fed by the enteral route, and this by itself is associated with an improvement in prognosis.

Acknowledgements. We would like to thank Professor Stuart Cameron of the Guy's Hospital Renal Unit for his advice, insight and continuing support.

References

1. Feinstein EI (1987) Nutrition in acute renal failure. Adv Exper Med Biol 212:297–301
2. Little RA, Campbell IT, Green CJ, Kishen R, Waldek S (1990) Nutritional support in acute renal failure in the critically ill. In: Bihari D, Neild G (eds) Acute renal failure in the intensive therapy unit, Springer-Verlag, Heidelberg, pp 347–357
3. Teschner M, Heidland A (1989) Hypercatabolism in acute renal failure: Mechanisms and therapeutic approaches. Blood Purif 7:16–27
4. Butkus DE (1983) Persistent high mortality in acute renal failure: Are we asking the right questions? Arch Intern Med 143:209–212
5. Chew SL, Lins RL, Daelemans R, De Broe ME (1993) Outcome in acute renal failure. Nephrol Dial Transplant 8:101–107
6. Maher ER, Robinson KN, Scoble JE, et al (1989) Prognosis of critically ill patients with acute renal failure: APACHE II score and other predictive factors. Quart J Med 72:857–866
7. Storck M, Hartl WH, Zimmerer E, Inthorn D (1991) Comparison of pump driven and spontaneous continuous haemofiltration in postoperative acute renal failure. Lancet 337:452–455
8. Cameron JS (1986) Acute renal failure in the intensive care unit today. Intensive Care Med 12:64–70
9. Turney JH, Marshall DH, Brownjohn AM, Ellis CM, Parsons FM (1990) The evolution of acute renal failure 1956–1988. Quart J Med 74:83–104
10. Turney JH (1990) Why is mortality persistently high in acute renal failure? Lancet 335:971
11. Walser M (1980): Determinants of ureagenesis with particular reference to renal failure. Kidney Int 17:709–721
12. Heidland A, Schaefer RM, Heidbreder E, Horl WH (1988) Catabolic factors in renal failure: Therapeutic approaches. Nephrol Dial Transplant 3:8–16
13. Panzetta GO, Rugiu C, Maschio G (1991) Metabolic alterations in acute renal failure: The hypermetabolism and the multiple organ failure syndrome. Int J Artif Organs 14:125–132
14. Bouffard Y, Viale JP, Annat G, Delafosse B, Guillaume C, Motin J (1987) Energy expenditure in the acute renal failure patient mechanically ventilated. Intensive Care Med 13:401–404

15. Manji S, Shikora S, McMahon M, Blackburn GL, Bistrian BR (1990) Peritoneal dialysis for acute renal failure: Overfeeding resulting from dextrose absorbed during dialysis. Crit Care Med 18:29–31
16. Cheung AK, Parker CJ, Wilcox LA, Janatova J (1990) Activation of complement by haemodialysis membranes: Polyacrylonitrile binds more C3a than cuprophan. Kidney Int 37:1055–1059
17. Bihari DJ, Beale RJ (1991) Renal support in the intensive care unit. Current Opinion Anaesth 4:272–278
18. Gutierrez A, Alvestrand A, Wahren J, Bergstrom J (1990) Effect of in vivo contact between blood and dialysis membranes on protein catabolism in humans. Kidney Int 38:487–494
19. Feinstein EI (1987) Nutritional haemodialysis. Kidney Int 32:S167–S169
20. Bellomo R, Martin H, Parkin G, Love J, Kearley Y, Boyce N (1991) Continuous arteriovenous haemodiafiltration in the critically ill: Influence on major nutrient balances. Intensive Care Med 17:399–402
21. Bartlett RH, Mault JR, Dechert RE, Palmer J, Swartz RD, Port FK (1986) Continuous arteriovenous haemofiltration: Improved survival in surgical acute renal failure? Surgery 100:400–408
22. Wendon J, Smithies M, Shepperd M, Bullen K, Tinker J, Bihari DJ (1989) Continuous high volume venous venous haemofiltration in acute renal failure. Intensive Care Med 15:358–363
23. Swartz RD, Flamenbaum W, Dubrow A, Hall JC, Crow JW, Cato A (1988) Epoprostenol (PGI2 – prostacyclin) during high risk haemodialysis – preventing further bleeding complications. J Clin Pharmacol 28:818–825
24. Bihari DJ, Smithies M, Gimson AES, Tinker J (1987) The effects of prostacyclin on oxygen delivery and uptake in critically ill patients. New Engl J Med 317:397–403
25. Abel RM (1983) Nutritional support in the patient with acute renal failure. J Am Coll Nutr 2:33–44
26. Koretz RL (1983) What supports nutritional support? Dig Dis Sci 29:577–588
27. Naylor CD, Detsky AS, O'Rourke K, Fonberg E (1987) Does treatment with essential amino acids and hypertonic glucose improve survival in acute renal failure? A meta-analysis. Renal Failure 10:141–152
28. Maynard ND, Bihari DJ (1991) Postoperative feeding. Br Med J 303:1007–1008
29. Beale RJ, Maynard ND, Smithies MN, et al (1992) Changing nutritional therapy in a general ICU. Intensive Care Med 18:S104 (Abs)

Nutritional Support in Liver Disease

E. Lerebours

Introduction

Most of the nutrients absorbed in the gastronintestinal (GI) tract undergo biochemical transformation on reaching the liver via the portal circulation. Hence, malnutrition, whether occurring before the onset of liver disease or developing as a consequence of the hepatic dysfunction, has important clinical and therapeutic implications [1, 2]. The two main therapeutic objectives of nutritional support for patients with liver diseases are to prevent further liver cell injury and to provide a favorable environment for repair and regeneration of liver cells.

Earlier studies on nutritional aspects of liver disease focused on the striking intolerance of patients to protein-containing meals. Over the last decades, more attention has been given to the nutritional problems of patients with liver disease. In this chapter, the clinical aspects of nutrition in liver disease and the underlying rationale for specific nutritional therapies will be reviewed.

Assessment of Nutritional Status

The presence of liver disease may affect many of the traditional indices utilized to evaluate the nutritional status. Thus, deficiencies in specific nutrients may be masked by the effects of hepatic inflammation, and conversely, abnormalities related primarily to liver injury may mimick depletion of nutrient's body stores. For instance, hypoproteinemia observed in advanced liver disease may be due either to a decrease in the intrinsic hepatic capacity for protein synthesis due to the liver disease or to visceral protein depletion.

From a clinical point of view, nutritional assessment should always include a complete medical and dietary history, physical examination, and evaluation of the fat stores and protein (somatic and visceral) compartments. A bedside evaluation by the clinician of muscle mass and subcutaneous fat stores usually provides a reliable initial nutritional assessment. Fat stores can be estimated by measurements of the triceps and subscapular skinfold thickness. The somatic protein compartment is often assessed by the relationship of body weight to height, and the measurement of the midarm muscle circumference. However, in patients with liver disorders, these anthropometric techniques may occasionally be misleading because of apparent or infraclinical edemas leading to possible underestimation of the severity of protein and fat store depletion. In patients with liver disease, the plasma protein levels are a poor indicator of the status of visceral protein stores [3, 4]. The creatinine-height index is generally a better indicator of lean body mass in patients with hepatic failure, if there is no associated renal dysfunction such as the hepato-renal syndrome. Similarly, impaired urea synthesis and intra- and extracellular accumulation of ammonia in liver diseases may result in considerable underestimation of negative nitrogen balance.

Recent improvements to quantitate whole body nitrogen, potassium, phosphorus, and body compartments by neutron activation analysis will be a useful tool for a better appreciation of body compositional changes in liver disease.

In clinical practice, most methods and formulae used to estimate energy requirements are based on data obtained from the study of large numbers of healthy individuals. Caution should be exercised when applying those formulae to patients with liver disease. Body weight may be normal or increased in decompensated cirrhosis because of water and sodium retention, although patients may have severe loss of muscle mass. The proportion of lean body mass and energy requirements may be altered by liver dysfunction, and reference values for normal subjects are inappropiate.

Frequency of Malnutrition

Malnutrition is a common feature in patients with advanced liver disease. In contrast with the considerable information on malnutrition in alcoholic liver disease, reports regarding the nutritional status of patients with non-alcoholic liver disease are limited [5, 6].

More recently, with the advent of liver transplantation, a systematic nutritional evaluation is often performed during the process of candidate selection. Consequently, the data base on nutritional changes in patients with end-stage, non-alcoholic liver disease has recently expanded [4, 7, 8]. Malnutrition is quite common in patient with end-stage liver disease waiting for orthotopic liver transplantation. Among the treatable factors influencing ultimate survival, protein-caloric malnutrition is potentially one of the most important, particularly in children. Therefore, critical evaluation of nutritional therapy is required.

Factors causing Malnutrition

The pathophysiology of malnutrition in liver disease is multifactorial [1, 2]. Major factors directly related to the hepatic injury include the energy and protein metabolism abnormalities discussed in the following section of this article. Impaired dietary intake is probably one of the principal causes for nutritional deficiencies in patients with chronic liver disease. Reduction in nutrient intake may arise as a result of associated anorexia and nausea and also because dietary protein intake is often restricted for therapeutic reasons as a part of the management of hepatic encephalopathy. However, some investigators have found that cirrhotic patients generally have a normal dietary intake, and therefore the role of poor dietary intake in the pathogenesis of malnutrition in liver disease remains controversial [6, 9]. Increasing data suggest that nutritional deficiencies could arise also because of impaired digestion and absorption of nutrients. Moderate steatorrhea is found in 40 to 50% of cirrhotics and is related to different factors: decreased delivery of bile acids into the intestinal lumen, impaired capacity for absorption of long chain fatty acids, interference between lipid absorption and neomycin, and in some but not all cases an exocrine pancreatic insufficiency. However, if we except occasional patients with primary biliary cirrhosis or primary sclerosing cholangitis complicated with celiac disease, GI malabsorption is probably not the main pathophysiologic abnormality underlying the development of protein-caloric malnutrition. The repeated occurrence of major complications may further contribute to the development of malnutrition because of the increased protein catabolism associated with the severe acute illness.

Metabolic Alterations

Controversy exists about the metabolic consequences of liver diseases. It must be emphasized that one of the most important aspects to consider when performing metabolic studies in liver disease is the selection and characterization of the patient groups. It is quite obvious that cirrhotic patients represent an heterogenous population, not only with respect to the etiology and state of the disease, but also with regard to the severity of alterations in intermediary metabolism. Elsewhere, the established success of orthotopic liver transplantation as a definitive treatment option for patients with end-stage liver disease and fulminant hepatic failure has redirected attention concerning the metabolic alterations present in such patients, but only scant information has been gathered.

By virtue of its oxydative and synthetic functions, the liver has a critical regulatory role in the amino acid homeostatis. Hepatocellular dysfunction is responsible for a number of metabolic disturbances that alter the body's utilization of numerous nutrients. Despite controversy on whole body protein synthesis and degradation in cirrhosis, changes in protein metabolism have been shown to be particularly prominent in the fasting state. One of the possible explantations for these apparent discrepant findings of amino acid tracer studies could be the choice of patient population. Protein turn-over and endogenous breakdown are elevated in malnourished patients with severe cirrhosis and fulminant hepatic failure [10, 11]. At the opposite, stable cirrhotic patients are not in a catabolic state. The accumulation of aromatic amino acids in blood is directly related to the increase of protein breakdown.

The effects of protein supplementation in cirrhotic patients are controversial. Swart and colleagues [11], using a single dose of 15 N labelled glycine, have shown that dietary proteins appear to be more efficiently handled in stable cirrhotic patients than in controls. In 17 cirrhotic patients of whom 13 had clinical and encephalographic evidence of hepatic encephalopathy, branched chain amino acids (BCAA) supplements significantly reduced protein oxydation and endogenous breakdown, but did not significantly after protein metabolism in stable cirrhotic patients with subnormal fasting plasma leucine concentration. In this latter group, the extra leucine infused was entirely oxidized and did not detectably contribute to protein synthesis [12].

Finally, cirrhotic patients seem characterized by an early development of a starvation type metabolism due to the liver's inability to store significant amounts of glycogen and to release glucose by glycogenolysis. This more rapid transition to glyconeogenesis from amino acids (AA) would fill the energy gap from low glycogen stores. Considering the controversial data about the increased oxydative losses of protein in patients with liver diseases, it may be hypothesized that the frequent protein deficiency observed in patients with liver disease is mainly a consequence of a decreased dietary intake.

An impaired glucose metabolism is a well recognized finding in cirrhotic patients [13]; most (60–80%) are glucose intolerant, and 10–15% eventually develop diabetes.

The pathogenetic factors responsible for this impaired glucose metabolism observed in cirrhosis could theoretically be a defect in insulin secretion and/or a deficit in insulin action. Since cirrhotic patients are characterized by hyper-insulism, both in the fasting state and after oral or IV glucose administration, resistance to the action of insulin was suggested some 20 years ago. The pathogenesis of insulin resistance in cirrhotic patients is complex [13]. Portasystemic shunts and reduced insulin hepatic clearance lead to a peripheral hyperinsulinism which in turn induces a down regulation of the intracellular events regulating insulin action in peripheral tissues. Suppression of hepatic glucose production by insulin does not appear to be impaired in cirrhotic patients. But, the normal compensatory hyperinsulinic response to insulin resistance is insufficient in cirrhosis to offset insulin resistance, and glucose intolerance develops. As for the other conditions of reduced insulin sensitivity (diabetes, obesity, essential hypertension), the cellular mechanism of the observed reduction in whole body glucose uptake is poorly understood.

One supposed mechanism for weight loss and malnutrition observed in alcoholic liver disease is a hypermetabolic state. Measurements of energy expenditure have been limited and somewhat conflicting. However, taking into account correction for lean body mass, most recent studies support the notion of a hypermetabolic state [14].

Nutritional Support

The literature concerning the nutritional support of patients with liver disease is not easy to assess because of the heterogeneity of the patient groups studied, the differences in the aims of the studies, the differences in regimens prescribed, and the disagreements about end-point objectives.

Five different situations may be analysed:

- Nutritional therapy in liver disease without hepatic encephalopathy;
- Alcoholic hepatitis;
- Nutritional support in the presence of hepatic encephalopathy;
- Fulminant hepatic failure;
- Orthotopic liver transplantation.

Nutritional Therapy in Liver Disease without Encephalopathy

Stable cirrhotic patients without hepatic encephalopathy tolerate well high protein intake. So, the aim of the treatment is to achieve an increased nutritional intake whenever possible either by encouraging the patients to eat more normal food with or without oral supplementation, or by instituting an enteral feeding. In such situation, conventional dietary proteins and standard amino acid mixture appear to be safe in patients with liver disease in most instances.

The evaluation of the nutritional effects of BCAA is controversial. This evaluation has been focused for many year on their effects of mental function. Few studies only have included a detailed nutritional assessment. This is remarkable since the primary rationale for the use of BCAA in hepatic encephalopathy has considerably weakened since first proposal in 1975 [15]. Leucine, valine and isoleucine have several properties that may be of potential benefit to malnourished patients with liver disease. BCAA inhibit muscle protein breakdown, and also increase the synthesis of hepatic and muscle proteins and serve well as an energy source for muscle tissue [16]. Those effects are independent from their possible therapeutic value in portal systemic encephalopathy. In most studies using BCAA preparation, the control group received no supplemental nitrogen, and therefore those investigations cannot be analysed further from a comparative nutritional prospective aspect [1, 2, 17]. In others, nitrogen was provided to the non-BCAA patients but there was no nutritional assessment. Only the recent study of Chin et al. [18] demonstrates in a well designed trial that a BCAA enriched formula has advantages over standard semi-elemental formula in improving nutritional status with end-stage liver disease. Present data do not support a role for BCAA supplementation as a primary therapy for malnutrition in liver disease. In most stable cirrhotic patients, the additional leucine provided by the enriched BCAA solution was essentially oxydized without significant effect on protein synthesis or catabolism [12].

Nevertheless, the optimal BCAA concentration of total amino acid for nutritional intervention has not been fully evaluated although BCAA concentration of 100% given intravenously appears to be detrimental [19]. Furthermore, the relative concentrations of individual BCAA may be more important than the total BCAA content, and leucine may be more critical than other BCAA because of its nitrogen sparing action [20].

Considering the cost of BCAA supplementation and the cost to benefit ratio, it is impossible to justify the use of BCCA in every malnourished patient with cirrhosis. BCAA supplementation sould be reserved as an alternative for the patients with demonstrated intolerance leading to sustained suboptimal protein intakes.

Alpha-keto-analogues of BCAA (BCKA) are the nitrogen free products derived from deamination of leucine, valine and isoleucine. BCKA are rapidly converted back to the corresponding BCAA by transamination of their carbon skeleton. Therefore, BCKA are potentially useful for disorders characterized by an accumulation of nutritional irrelevant nitrogen, mainly chronic renal failure and hepatic failure. BCKA have several metabolic effects with potentially beneficial nutritional consequences, including suppression of protein breakdown and stimulation of protein synthesis. Actually, there is no clear evidence for the use of BCKA in the nutritional therapy of patients with liver disorders [2]. Nevertheless further studies are needed.

Alcoholic Hepatitis

Alcoholic hepatitis is known to be a potential precursor lesion for development of an alcoholic cirrhosis even if in its earlier, precirrhotic stage, alcoholic hepatitis is potentially reversible. Severe alcoholic hepatitis can be fatal and be complicated by portal hypertension, fluid retention and hepatic encephalopathy. Several controlled trials have evaluated the different therapeutic approaches of alcoholic hepatitis. A recent meta-analysis [21] and a prospective controlled trial have demonstrated the efficacy of corticosteroids in the severe form of alcoholic hepatitis [22]. The rationale for the use of a nutritional supplementation is that patients with moderate to severe alcoholic hepatitis are uniformly malnourished, that liver lesions will heal more quickly, and that adverse complications will be reduced if the nutritional status of the patient can be improved. In one study, parenteral AA supplementation for 1 month in patients with alcoholic hepatitis resulted in a greater clinical and laboratory improvement and a reduced mortality than those of the control group. Four of 18 control patients died, all 17 patients receiving AA supplementation survived [23]. In all the other studies, enteral or parenteral amino acid supplementation does not affect immediate or delayed mortality in alcoholic hepatitis but resulting in a greater improvement of biochemical, metabolic and nutritional parameters [24–28]. The improvement in these parameters indicates that such a treatment is beneficial in patients with alcoholic hepatitis even though it may not be sufficient to alter death rate. Combination of nutritional supplementation and high dose corticosteroids should also receive further trials.

Nutritional Support in the Presence of Hepatic Encephalopathy

The pathogenesis of hepatic encephalopathy remains mainly controversial. Of particular relevance to the nutritional support of encephalopatic patients has been the demonstration of an increased plasma concentration of the aromatic amino acids phenylalanine and tyrosine as well as methionine and tryptophan. These changes are associated with a reduction in plasma concentrations of BCCA (valine, leucine, isoleucine). The pathogenesis of those changes have been discussed previously [29, 30].

The relationship between the disturbed plasma amino acid profile, the pathogenesis of hepatic encephalopathy and the development of the false neurotransmitters hypothesis have been discussed initially in 1971 by Fischer and Baldessanini [31]. The changes in circulating BCAA and aromatic AA were considered important in the pathogenesis of hepatic encephalopathy. The impairement of the blood brain barrier, demonstrated in humans, may also contribute to an increased uptake of amino acids.

Even if ammonia obviously plays an important role in the pathogenesis of hepatic encephalopathy, proof that it is the cause of this syndrome has never been established. Most of the recent studies related to pathogenesis of hepatic encephalopathy have been focused on the relationship between ammonia hypothesis and glutamine metabolism. Arterial ammonia concentration is elevated in patients with hepatic encephalopathy. Recent studies have raised the possibility that high brain ammonia levels have effects on brain water content. Increased brain water content was observed in normal dogs rendered hyperammoniemic by a 3-day urease treatment. Two observations link a role for ammonia and the development of brain edema in fulminant hepatic failure. Swelling of cortical astrocytes, a feature in several experimental models of fulminant hepatic failure [32], can be observed after infusion of ammonia in experimental models. Similarly, addition of ammonia to astrocytes in primary cultures resulted in an increased cell volume.

These effects could be mediated by products of ammonia metabolism rather than by ammonia itself. Glutamine synthesis is the major mechanism involved in ammonia removal by brain in both normal and hyperammoniemic conditions [33]. Glutamine synthetase is mainly located in astrocytes [34] where it catalyzes the formation of glutamine from ammonia and glutamate. There is no evidence suggesting that cerebral glutamine synthetase in brain is induced in conditions of either acute or chronic hyperammoniemia [35]. Recent studies have demonstrated in hyperammoniemic animals a correlation between the rise in brain glutamine and the brain water level, and have proposed that the ammonia-induced increase in brain water is mediated by the osmotic effect of glutamine [36, 37]. Administration of methionine sulfoxamine, an inhibitor of glutamine synthetase, prevents the increase of both glutamine and water. Under normal physiological conditions, glutamine transport participates to the regulation of water movement in the brain. A role for glutamine in the regulation of cell volume has also been proposed for other tissues; in the liver, glutamine uptake induces cellular swelling. By contrast with brain and liver findings, Girard and Butterworth [35] demonstrate a time dependent increase in glutamine synthetase in rat skeletal muscle in parallel with the degree of hyperammoniemia. Therefore, a therapeutic approach increasing glutamine synthetase activity in skeletal muscle could be potentially useful in hyperammoniemia conditions. It is conceivable that the administration of BCAA mixture might act by such a mechanism. One previous study reported that addition of BCAA to skeletal muscle homogenates *in vitro* resulted in a significantly increased synthetase activity [38]. Nevertheless, although it is generally assumed that muscle is the main glutamine releasing organ in normal situation, the *in vivo* quantitative role of muscle in ammonia detoxification during hyperammoniemia related to liver insufficiency, remains unclear. Dejong et al. [39] have demonstrated that net muscle glutamine efflux increased during porta-caval shunting, but decreased during liver ischemia. Those data suggest that the role of skeletal muscle in the detoxification of ammonia during severe acute hyperammoniemia induced by acute liver ischemia in the rat is limited.

The rationale of BCAA therapy in encephalopathic patients was based on the observation of an abnormal AA profile. It was postulated that the restoration of a normal plasma AA pattern might induce the return to a normal central nervous system neurotransmission. In healthy sujects, IV infusion of BCAA increases the peripheral levels of BCAA and results in a decrease in the concentration of tyrosine and phenylalanine [40, 41]. Similar findings were reported in cirrhotic patients [42, 43]. These data explain the publication of a large number of controlled trials concerning the use of BCAA alone, BCAA enriched and aromatic AA depleted mixtures of amino acids in the treatment of hepatic encephalopathy. The interpretation of these trials is rather difficult. Two meta-analysis of these trials have been published almost simultaneously [44, 45]. They reached very different conclusions! This discrepancy emphasizes the obvious difficulties arising when collecting data for meta-analysis. Even if meta-analysis consider the same trials with complicated designs, they may abstract dramatically different data for the same end-point and infer conflicting conclusions about treatment efficacy [27].

Three groups of clinical trials may be separated according to the encephalopathy grade:

- Therapy of acute hepatic encephalopathy;
- Therapy of chronic encephalopathy; and
- Therapy of subclinical encephalopathy.

BCAA treatment of acute hepatic encephalopathy. The seven published randomized controlled trials are diverse in design, heterogeneous in execution and variable in interpretation [44, 45]. Three studies compared BCAA with a non-specific therapy (glucose or conventional AA mixture) [47–49]. Four studies were designed to answer the question: "Is BCAA therapy better than conventional therapy (lactulose or neomycin)?" [50–53]. The amount of BCAA administered varied greatly, ranging from 22 to 57 g/day and treatment continued for periods ranging from 4 to 16 days. The overall conclusion drawn from these studies is that BCAA therapy, whether pure or combined with other AA, irrespective of the amount administered, does not affect significantly the outcome of patients with acute hepatic encephalopathy.

BCAA treatment of chronic hepatic encephalopathy. Four trials have been published [44, 45]. They attempt to answer two questions: "Can the neurologic state of patients be improved by BCAA?" "Are BCAA enriched diets better tolerated than regular protein diets?" In none of the 3 cross-over studies, the BCAA enriched diet was superior to the control diet. The fourth study compared 2 diets in 2 different groups of patients. Dietary protein was shown to be more comagenic than the BCAA enriched diet. It may be concluded that oral BCAA supplement is as effective as an equivalent amount of proteins in inducing positive nitrogen balance but without giving encephalopathy as frequently. These data suggest that the potential role of BCAA in chronic encephalopathy has shifted from a primary therapeutic agent to a safer mean of improving the nutritional status of the patients. Such solutions should be tried in patients in whom the minimal daily proteins requirements induce recurrent hepatic encephalopathy.

BCAA and subclinical encephalopathy. Encephalopathy is probably much more common in patients with cirrhosis than it is generally though. According to the psychometric or electrophysiologic tests used for the diagnosis, the incidence of hepatic encephalopathy may be as high as 60–70%. Only a few controlled studies about the efficacy of therapy have been performed in patients with sub-clinical encephalopathy [44–45]. The only conclusion that can be drawn from the two published studies is that BCAA enriched diets are well tolerated by cirrhotic patients without overt encephalopathy. These trials do not show that BCAA supplementation is of any value in cirrhotic patients with subclinical hepatic encephalopathy.

Fulminant Hepatic Failure

The dramatic syndrome of fulminant hepatic failure (FHF) is often associated with the rapid development of protein caloric malnutrition [1, 2]. The development of liver transplantation has dramatically modified the prognosis of these patients. It is very doubtful that nutritional support, in contrast with metabolic support, would have any major role in these patients; the only hope would be a timely liver transplantation. Metabolic alterations found in patients with FHF remain poorly understood. An essential aspect for the management of those patients is the need for a very close monitoring of blood glucose levels and an adequate dextrose infusion to prevent hypoglycemia. Hypoglycemia in FHF seems related to a profound decrease in hepatic glycogen store and an impairment of gluconeogenesis pathways. In patients with FHF complicated by cerebral edema, water-dextrose solutions should be used with caution, better at concentrations of 20 to 40% to avoid an increased brain swelling due to excess free water.

Because lipid emulsions are calorically dense, they may be more suitable as a fuel source in FHF patients. A preliminary report concluded that the use of IV lipids is safe in FHF [54]. Studies of protein metabolism have shown that FHF is often associated with an increased endogenous release of AA from protein breakdown, and a decreased albumin synthesis [10].

A major goal of therapy should be to reduce protein catabolism and to provide AA for hepatic regeneration. BCAA supplementation appear a reasonable option under these circumstances but further clinical studies are needed.

Liver Transplantation

Malnutrition is a common findings in patients with advanced liver diseases who are candidates for an orthotopic liver transplantation. A poor nutritional status increases mortality and morbidity in the postoperative period [55–57]. Nevertheless, it is difficult to clearly establish the impact of nutritional therapy in the results of liver transplantation. During the pretransplantation period, the nutritional management is not specific. The objective is the maintenance or the improvement of the nutritional status of the patient while avoiding the development or aggravation of hepatic encephalopathy.

The postoperative period is characterized by a non-specific severe state of high protein catabolism [10]. Administration of high doses of corticosteroids plays a significant role in this hypercatabolism.

Success of the liver transplantation is associated with a rapid correction of the prexisting abnormal AA profiles. Therefore, if a high protein intake is required in the postoperative period, there is probably no need for special AA mixtures. Only one randomized prospective study has evaluated the benefits of nutritional support in the postoperative period after liver transplantation [7]. TPN was associated with a better nitrogen balance and a reduction of the duration of stay in the ICU. BCAA did not appear to be superior to standard AA.

Conclusion

Malnutrition is frequent in patients with liver disease. Nutritional support seems to improve nutritional status. However, the real impact of nutritional support on patient's outcome or encephalopathy occurrence remains more debatable. Further researches are needed to improve our knowledge about the metabolic disturbances associated with liver diseases.

References

1. Silk DBA, O'Keefe SJD, Wicks C (1991) Nutritional support in liver disease. Gut 11:529–533
2. Munoz SJ (1991) Nutritional therapies in liver disease. Sem Liv Dis 11:278–291
3. Merli M, Romiti A, Riggio O, Capoccacia L (1987) Optimal nutritional indexes in chronic liver disease. JPEN 11 (Suppl):130S–134S
4. DiCecco SR, Wieners EJ, Weisner RH, et al (1989) Assessment of nutritional status in patients with end-stage liver disease undergoing liver transplantation. Mayo Clin Proc 65:95–102
5. O'Keefe SJ, EL-Zayadi AR, Carrher TE, et al (1980) Malnutrition and immunocompentence in patients with liver disease. Lancet 2:615–617
6. Morgan AG, Keller J, Walker BE, et al (1990) Nutrition in cryptogenic cirrhosis and chronic aggressive hepatitis. Gut 17:113–118
7. Reilly J, Mehta R, Teperman L, et al (1990) Nutritional support after liver transplantation: A randomized prospective study. JPEN 14:386–391
8. Hehir DJ, Jenkins RL, Bistrian BR, Blackburn G (1985) Nutrition in patients undergoing liver transplantation. JPEN 9:695–700
9. Munoz S, Heubi J, Deems RO, et al (1990) Vitamin D and E deficiency in primary sclerosing cholangitis: Mechanisms, frequency and relation to deficiency in other lipid soluble vitamins. Hepatology 12:958 (Abst)
10. O'Keefe SJD, Abraham RR, Davis M, Williams D (1991) Protein turnover in acute and chronic liver disease. Acta Chir Scand 507 (Suppl):91–101
11. Swart CR, Van Den Berg JWO, Wattimena JLD, Rietveld T, Van Vvume JK, Frenkel M (1988) Elevated protein requirement in cirrhosis of the liver investigated by whole body protein turnover studies. Clin Sci 75:101–107
12. Weber FL, Bagby BS, Licate L, Kelsen SG (1990) Effects of branched-chain amino acids on nitrogen metabolism in patients with cirrhosis. Hepatology 11:942–950
13. Petrides AS, Defronzo RA (1989) Glucose metabolism in cirrhosis: A review with some perspectives for the future. Diab Metabol Rev 5:691–709
14. Marsano L, Mc Clain CJ (1991) Nutrition and alcoholic liver disease. JPEN 15:337–344
15. Fischer JE, Funovics JM, Aguirre A, et al (1975) The role of plasma amino acids in hepatic encephalopathy. Surgery 78:276–290
16. Tischler ME, Desautels M, Goldberg AL (1982) Does leucine, leucyl-RNA, or some metabolite of leucine regulate protein synthesis and degradation in skeletal and cardiac muscle? J Biol Chem 257:1613–1621
17. Cabre E, Gonzalez-Huk F, Abad-Lacruz A, et al (1990) Effect of total enteral nutrition on the short-term outcome of severely malnourished cirrhotics: A randomized controlled trial. Gastroenterology 98:715–720
18. Chin SE, Sheperd RW, Thomas BJ, et al (1992) Nutritional support in children with end-stage liver disease: A randomized cross-over trial of a branched-chain amino acid supplement. Am J Clin Nutr 56:158–163
19. Wright PD, Holdsworth JD, Dionici P, Clague MB, James OFW (1986) Effect of branched-chain amino acid infusions on body protein metabolism in cirrhosis of liver. Gut 27:96–102
20. Bonau RA, Ang SD, Jeevanandam M, Daly JM (1984) High branched-chain amino acids solutions: Relationship of composition to efficacy. JPEN 8:622–627

21. Imperiale TF, Mc Cullough AJ (1990) Do corticosteroids reduce mortality from alcoholic hepatitis? A meta-analysis of the randomized trials. Ann Int Med 113:299–307
22. Ramond MJ, Poynard T, Rueff B, et al (1992) A randomized trial of prednisolone in patients with severe alcoholic hepatitis. N Engl J Med 326:507–512
23. Nasrallah SM, Galambos JT (1980) Amino acid therapy of alcoholic hepatitis. Lancet 2:1276–1277
24. Mendenhall C, Bongiovanni G, Goldberg S, et al (1985) VA cooperative study on alcoholic hepatitis. III: Changes in protein calorie malnutrition associated with 30 days of hospitalization with and without enteral nutrition therapy. JPEN 9:590–596
25. Naveau S, Pelletier G, Poynard T (1986) A randomized clinical trial of supplementary parenteral nutrition in jaundiced alcoholic cirrhotic patients. Hepatology 6:270–274
26. Mezgy E, Caballeria J, Mitchell MC, Pares A, Herlong HF, Rodes J (1991) Effect of parenteral amino acid supplementation on short-term and long-term outcomes in severe alcoholic hepatitis: A randomized controlled trial. Hepatology 14:1090–1096
27. Bonkovsky HL, Fiellin DA, Smith GS, Slaker DP, Simon D, Galambo S (1991) A randomized controlled trial of alcoholic hepatitis with parenteral nutrition and oxandrolone. I. Short-term effects on liver function. Am J Gastroenterol 86:1200–1208
28. Bonkovsky HL, Singh RH, Jafri IM, et al (1991) A randomized controlled trial of treatment of alcoholic hepatitis with parenteral nutrition and oxandrolone. II. Short-term effects on nitrogen metabolism, metabolic balance and nutrition. Am J Gastroenterol 86:1209–1218
29. Mullen KD, Weber FL (1991) Role of nutrition in hepatic encephalopathy. Sem Liver Dis 11:292–304
30. Fischer JE (1990) Branched-chain enriched amino acid solutions in patient with liver failure: An early example of nutritional pharmacology. JPEN 14:249S–256S
31. Fischer JE, Baldessarini MJ (1971) False neurotransmitters and hepatic failure. Lancet 2:75–79
32. Swain M, Butterworth RF, Blei AT (1992) Ammonia and related amino acids in the pathogenesis of brain edema in acute ischemic liver failure in rats. Hepatology 15:449–453
33. Cooper JP, Bachmann C, Peheim E, Beruter J (1985) Cerebral ammonia metabolism in hyperammoniemic rats. J Neurochem 44:1716–1723
34. Martinez-Hernandez A, Bell KP, Norember MD (1977) Glutamine synthetase: Glial localization. Science 195:1356–1358
35. Girard G, Butterworth RF (1992) Effect of porta-caval anastomosis on glutamine synthetase activities in liver brain, and skeletal muscle. Dig Dis Sc 37:1121–1126
36. Leven LH, Koehler RC, Brusilow SW, Jones J, Traystman RJ (1989) Elevated brain water during urease-induced hyperammoniemia in dogs. In: Hoff JT, Betz AL (eds). Intracranial pressure VII. Springer-Verlag Berlin pp 1032–1034
37. Takahashi H, Koehlem RC, Brusilow SW, Traystman RJ (1991) Inhibition of brain glutamin accumulation prevents cerebral edema in hyperammoniemic rats. Am J Physiol 281:H826–829
38. King PA, Goldstein L, Newsholme EA (1983) Glutamine synthetase activity of muscle in acidosis. Biochem J 216:523–525
39. Desong CHC, Kampman MT, Deutz NEP, Soeters PB (1992) Altered glutamine metabolism in rat portal drained viscera and hindquarter during hyperammoniema. Gastroenterology 102:936–948
40. Hagenfeldt L, Eriksson S, Wahren J (1980) Influence of leucine on arterial concentrations and regional exchange of amino acids in healthy subjects. Clin Sci 59:173–181
41. Eriksson S, Hagenfeldt L, Wahren J (1981) A comparison of the effects of intravenous infusion of individual branched-chain amino acids on blood amino acid levels in man. Clin Sci 60:95–100
42. Sato Y, Eriksson S, Hagenfeldt L, et al (1981) Influence of branched-chain amino acid infusion on arterial concentrations and brain exchange of amino acids in patients with hepatic cirrhosis. Clin Physiol 1:151–165

43. Rossi-Fanelli F, Angelic M, Cangiano C, et al (1981) Effect of glucose and/or branched-chain amino acid infusion on plasma amino acid imbalance in chronic liver failure. JPEN 5:414–419
44. Eriksson LS, Conn HO (1989) Branched-chain amino acids in the managment of hepatic encephalopathy: An analysis of variants. Hepatology 10:228–246
45. Naylor CD, O'Rourke K, Detsky AS, Baker JP (1989) Parenteral nutrition with branched-chain amino acids in hepatic encephalopathy: A meta-analysis. Gastroenterology 97:1033–1042
46. Der Simonian R (1990) Parenteral nutrition with branched-chain amino acids in hepatic encephalopathy: A meta-analysis. Hepatology 11:1083–1084
47. Wahren J, Denis J, Desurmont P, et al (1983) Is intravenous administration of branched-chain amino acids effective in the treatment of hepatic encephalopathy? A multicenter study. Hepatology 3:475–480
48. Michel H, Bories P, Aubin JP, et al (1985) Treatment of acute hepatic encephalopathy in cirrhotics with a branched-chain amino acids enriched versus a conventional amino acids mixture. Liver 5:282–289
49. Vilstrup H, Gluud C, Hardt F, et al (1985) Branched-chain enriched amino acid nutrition does not change the outcome of hepatic coma in patients with cirrhosis of the liver. J Hepatol 1 (Suppl. 2):347 (Abst)
50. Rossi-Fanelli F, Riggio O, Cangiano C, et al (1982) Branched-chain amino acids vs lactulose in the treatment of hepatic coma: A controlled study. Dig Dis Sci 27:929–935
51. Cerra FB, Cheung NK, Fischer JE, et al (1985) Disease-specific amino acid infusion (FO80) in hepatic encephalopathy: A prospective, randomized, double-blind controlled trial. JPEN 9:288–295
52. Strauss E, dos Santos WR, daSilva EC, et al (1986) Treatment of hepatic encephalopathy: A randomized clinical trial comparing a branched-chain enriched amino acid solution to oral neomycin. Nutr Supp Serv 6:18–21
53. Fiaccadori F, Ghinelli F, Pedretti G, et al (1985) Branched-chain enriched amino acid solutions in the treatment of hepatic encephalopathy: A controlled trial. Ital J Gastroenterol 17:5–10
54. Forbes A, Wicks C, Marshall W, et al (1987) Nutritional support in fulminant hepatic failure: The safety of lipid solutions. Gut 28:1347–1348
55. Porayko MK, Dicecco S, O'Keefe SJD (1991) Impact of malnutrition and its therapy on liver transplantation. Sem Liver Dis 11:305–314
56. Shaw B, Wood P, Gordon RD, Iwatsuki S, Gillquist WP, Starzl TE (1985) Influence of selected patient variable and operative blood loss on six-months survival following transplantation. Sem Liver Dis 5:385–393
57. Moukarzel AA, Nasm I, Varoas J, Mc Diarmid SV, Busuttic RW, Ament ME (1990) Effect of nutritional status on outcome of orthotopic liver transplantation in pediatric patient. Transpl Proceedings 22:1560–1563

Nutrition and Metabolism in Acute Respiratory Failure

J. Takala

Introduction

The vast majority of intensive care patients require mechanical ventilation (MV) and other forms of advanced life support for less than one week. Major metabolic disturbances are rare in these patients and nutritional support can usually be managed according to clinical nutrition routines without problems. Approximately 10% of general ICU patients require prolonged intensive care, and their treatment produces 40 to 50% of all intensive care days (J Takala, unpublished). Depending on the type of individual departments, these figures may somewhat vary, but in general, less than 15% of patients require MV for more than one week.

In prolonged intensive care, respiratory failure is the rule and infections and multiple organ dysfunction (MOF) are common. The metabolic problems of these patients are characterized by hypermetabolism and increased net protein losses, while the patients depend on artificial nutrition. Under these conditions, the nutritional status may deteriorate rapidly, and interfere with the recovery from critical illness.

Adequate nutritional support can reduce the losses of energy and protein, and prevent the development of severe nutritional depletion. The repletion of the losses that have occurred during the acute phase of the illness is usually possible only after the convalescence has begun and the full recovery of functional and nutritional status may take for weeks, even months.

Nutritional support may have a marked impact on ventilation. Clinicians dealing with nutritional support in patients with respiratory problems became aware of this in the late 1970s, when studies by Kinney and Askanazi in the United States, and by Iapichino and Gattinoni in Italy demonstrated that increased production of carbon dioxide during administration of parenteral nutrition (TPN) with hypercaloric amounts of glucose markedly increased ventilatory demand in the acutely ill patient, and occasionally caused respiratory distress [1–3].

The interactions between nutrient supply and gas exchange have been subsequently revealed in more detail [4–8]: TPN with large amounts of glucose increases the demand for minute ventilation by increasing the CO_2-production, especially if lipogenesis is induced [4]; hypermetabolic surgical patients tend to have larger increase in VCO_2 than depleted patients in response to high glucose TPN [4]; substituting part of the glucose with lipids during hypercaloric TPN may reduce the demand for minute ventilation [5, 6], and ventilator-dependent patients may benefit from high fat diets during weaning [7]; high protein intake and branched-chain amino acids (BCAA) may increase the ventilatory drive [8].

Most of these studies have been performed in spontaneously breathing patients, who despite severe illness are not comparable to the intensive care patient with acute respiratory failure (ARF) requiring MV. Indeed, the effects of nutrients on ventilatory demand and gas exchange in MV patients have not been systematically studied. Currently, high carbohydrate loads are avoided in the acutely ill patient, and the risk of inappropriate loading of the respiratory system by nutrition is therefore reduced. The effects of nutrition on gas exchange and ventilatory demand are still important in patients with severely impaired gas exchange and poor work performance, when even a minor change in ventilatory demand may facilitate weaning or prolonged ventilator dependency.

Malnutrition is associated with increased morbidity and mortality, and reduced diaphragmatic function and muscle mass in patients with chronic obstructive lung disease [9–11]. In addition, abnormalities in peripheral muscle function, including increased fatiguability, have been observed in nutritional depletion [10]. No clinical data are available on the interaction between nutrition and muscle function in patients with ARF. Nevertheless, it is reasonable to assume that the skeletal muscles, including the respiratory muscles, are susceptible to the effects of nutritional depletion also in ARF, though the clinical relevance of this interaction is not known presently.

This chapter reviews the interrelation of metabolic and nutritional demands with ventilatory demand and gas exchange in acute respiratory failure.

Energy Expenditure

Most conditions leading to severe ARF are characterized by hypermetabolism: sepsis and infections, major injuries, postoperative complications and MOF can all be expected to increase energy expenditure (EE). Relatively little data on EE in patients with ARF is available, and the observations are mostly limited to single or short-term measurements [12–17].

The typical patients requiring prolonged intensive care, e.g. due to septic respiratory failure, may be fully dependent on nutritional support for several weeks, while being septic, hypermetabolic, and catabolic. Despite this, published longitudinal data on the patterns of EE in patients requiring prolonged MV are scarce and largely anecdotal [12, 13, 15, 18]]. As demonstrated in Fig. 1 in a representative patient, ARF may be associated with prolonged, persistent hypermetabolism, which in its severity and duration is comparable to the pattern observed after major burn. In contrast to major burns, the presence of hypermetabolism in ARF is much less well recognized.

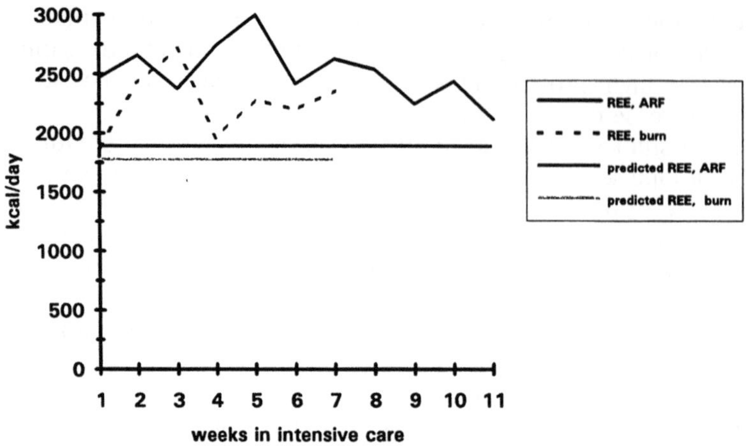

Fig. 1. Patterns of energy expediture during prolonged intensive care in acute respiratory failure and after major (50% of body surface area) burn injury

The most consistent finding in the longitudinal studies is the wide intraindividual variability of EE in respiratory failure [12, 13, 15, 18]. Further interpretation of the results is limited by the small [13, 15] or unspecified [12, 18] number of patients measured for more than one week, presentation of mean values for the whole duration of the study without the individual day-to-day variability [18], or expressing hypermetabolism for patient day only without taking into account the duration of individual treatments [12], and the lack of information on the clinical course of the patients; accordingly, the findings should be interpreted cautiously. Nevertheless, the results tend to suggest that in prolonged ARF, most patients are indeed hypermetabolic (EE 20–70% higher than predicted), and that prolonged negative energy balance and lack of hypermetabolism may both be related to poor prognosis.

The hypermetabolism tends to persist also during the recovery (Fig. 2), as shown for 14 patients with adult respiratory distress syndrome (ARDS) during the first week of MV and at the beginning of weaning 2 to 11 weeks (median 3 weeks) later. Since the clinical course of patients with severe ARF and ARDS is often associated with episodes of infection and alterations in vital functions, marked intraindividual day-to-day variation in the EE is bound to occur. Even in short-term, the variation can be upto 50% (Fig. 3) [13, 15].

Estimates of energy requirements are commonly based on formulae, such as the Harris-Benedict formula, with added energy to compensate for the estimated degree of hypermetabolism. The average degree of hypermetabolism can be relatively reliably estimated for characteristic groups of postoperative or injured patients. Attempts have been made to improve the predictions by correction factors, which take into account for each patient various components of metabolic stress, such as fever, the presence of severe infection, recent extensive operation, type of injury, and the presence of "respiratory distress syndrome" [19]. The use of correction factors slightly improves the prediction, but it has not been evaluated in longitudinal studies. If nutritional requirements are incorrectly estimated during prolonged hypermeta-

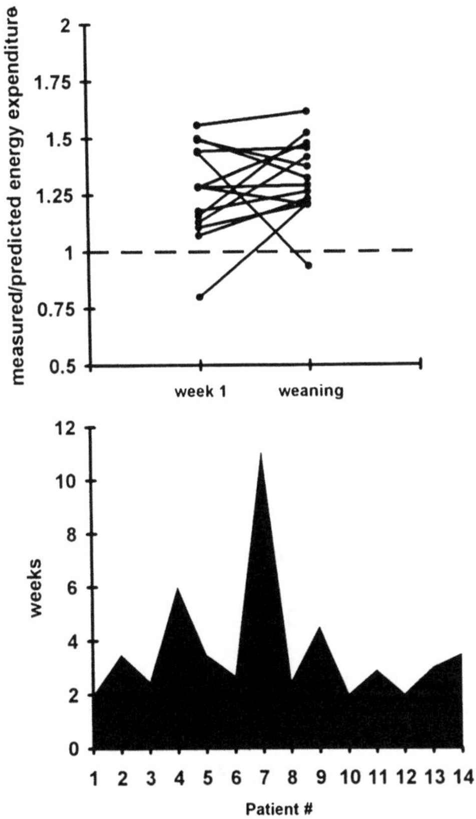

Fig. 2. Degree of hypermetabolism (top) in acute respiratory failure during the first week of intensive care and at the beginning of weaning. Energy expenditure is expressed as the ratio between measured and predicted (according to the Harris-Benedict formula) energy expenditure. The duration (weeks) of intensive care between the two measurements is shown for the individual patients (median three weeks; bottom)

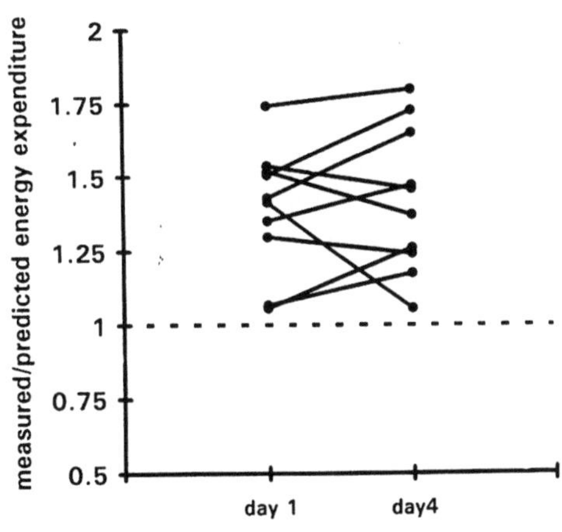

Fig. 3. Short-term variation in energy expenditure in patients with acute respiratory failure. Results indicate measurements at three-days interval

bolism, the cumulative net loss of nutrients can be severe enough to interfere with healing and recovery. The acute disorders of vital functions may also necessitate reduction of nutrient supply, with concomitant increased fluctuation of energy balance. It is evident that the patterns of hypermetabolism during ARF and MOF need to be described in more detail.

Components of Ventilatory Demand

The demand for alveolar ventilation is determined by the rate of CO_2-production from energy metabolism and the alveolar partial pressure of carbon dioxide ($PaCO_2$). The arterial carbon dioxide partial pressure ($PaCO_2$), a function of $PaCO_2$, is the major signal for the feed-back control of ventilation: the $PaCO_2$ is reflected in the pH at the brain stem respiratory center, and ventilation will be adjusted to oppose any change in the pH. The $PaCO_2$ is normally strictly controlled by this feed-back system, and resting $PaCO_2$ reflects the set-point of the respiratory control mechanism. The demand for minute ventilation (VE) required to maintain the body pool of CO_2 in a steady state depends on the alveolar ventilation and the efficiency of CO_2-removal. The efficiency of CO_2 removal is estimated as the ratio of physiological dead space to tidal volume (VD/VT) and it is a function of both lung function and breathing pattern. The relationship between these variables is defined by the Bohr equation:

$$VE = k \cdot VCO_2/[PaCO_2 \cdot (1\text{-}VD/VT)]$$

where k is a constant (k=0.1150, when VCO_2 is expressed in ml/min, STPD, VE in L/min, BTPS, and $PaCO_2$ in kPa). The relationship between ventilatory demand, CO_2 production and dead space to tidal volume ratio at a constant $PaCO_2$ can be presented graphically according to the Bohr equation (Fig. 4). Normal VE can be predicted using normal VCO_2 (obtained from the Harris-Benedict equation and the actual RQ) and normal VD/VT. When the x- and the y-axis represent VCO_2 and VE, respectively, the VD/VT is represented by diagonal lines. The VE demand caused by hypermetabolism can then be estimated as shown in Fig. 4. Using this approach, it has been estimated that hypermetabolism may contribute up to 50% of the increase in VE demand in patients with ARDS (Fig. 5) [20]. It is also evident that the impact of VCO_2 on the VE demand depends on the VD/VT: at higher VD/VT, more VE is required to compensate for an increase in VCO_2. Analogously, the $PaCO_2$ is also very important: at higher $PaCO_2$, less VE is required to compensate for an increase in VCO_2. The combination of high CO_2 production and VD/VT is common in ARF. The increase in VE demand is poorly tolerated in ARF, since the work of breathing is high and the work performance may be impaired.

The $PaCO_2$ set-point and the breathing pattern are crucial in determining the VE demand during spontaneous breathing and mechanical ventilatory

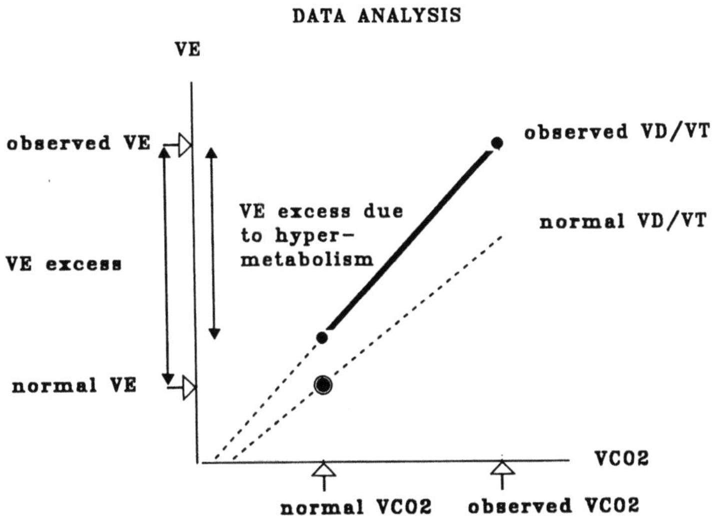

Fig. 4. Graphic representation of the Bohr equation at a constant arterial PCO_2. Minute ventilation (VE; y-axis) and CO_2 production (VCO_2; x-axis) and dead space to tidal volume ratio (VD/VT; diagonal dashed lines) are shown. For an observed level of ventilation and CO_2 production, the contribution of hypermetabolism to the ventilatory demand is demonstrated

support with a spontaneous breathing component. The $PaCO_2$ set-point can be substantially and inappropriately reduced in patients with ARF [21].

Hypermetabolism *per se* increases CO_2 production and accordingly, the demand for alveolar gas exchange. In ARF, hypermetabolism is associated with reduced efficiency of CO_2 removal, which amplifies the effect of CO_2 production on the VE demand (Fig. 6). An increased VD/VT will increase both the VE for a given level of CO_2 production and the amount of VE required to compensate for an increase in CO_2 production at a constant

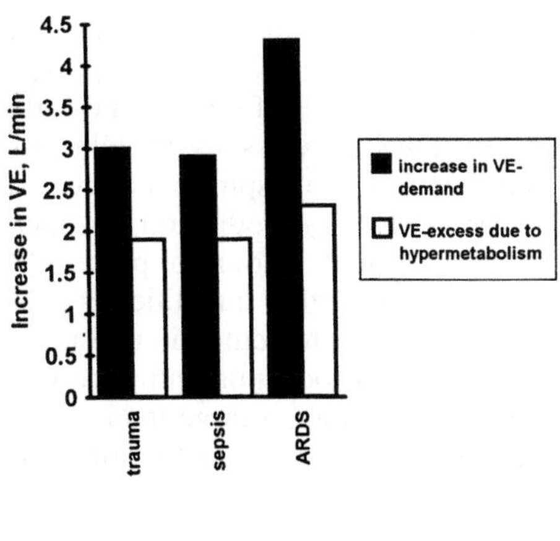

Fig. 5. The increase in ventilatory demand and the contribution of hypermetabolism to the increase is shown for patients with acute respiratory failure due to multiple injury, sepsis and ARDS. (Adapted from [20] with permission)

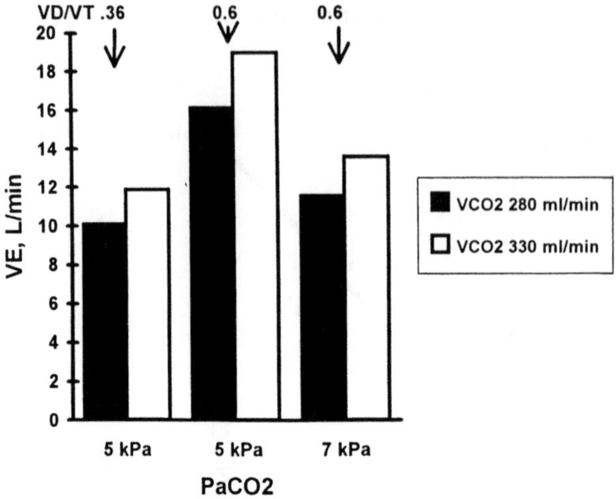

Fig. 6. Interaction between ventilatory demand, dead space to tidal volume ratio, arterial PCO_2, and CO_2 production. The effect of a moderate increase in CO_2 production is shown. With an increased VD/VT, the ventilatory demand is higher and increases more in response to the increase in CO_2 production. If moderate hypercapnia is allowed, most of the impact of increased VD/VT can be eliminated

$PaCO_2$ level. On the other hand, the ventilatory demand can be effectively reduced by an increase in $PaCO_2$ level.

In ARF, moderate hypercapnia is in general well tolerated. The reduction in ventilatory demand by adapting the patient to a higher $PaCO_2$ level may help to reduce ventilator-induced lung injury, reduce the work of breathing during weaning, and, by reducing the ventilatory cost of increased CO_2 production, allow the use of higher nutrient intakes during nutritional repletion.

Interactions of Nutrition and Ventilation

The concept of a link between nutrition and ventilatory demand is not a new one. In the early 1920s, Lusk [22] suggested that in patients with active tuberculosis, the intakes of protein and carbohydrate should be limited in order to put the lungs at rest, since protein and carbohydrate increase metabolic rate and therefore the respiratory activity. He also observed that in patients with tuberculosis, CO_2 production was increased by 17% and minute ventilation by 94%. A small amount of protein (21 g) had no effect on EE and ventilation, whereas higher quantities of protein induced distinct parallel increases in EE and minute ventilation. Glucose (100 g) had no effect on EE but increased CO_2 production with a consequent 17% increase in minute ventilation. Furthermore, a large load of lipids (140 g), despite a 12% increase in EE, increased minute ventilation by only 14.5%. The patients were moderately hypermetabolic and their protein losses were not large. These observations led to the conclusion that "fat, with little carbohydrate, together with a low protein intake, constitutes a rational diet for the man ill with pulmonary tuberculosis" [22]. For the hospitalized patient with tuberculosis, a diet containing 2500 kcal (total) with 60 to 90 g of protein was recommended.

In fact, these principles, established 70 years ago, can well be applied with minor modifications also for the ICU patient with respiratory failure. The rate of CO_2 production depends both on the EE and the mixture of substrates metabolized by the body. The substrate mixture will be reflected in the ratio between the amount of CO_2 produced and oxygen consumed (respiratory quotient, RQ). The amount of CO_2 produced per unit of energy is smallest during fat oxidation [23]. As compared to the oxidation of fat, protein oxidation produces approximately 20% and that of carbohydrate 37% more CO_2 per unit of energy. At a given EE, these differences will be directly reflected in the demand for minute ventilation, if the other components of the Bohr equation remain constant.

Clinical studies have demonstrated that the CO_2 production at a given energy intake is lower, when energy is administered as both lipids and glucose [5, 6, 24, 25]. The RQ normally varies between the extremes of 0.7 for pure lipid oxidation and 1.0 for pure glucose oxidation (with 0.8 for protein oxidation). While changes in RQ from 0.7 to 1.0 at a constant EE would increase CO_2 production by 37%, the variation of RQ during artificial nutrition is much smaller in most ICU patients.

The CO_2 production can be markedly reduced in the rare instances when net lipid synthesis has been induced, either by switching from glucose to a mixture of glucose and lipids, or by substantially reducing the energy intake. Net lipogenesis is a rarity in the acutely ill patients, but may occur as a result of hypercaloric feeding during convalescence.

The studies that originally alerted the clinicians of the adverse effects of nutrition on ventilation were mostly performed in spontaneously breathing patients using energy intakes, which were 50–100% higher than the EE, and consisted predominantly of glucose [1, 2, 4, 6]. These observations have often been extrapolated as such to ICU patients with ARF.

When energy intakes corresponding to or moderately exceeding EE are given to ICU patients with respiratory failure, the composition of the diet appears to have only a minor effect on respiratory quotient, and the changes in CO_2 production and oxygen consumption are related more to the energy content of the diet than to its composition [17, 27, 28]. Talpers et al. [27] recently demonstrated that, in stable mechanically ventilated patients receiving parenteral nutrition with an average energy intake of 1.3 times predicted EE, variation of the energy composition from 40 to 75% carbohydrate had no consistent impact on CO_2 production (Fig. 7). In contrast, when the intake of a mixed parenteral diet was increased from the level of predicted EE to twice the predicted EE, CO_2 production increased substantially. Unfortunately, oxygen consumption and actual EE were not measured. In addition, the use of patients as their own controls in treatments lasting for days must

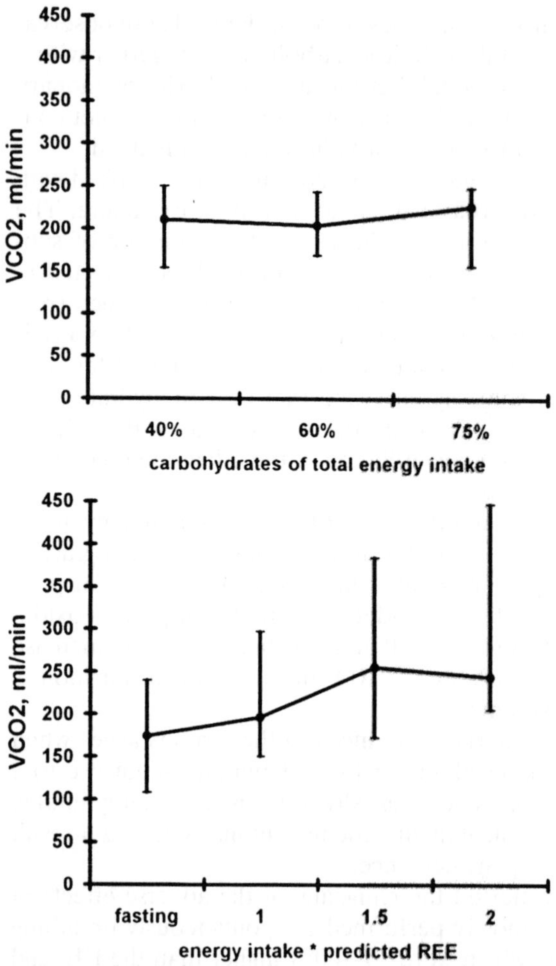

Fig. 7. At an energy intake of 1.3 times predicted energy expenditure, the composition of diet has little effect on CO_2 production in stable mechanically ventilated patients (top). Increased energy intake induces a marked increase in CO_2 production (bottom). Values are median and range (Adapted from [26] with permission)

have contributed to the wide variation between individual responses. Nevertheless, the results support the concept that at moderate intakes, energy substrate composition has a limited impact on the oxidized substrate mixture. It is likely that the composition of the diet may modify the contribution of exogenous versus endogenous substrates in the overall substrate oxidation.

Similar results have been observed in enterally fed patients with ARF (Fig. 8). Enteral feeding at an energy intake of 1.3 times measured energy expenditure with either 23 or 48% of the total energy intake as lipids resulted in minor changes in CO_2 production and no consistent differences between the diets were observed in gas exchange variables. Furthermore, a recent study in infected patients, half of them with ARF, demonstrated that modifying the carbohydrate content of enteral feeding from 50 to 28%, and

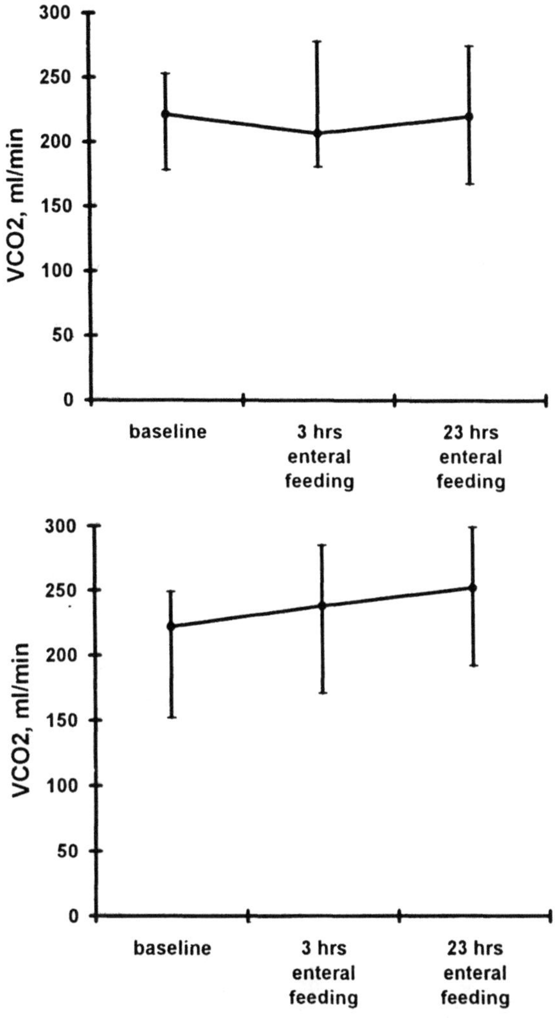

Fig. 8. Effect of diet composition on CO_2 production during enteral feeding with an energy intake of 1.3 times measured energy expenditure. No differences are observed between diets with either 23% (top) or 48% (bottom) of the total energy intake as lipids. Values are median and range, n=11 for the low fat diet and n=9 for the higher fat diet (Takala J, unpublished)

fat content from 30 to 55%, only slightly reduced carbohydrate oxidation while fat oxidation persisted at a relatively constant rate [27].

A striking finding in the study by Askanazi et al. [4] was the increase in oxygen consumption (29%) that accompanied the large increase in CO_2 production (56%) during the hypercaloric TPN in the acutely ill injured and septic patients, and which was not observed in the depleted patients. The increase in oxygen consumption was attributed to increased sympathetic activity, reflected as increased urinary excretion of norepinephrine. In contrast, when 50% of the non-protein energy was infused as fat, the increases in both oxygen consumption and CO_2 production were considerably smaller. In mechanically ventilated patients with ARF, increases in oxygen consumption in response to nutrient administration up to rates corresponding to 1.5 · measured energy expenditure appear to be small, usually less than 15% [5, 17, 29]. The use of slightly lower dietary intakes almost certainly contributes to the smaller increases in oxygen consumption. Another contributing factor is most likely the oxygen cost of breathing. When CO_2 production increases in response to nutrition, the consequent increase in ventilation will increase the work of breathing in spontaneously breathing patients. In normal subjects, the work of breathing represents less than 5% of whole body oxygen consumption. The spontaneously breathing injured and septic patients are likely to have increased work of breathing, and therefore an increase in ventilatory demand by any mechanism will have a larger impact on whole body oxygen consumption. In addition, if ventilatory demand increases in patients with marginal ventilatory reserves, the imminent respiratory distress will activate the sympathetic nervous system.

The increase in energy expenditure due to the diet-induced thermogenesis will also increase CO_2 production and ventilatory demand. During TPN with energy intake at 1.5 · measured EE, the combined effect of the diet-induced thermogenesis and increase in RQ increased the CO_2 production by 43%, when the RQ was very low before the commencement of TPN with glucose as the energy source in patients with ARF [5]. When half of the non-protein energy was given as lipids, the increase in CO_2 production was 21%. This observation emphasizes the fact that while during hypocaloric feeding and at energy intakes close to EE, dietary composition has little impact on CO_2 production (Fig. 9), during hypercaloric feeding an increased proportion of lipids may reduce the CO_2 production to a clinically relevant extent.

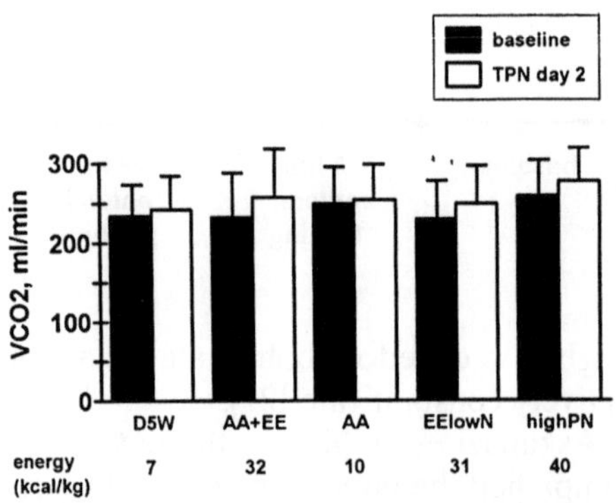

Fig. 9. Effect of various parenteral nutrient infusions on CO_2 production. The total energy intake on the second infusion day is shown below the x-axis. D5W = 5% glucose; AA + EE = 1.5 g/kg/day of amino acids and energy (glucose and lipids) at a rate corresponding to the measured baseline energy expenditure; AA = 1.5 g/kg/day of amino acids; EElowN = 0.6 g/kg/day of amino acids and energy (glucose and lipids) at a rate corresponding to the measured baseline energy expenditure; highPN = a fixed program with 120 g of amino acids and 2200 kcal of non-protein energy (glucose and lipids). At energy intakes close to actual energy expenditure or clearly less, only minor changes in CO_2 production occur. (Adapted from [17] with permission)

High protein intake and amino acid infusions appear to have an effect on the respiratory control mechanism and may reduce the $PaCO_2$ set-point, which further increases the ventilatory demand. Increasing the amino acid content of TPN lowers the arterial PCO_2 and enhances the ventilatory response to hypercapnia in spontaneously breathing depleted patients [30]. A similar change has been demonstrated in healthy subjects, when amino acids alone are infused after a period of semistarvation [31]. BCAA may have a pharmacologic effect on ventilatory control. A short-term infusion of BCAA may have a pharmacologic effect on ventilatory control. A short-term infusion of BCAA lowers the arterial PCO_2 both in the sleep state in healthy volunteers [32, 33] and in spontaneously breathing patients after open heart surgery [34]. These effects have been observed with intakes clearly higher than relevant for nutritional support, and do not presently have clinical application. When the intake of protein and the proportion of BCAA in TPN was increased during postoperative pressure support ventilation, no alteration in gas exchange and ventilatory control was observed [35]. The lack of effect of protein intake on ventilation in the study of Delafosse et al. [35] may have been related to an abnormally low PCO_2 throughout the study and the use of relatively high level of pressure support ventilation.

Nutritional Implications and Therapeutic Strategy

From the therapeutic point of view, it is crucial to recognize the pattern of persistent hypermetabolism and increased protein losses, and the fact that, due to the naturally complicated course of severe ARF, the day-to-day variation of EE is wide and the degree of hypermetabolism unpredictable. Net loss of protein is unavoidable during the most acute phase of the illness, and nutritional repletion can be achieved once convalescence has begun.

The goal of nutritional support during the acute phase of the illness should be to reduce the nutrient losses to a reasonable level without inappropriate loading of the respiratory system. Careful monitoring of EE, nitrogen losses and their response to nutrition, in addition to the clinical status, will aid in recognizing the transition from the hypermetabolic flow phase to convalescence. During convalescence, the goal should be to start nutritional repletion in conjunction with the functional rehabilitation of the patient. Since nutrition with energy intakes exceeding the energy expenditure are necessary during nutritional repletion, the risk for an inappropriate increase in ventilatory demand is increased, and unexpected individual responses may occur.

The strategy for avoiding unnecessary loading of the respiratory system during the acute phase of the disease should be based on an energy intake exceeding the actual EE by 15–25%. The slight energy excess takes into account the spontaneous variation of EE and the thermogenic response to nutrition. In addition, part of the energy (30–60%) should be given as lipids. During convalescence, the energy intake may be increased by 50% above the EE in order to facilitate nutritional repletion. In these circumstances, it is probably advantageous to administer roughly 50% of the energy as lipids. Very high protein intakes may inappropriately increase the ventilatory drive. If increased ventilatory demand due to nutrition is suspected, the following steps may help to reduce the ventilatory demand:

- If the RQ is high, the proportion of lipids in the diet should be increased;
- The total energy intake should be reduced to match the EE; and
- If the protein intake is high, it should be reduced to 1.0–1.5 g/kg/day.

The response in gas exchange will take place in a matter of hours, and the attempt to reduce the ventilatory demand should not be unnecessarily prolonged. If an effect is not obvious in 12 h, it is unlikely to occur. A representative example is shown in Fig. 10. A patient recovering from severe ARF due to acute hemorrhagic pancreatitis had difficulties in weaning. A relatively high carbohydrate enteral and parenteral feeding program (65% of total energy as carbohydrates) at 50% in excess to EE was given. The hypercaloric diet was given in order to enhance nutritional repletion and the low proportion of lipids selected due to persistent hypertriglyceridemia. Measurement of gas exchange and ventilation (Fig. 10) revealed high minute ventilation with normal arterial PCO_2 and oxygenation and a respiratory quotient approaching 1. The CO_2 production and oxygen consumption were both high and the patient appeared clearly dyspneic. A reduction of the total energy intake to 1.2 · energy expenditure and a reduction of the proportion of carbohydrate to 35% of the total energy intake reduced the minute ventilation by approximately 30% in 6 h, with a concomitant reduction of CO_2 prodution, oxygen consumption and respiratory quotient.

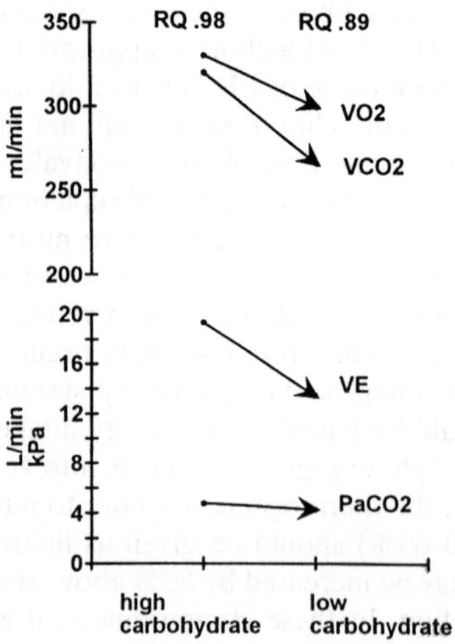

Fig. 10. Reduction of ventilatory demand by reduction of the total energy intake and the proportion of carbohydrates. For details, see text

In order to define the appropriate therapeutic approach for the reduction of nutrient losses during the acute phase of respiratory failure, consideration of the relationship between energy and nitrogen balance is useful. Studies in nutritionally depleted patients have clearly demonstrated that nitrogen equilibrium can be achieved with different combinations of nitrogen intakes and energy balances [36, 37]. Larsson et al. [38] have demonstrated that in injured patients, some with ARF, N equilibrium cannot be obtained despite high energy intake and N intakes up to 0.3 g/kg/day; an optimum N sparing was obtained with an intake of approximately 0.2 g/kg/day and a further increase had no beneficial effect.

The only study so far on the relationship between energy and N balance in ICU patients, the majority with ARF, was performed by Pitkänen et al. [17] (Fig. 11). Using a two-day feeding model, an optimum nitrogen sparing was obtained by a non-protein energy intake corresponding to prenutrition EE and 1.5 g/kg/day of amino acids. This is in accordance with the results of previous studies [5, 38].

The above recommendations are based on short-term studies; no long-term studies are presently available. Accordingly, in patients with ARF these guidelines may applied as the basis for nutritional support; in addition, careful monitoring of individual patients for efficacy and unexpected responses is the key to successful clinical management of these patients.

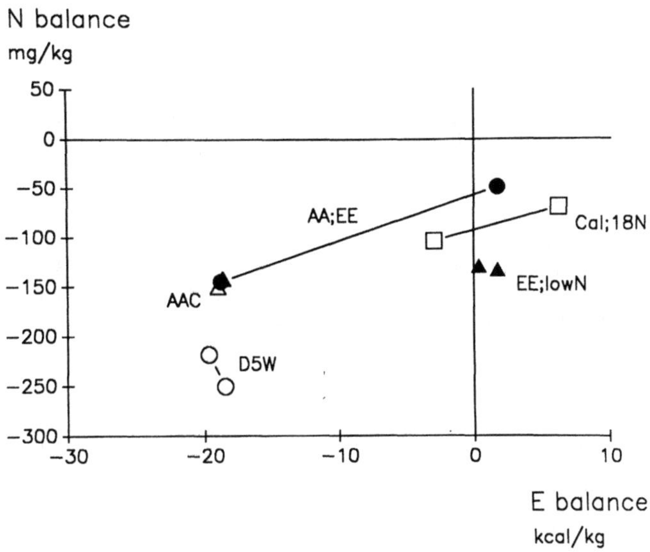

Fig. 11. Relationship between energy and nitrogen balance in patients with acute respiratory failure receiving the diets explained in Fig. 9. (From [17] with permission)

Conclusion

The therapeutic strategy for nutritional support in acute respiratory failure can be summarized as follows:

- In severe acute respiratory failure with prolonged need for intensive care, a pattern of hypermetabolism and increased protein losses will persist until convalescence. The nutritional support should aim at energy equilibrium and reasonable reduction of the losses of nitrogen. The energy expenditure may vary widely and careful monitoring in order to avoid inappropriate extensive nutrient losses during the acute phase of the disease is mandatory.
- The repletion of the obligatory losses of nutrients, concomitantly with functional rehabilitation should be commenced after convalescence has begun.
- The nutrition-induced increase in ventilatory demand can be minimized by limiting the energy intake during the acute phase of the disease to close to energy expenditure, by administering 30–60% of the energy as lipids, and by allowing moderate hypercapnia.

References

1. Askanazi J, Elwyn DH, Silverberg PA, et al (1980) Respiratory distress secondary to a high carbohydrate load: A case report. Surgery 87:596–598
2. Askanazi J, Rosenbaum SH, Hyman AI, et al (1980) Respiratory changes induced by the large glucose loads of total parenteral nutrition. JAMA 243:1444–1447
3. Gattinoni L, Iapichino G, Moise G, Bernasconi C (1974) Bilancio energerico nel politraumatizzato durante alimentazione parenterale: Osservazioni preliminari. Anesteziol Reanimatol 15:353–354
4. Askanazi J, Carpentier YA, Elwyn DH, et al (1980) Influence of total parenteral nutrition on fuel utilization in injury and sepsis. Ann Surg 191:40–46
5. Roulet M, Detsky AS, Marliss E, et al (1983) A controlled trial of the effect of parenteral nutritional support on patients with respiratory failure and sepsis. Clin Nutr 2:97–105
6. Askanazi J, Nordenström J, Rosenbaum SH, et al (1981) Nutrition for the patient with respiratory failure: Glucose vs fat. Anesthesiology 54:373–377
7. Al-Saady NM, Blackmore CM, Bennett ED (1989) High fat, low carbohydrate, enteral feeding lowers $PaCO_2$ and reduces the period of ventilation in artificially ventilated patients. Int Care Med 15:290–295
8. Takala J (1989) Branched-chain amino acids and respiratory function in man. In: Kinney JM, Borum PR (eds) Perspectives in clinical nutrition. Urban and Schwarzenberg, Baltimore-Munich, pp 221–229
9. Schols A, Mostert R, Soeters P, Greve LH, Wouters EFM (1989) Inventory of nutritional status in patients with COPD. Chest 96:247–249
10. Whittaker JS, Ryan CF, Buckley PA, Road JD (1990) The effects of refeeding on peripheral and respiratory muscle function in malnourished chronic obstructive pulmonary disease patients. Am Rev Respir Dis 142:283–288
11. Braun SR, Dixon RM, Keim NL, Luby M, Anderegg A, Shrago ES (1984) Predictive clinical value of nutritional assessment factors in COPD. Chest 85:353–357

12. Bartlett RH, Dechert RE, Mault JR, Ferguson SK, Kaiser AM. Erlandson EE (1982) Measurements of metabolism in multiple organ failure. Surgery 92:771–779
13. Carlsson M, Nordenström J, Hedenstierna G (1984) Clinical implications of continuous measurements of energy expenditure in mechanically ventilated patients. Clin Nutr 3:103–110
14. Lanschot JJB van, Feenstra BWA, Vermeij CG, et al (1988) Accuracy of intermittent metabolic gas exchange recordings extrapolated for diurnal variation. Crit Care Med 16:737–742
15. Vermeij CG, Feenstra BWA, van Lanschot JJB, Bruining HA (1989) Day-to-day variability of energy expenditure in critically ill surgical patients. Crit Care Med 17:623–626
16. Swinamer DL, Phang PT, Jones RL, Grace M, King EG (1987) Twenty-four hour energy expenditure in ciritically ill patients. Crit Care Med 15:637–643
17. Pitkänen O, Takala J, Pöyhönen M, Kari A (1991) Nitrogen and energy balance in septic and injured patients: Response to parenteral nutrition. Clin Nutr 10:258–265
18. Forsberg E, Soop M, Thörne A (1991) Energy expenditure and outcome in patients with multiple organ failure following abdominal surgery. Intensive Care Med 17:403–409
19. van Lanschot JJB, Feenstra BWA, Vermeij CG, Bruining HA (1986) Calculation versus measurement of total energy expenditure. Crit Care Med 14:981–985
20. Kiiski R, Takala J (1991) Increased ventilatory demand due to hypermetabolism in acute respiratory failure. Crit Care Med 19:S92
21. Ravenscraft SA, McArthur CD, Path MJ, Iber C (1991) Components of excess ventilation in patients initiated on mechanical ventilation. Crit Care Med 19:916–925
22. Lusk G (1928) Metabolism in fever. In: Lusk G (ed) The elements of the science of nutrition. WB Saunders, Philadelphia and London, pp 716–721
23. Swift RW, French CE (1954) Energy metabolism and nutrition. The Scarecrow Press, Washington DC
24. Giovannini I, Chiarla C, Boldrini G, Gastagneto M (1989) Impact of fat and glucose administration on metabolic and respiratory interactions in sepsis. JPEN 13:141–146
25. Angelillo VA, Sukhdarshan B, Durfee S, Dahl J, Patterson AJ, O'Donohue J (1985) Effects of low and high carbohydrate feedings in ambulatory patients with chronic obstructive pulmonary disease and chronic hypercapnia. Ann Intern Med 103:883–885
26. Iapichino G, Radrizzani D, Leoni L, et al (1987) A comparison of mixed and glucose systems in the total parenteral nutrition of malnourished patients. Clin Nutr 6:1–4
27. Talpers SS, Romberger DJ, Bunce SB, Pingleton SK (1992) Nutritionally associated increased carbon dioxide production: Excess total calories vs high proportion of carbohydrate calories. Chest 102:551–555
28. Schneeweiss B, Graniger W, Ferenci P, et al (1992) Short-term energy balance in patients with infections: Carbohydrate-based versus fat-based diets. Metabolism 41:125–130
29. Laaban JP, Lemaire F, Baron JF, et al (1985) Influence of caloric intake on the respiratory mode during mandatory minute volume ventilation. Chest 87:67–72
30. Askanazi J, Weissman C, LaSala P, et al (1984) Effect of protein intake on ventilatory drive. Anesthesiology 60:106–110
31. Weissman C, Askanazi J, Rosenbaum S, et al (1983) Amino acids and respiration. Ann Intern Med 98:41–44
32. Takala J, Askanazi J, Weissman C, et al (1988) Changes in respiratory control induced by amino acid infusions. Crit Care Med 16:465–469
33. Kirvelä O, Thorpy M, Takala J, Askanazi J, Singer P, Kvetan V (1990) Respiratory and sleep patterns during nocturnal infusions of branched-chain amino acids. Acta Anaesthesiol Scand 34:645–648
34. Takala J, Kiiski R, Kari A (1989) Ventilatory stimulation by branched-chain amino acids after weaning from mechanical ventilation. Clin Nutr 8 (Suppl):36
35. Delafosse B, Bouffard Y, Bertrand O, Viale JP, Annat G, Motin J (1989) Effects of protein intake on pulmonary gas exchange and ventilatory drive in postoperative patients. Anesthesiology 70:404–407

36. Shaw SN, Elwyn DH, Askanazi J, Iles M, Schwarz Y, Kinney JM (1983) Effects of increasing nitrogen intake on nitrogen balance and energy expenditure on nutritionally depleted adult patients receiving parenteral nutrition. Am J Clin Nutr 37:930–940
37. Pitkänen O, Takala J, Pöyhönen M, et al (1991) Nitrogen and energy balance in depleted patients undergoing major gastrointestinal surgery: Response to TPN. Clin Nutr 10:36–42
38. Larsson J, Lennmarken C, Mårtensson J, et al (1980) Nitrogen requirements in severely injured patients. Brit J Surg 77:413–416

Nutritional Complications associated with Chemotherapy and Irradiation in Cancer Treatment

T. R. Ziegler

Introduction

Multiple factors contribute to weight loss and depletion of body protein and fat in many individuals with cancer, a wasting state known as cancer cachexia. Malnutrition may occur in cancer patients due to diminished oral food intake (e.g. secondary to anorexia or mechanical factors such as obstruction of the gastrointestinal (GI) tract); abnormal nutrient losses from the body (vomiting, diarrhea and malabsorption); abnormalities in protein, fat, carbohydrate and energy metabolism with defective nutrient assimilation related malignancy itself; possible competition by the tumor for nutrients; and catabolic effects of operations, infection and other associated illnesses. Cancer treatment with chemotherapy and radiotherapy also contributes to protein-energy malnutrition wasting in oncologic patients and may interrelate with factors noted above (Table 1).

This chapter will review nutritional complications associated with administration of chemotherapeutic drugs and radiotherapy in the cancer patient. The incidence of malnutrition and data on altered substrate metabolism in cancer patients will be considered initially, followed by a review of available data on the effects of chemo- and radiotherapy on nutrient metabolism.

Malnutrition in Cancer Patients

The incidence, severity and clinical impact of malnutrition in cancer patients is highly variable. In addition to the factors cited above, the incidence of

Table 1. Major factors which contribute to malnutrition in cancer patients

- Diminished food intake (e.g. anorexia, pain, GI tract obstruction)
- Abnormal nutrient losses (emesis, diarrhea, malabsorption)
- Altered nutrient metabolism (fat, protein, carbohydrate, energy)
- Possible host-tumor competition for nutrients (? related to tumor mass or tumor metabolic activity)
- Catabolic effects of infection, operation, other illnesses
- Chemotherapy and irradiation (alone and in combination)
- Availability of specialized nutritional support

nutritional depletion is also related to patient age, pre-morbid nutritional status, tumor type, tumor burden and the aggressiveness of treatment. However, several studies indicate that malnutrition is common in both hospitalized and non-hospitalized cancer patients [1–4]. Nixon et al. [1] studied nutritional status in 54 hospitalized adults (average age 57 years) using body weight (BW) pattern and other anthropometric data, creatinine excretion and serum albumin as nutritional indicators. Almost all patients in this study exhibited evidence of protein-calorie malnutrition; however, the relative diminution of body fat, skeletal muscle and circulating proteins was highly variable in these patients with a variety of tumor types. The creatinine to height ratio was below 80% of standard in 88% of patients, and was found to be the most sensitive indicator of malnutrition. Plasma folate, vitamin C and vitamin A levels were below normal in 20 to 45% of patients. The basal metabolic rate and caloric intake were similar to values from normal adults of similar size. Importantly, the degree of malnutrition correlated inversely with the length of patient survival.

In a study of 3,047 patients enrolled in 12 chemotherapy protocols of the Eastern Cooperative Oncology Group, DeWys et al. [2] found that some degree of weight loss was common and was significantly associated with patient survival. The frequency of any weight loss ranged from 31% in patients with favorable non-Hodgkin's lymphoma to 87% in patients with gastric cancer. Within treatment groups, median survical was shorter in patients who had lost 6% or more of pre-illness weight versus those without any weight loss. Within performance status and tumor burden catagories, weight loss independently affected prognosis and survival. In most patient subgroups, a history of weight loss was associated with decreased performance status, and reduced chemotherapy response rates, particularly in patients with breast cancer [2].

In a group of 280 cancer patients with several different tumor types receiving several forms of treatment, malnutrition was primarily related to the type of tumor (being more severe in those with esophageal and gastric cancer) and was generally more severe in those with advanced disease [3]. A study of 120 men with head and neck malignancies evaluated the impact of age and nutritional status on operative outcomes. In these patients, the severity of malnutrition alone correlated with the incidence of postoperative complications and the length of hospital stay [4]. Further, older patients (>60 years) with evidence of preoperative malnutrition had the highest complication and one year mortality rates versus older normally nourished patients or young (<60 years) patients with any degree of malnutrition. Only 20% of the older malnourished patients received preoperative enteral or parenteral nutritional support versus 60% of the younger malnourished individuals [4].

Taken together, the available studies document that some degree of malnutrition is relatively common in various categories of cancer patients and also has an important role in clinical outcome. Thus, considering the possible impact of chemotherapy and radiation therapy on nutritional status is important in the care of patients with malignancy.

Altered Substrate Metabolism

A number of abnormalities in protein, carbohydrate, fat and energy metabolism have been identified in subgroups of cancer patients which appear to be due to the presence of the malignancy itself [5–24]. Although the exact mediators and molecular mechanisms of these metabolic alterations remain largely unknown, they appear to be common. It is likely that these metabolic alterations contribute, at least in some patients, to a relative inability to efficiently utilize enteral or parenteral nutrients.

Abnormal Carbohydrate Metabolism

Alterations in glucose metabolism have consistently been identified in cancer patients with a variety of tumor types. In a study of 44 lung cancer patients (average weight loss 16% of usual BW), Heber et al. [5] found significantly greater whole body glucose production rates in the patients compared to matched controls (3.4 ± 0.2 versus controls 2.3 ± 0.1 mg/kg/min; $P < 0.005$). Although fasting blood glucose was unchanged, insulin resistance and abnormal glucose disposal after an oral glucose load were documented. Additional studies by these and other investigators document glucose intolerance, reduced first-phase insulin secretion after a glucose challenge, insulin resistance and diminished peripheral glucose uptake, increased glucose turnover, and increased glucose production via gluconeogenesis and recycling via lactate (Cori cycle) in other types of cancer [6–10]. While the mechanisms for these effects on carbohydrate metabolism are unknown, they do not appear to be related to changes in the circulating classical counter-regulatory hormones such as cortisol, glucagon, or catecholamine [6]. Additional studies showed malnourished patients with lung or colon cancer to exhibit elevated growth hormone levels; however, the role of this anti-insulin hormone in the underlying glucose metabolism of these individuals is unclear [7].

Abnormal Protein Metabolism

Skeletal muscle wasting and hypoalbuminemia are characteristic clinical and biochemical features of cancer cachexia. Malignant disease alters protein metabolism in humans in a manner which contributes to net loss of lean body mass [5, 7–12].

Shaw and Wolfe [10] using isotopic techniques documented a blunted effect of glucose infusion to diminish net body protein catabolism in patients with advanced weight loss and upper GI tract cancer. Cancer patients with weight loss exhibited higher rates of whole-body protein catabolism which contributed to the relative inability of glucose infusion to improve net protein catabolism. A normal response to glucose infusion on protein kinetics was observed in patients with cancer but no significant weight loss.

Other studies in patients with a variety of tumors documented increased whole body protein turnover, increased rates of protein breakdown, reduced rates of protein synthesis in skeletal muscle and increased hepatic protein synthesis [5, 9, 11–12]. Limited data are available on amino acid levels in cancer patients; however, branched-chain amino acid (BCAA) concentrations are maintained in cachectic cancer patients in contrast to lower levels seen in simple starvation. Lung cancer patients have reduced fasting alanine levels [5], while patients with different tumor types (breast versus GI versus head and neck) had significantly different levels of plasma arginine, phenylalanine, tryptophan, valine and taurine [11]. In as study of 55 cancer patients with esophageal cancer, lymphoma or sarcoma, Norton et al [12] found only proline levels to be reduced from the normal range in the lymphoma and sarcoma patients whom had not lost significant BW; those with some weight loss had reduced histidine and arginine levels. However, in the weight-losing esophageal cancer patients, a marked reduction in plasma levels of 12 of 15 amino acids (except leucine, valine and ornithine) was observed. Thus, the type of tumor and the underlying nutritional status may both influence circulating amino acid profiles.

Abnormal Fat Metabolism

Hyperlipidemia and erosion of endogenous fat stores are commonly observed in cancer patients. Excess depletion of the body fat compartment relative to the depletion of lean tissue has also been documented [9–10, 13–14]. Stable isotope studies demonstrated increased rates of free fatty acid and glycerol turnover in patients with GI malignancies whom had experienced weight loss, and glucose infusion failed to normally inhibit lipolysis in such patients [9–10]. In other studies, patients with various tumor types had decreased levels of circulating lipoprotein lipase, and thus were less able to promote storage of fat from circulating lipoproteins compared to normals [9, 13]. Although increased rates of lipolysis and diminished rates of lipogenesis have been noted, circulating plasma free fatty levels are variable in cancer patients [9–10, 13–14].

Alterations in Resting Energy Expenditure

Although alterations in resting energy expenditure (REE) in cancer patients have been well documented, the findings in various types of patients have been extremely variable [9, 15–18]. For example, in weight-losing cancer patients, elevated energy expenditure is not uniformly observed, while other individuals with stable weight or weight loss demonstrate hyper- or even hypometabolism [9, 15–18].

Arbeit et al. [15] studied 9 patients with localized sarcomas and 4 patients with diffuse sarcoma or carcinoma. Those with localized disease (and less weight loss) had significantly greater REE than matched controls (controls 18.1±2.9 versus localized 21.4±3.7 kcal/kg/day); however, REE in those with diffuse disease was greater than either of the previous groups (25.6±3.7 kcal/kg/day). Patients studied both before and after tumor excision (n=4) demonstrated a significant drop in REE after tumor removal, and the percent fall in REE was significantly correlated with tumor volume. In a larger study of 136 individuals (largely composed of patients with gastric, colorectal and bronchial neoplasms), Hansell et al. [16] found REE to correlate significantly with BW and lean body mass, and not with type of tumor or the presence of metastases. The closest correlation was between REE and lean body mass, but no difference was found when the data were expressed as kcal/kg LBM/day between groups when separated into weight stable, weight-losing, malignant, and nonmalignant categories. These authors concluded that REE was not elevated as a function of these tumor types and that weight loss in cancer patients is not explained by an increase in REE [16].

In a study of 73 patients with colorectal cancer, 49% had an abnormal REE (outside 10% of predicted) [17]. However, approximately one half of these patients were hypometabolic and the other half of those with abnormal REE were hypermetabolic. REE did not correlate with tumor burden or nutritional status of the patients [17].

Another study in patients with lung and colon cancer found no difference in mean REE between cancer patients, patients with GI disease, or those with chronic lung disease, and no difference in REE in cancer patients with weight loss versus controls with weight loss [18]. Weight loss correlated with REE only in female lung cancer patients in this study [18]. Therefore, the available data suggest that changes in EE are generally not sufficient to explain cachexia or restoration of BW in many patients with cancer. Table 2 lists alterations in substrate and energy metabolism identified in cancer patients.

Body Composition in Cancer Patients

A number of studies have evaluated the protein, fat, lean body mass and water compartments of the body in cancer patients compared to healthy controls or patients with non-malignant disease. Additional studies have determined changes in body composition after chemotherapy or radiation therapy as discussed below.

Cohn et al. [19] determined serial body composition in 37 cancer patients over a 6 month period using prompt neutron activation to measure total body nitrogen (N); total body potassium was determined by whole body counting and total body water (TBW) was measured with tritiated isotope methods. The patients had a mixture of hematologic and solid tumors. Results showed a marked heterogeneity in N balance, ranging from negative to positive. Weight loss was common, and was a function of reductions in body

Table 2. Alterations in substrate and energy metabolism in cancer

Carbohydrate metabolism
Increased glucose production rate by liver (gluconeogenesis)
Insulin resistance
Reduced first-phase insulin secretion after glucose challenge
Diminished peripheral glucose uptake
Increased glucose turnover
Increased glucose recycling (Cori cycle)
Glucose intolerance
Fat metabolism
Erosion of endogenous fat stores (increased lipolytic rate)
Increased free fatty acid and glycerol turnover
Decreased rate of lipogenesis
Diminished ability of glucose to suppress lipolysis
Decreased lipoprotein lipase activity
Hyperlipidemia
Protein metabolism
Increased skeletal muscle protein catabolism
Reduced protein synthetic rate in muscle
Blunted effect of glucose to inhibit protein breakdown
Increased rates of whole-body protein catabolism
Increased hepatic protein synthesis
Reduced amino acid levels in plasma
Negative nitrogen balance
Energy metabolism
Variable effects (hyper, hypo or normometabolism) with different tumor types, tumor burdens and stage on resting energy expenditure

fat, lean body mass (as measured by total body potassium) and body water. Patients whom had lost weight had markedly low calorie and N intakes during the course of study. Heymsfield et al. [20] found that weight loss in cancer patients and in non-cancer patients with anorexia nervosa was accounted for by changes in both body fat and skeletal muscle. Cancer patients lost relatively less BW than the anorexics due to the presence of ascites, tumor volume and a lower proportional loss of visceral organ mass (heart, kidney, liver and spleen). Thus, BW changes may be misleading in some patients and may mask significant diminution in body fat and skeletal muscle [20].

Lundholm [21] reviewed studies indicating that protein-calorie malnutrition is common in those with advanced cancer; however, relative loss of adipose tissue, visceral protein and skeletal muscle varied considerably from patient to patient. MacFie and Burkinshaw [22] tested the hypothesis that patients with malignant disease may adapt differently to malnutrition than patients without cancer by utilizing neutron activation and anthropometric measurements to study 49 patients with GI cancer and 91 patients with non-malignant GI disease who had lost greater than 10% of pre-illness weight. Body composition and the tissue composition of weight loss was evaluated.

The loss of BW in both cancer and benign disease patients was primarily accounted for by loss of muscle mass and body fat. Non-muscle protein in each group was generally maintained and with progressive weight loss, a progressive loss of fat, muscle protein and water was observed. Because changes in body composition and tissue compartments were similar in cancer and non-cancer patients with similar degrees of weight loss, these authors concluded that cancer patients do not exhibit a unique adaptation to malnutrition as a function of the malignancy [22].

The Role of Cytokines in Cancer Cachexia

Endogenous cytokines such as tumor necrosis factor (TNF), IL-1, IL-6, and interferon-γ may play a role in cancer cachexia and alterations in substrate metabolism identified in these patients. Altered cytokine production in cancer may contribute to reduced spontaneous food intake, skeletal muscle wasting, body protein redistribution, altered liver protein synthesis and abnormalities in fat and carbohydrate metabolism; however, the possible effects of cytokines on these processes remain poorly defined [23–24]. For example, elevated levels of the various cytokines in plasma are rarely detected in cancer patients, and no one cytokine has been consistently implicated in cancer cachexia or specific metabolic abnormalities in cancer patients. On the other hand, some studies show a slight to modest increase in food intake and lean tissue retention in animals with administration of antibodies directed against specific cytokines [22–23]. The complex and overlapping effects of circulating and local tissue cytokines make study of specific nutritional effects difficult. Determination of the role of various cytokines in the nutritional complications of cancer requires further study.

Nutritional Complications associated with Chemotherapy

The administration of chemotherapeutic agents may have profound effects on the nutritional status of the host. Nutritional complications associated with chemotherapy are multifactorial in etiology and include alterations in nutrient intake, absorption and metabolism. It is important to consider effects of chemotherapy in the context of the preexisting alterations in nutritional status and substrate/energy metabolism due to the tumor-bearing state itself, as outlined above.

Although several studies on nutritional complications of chemotherapy have been performed to date, the type of chemotherapeutic drugs used, their doses and the timing of administration for various tumor types are consistently revised as studies proceed. Thus, although the studies reviewed in this section are applicable to current patients receiving chemotherapy, additional studies in this area are warranted.

Altered Food Intake during Chemotherapy

Nearly all drugs used for the therapy of cancer are associated with anorexia, which represents a major factor limiting dietary intake during chemotherapy [25–29]. Anorexia may, in part, have a psychological basis (e.g. due to depression or to learned food aversions in anticipation of nausea and emesis [28]), but may also be secondary to direct effects of chemotherapeutic agents on brain centers which influence the sensation of hunger. Nausea and vomiting are extremely common with certain types of chemotherapeutic agents, particularly nitrogen mustards, cis-platinum, imidiazole carboxamide, streptozotocin, adriamycin and cyclosphosphamide [26–27]. Of these agents, nausea and vomiting is severe but not usually prolonged with nitrogen mustards, and may be lessened by administration of longer drug infusions. These symptoms may still persist for several days with the use of cis-platinum. Nausea and vomiting are generally more severe when drug combinations are given, in particular adriamycin and cyclophosphamide [25–27]. Adriamycin and 5-fluorouracil are reported to induce vomiting in 50 to 65% of cases, depending on drug dose and frequency of dosing [27]. These effects probably occur via direct effects on central nervous system centers such as the medullary reticular formation and the chemoreceptor trigger zone [26–27]. Some chemotherapeutic drugs cause a metallic taste or other abnormal tastes in the mouth which may reduce subsequent food intake [25–26].

Anorexia, nausea and vomiting is dependent to some degree on drug dose, the agents used, other associated symptoms (e.g. fever, pain) and the antiemetic protocol employed. The severity of these symptoms may influence when food is ingested and the type of food eaten. Recent aggressive use of parenteral anti-emetics has greatly diminished the incidence and severity of nausea and vomiting during chemotherapy.

Learned food aversions were tabulated before and for 6 months after the initial course of chemotherapy in a study of 76 patients with lung or breast cancer [28]. A pre-treatment reduction in appetite occurred in 40% of the total sample, and was higher in lung versus breast cancer patients (57 versus 19%). Twenty-four percent of the study group reported abnormalities in taste function prior to therapy, and pre-treatment food aversions were noted by approximately 30% of patients. New treatment-related food aversions involving all food groups were formed in 55% of the patients after initiating chemotherapy [28]. These aversions usually occurred shortly after the first chemotherapy course, were food specific (especially sweets, meat, caffeinated beverages, and high-fat foods) and of short duration (median duration less than one month). Food aversions decreased with successive rounds of chemotherapy, and no one drug out of the 21 different agents used was associated with specific food aversions. Although patients with emesis had a higher incidence of food aversions, 46% without emesis had at least one new aversion to a specific food during the study [28]. Another study examined diet intake in 32 patients with small cell lung cancer receiving cisplatin, vincristine and tenoposide at the initiation of chemotherapy and again after 1 and 3 months of therapy [29]. Enteral energy and protein intake decreased during the first 2 days of cyclical drug therapy, but returned to pretreatment levels by the third day. Of the patients who lost weight, dietary intake was lower during chemotherapy versus pre- and post-treatment intake values in weight-stable patients [29].

Mucosal Abnormalities

Ulceration of the oral, esophageal and gastric mucosa is common with administration of certain chemotherapeutic agents because of the rapid turnover and chemosensitivity of cells of the GI mucosa [25–27]. Mucosal ulcerations and inflammation may present as mucositis, stomatitis, cheilosis, glossitis and esophagitis, and interfere with nutrient ingestion due to local discomfort and pain with ingestion of certain foods, especially solids. The drugs most commonly associated with mucosal ulceration and inflammation include methotrexate, 5-fluorouracil, bleomycin, adriamycin, vinblastine and actinomycin D [25–27]. The mucositis produced by methotrexate, actinomycin D and adriamycin is enhanced when combined with concurrent radiation treatment. In addition, chemotherapeutic agents, particularly methotrexate and 5-fluorouracil, may have more generalized effects on the intestinal mucosa leading to diarrhea, mucosal ulceration and mucosal hemorrhage in both the small and large bowel; these effects may lead to secondary malabsorption in severe cases.

Daenen et al. [30] studied intestinal permeability to lactulose and mannitol, and intestinal protein leakage (gut clearance of α-1-antitrypsin) in 37 patients with acute leukemia receiving vincristine, doxorubicin, and prednisone, cytarabine and daunorubicin, or cytarabine and amsacrine [30]. The patients were studied 10–12 days after aggressive induction chemotherapy. Although mucosal damage as measured by these tests was variable from patient to patient, 81% demonstrated abnormalities in one or both tests. Gut protein leakage was abnormally increased in 74%, and gut permeability to the poorly absorbable, non-metabolizable sugar lactulose was abnormally high in 44% of patients. Results were normal when the tests were repeated after hematologic recovery. Thus, these chemotherapy protocols appeared to increase protein loss from the gut and increase paracellular permeability in the small intestine. These effects may contribute to protein malnutrition as well as increased movement to bacteria and endotoxin across damaged gut mucosa.

In most cases, the mucosal abnormalities after chemotherapy are short-lived (lasting days to weeks) as the mucosa has a rapid renewal rate in individuals able to take enteral nutrition. However, if enteral intake is limited, the mucosa may continue to atrophy and healing will be delayed following chemotherapy.

Additional GI toxicities reported with chemotherapeutic agents include adynamic ileus associated with vinblastine; ileus, constipation and abdominal pain associated with vincristine; hepatocellular damage with mithramycin; glutamine depletion, hepatic dysfunction and pancreatitis with asparaginase, and cirrhosis with methotrexate administration [25–27]. Chemotherapy and cancer are also associated with an increased incidence of secondary infections; when these effect the GI tract (e.g. oral or esophageal candidiasis), odynophagia and dysphagia may contribute to diminished food intake.

Protein Metabolism and Nitrogen Balance

Most studies on the effects of chemotherapy and protein metabolism demonstrate that commonly used agents induce negative N balance and net body protein catabolism during and shortly after therapy [31–35]. This protein catabolism is of particular concern because loss of lean tissue is associated with poorer outcomes in cancer patients [1–2].

The effects on body protein are not solely due to insufficient nutrient intake, because protein loss occurs even in the face of adequate intake provided parenterally [31–35]. Thus, Herrmann [31] studied protein metabolism in 7 adult males with metastatic testicular cancer receiving combination chemotherapy with vinblastine, cis-platinum and bleomycin with adequate calorie and N intake provided via TPN during chemotherapy. Labelled glycine tracer was infused to measure the rates of protein synthesis, catabolism and turnover on days 5 to 7 after the initiation of chemotherapy. Negative N balance occurred during chemotherapy ($\approx$2 g/d), and was associated with a 23% decrease in whole body protein turnover, a 34% decrease in protein synthesis, and a 30% decrease in protein catabolism. The impaired protein synthesis observed in these patients may have inhibited protein-anabolic effects of IV nutrition, and may be due, in part, to the ability of these agents to inhibit DNA synthesis.

In another report, nutrient intake and N metabolism was studied during chemotherapy in 7 patients with leukemia (receiving cytarabin, daunorubicin and vincristine) and 6 patients with a variety of solid tumors and receiving other chemotherapeutic protocols [32]. The patients were normally nourished prior to therapy; however, the tumor patients as a group demonstrated reduced N and energy intakes, N balance, urinary N and fecal N versus matched control individuals. Of interest, these differences were largely accounted for by patients with weight loss during chemotherapy; data on those who maintained BW (n = 7) were similar to the controls. The decrease in the creatinine-height index in weight-losing patients suggested that losses in muscle mass occurred in this group.

The protocols employed in bone marrow transplantation (BMT) regimens have been shown to cause massive net losses of body protein, even when presumably adequate nutrients were provided by the parenteral route to replace diminished enteral intake [33–35]. These protocols often employ large doses of chemotherapy combined with total body irradiation. Cheney et al. [33) studied body composition in patients with acute lymphocytic leukemia receiving allogeneic BMT after conditioning therapy with cyclophosphamide, methotrexate and total body irradiation. TPN was begun 5–6 days prior to transplantation (during the chemotherapy regimen) at a dose to provide 160% of estimated basal energy needs/day and 1.5 g/kg/day protein. Body composition analysis was performed using N balance methods, tracer dilution techniques, and anthropometry at weeks 1 and 4 after BMT. These studies demonstrated negative N throughout the post-BMT period, an expansion of the extracellular fluid compartment, a contraction of the intracellular fluid compartment, a significant loss of body cell mass, and no significant change in body fat. In a study in similar patients receiving adequate calories and protein with a BCAA enriched TPN solution or a standard TPN solution after BMT, variable (−2 to −18 g/day) but markedly negative N balance occurred in both TPN groups during the entire 4 weeks of observation [34]. Increased urinary excretion of 3-methylhistidine, a marker of myofibrullar protein breakdown, was also noted in each diet group.

In a recent randomized, double-blind controlled trial of 45 patients with hematologic malignancies receiving allogeneic BMT, Ziegler et al. [35] documented negative N balance (averaging ≈ −4 g/d) during day 4 to 11 after BMT and high dose cytosine arabinosidem cyclophosphamide and total body irradiation, despite aggressive TPN providing a standard dose of ≈35 kcal/kg/day and 1.5 g protein/kg/day [35]. Use of an isonitrogenous, isocaloric TPN solution supplemented with the amino acid glutamine significantly diminished the degree of N loss (to −1.4 g nitrogen/day) and the 3-methylhistidine excretion in these patients, in association with an increase in blood glutamine levels of 40%. Importantly, the alterations in protein metabolism with glutamine supplementation were associated with a significant reduction in the rate of microbial colonization, the incidence of clinical infection and the length of hospital stay (from 36 days in the controls to 29 days in the glutamine-supplemented group). In a study of a subgroup of these patients, those randomized to standard glutamine-free TPN demonstrated a 20% expansion of the extracellular fluid space during the period from the BMT until hospital discharge; this fluid expansion was significantly attenuated in the glutamine group [36]. The observed increase in extracellular water noted in BMT patients receiving standard TPN (without the addition of glutamine) is classically accompanied by a decrease in the intracellular fluid volume as erosion of lean body mass occurs.

Effect of Chemotherapy on Energy and Non-Protein Substrate Metabolism

The effect of chemotherapy on EE and fat and carbohydrate metabolism have not been extensively studied. Delarue et al. [37] studied REE in patients with non-Hodgkin's lymphoma receiving three 5-day courses of high-dose adriamycin, cyclophosphamide, vindesine and bleomycin. REE was measured prior to chemotherapy and again on days 2, 3 and 5 of each drug course. After the first course of chemotherapy, a significant decrease in REE occurred on days 3 and 5; during course 2, REE remained stable during the 5-day measurement period (but was lower than the first course), while in course 3, REE increased significantly from baseline on days 2, 3 and 5. These authors concluded that reduced REE during course 1 and the lower values in course 2 relative to course 1 were related to reduced tumor volume following chemotherapy. During course 3, as the reduction in tumor mass is diminished, the differential increase in REE is due to the effects of chemotherapy.

Tayek and Chlebowski [38] studied the metabolic response to 5-fluorouracil chemotherapy in patients with colon cancer. Prior to chemotherapy, plasma growth hormone levels were significantly increased and fasting hepatic glucose production and leucine appearance rates were slightly, but not significantly increased versus control values. With 5 days of continuous 5-fluorouracil infusion, the patients demonstrated a significant elevation in fasting glucose levels and hepatic glucose production associated with insulin resistance. The rate of leucine oxidation was significantly increased and leucine incorporation into protein was significantly reduced during chemotherapy.

Changes in lipid and lipoprotein metabolism with chemotherapy have been little studied. In one study, total cholesterol and low density lipoprotein values increased after chemotherapy in patients with small cell lung cancer who responded to anti-neoplastic treatment. In contrast, breast cancer patients who responded did not demonstrate changes in serum lipid levels, with the exception of serum triglycerides, which rose significantly with successful chemotherapy [39]. In another study, patients with head and neck or GI cancer requiring operations and those with solid tumors (with or without metastatic disease) requiring chemotherapy did not demonstrate alterations in stearic, linoleic, linolenic or arachadonic acid levels versus control values [40].

Alterations in Micronutrients

A few studies have determined changes in circulating vitamin levels with chemotherapy [41–44]. Administration of 5-fluorouracil was associated with lowered levels of thiamin [41], while combined cytostatic therapy was associated with reduced blood folate levels in patients with malignant lymphoma [42]. In another study, patients with cancer of the colon and stomach received combined therapy with cytoxan, oncovin, methotrexate and 5-fluorouracil during a 5-day treatment period which was repeated at 4 week intervals for 1 year [43]. Levels of thiamine, pyridoxine and riboflavin decreased significantly over time with chemotherapy. Other authors have suggested that thiamine and folate deficiency are associated with other forms of chemotherapeutic agents [44].

Studies of amino acid levels after chemotherapy in humans are also limited. In one study, cancer patients with hepatic metastases received chemotherapy and enteral or parenteral nutrition support as tolerated [40]. Abnormally low levels of leucine, threonine, serine, proline and glycine were observed during chemotherapy. Most amino acid levels returned to normal with nutritional support, especially with parenteral feeding; however, leucine levels remained depressed throughout chemotherapy despite nutritional support. In a study of BMT patients receiving TPN after high-dose chemotherapy and irradiation, no abnormally low amino acid levels were observed as amino acid levels generally reflected the composition of the infused amino acid solution [35].

The nutritional complications associated with administration of chemotherapeutic agents are summarized in Table 3.

Table 3. Nutrition-related complications associated with administration of cancer chemotherapy[a]

Diminished food intake
Anorexia
Nausea and emesis
Alteration in taste and learned food aversions
Mucositis, stomatitis, glossitis, esophagitis
Oral and esophageal candidiasis
Adynamic ileus, abdominal pain
Decreased nutrient absorption
Enteritis, colitis, mucosal ulceration, diarrhea
Diminished rates of mucosal regeneration
Diminished levels of absorptive enzymes
Protein-losing enteropathy
Altered protein metabolism
Decreased protein synthetic rates
Increased myofibrillar protein breakdown
Increased leucine oxidation and reduced incorporation into protein
Reduced amino acid levels in plasma
Net body protein catabolism and negative nitrogen balance
Altered energy and substrate metabolism
Increased energy expenditure
Increased hepatic glucose production and insulin resistance
Variable changes in circulating lipids and lipoproteins
Vitamin deficiency
Lowered levels of thiamine, folate, riboflavin in plasma

[a] The effects of different agents on the above parameters are highly variable in individual patients, due to factors such as underlying illnesses and nutritional status, tumor type, stage of disease, specific agent(s) used and the dosage and timing of chemotheraphy administration.

Nutritional Complications associated with Irradiation Therapy

Therapeutic irradiation therapy is associated with acute and chronic effects which may significantly impact nutritional status. In a study by Decosse et al. [45] published in 1969, over 20% of patients with irradiation-induced enterocolitis died from complications related to radiation therapy, even though the primary tumor was thought to be controlled.

Gastrointestinal Complications

As in chemotherapy dosing, toxicity associated with irradiation therapy is a major factor determining the dose of radiation utilized. The toxicity of irradiation commonly involves the GI tract; mucosal injury is the most common complication of radiation therapy which affects nutrition.

As reviewed by Donaldson, about 60% of cancer patients require some form of radiation treatment; the GI complications of radiotherapy are largely a function of the area of the body irradiated, the doses employed and the site of the tumor, as well as the performance status of the patient and the use of chemotherapy [26, 47]. Thus, in patients with CNS tumors, decreased oral intake may occur initially as a complication of the tumor itself (causing altered mentation, nausea and vomiting); cranial radiation may worsen these symptoms [26, 47]. In patients with head and neck tumors, mucositis is common after radiation, and associated xerostomia and dysphagia decrease oral food intake. Progressive ulceration and bleeding may also occur and these individuals frequently report loss of taste sensation and smell [47]. Irradiation which involves the salivary glands may lead to thickened saliva and secondary dysphagia.

In a study of 122 adults with squamous cell carcinoma of the oral cavity and oropharynx undergoing curative radiation, 93% lost weight during the 6–8 week course of therapy, and 9% of patients lost more than 10% BW [47]. Organs in the thorax, such as the lung, esophagus or mediastinum may be irritated by radiation therapy and give rise to dysphagia; these symptoms may last for several weeks after therapy. Chronic esophageal stenosis, ulceration and even perforation may occur several weeks after completion of treatment to this area, but usually only after prolonged radiation therapy associated with severe mucosal inflammation.

The gastric mucosa is relatively resistant to radiation-induced injury; however, mucosal alterations of the small and large bowel are relatively common. The intestinal mucosa exhibits shortening of villi, reduced mitosis after irradiation, and abnormal rates of mucosal regeneration. Recovery of the epithelium often takes weeks after the inital insult, especially in patients with diabetes, vascular disease and hypertension [26, 47]. Patients receiving radiation to the small bowel and/or colon commonly exhibit nausea, emesis and diarrhea; malabsorption of glucose, fat and protein as well as micronutrients may occur in association with reduced functional surface area and absorptive enzyme deficiencies [26, 47]. The potential for nutritional complications of abdominal radiation is illustrated in a study of patients with non-Hodgkin's lymphoma; 88% suffered weight loss in the 6-week treatment period, including 13% who lost more than 10% of pre-treatment weight [26].

Nutrition-related complications were evaluated in a study of 74 head and neck cancer patients treated with curative doses of radiation for 6 weeks [47]. Subjective assessment of the patients over time revealed that ≈25% experienced oral complications including loss of taste, dry mouth, swallowing difficulties and anorexia prior to therapy. By the fourth week of irradiation, 80% complained of dry mouth and the percentage of the diet taken as liquids increased significantly [47]. The percentage of those reporting changes in taste increased sixfold (especially for meats, fruits, vegetable and sweets), anorexia increased 3-fold, and patients with swallowing difficulties increased by 40% [47].

The size of the radiation field has a major impact on the ultimate weight loss due to diminished food intake. In patients with larynx cancer, only 19% of patients lost weight (mean = 1.5 kg) when the therapeutic field was 7 by 7 cm or less, while 67% lost weight (mean loss = 5.3 kg) when the radiation field was larger [48].

Another study evaluated the clinical presentation, operative findings and outcome in 40 patients requiring surgery for bowel complications after radiation therapy for cervical and bladder carcinoma [49]. The most common complication was radiation-induced bowel ischemia (n=20) which occurred between 3 and 18 months after radiotherapy and required operation; 12 of these patients had chronic perforation, 6 had rectal bleeding and 2 anorectal ulcerations. Late complications were noted in 15 patients presenting between 2 and 24 years after therapy, most often with partial bowel obstruction due to fibrous strictures [49]. Other studies suggest that similar late radiation effects (obstruction, enteritis, colitis or fistula) occur in 0.5–15% of patients [27]. In a retrospective review of 57 patients requiring hospitalization for intestinal injuries after radiotherapy (primarily for cervical, endometrial, rectal and bladder carcinoma), operations were required in 33 (58%) [50]. Twenty seven of the patients (47%) had multiple intestinal complications. Reasons for operation in the study group included bowel resection (32%), colostomy alone or lysis of adhesions (9% each), as well as a number of miscellaneous causes [50]. Five anastomotic leaks and 6 postoperative deaths occurred, and a number of postoperative complications such as fistula, short-bowel syndrome and wound disruption were noted [50]. Thus, patients who receive abdominal radiation are a high-risk group for subsequent operative complications which may further worsen their nutritional status due to GI tract dysfunction, infection and other sequelae.

Silvain [51] reviewed the outcomes of 31 patients with severe radiation enteritis requiring TPN due to intestinal dysfunction. Prior to TPN initiation, 13 of these patients had required either intestinal resection or bypass. Median follow-up in this study was 2.5 years (range 1 month to 12 years) from the time of TPN initiation. Oral feeding was able to be resumed in only 36% of these patients. A total of 18 patients died, 13 from complications associated with radiation enteritis. Survival probability was 58% at one year and 36% at five years and was related to patient age, the presence of vascular disease and occurrence of enteric fistula or perforation [51].

Limited data are available in humans on malabsorption induced by radiation, although this complication is observed clinically. Absorption of glucose and fat was diminished after large doses of abdominal radiation in rats [52]. In another animal study, rats receiving a single dose of abdominal radiation (6 Gy) demonstrated diminished jejunal active transport of D-glucose and maximal water uptake at 3 days with a return to normal by 7 days; L-leucine uptake was abnormally low and mucosal permeability to poorly absorbed solutes was elevated for more than 7 days after injury [53]. In a study of patients receiving combined chemotherapy and irradiation for unresectable pancreatic cancer, fat absorption worsened after therapy; however D-xylose absorption (a measure of upper small intestinal carbohydrate absorption) was unaltered after therapy [54]. Of interest, a group of 11 patients with debilitating diarrhea after radiation demonstrated elevated (2-6-fold) stool bile acid levels, which responded promptly to therapy with oral cholestyramine [55].

Little information is available on possible direct protein-catabolic effects of irradiation on human skeletal muscle or whether radiation may cause other metabolic abnormalities related to nutrition, other than those related to GI toxicity. Complications associated with irradiation therapy relevant to nutrition are listed in Table 4.

Effects of Combined Chemotherapy and Radiation Therapy

Multimodality therapy is increasingly being utilized in cancer treatment. It is to be expected that the more intensive therapeutic protocols are associated with greater risks for nutritional complications. It is known, for example, that radiation esophagitis is enhanced when agents such as actinomycin, vinblastine, and hydroxyurea are given concurrently. Toxicity of the intestinal mucosa with radiation is more common and severe when actinomycin-D, adriamycin or 5-fluorouracil are given [26]. The toxic effects of radiation and chemotherapy on the GI tract may be additive or synergistic depending on the agents and dosages utilized [26, 46].

As noted above, protocols commonly used in bone marrow transplantation incorporating high-dose chemotherapy and radiation commonly result in massive losses of body protein, even when presumably adequate parenteral nutrition is provided [33–35]. This protein loss is associated with skeletal muscle weakness, an increased rate of infection and delayed convalescence.

In a study of 44 children receiving aggressive abdominal radiation and/or chemotherapy, severe weight loss was observed only in patients receiving the combined therapy, and 69% of these received actinomycin-D [26]. Further study on nutritional complications associated with many of the newer therapeutic modalities being utilized in cancer patients is clearly needed.

Table 4. Nutrition-related complications associated with administration of radiation therapy[a]

Region irradiated	Acute	Chronic
Head and neck	Mucositis Dysphagia Anorexia Altered taste Thickened saliva	Mucosal Ulceration Xerostomia Trismus
Thorax	Dysphagia Inflammation	Pharyngeal and esophageal ulceration, esophageal stenosis and perforation
Abdomen and pelvis	Anorexia Nausea Vomiting Pain Mucosal hemorrhage Diarrhea Enteritis, colitis Reduced mucosal regeneration Malabsorption	Mucosal ulceration Diarrhea Malabsorption Enteritis, colitis Stricture, obstruction Fistula Chronic perforation Poor wound healing

[a] Complications risks are variable in individual patients and dependent on factors such as underlying illnesses and nutritional status, radiation dosage, location and size of radiation field, timing of administration, tumor type and tumor bulk.

Conclusion

Protein-energy malnutrition is not uncommon in cancer patients and is associated with poor clinical outcomes. A number of metabolic abnormalities in carbohydrate, fat and protein metabolism have been identified in cancer patients, which favor protein and energy wasting. The hormonal, cytokine and molecular mechanisms for these are poorly understood.

Both chemotherapy and irradiation therapy have profound effects on the nutritional status of patients with cancer and may contribute to malnutrition in cancer patients. The systemic nutritional effects of these therapies depend on patient characteristics including age and associated illnesses, as well nutrient intake, digestion, absorption and nutrient utilization are influenced by the dose used, the site and size of the tumor, the frequency of drug and/or radiation administration, and the nature of the underlying metabolic abnormalities in energy and substrate utilization associated with the tumor itself. Additionally, psychological factors undoubtedly play a major role in food intake in these patients. Thus, nutritional complications associated with chemotherapy and irradiation are common and are usually multifactorial. These need to be considered when planning nutritional support strategies for individuals with cancer.

References

1. Nixon DW, Heymsfield SB, Cohen AE, et al (1980) Protein-calorie undernutrition in hospitalized cancer patients. Am J Med 68:683–690
2. Dewys WD, Begg C, Lavin PT, et al (1980) Prognostic effect of weight loss prior to chemotherapy in cancer patients. Am J Med 69:491–497
3. Bozzetti F, Migliavacca S, Scotti A, et al (1982) Impact of cancer, type, site, stage and treatment on the nutritional status of patients. Ann Surg 196:170–179
4. Linn BS, Robinson DS, Klimas NG (1988) Effects of age and nutritional status on sugical outcomes in head and neck cancer. Ann Surg 207:267–273
5. Heber D, Byerly LO, Chlebowski RT (1985) Metabolic abnormalities in the cancer patient. Cancer 55:225–229
6. Chlebowski RT, Heber D (1986) Metabolic abnormalities in cancer patients: Carbohydrate metabolism. Surg Clin N Am 66:957–967
7. Heber D, Byerly LO, Tchekmedyian NS (1992) Hormonal and metabolic abnormalities in the malnourished cancer patient: Effect on host-tumor interaction. JPEN 16 (Suppl):60S–64S
8. Holroyde CP, Reichard GA (1986) General metabolic abnormalities in cancer patients. Anorexia and cachexia. Surg Clin N Am 66:947–955
9. Kern KA, Norton JA (1988) Cancer cachexia. JPEN 12:286–298
10. Shaw JHF, Wolfe RR (1988) Whole-body protein kinetics in patients with early and advanced gastrointestinal cancer: The response to glucose infusion and total parenteral nutrition. Surgery 103:148–155
11. Kurzer M, Mequid MM (1986) Cancer and protein metabolism. Surg Clin N Am 66:969–1001
12. Norton JA, Gorschboth CM, Wesley RA, Burt ME, Brennen MF (1985) Fasting plasma amino acid levels in cancer patients. Cancer 56:1181–1186
13. McAndrew PF (1986) Fat metabolism and cancer. Surg Clin N Am 66:1003–1011
14. Legaspi A, Jeevanandam M, Starnes HF, Brennan MF (1987) Whole body lipid and energy metabolism in the cancer patient. Metabolism 36:958–963
15. Arbeit JM, Lees DE, Corsey R, Brennen MF (1984) Resting energy expenditure in controls and cancer patients with localized and diffuse disease. Ann Surg 199:292–298
16. Hansell DT, Davies JWL, Burns HJG (1986) The relationship between resting energy expenditure and weight loss in benign and malignant disease. Ann Surg 203:240–245
17. Dempsey DT, Knox LS, Mullen JL, Miller C, Feurer ID, Buzby GP (1986) Energy expenditure in malnourished patients with colorectal cancer. Arch Surg 121:789–795
18. Nixon DW, Kutner M, Heymsfield S, et al (1988) Resting energy expenditure in lung and colon cancer. Metabolism 37:1059–1064
19. Cohn SH, Gartenhaus W, Vartsky D, et al (1981) Body composition and dietary intake in neoplastic disease. Am J Clin Nutr 34:1997–2004
20. Heymsfield SB, McManus CB (1985) Tissue components of weight loss in cancer patients. Cancer 55:238–249
21. Lundholm KG (1986) Body compositional changes in cancer patients. Surg Clin N Am 66:1013–1023
22. MacFie J, Burkinshaw L (1987) Body composition in malignant disease. Metabolism 36:290–294
23. Moldawer LL, Rogy MA, Lowry SF (1992) The role of cytokines in cancer cachexia. JPEN 16 (Suppl):42S–49S
24. McNamara MJ, Alexander HR, Norton JA (1992) Cytokines and their role in the pathophysiology of cancer cachexia. JPEN 16 (Suppl):50S–55S
25. Costa G, Donaldson SS (1979) Effects of cancer and cancer treatment on the nutrition of the host. N Engl J Med 300:1471–1474
26. Donaldson SS, Lenon RA (1979) Alterations of nutritional status: Impact of chemotherapy and radiation therapy. Cancer 43:2036–2052

27. Kokal WA (1985) The impact of antitumor therapy of nutrition. Cancer 55:273–278
28. Mattes RD, Arnold C, Boraas M (1987) Learned food aversions among cancer chemotherapy patients: Incidence, nature and clinical implications. Cancer 60:2576–2580
29. Ovesen L, Hannibal J, Allingstrup L (1992) Dietary intake in patients with small cell lung cancer: The effect of aggressive chemotherapy. Eur J Clin Nutr 46:535–537
30. Daenen S, Muskiet FAJ, Marrink J, Halie MR (1991) Aggressive chemotherapy for acute leukemia frequently causes intestinal protein leakage. Eur J Cancer 27:552–556
31. Herrmann VM, Garnick MB, Moore FD, Wilmore DW (1981) Effect of cytotoxic agents on protein kinetics in patients with metastatic cancer. Surgery 90:381–387
32. Ollenschlaeger G, Konkol K, Wickrammanayake PD, Schrappe-Baecher M, Mueller JM (1989) Nutrient intake and nitrogen metabolism in cancer patients during oncological chemotherapy. Am J Clin Nutr 50:454–459
33. Cheney CL, Abson KG, Aker SN, et al (1987) Body composition changes in marrow transplant recipients receiving total parenteral nutrition. Cancer 59:1515–1519
34. Lenssen P, Cheney CL, Aker SN, et al (1987) Intravenous branched chain amino acid trial in marrow transplant recipients. JPEN 11:112–118
35. Ziegler TR, Young LS, Benfell K, et al (1992) Clinical and metabolic efficacy of glutamine-supplemented parenteral nutrition after bone marrow transplantation: A randomized, double-blind, controlled study. Ann Int Med 116:821–828
36. Scheltinga MR, Young LS, Benfell K, et al (1991) Glutamine-enriched intravenous feedings attenuate extracellular fluid expansion after a standard stress. Ann Surg 214:385–395
37. Delarue J, Lerebours E, Tilly H, et al (1990) Effect of chemotherapy on resting energy expenditure in patients with non-Hodgkin's lymphoma. Cancer 65:2455–2459
38. Tayek JA, Chlebowski RT (1992) The metabolic response to chemotherapy in colon cancer patients. JPEN 16 (Suppl):65S–71S
39. Alexopoulos CG, Poournaras S, Vaslamatzis M, Avgerinos A, Raptis S (1992) Changes in serum lipids and lipoproteins in cancer patients during chemotherapy. Cancer Chemother Pharmacol 30:412–416
40. Ching N, Grossi C, Jham G, et al (1984) Plasma amino acid and serum unesterified fatty acid deficits and the effect of nutritional support in chemotherapy treatment. Surgery 95:730–737
41. Dickerson JWT, Basu TK (1977) Specific vitamin deficiencies and their significance in patients with cancer and receiving chemotherapy. In: Winick M (ed) Nutrition and Cancer, John Wiley and Sons, New York, pp 95–104
42. Schreurs WHP, Odink J, Egger RJ, Wedel M, Bruning PF (1985) The influence of radiotherapy and chemotherapy on the vitamin status of cancer patients. Internat J Vit Nutr Res 55:425–432
43. Henquin N, Havivi E, Reshef A, Barak F, Horn Y (1989) Nutritional monitoring and counselling for cancer patients during chemotherapy. Oncology 46:173–177
44. Dreizen S, McCredie KB, Keating MJ, Andersson BS (1990) Nutritional deficiencies in patients receiving cancer chemotherapy. Postgrad Med 87:167–170
45. Decosse JJ, Rhodes RD, Wentz WB, et al (1969) The natural history and management of radiation-induced injury of the gastrointestinal tract. Ann Surg 170:369–376
46. Donaldson SS (1984) Nutritional support as an adjunct to radiation therapy. JPEN 8:302–310
47. Chencharick JD, Mossman KL (1983) Nutritional consequences of the radiotherapy of head and neck cancer. Cancer 51:811–815
48. Pezner R, Archambeau JO (1985) Critical evaluation of the role of nutritional support for radiation therapy patients. Cancer 55:263–267
49. Schofield PF, Holden D, Carr ND (1983) Bowel disease after radiotherapy. J R Soc Med 76:463–466
50. Deitel M, To TB (1987) Major intestinal complications of radiotherapy. Arch Surg 122:1421–1424
51. Silvain C, Besson I, Ingrand P, et al (1992) Long-term outcome of severe radiation enteritis treated by total parenteral nutrition. Dig Dis Sci 37:1065–1071

52. Thomson ABR, Cheeseman CI, Walker K (1986) Late effects of abdominal radiation on intestinal uptake of nutrients. Rad Res 107:344–353
53. Baer AR, Cheeseman CI, Thomson ABR (1987) The assessment of recovery of the intestine after acute radiation injury. Rad Res 109:319–329
54. Barkin JS, Kalser MH, Thomsen S, Redlhammer D (1982) Defect in assimilation following combined radiation and chemotherapy in patients with locally unresectable pancreatic carcinoma. Cancer 50:2189–2192
55. Arlow FL, Dekovich AA, Priest RJ, Beher WT (1987) Bile acids in radiation-induced diarrhea. South Med J 80:1259–1261

Nutrition in Sepsis

F. B. Cerra

Introduction

The term "sepsis" has many meanings in the intensive care unit (ICU). It has been applied to ICU patients with and without demonstrable infection who manifest a constellation of signs, symptoms and laboratory data that generally characterize the patients as "sick". A multitude of other labels have been applied such as sepsis syndrome, hypermetabolism and the hyperdynamic state. Because of the confusion surrounding this terminology, a consensus conference and standardized definitions were developed [1]. For clarity in this presentation, these definitions will be used. Thus, the systemic inflammatory response will describe those ICU patients with alterations in temperature and white blood count who are also manifesting a hyperdynamic, hypermetabolic state. Sepsis will refer to patients with the same characteristics who also have a demonstrated source of infection.

This discussion will focus on those ICU patients who have had an injury and are manifesting the systemic inflammatory response with or without sepsis and who are at risk for developing multiple organ dysfunction and the progressive multiple organ failure syndrome (MOF). Fig. 1 summarizes these patterns of post-injury response [2]. The injuries identified as being associated with this response include hypovolemic shock, septic shock, polytrauma (soft tissue injury, fractures, burns), and such diseases as pancreatitis [3]. The injury is associated with an interval of reduced microcirculatory perfusion followed by resuscitation. Some patients expire in shock and some shortly following resuscitation. These groups are not the patients under discussion in this chapter. The shock-resuscitation is frequently associated with clinically relevant single organ failures such as lung and kidney. With a single uncomplicated injury, most patients rapidly recover. This group of patients is also not the subject of this discussion. The remaining patients, approximately 20% of surgical ICU admissions, persist in the systemic inflammatory response and are at risk for developing secondary organ dysfunction (liver, kidney) and progressive organ failure and death. After 3 to 4 days, this group of patients cannot be statistically subdivided on the basis of clinical parameters, physiologic responses, metabolic responses, or type of infecting organism. It is this group of patients on which this chapter will focus.

The mainstay in management in this setting remains source control, effective microcirculatory resuscitation, and the use of nutrients to support meta-

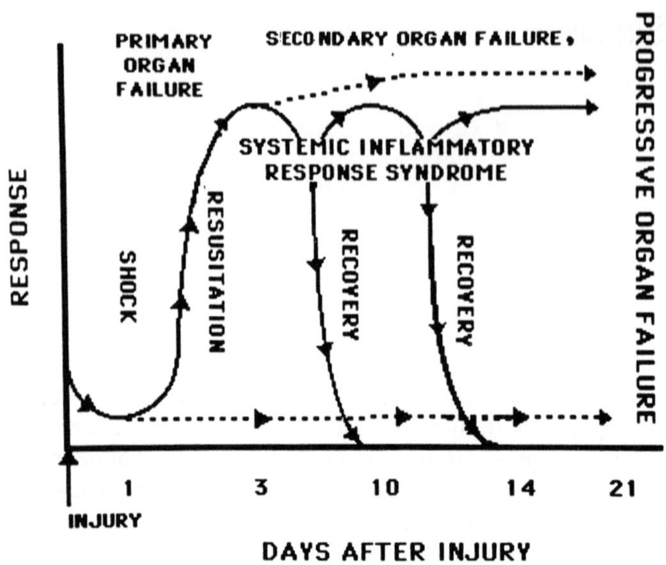

Fig. 1. The figure depicts the patterns of clinical response after an injury is sustained. Four phases of response occur in the patients: shock, resuscitation, systemic inflammatory response, and organ dysfunction and failure. The effects of nutrition/metabolic support are discussed in this context

bolism. This latter modality, that of nutrition/metabolic support, will be the topic of discussion. Three classes of outcomes have been studied in this setting: those relating to the effects of the therapy on body composition and protein metabolism such as levels of visceral proteins, nitrogen (N) balance, and energy expenditure (EE), those related to effects on disease processes such as acute lung injury or the metabolic response to injury, and those related to relevant patient outcomes such as mortality, morbidity, length of stay, and resource utilization. This discussion will utilize these classes of outcomes in evaluating the nutrition/metabolic support of the systemic inflammatory response and sepsis.

Within this framework, 4 major questions require discussion:

1. Is the use of nutrition/metabolic support associated with improved outcomes?
2. Is enteral nutrition more efficacious than total parenteral nutrition?
3. Is enteral nutrition early postinjury more efficacious than late postinjury?
4. Is the type of nutritional formulation important?

Is the Use of Nutrition/Metabolic Support associated with Improved Outcomes?

To answer this question, a non-nutrition control group is required. No such studies are to be found in the literature. In the studies available, glucose solutions were used in the control group, creating a setting of semistarvation. Two studies that evaluate patient outcomes are available.

The first study was a multicenter, randomized prospective clinical trial of nutrition support in ICU patients with liver failure [4]. The control patients received glucose and neomycin; the experimental group received glucose and amino acids at a dose of 1–1.5 g/kg/day. The primary outcome variables were recovery from encephalopathy and 28-day mortality. The group that received glucose and amino acid support recovered faster and more completely from encephalopathy by clinical and electroencephalographic criteria, and had a significant reduction in 28-day mortality.

The second study was also a randomized, prospective clinical trial performed in 300 patients undergoing major general surgical procedures [5]. The control group received a fixed amount of glucose, 250–300 g/day. The experimental group received total parenteral nutrition (TPN) with non-protein calories as 70% glucose and 30% IV fat (20% Intralipid) provided at 120% of measured resting EE; and amino acids to replace measured N losses (approximately 1.5 g/kg/day). This intent to treat study did not provide therapy only to the group of patients under discussion, and did not discern an outcome benefit in the treatment arm. There is, however, an important observation in the control arm that does have relevance to this discussion.

Approximately 20% of the control group was still on IV glucose therapy 14 days postoperatively. At this point, there were significant alterations in body composition consistent with malnutrition and the patients were switched to TPN. This group required a much more ICU treatment such as ventilator days, oxygen support and antibiotics, and experienced a significant increase in such complications as wound failure, infections, and mortality.

One of the parameters of concordance in these two studies was the lack of nitrogen retention in the control groups, and a large cumulative net N loss over the disease course. Another was the significant net negative energy balance. In both studies, the TPN arms were not associated with an increase in TPN related complications, a phenomenon that has not been so in other studies attempting to evaluate the efficacy of TPN in similar settings. It would also appear that the prolonged use of just energy support as glucose is associated with marked alterations in body composition consistent with malnutrition and poorer patient outcomes that are clinically relevant.

Several clinical studies have evaluated the effect of nutrition therapy, primarily TPN, on the protein catabolism that is characteristic of the systemic inflammatory response [6–12]. Nutrition support is able to improve N retention. This effect, however, appears to occur by an improvement in protein synthetic rate and not by a substantial reduction in the absolute rate of catabolism. Thus, the net catabolism is reduced by an increase in synthetic rate.

The clinical correlate of these observations is the continued loss of lean body mass characteristic of a prolonged systemic inflammatory response [11].

Is the Enteral Route more Efficacious than the Parenteral One?

Only a few studies have evaluated patients with the systemic inflammatory response using patient outcomes as the focus of the studies. A second issue evaluated in these studies is the effect of the timing of the nutrition support relative to the injury event.

The series of studies most applicable to the present discussion were performed in patients who sustained abdominal trauma, either blunt or penetrating [13–15]. All three studies required an abdominal trauma index of 15 or greater on admission; and all were randomized, prospective studies with feeding started 12 to 24 h post-injury. The first study evaluated 98 trauma patients with the primary outcome being infectious complications over a 15-day study period [13]. The septic complications included pneumonia, abdominal abscess formation, line sepsis, empyema, fasciitis and wound dehiscence. The patients received 1.5–2.0 g/kg/day of protein or amino acids, and approximately 30 Kcal/kg/day of non-protein calories as glucose and fat. The major statistically significant results of the study are summarized in Table 1.

The second study evaluated 75 patients who had sustained abdominal trauma [14]. The primary outcome analysis was septic complications. Feedings were adjusted to achieve maximum nitrogen retention and consisted of 1.2–1.5 g/kg/day of amino acids, and approximately 30 Kcal/kg/day of non-protein calories mostly as glucose but with some fat. The investigators observed a substantial early improvement in visceral proteins and a reduction in infectious complications from 37 to 17% in the enterally fed group. They also observed a reduction in total septic morbidity from 20 (2 abdominal abscesses and 6 pneumonia's) to 3% (1 abdominal abscess) in the enterally fed group over the 10-day study interval.

The third study is a meta-analysis of 8 prospective, randomized clinical trials performed in different institutions where the same enteral and parenteral formulae were used in all studies and feedings were begun within 30 h

Table 1. Effect of route of nutrition on infectious complications

Parameter	Enteral (%)	Parenteral (%)
Pneumonia	11.8	31
Abdominal abscess	1.9	13.3
Line sepsis	1.7	13.3
Total infections/patient	0.25±0.06	1.6±0.8
Total infections/infected patient	1.08±0.08	1.6±0.8

There were no differences in nitrogen retention, days of nutrition, ventilator days, mortality, length of stay, number of and days on antibiotics.

of injury on the mean [15]. Four studies were performed exclusively in trauma patients with an abdominal trauma index of 15 or greater; and 4 studies were performed in trauma/general surgery patients. A total of 118 patients received enteral nutrition with 26 dropouts; and a total of 112 patients received TPN with 10 dropouts. Nutrition therapy failures were greater in the enteral than the TPN group. The occurrence of infectious complications was the primary outcome analyzed. The first analysis excluded all dropouts. The analysis resulted in a difference in infectious complications of 17% (18% enteral and 35% TPN). The second analysis included all patients (intent to treat) and confirmed the first analysis. There were no observed differences in mortality, length of stay and cost. This analysis also did not confirm the early improvement in visceral protein levels in the enteral nutrition group observed in the previous studies. There were also increases in the prevalence of abdominal distention and diarrhea in the enterally fed group (46 vs 24% for distention; 34 vs 9% for diarrhea).

The last pertinent study evaluated the patient outcome when either EN or TPN was begun after the systemic inflammatory response was established [16]. The study was performed in 66 general surgery ICU patients who were randomized to receive either EN or TPN starting approximately 4 days after ICU admission when the systemic inflammatory response was established. The nutrition support consisted of 1.5–2.0 g/kg/day of amino acids and, approximately 30 Kcal/kg/day of calories as glucose and fat. Nutrition intake was adjusted to achieve maximum N retention. There were no demonstrable effects of the route of nutrition administration on nutrition outcomes or on such patient outcomes as the incidence or organ failure or mortality.

Thus, there appears to be a window within which the enteral route can improve patient outcome in those patients in whom EN can be performed. This window appears to be the initiation of EN sometime between the injury event and the establishment of the systemic inflammatory response approximately 4 days after injury. The nutritional outcomes appear to be comparable between the 2 routes of administration irrespective of the time of initiation of nutrition support. The patient outcome where there was some demonstration of efficacy was a reduced incidence of infectious complications in the enterally fed group when the nutrition support was initiated within the first 1–2 days after injury. This reduction in infection rate appears to be for both line sepsis and for infections other than line sepsis. Statistical significance was not reached for other outcome parameters such as mortality, length of stay, and critical care services.

Is Enteral Nutrition early Postinjury more Efficacious?

To evaluate this question, the same enteral feeding needs to be used in each group; and the primary difference between groups should be in the time after injury that EN is initiated. Two studies are relevant, one in patients sustaining burn injury and the other in patients sustaining polytrauma [17, 18].

In the burn study, 10 patients received very early EN within 4.4±0.5 h of injury, and 10 patients had initiation of EN late after injury, 57.5±2.6 h [17]. The patients were a matched cohort with respect to age, sex ratio, burn size, and survival probability. The enteral formula consisted of blenderized food and was administered in an amount to meet estimated energy requirements. The early enteral group achieved more rapid and more effective N retention, achieving positive balance in 8.8±4.1 vs 24.1±6.9 days. There were no differences demonstrable in the visceral protein concentrations. The very early EN patients also were observed to have less urinary catecholamine excretion and plasma glucagon concentrations during the first 2 weeks of the study; there were no differences observed in the plasma cortisol concentrations.

The second study was a double-blinded, randomized, prospective clinical trial in patients who had sustained blunt trauma [18]. Following resuscitation and control of bleeding, 49 patients were randomized to receive early feeds (target 24 h) or late feeds (72 h) [18]. Feeds were given via nasoduodenal feeding tube with a rapid advance technique to achieve full volume within 24–36 h. The same enteral feeding was used in all patients (Riabilan HN, O'Brian Pharmaceuticals). At least 7 days of therapy had to be given to be considered a completer for the study. 39 patients completed the study, 20 early and 19 late feeds. Outcome variables for the study included catecholamine and cortisol response, total urine N, and 3-methylhistidine excretion, and infection and acute lung injury incidence over the 7–10 day study interval. The results are summarized in Table 2. In age, sex and injury matched patients, there were no observed differences in either nutrition parameters or patient outcome parameters, including the acute phase hormone response.

It is difficult to draw conclusions from these studies due to differences in patient type and study design. When combined with the previous section, however, there is a general impression that early EN (less than 3–4 days after

Table 2. Effect of timing of enteral nutrition on patient outcome

Parameter	Early	Late	P-value
Age, years	43.8±21.6	40.6±18.4	NS
ISS	33.2±10.9	31.3±9.1	NS
Initiation of feeding-hours after injury	30.5±12.7	81.7±11.3	NS
ICU days	11.4±8	9.9±6.7	NS
Ventilator days	9.7±8.2	8.1±6.8	NS
Acute lung injury	11 patients	3 patients	<0.025
Infections	29	14	0.065
Mortality	2	2	NS
Organ failure syndrome	2	2	NS

NS = not significant

There were no differences in catecholamine excretion, cotisol response, visceral protein concentrations, or 3-methylhistidine excretion. The early feeding group achieved earlier nitrogen retention.

injury) is associated with a reduction in clinically relevant infectious complications in trauma patients, and that this reduction is in excess of that accountable by the infectious complications directly attributable to the administration of TPN. Effects on other patient outcome parameters have not been demonstrated. On the down side, EN seems to be accompanied by an increased incidence of GI side effects and a higher failure rate in achieving targeted nutrition support goals.

Is the Type of Nutrition Formulation Important?

The last consideration pertains to the role of the formulation of the nutritional product on both nutrition-related, disease-specific, and patient-related outcomes in patients with the post-resuscitative inflammatory response. Individual vitamin and mineral deficiencies will not be discussed as their efficacy has been demonstrated and current nutrition support regimens work well to control these problems. A number of studies have evaluated nutrition or disease specific outcomes as they relate to product formulation.

One study evaluated the effect of calorie/nitrogen ratio in 35 patients with the persistent inflammatory response and sepsis in a general surgery ICU [19]. This study focused on enteral products as they are premixed to provide, in a predetermined volume of formula, the daily energy and nutrient requirements. The emphasis in much of EN practice has been to provide a given formula in an amount to achieve energy equilibrium. Thus, isocaloric amounts of three different formulas were provided to meet the patients energy requirements and nutritional outcomes were assessed. Three different calorie/N ratios were prospectively delivered to a matched cohort of patients. Only those patients receiving a full dose of formula for a minimum of 8 days were included in the study. The patients who received the low calorie/N ratio (97/1) were observed to have much better N retention and improvements in visceral protein concentrations, and to experience a lower respiratory quotient. In addition, a strong inverse correlation was observed between these parameters and an increasing calorie/N ratio. Much of this effect was probably related to the differences in protein (amino acid) content of the formulae. Nonetheless, formula composition was observed to be an important determinant of nutrition outcomes. Energy equilibrium *per se* was not observed to be an adequate indicator of nutritional efficacy.

A number of studies have evaluated whether or not the metabolic pathways of protein (amino acid) metabolism can be modulated by nutrients, i.e. whether or not the efficiency of protein (amino acid) utilization can be improved [12, 20, 21]. The criteria for efficiency were N retention, ureagenesis, and visceral protein synthesis. The formulations used were enriched with the branched-chain amino acids (BCAA) with lesser amounts of the remaining amino acids present in the final product. The major study was a randomized, prospective, blinded clinical trial in metabolically stressed surgical ICU patients [12]. The study evaluated the effects of stress level, amino acid formulation (BCAA enriched or standard), and dose of amino acids on the N economy in an isocaloric, isonitrogenous study design. On a per kilogram patient weight basis, the BCAA enriched solution were correlated with more N retention, with less ureagenesis, and higher levels of visceral proteins. These nutrition outcome effects were present on an intent-to-treat basis and were more promiment in the higher levels of metabolic stress. The formulation, dose administered, and the stress levels functioned as independent variables.

Studies with smaller numbers of patients have been interpreted not to demonstrate these effects [20]. When the data was reviewed, however, the effect on cumulative N retention was present. A recent study in 80 general surgery ICU patients with sepsis using a prospective, randomized design with 14 days of therapy, confirmed the findings of the multicenter trial on nutrition and disease-related outcomes. In addition, this study again demonstrated the underlying disease (tissue injury, sepsis and the inflammatory response) to be an independent variable effecting outcome [21].

Another study evaluated the effect of glutamine enriched (approximately 40 g/day) TPN in 20 bone marrow transplant recipients [22]. The study was prospective, randomized and blinded with the TPN provided over a 3 to 4 week study duration. This group of patients did not undergo surgical stress. Nonetheless, recipients of bone marrow transplants have significant disruption of their gut barrier, are usually quite catabolic, and are frequently hypermetabolic. For these reasons, the data may be applicable to the present discussion. The group that received the glutamine supplementation did not experience the expansion of the extracellular fluid compartment observed in the patients receiving the standard amino acid formulation (a 20% expansion). Data evaluating bacterial colonization and clinical infection was also collected (blood, throat, urine, stool). This data is somewhat difficult to evaluate, but was interpreted by the authors to be consistent with a reduction in bacterial colonization and infection rate in the patients who received the glutamine enriched formula.

Other studies have evaluated the effects of enteral peptide formulations and soy-polysaccharide fiber in critically ill patients [23, 24]. To date, clinically relevant effects on nutrition, disease-related or patient-related outcomes have not been demonstrated.

The final group of studies evaluates the influence of dietary formulation on patient related outcomes [25–28]. These studies have primarily altered the polyunsaturated fatty acid (PUFA), arginine and purine content of the formulations. Since all these nutrients were present in the enteral formulae, an evaluation of the effects of the components was excluded from the analyses. The scientific focus of these studies was on modulating the inflammatory and immune response to tissue injury. The study designs were randomized, prospective and, in most cases, blinded and utilized early enteral feeding techniques.

One study was performed in patients sustaining burn injury [25]. The study diet consisted of a modular tube feeding formula of whey protein enriched with arginine, cysteine and histidine (total protein of 54 g/L), low in total fat (14 g/L) and restricted in linoleic acid, and enriched with Ω3 PUFA (50% fish oil and 50% safflower oil). This diet was compared to Osmolite (Ross Laboratories, Columbus, Ohio) and TraumaCal (Mead Johnson, Evansville, Indiana). The latter two formulae were adjusted so all three formulae were isonitrogenous and isocaloric on a per liter basis; additional protein was added to the Osmolite, and the TraumaCal was diluted. Fifty patients normalized for burn size and severity were studied on a 3 to 4 week period. The patient outcome results are summarized in Table 3. The experimental formula was associated with significant reductions in wound infection and length of stay adjusted for percent burn.

Another series of studies evaluated an enteral formula fortified with menhaden oil, arginine and ribonucleic acid (Impact, Sandoz Nutrition, Minneapolis, Minnesota). The control enteral product was Osmolite. The first study evaluated the effects of this formula on *in vitro* tests of immune function in surgical ICU patients who were manifesting a persistent inflammatory response and sepsis 7–10 days after injury [26]. The effects were compared at baseline, after 3–4 days of feeding, and after 7–8 days of feeding. The experimental formula consistently enhanced these tests. The control formula was associated with no improvement in all cases and continued suppression of *in vitro* responsiveness in most cases. Another study evaluated these same formulae in 88 patients undergoing upper GI surgery for malignancy [27]. The results of this study confirmed the observations made with the *in vitro* tests of immune function. In addition, a significant reduction in length of stay was observed in the experimental group (20 ± 0.4 vs 15.8 ± 5.1 days, $p = 0.01$). There was also a reduction in total complications associated with the administration of the experimental formula (37 vs 11, $p = 0.02$). The last study was a multicenter comparison of the same two formulae [28]. The primary outcome variable was length of stay. The study entered all ICU admissions who qualified for the protocol (326 patients). The dominant patient group was patients who sustained polytrauma. There were 296 patients eligible for anal-

Table 3. Effect of formula type on patient outcomes in burn patients

Parameter	Experimental formula	Osmolite	Traumacal	P-value
Number of patients	17	14	19	NS
Wound infection	2	8	8	0.03
Pneumonia	2	6	9	0.06
Total infections	7	16	21	0.07
Length of stay/% burn (days)	0.83	1.21	1.21	0.02
Deaths	2	1	7	0.06

There were no differences observed in antibiotic days, ventilator days, or in the number of surgeries performed.

ysis on an intent to treat basis; and in whom there was a median reduction in length of stay of 4 days. Patients who received at least 7 days of therapy (151 patients) had an observed reduction in median length of stay of 6 days ($p = 0.01$). Patients who completed the protocol (85 patients), experienced a median reduction in length of stay of 8 days (a 26.7% reduction, $p = 0.05$). The length of stay effect of the diet was an independent variable and was more dominant the earlier post-injury the EN was initiated. There were no observed differences in mortality or in overall complication rate. The mortality observed was much less than that predicted by the APACHE II score or TISS score, perhaps reflecting the use of early enteral feeding. The experimental formula appeared to help those patients who were going to survive more rapidly.

Thus, the type of diet provided effects nutrition- and, for some parameters, disease-related outcomes. In the latter instances, nutrients appear to be able to modulate metabolic pathways and the metabolic response to injury. It also appears as if nutrients can favorably alter clinically relevant patient outcomes such as length of stay, but are unable to significantly alter those metabolic processes leading to death.

Conclusions

This chapter focuses on 4 important questions concerning the therapeutic use of nutrition/metabolic support in critically ill patients who sustain the systemic inflammatory response syndrome following tissue injury and infection. The use of this technology appears to improve nutritional and patient outcomes, provided the complication rate of the technology is maintained within an acceptable range. The enteral route appears to be more efficacious than the parenteral route in achieving relevant patient outcomes. There remains, however, a reasonably large group of patients in whom the enteral route cannot be used. TPN remains a relatively safe and efficacious technology in these settings. The timing of the initiation of enteral nutrition/metabolic support appears to be an important consideration. The beneficial effects were observed in those patients who received enteral nutrients early after injury and prior to the onset of a well-established inflammatory response. The formulation of the nutrition/metabolic support also appears to be a critical determinant of nutritional, disease-related and patient-related outcomes. Nutrients appear to be able to modulate the metabolic response to injury and to improve patient outcome in those patients who will ultimately survive surgical trauma. They appear unable to alter those metabolic processes that ultimately lead to death. Clearly, much more research is necessary.

References

1. ACCP - SCCM Consensus Conference (1993) Definitions for sepsis and organ failure and guidelines for the use of innovative therapies in sepsis. Chest (in press)
2. Cerra FB (1992) Multiple Organ Failure Syndrome. Disease of the Month 38:843–947
3. Cerra FB (1987) Hypermetabolism, organ failure, and metabolic support. Surgery 101:1–14
4. Cerra FB, Cheung NK, Fischer JE, et al. (1985) Disease-specific amino acid infusion (FO80) in hepatic encephalopathy: A prospective, randomized, double-blind controlled trial. JPEN 9:288–295
5. Sandstrom R, Drott C, Hytlander A, et al. (1993) The effect of postoperative intravenous feeding (TPN) on outcome following major surgery evaluated in a randomized study. Ann Surg 217:185–195
6. Cerra FB, Siegel JH, Coleman B, et al. (1980) Septic autocannibalism, a failure of exogenous nutritional support. Ann Surg 192:570–580
7. Long CL, Jeevenaudan M, Kinney JM (1977) Whole body protein synthesis and catabolism in septic man. Am J Clin Nut 30:1340–1345
8. Shaw JHF, Wolfe RR (1987) Glucose and urea kinetics in patients with early and advanced gastrointestinal cancer: The response to glucose infusion, parenteral feeding, and surgical resection. Surgery 101:181–191
9. Bower RH, Talamini MA, Sax HC, et al. (1986) Postoperative enteral vs parenteral nutrition: A randomized controlled trial. Arch Surg 121:1040–1045
10. Iapichino G, Gattinoni L, Solca M, et al. (1982) Protein sparing and protein replacement in acutely injured patients during TPN with and without amino acid supply. Intensive Care Med 8:25–31
11. Cerra FB, Hirsch J, Mullen K, et al. (1987) The effect of stress level, amino acid formula, and nitrogen dose on nitrogen retention in traumatic and septic stress. Ann Surg 205:282–287
12. Kudsk KA, Croce MA, Fabian TC, et al. (1992) Enteral vs parenteral feeding. Ann Surg 215:503–513
13. Moore FA, Moore EE, Jonew TN, et al. (1989) TEN vs TPN following major abdominal trauma-reduced septic morbidity. J Trauma 29:916–923
14. Moore FA, Feliciano DV, Andrassy RJ, et al. (1992) Early enteral feeding, compared with parenteral, reduces postoperative septic complications. Ann Surg 216:172–183
15. Cerra FB, McPherson J, Konstantinides FN, et al. (1988) Enteral nutrition does not prevent multiple organ failure syndrome after sepsis. Surgery 104:727–733
16. Chiarelli A, Enzi GE, Casadei A, et al. (1990) Very early nutrition supplementation in burned patients. Am J Clin Nutr 51:10035–10039
17. Eyer S, Cipolle M, Rosenberg S, Cerra FB (1993) Enteral nutrition does not improve outcome in blunt trauma. J Trauma (in press)
18. Cerra FB, Shronts EP, Raup S, et al. (1980) Enteral nutrition in hypermetabolic surgical patients. Crit Care Med 17:619–622
19. Kuhl DA, Brown RO, Vehe KL, et al. (1990) Use of selected visceral protein measurements in the comparison of branched-chain amino acids with standard amino acids in parenteral nutrition support of injured patients. Surgery 107:503–510
20. Jimenez FJJ, Leyba CO, Mendez SM, et al. (1991) Prospective study on the efficacy of branched-chain amino acids in septic patients. JPEN 15:252–261
21. Scheltinga MR, Young LS, Benfell K, et al. (1991) Glutamine-enriched intravenous feedings attenuate extracellular fluid expansion after a standard stress. Ann Surg 214:385–395
22. Mowatt Larssen CA, Brown RO, Wotysiak SL, Kudsk KA (1992) Comparison of tolerance and nutritional outcome between a peptide and a standard enteral formula in critically ill hypoalbuminemic patients. JPEN 16:20–24
23. Frankenfield DC, Beyer PL (1989) Soy-polysaccharide fiber: Effect on diarrhea in tube-fed head-injured patients. Am J Clin Nutr 50:533–538

24. Gottschlich MM, Jenkins M, Warden GD, et al. (1990) Differential effects of three enteral dietary regimens on selected outcome variable in burn patients. JPEN 14:236–255
25. Cerra FB, Lehman S, Konstantinides N, et al. (1990) Effect of enteral nutrient on *in vitro* tests of immune function in ICU patients: A preliminary report. Nutrition 6:84–87
26. Daly JM, Lieberman D, Goldfine MS, et al. (1992) Enteral nutrition with supplemental arginine, RNA and omega-3 fatty acids in patients after operation: Immunologic, metabolic, and clinical outcome. Surgery 112:56–67
27. Bower RH, Lavin PR, Cerra FB, et al. (1993) Early enteral administration of a formula supplemented with arginine, nucleotides and fish oil reduces length of stay of ICU patients: A randomized prospective trial (in press)

Subject Index

MIX
Papier aus verantwortungsvollen Quellen
Paper from responsible sources
FSC® C105338

If you have any concerns about our products,
you can contact us on
ProductSafety@springernature.com

In case Publisher is established outside the EU,
the EU authorized representative is:
Springer Nature Customer Service Center GmbH
Europaplatz 3, 69115 Heidelberg, Germany

Printed by Libri Plureos GmbH
in Hamburg, Germany